Property of LifeSource Dept.

T5-DHA-085

Transplantation of Composite Tissue Allografts

Charles W. Hewitt and W. P. Andrew Lee
Editors

Chad R. Gordon
Associate Editor

Transplantation of Composite Tissue Allografts

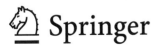

Editors
Charles W. Hewitt, Ph.D.
Professor of Surgery
Head, Division of Surgical Research
UMDNJ-Robert Wood Johnson
 Medical School
Cooper University Hospital
Camden, New Jersey

W. P. Andrew Lee, M.D.
Professor of Surgery and Orthopedic Surgery
Chief, Division of Plastic Surgery
University of Pittsburgh School of Medicine
Pittsburgh, Pennsylvania

Associate Editor
Chad R. Gordon, D.O.
Chief Resident
Department of Surgery
UMDNJ-Robert Wood Johnson Medical
 School
Cooper University Hospital
Camden, New Jersey

Cover illustration: The image depicts Saints Cosmas and Damian transplanting a lower extremity composite tissue allograft in place of an elder's amputated limb (c. 286 A.D.)

ISBN: 978-0-387-74681-4   eISBN: 978-0-387-74682-1
DOI: 10.1007/978-0-387-74682

Library of Congress Control Number: 2007937088

© 2008 Springer Science+Business Media, LLC
All rights reserved. This work may not be translated or copied in whole or in part without the written permission of the publisher (Springer Science+Business Media, LLC, 233 Spring Street, New York, NY 10013, USA), except for brief excerpts in connection with reviews or scholarly analysis. Use in connection with any form of information storage and retrieval, electronic adaptation, computer software, or by similar or dissimilar methodology now known or hereafter developed is forbidden.
The use in this publication of trade names, trademarks, service marks, and similar terms, even if they are not identified as such, is not to be taken as an expression of opinion as to whether or not they are subject to proprietary rights.

Printed on acid-free paper.

9 8 7 6 5 4 3 2 1

springer.com

This book is dedicated to the next generation; namely, Nicole, Ryan, Noah, and Zachary, along with my former students, residents, and fellows. They represent the future in terms of yet unrealized accomplishments and discoveries that await fruition.

CHARLES W. HEWITT

This book is dedicated to the research fellows, surgical residents, and medical students who have worked in our laboratories at Hopkins, Mass. General, and Pittsburgh in the last two decades. Their intellect, enthusiasm, and achievements are inspirational for future generations of contributors in composite tissue allotransplantation.

W. P. ANDREW LEE

I would like to dedicate this book to my dearest wife, Abbey, in gratitude for her everlasting encouragement and support. And to our precious son, Austin, who has provided endless nights of laughter and smiles.

CHAD R. GORDON

Foreword: The Import of Composite Tissue Transplantation

Four decades have passed since allogeneic transplantation first became a clinical reality. Although I have been passionate throughout my career in regards to solid organ transplantation, it gives me great pleasure to observe the success in the transplantation of composite tissue allografts, such as the first successful human hand transplant. I, along with many of my colleagues, have witnessed numerous patients who had suffered life-changing injuries benefit dramatically from successful composite tissue transplantation.

In order to fully appreciate these recent accomplishments, one must realize that a "composite tissue transplant" entails a significant challenge, encompassing a unique tissue combination in each specific case. For comparison, when performing a kidney or liver transplant, the transplanted organ's function can be quantified by several physiologic and biochemical metabolic processes. In this field, however, defining post-operative allograft function, in terms of its various components, can easily become quite puzzling.

This book, *Transplantation of Composite Tissue Allografts*, is wonderfully detailed, containing a thorough overview of important related subjects in the section of Composite Tissue Transplantation. This blossoming field, driven by some of the world's most compelling physicians, scientists, and surgeons, is quite inspiring to all. And it is our hope that this book will both inform and excite all who are interested in helping those patients benefit from transplantation of composite tissue allografts.

Thomas E. Starzl

Preface

This book reviews, updates, and synthesizes the recent accomplishments and ongoing research in the field of composite tissue allotransplantation (CTA). The volume focuses on the immunology, biotechnology, and bioengineering of CTA, as these areas have demonstrated the most growth within the field in the last five years.

The text presents the entire scope of CTA in a comprehensive format. This effort details the state-of-art advances of CTA and includes the numerous accomplishments of premier scientists and physicians from around the world engaged in the field. Significant advancements in the evolution of CTA are detailed from the historic legend of "Cosmas and Damian" through the most recent controversial topics of hand and face transplantation.

Transplantation of Composite Tissue Allografts is an ideal and valuable resource for a diverse group of physicians, scientists, researchers, residents, and students. This book will both inform and excite all who are interested in helping patients benefit from transplantation of composite tissue allografts.

Charles W. Hewitt
W. P. Andrew Lee
Chad R. Gordon

Contents

Section I

Chapter 1 The Establishment of Composite Tissue Allotransplantion as a Clinical Reality. 3
Joseph E. Murray

Chapter 2 The Evolution of Composite Tissue Allotransplantation: the Twentieth Century Realization of "Cosmas and Damian". 13
Chad R. Gordon, Joseph M. Serletti, Kirby S. Black, and Charles W. Hewitt

Chapter 3 The Impact of the Discovery of Cyclosporine on Transplantation of Composite Tissue Allografts. 26
Zsolt T. Csapo, Bence Forgacs, and Barry D. Kahan

Chapter 4 The First Limb Transplants with Cyclosporine. 36
Christopher J. Salgado, Samir Mardini, and Charles W. Hewitt

Section II

Chapter 5 Translational Research in Composite Tissue Allotransplantation 43
Linda C. Cendales, David E. Kleiner, and Allan D. Kirk

Chapter 6 Relative Antigenicity of Allograft Components and Differential Rejection. 55
Jignesh Unadkat, Justin M. Sacks, Stefan Schneeberger, and W. P. Andrew Lee

Chapter 7 On the Road to Tolerance Induction in Composite Tissue Allotransplantation 70
Mark A. Hardy

Chapter 8	**Donor-Specific Tolerance**	88
	Au H. Bui, Gerald Lipshutz, and Jerzy Kupiec-Weglinski	
Chapter 9	**Immune Tolerance Induction: Basic Concepts for Composite Tissue Allotransplantation**	105
	Patricio Andrades, Clement Asiedu, and Judith M. Thomas	

Setion III

Chapter 10	**Allograft Survival with Calcineurin Inhibitors**	121
	Neil F. Jones and Esther Voegelin	
Chapter 11	**Long-Term Prevention of Rejection and Combination Drug Therapy**	150
	Thomas H. Tung	
Chapter 12	**Locoregional Immunosuppression in Composite Tissue Allografting**	164
	Scott A. Gruber	
Chapter 13	**New Approaches to Antibody Therapy**	172
	Dalibor Vasilic, Moshe Kon, and Cedric G. Francois	

Setion IV

Chapter 14	**World Experience of Hand Transplantation-Independent Assessment**	193
	W. P. Andrew Lee, Justin M. Sacks, and Elaine K. Horibe	
Chapter 15	**Hand Transplantation: Lyon Experience**	209
	Palmina Petruzzo, Emmanuel Morelon, Jean Kanitakis, Lionel Badet, Assia Eljaafari, Marco Lanzetta, Earl Owen, and Jean-Michel Dubernard	
Chapter 16	**Hand Transplantation: The Louisville Experience**	215
	Vijay S. Gorantla and Warren C. Breidenbach III	
Chapter 17	**Hand Transplantation: The Innsbruck Experience**	234
	Stefan Schneeberger, Marina Ninkovic, and Raimund Margreiter	

Section V

Chapter 18	**Vascularized Bone Marrow Transplantation**	253
	Chau Y. Tai, Louise F. Strande, Hidetoshi Suzuki, Martha S. Matthews, Chad R. Gordon, and Charles W. Hewitt	

Contents

| Chapter 19 | Vascularized Bone Marrow Transplantation: Pathology of Composite Tissue Transplantation-Induced Graft-Versus-Host-Disease .... 272 |
Rajen Ramsamooj and Charles W. Hewitt

Chapter 20 Immune Cell Redistribution After Vascularized Bone Marrow Transplantation............................. 278
Waldemar L. Olszewski and Marek Durlik

Section VI

Chapter 21 Vascularized Knee Transplantation................... 293
Michael Diefenbeck and Gunther O. Hofmann

Chapter 22 Tracheal Transplantation 307
Gabriel M. Marta and Walter Klepetko

Chapter 23 Laryngeal Transplantation.......................... 330
Robert R. Lorenz and Marshall Strome

Chapter 24 Face Transplantation................................ 344
Maria Siemionow and Galip Agaoglu

Chapter 25 The Role of Allografts in Lower Extremity Reconstruction....................................... 355
Milton B. Armstrong, Ricardo Jimenez-Lee, and Eddie Manning

Chapter 26 Skin Allografts in Scalp Reconstruction 367
Peter C. Neligan

Chapter 27 Abdominal Wall Transplantation 374
David M. Levi and Andreas G. Tzakis

Chapter 28 Peripheral Nerve Allotransplantation.................. 382
Chau Y. Tai and Susan E. Mackinnon

Chapter 29 Live-Donor Nerve Transplantation 407
Scott A. Gruber and Pedro Mancias

Section VII

Chapter 30 Ethical and Policy Concerns of Hand/Face Transplantation 429
Rhonda Gay Hartman

Chapter 31	Ethical Debate on Human Face Transplantation 443
	François Petit
Chapter 32	Psychosocial Issues in Composite Tissue Allotransplantation 452
	Barckley Storey, Allen Furr, Joseph C. Banis, Michael Cunningham, Dalibor Vasilic, Osborne Wiggins, Serge Martinez, Christopher C. Reynolds, Rachael R. Ashcraft, and John H. Barker
Chapter 33	Composite Tissue Transplantation in the Twenty-First Century 460
	Kirby S. Black and Charles W. Hewitt
Index... 467	

Contributors

Galip Agaoglu, M.D.
Division of Plastic Surgery,
The Cleveland Clinic Foundation,
Cleveland, Ohio

Patricio Andrades, M.D.
Division of Plastic and Reconstructive
Surgery, Department of Surgery,
Jose Jaoquin Aquirre Clinical
Hospital, University of Chile
School of Medicine, Santiago,
Chile

Milton B. Armstrong, M.D.
Division of Plastic Surgery,
Department of Surgery, University
of Miami, Miami, Florida

Rachael R. Ashcraft, M.D.
University of Louisville, Division of
Plastic Surgery Research, Louisville,
Kentucky

Clement K. Asiedu, Ph.D.
Clinical Instructor of Surgery,
University of Alabama at Birmingham,
Department of Surgery, Birmingham,
Alabama

Lionel Badet, M.D., Ph.D.
Department of Transplant Surgery,
Edouard Herriot Hospital,
Université Claude Bernard Lyon,
Lyon, France

Joseph C. Banis, M.D.
Clinical Associate Professor,
University of Louisville, Division
of Plastic and Reconstructive Surgery,
Department of Surgery, Louisville,
Kentucky

John H. Barker, M.D., Ph.D.
Professor of Surgery, University
of Louisville, Director, Plastic Surgery
Research, Louisville, Kentucky

Kirby Black, Ph.D.
Department of Biotechnology,
Kennesaw State University, Kennesaw,
Georgia

Warren Breidenbach, III, M.D.
Assistant Clinical Professor of Surgery,
University of Louisville, Kleinert,
Kutz Hand Care Center, Louisville,
Kentucky

Au H. Bui, M.D.
Division of Transplantation,
Department of Surgery, David Geffen
School of Medicine at UCLA, Los
Angeles, California

Linda C. Cendales, M.D.
Hand and Microsurgery and Composite
Tissue Allotransplantation, Orthopedic
Section, NIAMS, National Institutes of
Health, Bethesda, Maryland

Zsolt T. Csapo, M.D.
Visiting Assistant Professor, University of Texas at Houston School of Medicine, Division of Immunology and Organ Transplantation, University of Texas Health Science Center at Houston, Houston, Texas

Michael R. Cunningham, Ph.D.
Professor of Psychology, University of Louisville, Department of Communications, Louisville, Kentucky

Michael Diefenbeck, M.D.
Assistant Professor of Surgery, University of Munich, Munich, Germany

Jean-Michel Dubernard, M.D., Ph.D.
Professor of Surgery, Université Claude Bernard Lyon, Department of Transplantation Surgery, Edouard Herriot Hospital, Lyon, France

Marek Durlik, M.D.
Polish Academy of Sciences, Division of Transplantology, Department of Surgical Research and Transplantology, Medical Research Center, Central Clinical Hospital, Ministry of Internal Affaires, Warsaw, Poland

Assia Eljaafari, M.D., Ph.D.
Department of Transplantation Surgery, Université Claude Bernard Lyon, Edouard Herriot Hospital, Lyon, France

Bence Forgacs, M.D., Ph.D.
Division of Immunology and Organ Transplantation, University of Texas Health Science Center, Houston, Texas

Cedric G. Francois, M.D., Ph.D.
Senior Research Associate, Department of Physiology & Biophysics, University of Louisville, Louisville, Kentucky

Allen Furr, Ph.D.
Associate Professor of Sociology, Department Chair, University of Louisville, Louisville, Kentucky

Vijay Gorantla, M.D.
Research Fellow, Division of Plastic Surgery, Department of Surgery, University of Pittsburgh School of Medicine, Pittsburgh, Pennsylvania

Chad R. Gordon, D.O.
Chief Resident, Department of Surgery, UMDNJ-Robert Wood Johnson Medical School, Cooper University Hospital, Camden, New Jersey

Scott A. Gruber, M.D., Ph.D., M.B.A.
Professor of Surgery, Chief, Section of Transplant Surgery, Wayne State University School of Medicine, Harper University Hospital, Detroit, Michigan

Mark A. Hardy, M.D.
Professor of Surgery, Columbia University, New York, New York

Rhonda Gay Hartman, J.D., Ph.D.
Center for Bioethics and Health Law, Visiting Professor, University of Pittsburgh School of Medicine, Pittsburgh, Pennsylvania

Charles W. Hewitt, Ph.D.
Professor of Surgery, Head, Division of Surgical Research, UMDNJ-Robert Wood Johnson Medical School, Cooper University Hospital, Camden, New Jersey

Gunther O. Hofmann, M.D., Ph.D.
Department of Surgery, Klinikum Grosshadern, Ludwig-Maximilians-University Munich, Munich, Germany

Elaine K. Horibe, M.D.
Research Fellow, Division of Plastic Surgery, Department of Surgery, University of Pittsburgh School of Medicine, Pittsburgh, Pennsylvania

Contributors

Ricardo Jimenez-Lee, M.D.
Chief Resident, Division of Plastic Surgery, University of Miami, Miller School of Medicine, Miami, Florida

Neil F. Jones, M.D.
Professor of Surgery, David Geffen School of Medicine at UCLA, Division of Plastic & Reconstructive Surgery, Department of Orthopaedic Surgery, UCLA Medical Center, Los Angeles, California

Barry D. Kahan, M.D., Ph.D.
Professor of Surgery, University of Texas at Houston School of Medicine, Director, Division of Immunology and Organ Transplantation, University of Texas Health Science Center at Houston, Houston, Texas

Jean Kanitakis, M.D.
Université Claude Bernard Lyon, Edouard Herriot Hospital, Lyon, France

Allan D. Kirk, M.D., Ph.D.
National Institute of Diabetes & Digestive & Kidney Diseases, National Institutes of Health, Bethesda, Maryland

David E. Kleiner, M.D.
Staff Surgical Pathologist, Laboratory of Pathology, National Cancer Institute, Bethesda, Maryland

Walter Klepetko, M.D.
Professor of Surgery, University of Vienna, Department of Cardiothoracic Surgery, Vienna, Austria

Jerzy W. Kupiec-Weglinski, M.D., Ph.D.
Professor of Surgery, David Geffen School of Medicine at UCLA, Division of Liver and Pancreas Transplantation, Department of Surgery, Los Angeles, California

Marco Lanzetta, M.D.
Director, Hand Surgery & Reconstructive Surgery, San Gerardo Hospital, Monza, Italy

W. P. Andrew Lee, M.D.
Professor of Surgery and Orthopedic Surgery, Chief, Division of Plastic Surgery, University of Pittsburgh School of Medicine, Pittsburgh, Pennsylvania

David M. Levi, M.D.
Assistant Professor of Clinical Surgery, University of Miami, Division of Transplant Surgery, Jackson-Memorial Hospital, Miami, Florida

Gerald S. Lipshutz, M.D., D.D.S., M.S.
Assistant Professor of Surgery, David Geffen School of Medicine at UCLA, Departments of Surgery and Urology, UCLA Medical Center, Los Angeles, California

Robert R. Lorenz, M.D.
Assistant Professor of Surgery, Cleveland Clinic Lerner College of Medicine of Case Western Reserve University, Section Head, Head & Neck Surgery, The Cleveland Clinic Foundation, Cleveland, Ohio

Susan E. Mackinnon, M.D.
Shoenberg Professor of Surgery, Washington University School of Medicine in St. Louis Chief, Division of Plastic and Reconstructive Surgery, Washington University Medical Center, St. Louis, Missouri

Pedro Mancias, M.D.
Division of Pediatric Nephrology, Department of Pediatrics, University of Texas Health Science Center at Houston, Houston, Texas

Eddie Manning, M.D.
Resident, General Surgery,
Department of Surgery, University
of Miami, Miller School of Medicine,
Miami, Florida

Samir Mardini, M.D.
Division of Plastic Surgery,
Department of Surgery, Mayo Clinic
College of Medicine, Rochester,
Minnesota

Raimund Margreiter, M.D.
Surgical Director, Department for
Transplantation Surgery, Medical
University of Innsbruck, Innsbruck,
Austria

Steven Marra, M.D.
Assistant Professor, Division of
Cardiothoracic Surgery, Department
of Surgery, Robert Wood Johnson
Medical School, Cooper University
Hospital, Camden, New Jersey

Gabriel M. Marta, M.D.
Department of Cardiothoracic Surgery,
Medical University of Vienna, Vienna,
Austria

Serge A. Martinez, M.D., J.D.
Professor of Surgery, University of
Louisville School of Medicine,
Division of Otolaryngology-Head and
Neck Surgery, Department of Surgery,
Louisville, Kentucky

Martha S. Matthews, M.D.
Associate Professor of Surgery, Head,
Division of Plastic Surgery, Department
of Surgery, Robert Wood Johnson
Medical School, Cooper University
Hospital, Camden, New Jersey

Emmanuel Morelon, M.D., Ph.D.
Division of Kidney Transplantation,
Department of Surgery, Université
Claude Bernard, Hôpital Edouard
Herriot, Lyon, France

Joseph E. Murray, M.D.
Nobel Prize Winner, 1990,
Professor of Surgery Emeritus,
Harvard Medical School, Boston,
Massachusetts

Peter C. Neligan, M.D.
Professor of Surgery, University of
Toronto School of Medicine,
Head, Division of Plastic Surgery,
Toronto General Hospital,
Toronto, Canada

Marina Ninkovic, M.D.
Department of Plastic and
Reconstructive Surgery, Ludwig
Boltzmann Institute for Quality
Control, Leopold-Franzens University,
Innsbruck, Austria

Waldemar L. Olszewski, M.D.
Professor of Surgery, Polish Academy
of Sciences, Department of Surgical
Research and Transplantology, Medical
Research Center, Central Clinical
Hospital, Ministry of Internal Affaires,
Warsaw, Poland

Earl Owen, M.D.
Microsearch Foundation of Australia,
Outer Sydney Hand and Microsurgery
Unit, Sydney, Australia

Francois Petit, M.D.
Professor of Surgery, University
Patis-XII, Department of Plastic
Surgery, Hospital Henri-Mondor,
Créteil, France

Palmina Petruzzo, M.D.
Hand Surgery and Reconstructive
Microsurgery, San Gerardo Hospital,
Monza-University, Monza, Italy

Rajen Ramsamooj, M.D.
Associate Professor, U.C.-Davis School
of Medicine, Director of Transplant
Pathology, Department of Pathology,
Sacramento, California

Contributors

Christopher C. Reynolds, M.D.
University of Louisville, Division of Plastic Surgery Research, Louisville, Kentucky

Justin M. Sacks, M.D.
Research Fellow, Division of Plastic Surgery, Department of Surgery, University of Pittsburgh School of Medicine, Pittsburgh, Pennsylvania

Chris J. Salgado, M.D.
Assistant Professor of Surgery, Division of Plastic Surgery, Department of Surgery, Robert Wood Johnson Medical School, Cooper University Hospital, Camden, New Jersey

Stefan Schneeberger, M.D.
Research Assistant Professor of Surgery, Division of Plastic Surgery, University of Pittsburgh, Pittsburgh, Pennsylvania

Joseph Serletti, M.D.
Professor of Surgery, University of Pennsylvania School of Medicine, Chief, Division of Plastic Surgery, Department of Surgery, Hospital of The University of Pennsylvania, Philadelphia, Pennsylvania

Maria Siemionow, M.D., Ph.D., D.Sc.
Professor of Surgery, Cleveland Clinic Lerner College of Medicine of Case Western Reserve University, Director of Plastic Surgery Research, Head, Microsurgery Training, The Cleveland Clinic Foundation, Cleveland, Ohio

Thomas E. Starzl, M.D., Ph.D.
Director, Thomas E. Starzl Transplantation Institute, University of Pittsburgh School of Medicine, Pittsburgh, Pennsylvania

Barckley Storey, M.D.
University of Louisville, Division of Plastic Surgery Research, Louisville, Kentucky

Louise Strande, M.S.
Division of Surgical Research, Department of Surgery, UMDNJ-Robert Wood Johnson Hospital, Cooper University Hospital, Camden, New Jersey

Marshall Strome, M.D., M.S.
Professor of Surgery, Cleveland Clinic Lerner College of Medicine of Case Western Reserve University, Chairman, The Head and Neck Institute, The Cleveland Clinic Foundation, Cleveland, Ohio

Hidetoshi Suzuki, M.D.
Second Department of Anatomy, Hamamatsu University School of Medicine, Shizuoka, Japan

Chau Y. Tai, M.D.
Department of Surgery, Kern Medical Center, Bakersfield, California

Judith M. Thomas, Ph.D.
Professor of Surgery, University of Alabama at Birmingham School of Medicine, Departments of Surgery and Microbiology, Birmingham, Alabama

Thomas H. Tung, M.D.
Assistant Professor of Surgery, Washington University School of Medicine, Division of Plastic and Reconstructive Surgery, Washington University Medical Center, St. Louis, Missouri

Andreas G. Tzakis, M.D., Ph.D.
Medical Director, Transplant Services, Broward General Medical Center, Fort Lauderdale, Florida

Jignesh Unadkat, M.D.
Research Fellow, Division of
Plastic Surgery, Department of
Surgery, University of Pittsburgh
School of Medicine, Pittsburgh,
Pennsylvania

Dalibor Vasilic, M.D.
University of Louisville, Louisville,
Kentucky

Esther Voegelin, M.D.
Department of Orthopaedic Surgery,
University of Bern, Inselspital, Bern,
Switzerland

Osborne Wiggins, Ph.D.
Department of Philosophy, University
of Louisville, Louisville, Kentucky

Section I

Chapter 1
The Establishment of Composite Tissue Allotransplantion as a Clinical Reality

Joseph E. Murray*

1.1 Introduction

My rewarding career has combined two major professional disciplines, plastic/reconstructive surgery and transplantation biology. This chapter discusses my connection to these two specialties and my fascination with composite tissue allotransplantation (CTA).

Now in my 88th year, I am eager to keep up with current surgical techniques as in the case of CTA. As Stuart Brand said, "Once a new technology rolls over you, if you're not part of the steamroller, you are part of the road."

I, as in the case of many of my colleagues, do not wish to spend the rest of our lives being part of the road. As I demonstrated throughout my career, we as plastic surgeons are in the position to make significant biological advances.

A recent issue of *Plastic and Reconstructive Surgery* featured an article entitled "Face transplantation: an extraordinary case with lessons for ordinary practice."* This face transplant operation was performed in September 2005 by Dr. Dubernard and his team in France. This partial face allotransplant represents a giant step forward in both the area of CTA and modern surgical technique. Personally, it represents the ultimate merging of plastic/reconstructive surgery and transplantation biology, which again, are the two major professional disciplines of my career.

Face transplantation has been much discussed in the current literature, encompassing both praise and criticism. Dr. Dubernard and colleagues thankfully presented their work in Tuscon, Arizona in January 2006. Dr. Thomas Starzl and Sir Roy Calne were just two of the many illustrious attendees to applaud Dubernard's work.

Dr. Dubernard, who worked in our laboratory at the Harvard Medical School, has now advanced CTA towards unexpected directions. I feel whole-heartedly that these advances are worth pursuing!

When I entered the Harvard Medical School in 1940, my plan upon graduation was to return home to mid-Massachusetts as a general surgeon. When World War II intervened, medical students were unexpectedly drafted. Surgical internship, at

---

*Presented, in part, at the 75th annual meeting of the American Society of Plastic Surgeons, October 8th, 2006.

this time, had been reduced to 9 months. My first permanent assignment was to the Valley Forge Army Hospital in Phoenixville, Pennsylvania. It was there that I treated battle causalities from Europe, Africa and the Pacific.

It was at Valley Forge where I first saw a severely burned Air Force pilot named Charles Woods. He was the first patient I ever cared for, whose life was saved and whose face was reconstructed by using tissues from another person.

Included is a picture of Mr. Woods before his terrible injury and then after multiple surgeries (Fig. 1.1). This event would serve as my first introduction into the world of transplantation biology. In addition, Charles Woods went on to become a successful business entrepreneur, politician and father.

When I returned to Boston in 1951, we began studying human skin grafts. There was a patient (c. 1952) cared for at the Chelsea Naval Hospital. She had extensive third degree burns over her entire body, requiring the use of both skin allografts and autografts. Here we are placing allografts into position (Fig. 1.2) Soon after, the autografts survived and expanded while the allografts melted away (Fig. 1.3).

This patient went on to heal completely without any contractures, presumably due to the survival of dermal remnants from the allografts. This was an important physiological discovery. Unexpectedly, we also found normal breast development, a salutary biological observation (Fig 1.4).

After World War II, the study of composite tissue transplantation expanded tremendously and began to embrace multiple disciplines. It was mainly because skin grafts were frequently and commonly used in design of experimental methodology that plastic surgeons were mainly those involved.

Around 1951, Dr. Brad Cannon became the first chairman of the American College of Surgeon's Plastic Surgical Forum Committee (Fig.1.5). He gathered together several related subject areas, including the surgical treatment of congenital deformity, cleft lip and palate, hypospadius, wound healing and skin cancers.

In the early 1950s, there was also confusion about what to call various kinds of skin grafts. Zoologist, Sir Peter Medawar clarified our terminology into familiar

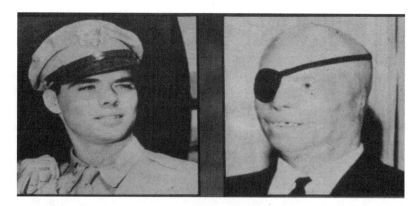

Fig. 1.1 Photographs of Charles Woods before and after his severe burn injury

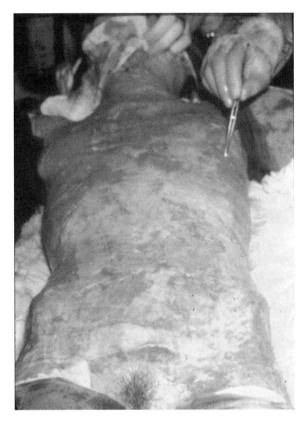

Fig. 1.2 Patient with extensive third degree burn

terms; those being autograft, allograft, and isograft. At that time, there was no existing medical journal dedicated solely to transplantation. Enthusiasts in tissue and organ transplantation had extreme difficulty in finding venues for publishing their material. Reports were scattered in embryology, anatomy, physiology and histology journals and symposia. Accordingly, the editors of *The Journal of Plastic Surgery* decided to include transplantation papers as an added bulletin in their journal. This continued for 10 years (Fig.1.6). The three editors at this time were Herbert Conway (Plastic surgeon, NY hospital), Ernest Eichwald (Pathologist, Great Falls, Montana), and Nathan Kaliss (Geneticist, Bar Harbor, Maine). In the 1970s, with the spectacular increase in transplantation, an independent journal, called the *American Journal of Transplantation*, was started. Today this journal is fourth among American surgical citations.

Since the first successful kidney transplant in 1954, hundreds of thousands of transplants have been performed worldwide. These include transplants of skin,

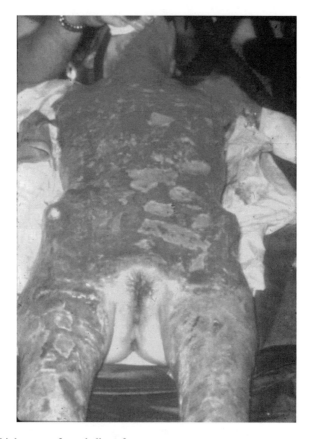

Fig. 1.3 Multiple autografts and allografts

bone and cartilage, cornea, endocrine glands, blood vessels, whole organ clusters and most impressively, composite tissue allografts. This growing field incorporates many disciplines, such as tissue engineering, oncology, genetics and immunology.

Some of the pioneering plastic surgeons involved in transplantation include John Converse, who was the second president of the transplantation society, J. Herbert Conway, and Fernando Monastario. Others include nationally recognized burn expert Truman Blocker who practice in Galveston, Texas. Lyndon Peer (Newark, New Jersey) published one of the first books on transplantation, while Bernard Sarnat became an expert in cartilage transplantation in southern California. John Woods became the first plastic surgical Chief and head of transplantation at the Mayo Clinic. Milt Edgerton and his wife, zoologist Patricia Edgerton, performed experimental work on transplantation at the Johns Hopkins Hospital.

Blair Rogers, Richard Stark, Peter Randall, and Erle Peacock were all clinical plastic surgeons performing transplantation experiments. This period was an exhilarating time. The war was now over and we were free to pursue our curiosity

The Establishment of Composite Tissue Allotransplantion as a Clinical Reality

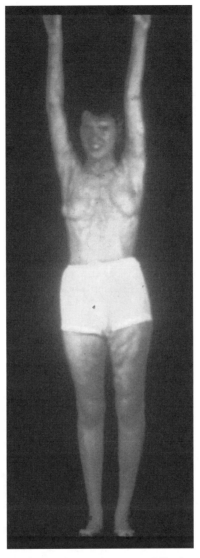

Fig. 1.4 Normal breast development without contractures following skin grafting for extensive third degree burns

and professional goals (Fig.1.7). A rare camaraderie developed which continues to exist to this day.

Successful transplantation led to the need for new definition of "death" based on the loss of brain function. It also led to the increased participation of the public and media in ethical decision-making in relation to the use of living donors.

During our original transplant operations, we conferred with physicians from other hospitals, lawyers, clergy of all denominations and the general public. We approached the Dean of Harvard medical school with aspirations to set up a

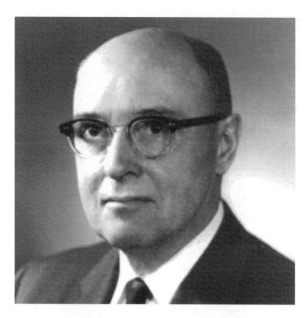

Fig. 1.5 Picture of Dr. Brad Cannon

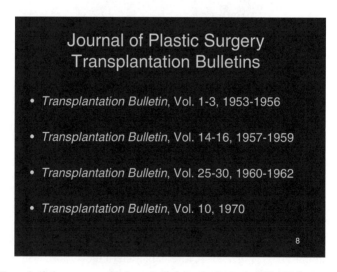

Fig. 1.6 Transplantation papers added as a bulletin to the Journal of Plastic Surgery

commission to define death in terms of loss of brain function, rather than loss of respiratory or cardiac activity. This commission report was published in the *Journal of the American Medical Association* (*JAMA*) in the late 1960s and these standards have been used nationally ever since.

From the 1950s to 1980s, I continued to work with skin grafts in mice, rabbits, dogs and human volunteers. This picture (Fig. 1.8) from 1955 shows four postage

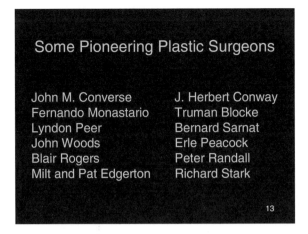

Fig. 1.7 Some pioneering plastic surgeons

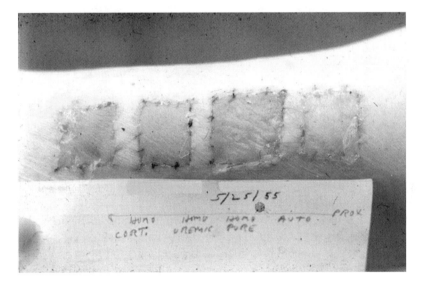

Fig. 1.8 Skin grafts to the upper arm of a uremic patient. From far right: autograft, pure homograft, from another uremic patient, from a patient on steroids

stamp-size grafts applied to the upper arm of a uremic patient. To the far right is the autograft. The second from the right is a pure homograft. The third from the right is from another uremic patient. Finally, the far left skin graft is from a patient on steroids due to another pre-existing medical condition. From these experiments, we learned that there is a differential strength of immune rejection.

In 1959, we were still testing the strength of the immune response in uremic patients. On the left (Fig. 1.9), we see the uremic twin's forearm. It shows a well-healed allograft received from his fraternal (dizygotic) healthy twin. On the right

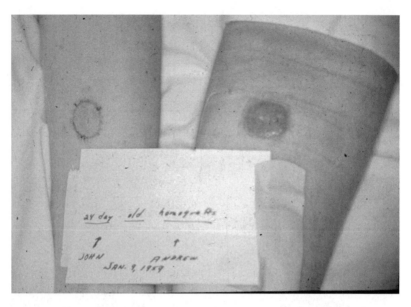

Fig. 1.9 Forearms of the uremic patient's twin brother with skin graft from dizygotic healthy twin on right forearm and from sick uremic patient on the left forearm

side we see the healthy twin's forearm showing acute rejection of the allograft received from his sick twin brother, indicating that they were not identical twins.

The kidney transplant from the healthy-to-sick twin was performed after subjecting the uremic patient to total body irradiation to suppress his immune response. The kidney transplant was successful, and it was the first successful kidney transplant between brothers.

We also experimented with maternal skin allografts, mother-to-child. Figure 1.10 (picture taken in 1958) shows the daughter's arm with a homograft from her mother on the right and an autograft on the left. This photograph was taken on the seventh postoperative day.

Figure 1.11 shows the mother and daughter grafts 2 years later, showing thinning of the allograft without contracture. Four years later in 1961, the homograft on the right is still intact but now thinner in respect to the autograft. We now learned that maternal allografts can last longer and survive well, but not completely (Fig. 1.12).

Figure. 1.13 (picture taken in 1963) shows me at the Harvard Medical School with four dogs, all of which underwent solitary kidney transplants. These renal allografts all survived over 1 year using immunosuppressive drugs.

Possibly, the best summation of the current status of CTA is a report in the June, 2006 issue of the *American Journal of Transplantation* entitled "Bilateral hand transplantation: six years after the first case." This report represents advancement in microsurgery, successful regeneration of nerves and muscles of the hand and the

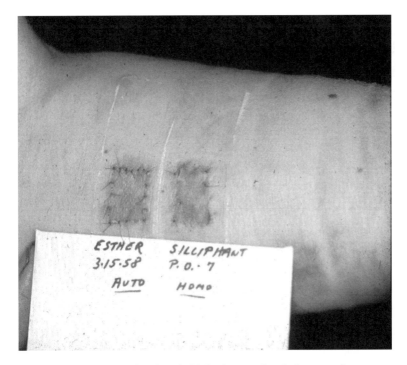

Fig. 1.10 Mother to daughter skin allograft. Right: from mother. Left: autograft

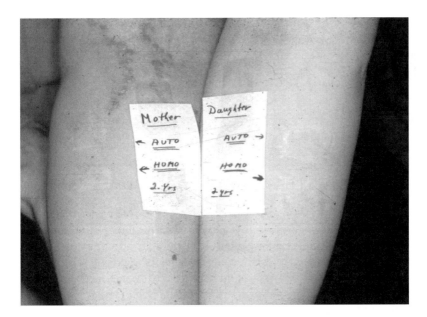

Fig. 1.11 Mother to daughter skin allograft. 2 years later

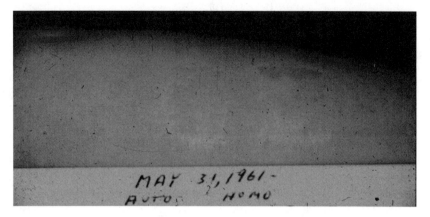

Fig. 1.12 Mother to daughter skin allograft. 4 years later

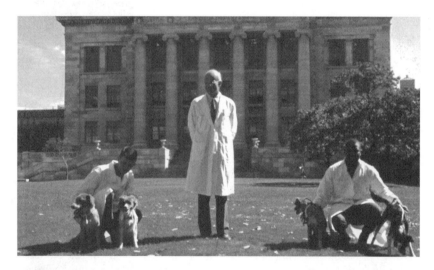

Fig. 1.13 Dr. Murray with 4 dogs who underwent solitary kidney transplants

complete healing of allogeneic skin. It also discusses the difficulty of implementing life-long immunosuppression for nonlethal conditions.

The past was great and the future will be even more exciting. I wish that I could be with you all – I will be with you in spirit on that wonderful steamroller ride! Thank you.

"Once a new technology rolls over you, if you're not part of the steamroller, you are part of the road." Stewart Brand, Amer J Transp, September 2006.

# Chapter 2
The Evolution of Composite Tissue Allotransplantation: the Twentieth Century Realization of "Cosmas and Damian"

Chad R. Gordon, Joseph M. Serletti, Kirby S. Black, and Charles W. Hewitt

Abstract The purpose of this article is to review the historical background and clinical status of composite tissue allotransplantation and to discuss the scientific evolution of composite tissue allotransplantation.

Composite tissue allotransplantation rapidly progressed in the 1980s with the discovery of cyclosporine. Although most success has been achieved with hand transplantation, others have made progress with allografts of trachea, peripheral nerve, flexor tendon apparatus, vascularized knee, larynx, abdominal wall, and most recently, partial face.

As a symbol of great success, the world's first partial face allotransplantation occurred in November 2005 in France. In April 2006, the second was performed in China. There are now multiple institutions with plans to attempt the world's first full facial/scalp transplant.

Composite tissue allotransplantation offers a viable alternative for unfortunate individuals suffering severe disfigurement and is a product of many decades of experimental research, beginning with rat hindlimb allografts.

2.1 Historical Background

Composite tissue allotransplantation (CTA) involves "transplanting a graft, composed of a variety of heterogeneous antigenic tissues, across a genetic mismatch," as in the case of a hand (i.e. skin, muscle, bone, tendon, nerve, vessels). This challenge presents multiple barriers and complexities in comparison to a more homogeneous organ such as kidney or liver.

The first historical mention of CTA dates back to the year AD 348, where legend has it that twin brothers from Arabia, Saints Cosmas and Damian (circa AD 286), posthumously transplanted an Ethiopian Moor's limb in place of an elder's amputated gangrenous limb.[1] According to Jacques de Vorágine's (XIII century, AD 1270) manuscript entitled "Leyenda Aúrea de la vida de los Santos" (Aureus Legend of the Saints life), "...the guard in charge of taking care of the temple dedicated to both Saints, suffered enormously because of a tumor in his leg; and one morning he woke up without pain and with a leg obtained from the corpse of a Ethiopian gentleman who passed away the day before (Fig. 2.1)."

The milestones achieved in transplantation of solid organs (primarily kidney and heart) motivated surgeons in 1964 to attempt the world's first hand transplant.[2,3] This unprecedented surgery was performed by a team led by Robert Gilbert in Ecuador on a young male patient who had lost both hands in an explosion. Immunosuppressive options were limited to azathioprine and hydrocortisone. Unfortunately, severe rejection to the hand was present 2 weeks after surgery and re-amputation was indicated soon thereafter. A trial of increment doses of immunosupression was not advised since previous animal experiments demonstrated severe toxicity.[4] This complication delayed the clinical dream of hand transplantation and decades would pass before the next attempt.

During this same year, the first clinical trials by Calne began using cyclosporine (CsA) in renal, pancreatic and liver transplantation.[5–7] Once the clinical efficacy of CsA had been demonstrated in solid organ transplantation, multiple research teams began investigating limb allograft transplant models in rats, dogs and rabbits. It was Hewitt (1985) who provided the groundbreaking results demonstrating successful rat limb allotransplants with CsA.[8–10]

These rat limb allografts showed a significant improvement in mean survival time with CsA during a period of 20 days (101 versus 18 days). Higher acceptance rates were subsequently reported when using a maintenance dose of CsA twice-per-week for in-definitive time (400 days survival). It was also shown that the transplanted limb's marrow and stroma functioned as a new type of bone marrow transplant, resulting in immune chimerism and potential tolerance induction without graft-versus-host disease (GVHD).[11]

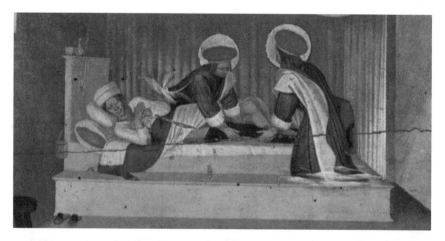

Fig. 2.1 Saints Cosmas and Damian performing a posthumous limb allograft transplant. (With permission from Gordon CR, Nazzal J, Lozano-Calderan SA, et al. "From experimental rat hindlimb to clinical face composite tissue allotransplantation: historical background and current status." Microsurgery 26(8):566–72, 2006.) (*See Color Plates*)

Many studies followed some tested combinations of steroids and CsA, while others evaluated different routes of administration. Most transplant researchers at this time were convinced that CsA was effective in avoiding limb allograft rejection in rats.[12-14] It was at this time, that the potential option of "using allografts of facial structures" was introduced by Achauer and colleagues in 1985.[15]

In 1987, Gunman-Stein and Shons confirmed the advantages of CsA by transplanting immature limbs in rats. These allografts experienced significant recovery of posterior limb function.[16] Kniha (1989) further demonstrated an acceptable limb growth rate while using CsA in a similar model in rabbits.[17] These investigational accomplishments not only confirmed adequate tissue integration of CsA, but also demonstrated the unexpected recovery of function and tissue growth.[18]

Pharmalogical research continued and new drugs were soon added to the list of available immunosuppressive agents. These included FK-506 (tacrolimus) and mycophenolate mofetil (MMF). In 1993, Benhaim demonstrated that rat limb allotransplants treated with MMF did not suffer rejection up to 32 weeks, versus those who had received CsA having mild-to-moderate acute graft rejection within 6 months. In addition, these limb allografts recovered full sensation and partial motor function.[19]

Three years later, the same group demonstrated more impressive postoperative limb function with the combination of both MMF and CsA. Again in 1999, they tested the combination of tacrolimus and MMF versus CsA and showed the former combination provided a superior antirejection effect without significant toxicity.[20]

By 2003, Siemionow provided the first and only rat transplant model to achieve life-long (720 days) donor-specific tolerance using fully major histocompatibility-mismatched hindlimb allografts. The immunosuppression was limited to a 7-day protocol of anti-alpha/beta T-cell receptor monoclonal antibody and CsA.[21-23]

In September 1991, Hewitt and Black co-chaired a conference sponsored by the Service for Rehabilitation Research and Development (a division of the Department of Veterans Affairs) held in Seattle, Washington. Its purpose was to entertain the feasibility of extremity (CTA) transplantation in patients with limb loss. Attendees concluded that the clinical reality of limb transplantation was quite possible, and many, in fact, expected the first attempts at hand transplantation to occur within the next 5 years.[24]

Six years later, in November 1997, the second conference was held in Louisville, Kentucky, known as the *First International Symposium on Composite Tissue Transplantation*. Various surgeons and transplant immunologists from around the world gathered to discuss numerous ethical, clinical, and research dilemmas in relation to hand transplantation.[25,26]

It was not until the researchers at Louisville released their (1998) revolutionary work demonstrating for the first time, in large animal CTA experimentation, that graft rejection could be prevented (including skin) using a clinically relevant immunosuppressive protocol consisting of cyclosporine and MMF. This achievement immediately called into question previous results which showed graft rejection in primate models and the validity of the primate model in representing composite tissue transplantation. More importantly, it provided the rationale for proceeding with the first modern-day hand transplant.[27]

Shortly thereafter, Jean-Michel Dubernard transplanted a right-hand-distal forearm allograft from a brain-dead donor to a 48-year-old New Zealand businessman in 1998 (Lyons, France). This individual had suffered a traumatic circular saw amputation of his right arm while being incarcerated (1984). In addition, his native arm had been reimplanted but electively amputated 5 years later by his request due to lack of function. Of note however, many critics since then have questioned and criticized this team's poor process of patient selection.

This inaugural patient received antithymocyte globulin, tacrolimus, MMF, and prednisone to prevent acute graft rejection. Chronic therapy consisted of tacrolimus, MMF, and prednisone. At 6 months, the motor and sensorial function of the patient was reported as "satisfactory" and the authors described the immunosuppressive therapy as "well-tolerated."[28]

A second hand transplant occurred in Louisville, Kentucky in January 1999. A team led by Breidenbach, Jones, and Gruber operated on a 37-year-old male who had lost his left hand at age 23 during a firecracker accident. His postoperative immunosuppression consisted of intravenous basiliximab, tacrolimus, MMF, and prednisone. The authors were pleasantly surprised with the quick return of neuromuscular function and minimal postoperative edema. These encouraging results were unexpected compared to previously replanted limbs, which had been described as "sub-optimal."[29]

Two separate hand transplants followed at Nanfang Hospital in Guangzhou, China in September of 1999. Unlike the previous two examples, these patients experienced a relatively short period of time (approximately 2 years) between their injury and operation. (The average interval period for the previous two cases was 12 years). The Chinese protocol followed the immunosuppression from Louisville, except for the amount of prednisone, which was significantly higher. Both transplants where done simultaneously, reporting no complications or events of rejection. No adverse effects of immunosuppression were documented. Functional evaluations in terms of motion and sensibility were done at 7 months, showing "fair" results in both subjects.[30]

In January 2000, an international team of 18 surgeons, including Dubernard (France), Hakim (England), and Owen (Australia) performed the first bilateral hand transplant at the Edouard-Herriot Hospital in France. The patient was a 33-year-old male who had both arms amputated below the elbow after an accident involving an amateur rocket. The immunosuppression protocol used was the same as the first hand transplant in France in 1998.[31]

Within that same month, another two unilateral transplants were performed in China. Two months later (March 2000), a second bilateral hand transplant took place at the University Clinic in Innsbruck, Austria on a 45-year-old male who had lost both hands after a pipe explosion 6 years prior to his surgery.[32]

The first female hand transplant was performed in China in May 2000. The patient was born with a severely deformed identical twin sister who died at birth. This case was quite different however, since no immunosuppressive therapy was indicated due to the obvious identical histocompatibility. There were no complications and outcomes were reported as "satisfactory." Following this chain of bilateral transplants, the Chinese transplanted another patient without any significant complications. As we approached the twenty-first century, many surgeons felt confident that all obstacles of hand transplantation had been overcome.[33]

Unfortunately, in February 2001, surgeons in London demonstrated the dramatic impact of noncompliance. This day entailed the elective amputation of the world's first successful hand transplant due to this inadequate compliance regarding immunosuppression and physical therapy. This frustrating event confirmed the importance of proper patient selection and compliance.[34]

Due to the results and the necessity of further evidence, the American Society for Surgery of the Hand (ASSH) urged investigators to withhold clinical trials until further research was completed to guarantee more promising results. The last reported cases include unilateral hand transplants in Milan, Italy (October 2001, November 2002), Brussels, Belgium (January 2002),[35] and most recently, Trzebnica, Poland (2006); and two bilateral hand transplants performed in Austria (February 2003) and France (May 2003).

In total, there have been 25 distal upper extremity allotransplants reported (12 unilateral and 4 bilateral hand transplants, 2 bilateral forearm transplants, and 1 thumb transplant). Hand transplantation has proven its feasibility, in spite of being technically challenging. However, the risk–benefit ratio remains quite complicated with respect to its required lifelong immunosuppression. Since the hand is considered "nonvital" in comparison to a heart or liver, for example, many challenging issues remain.[36]

As of today, there are few absolute indications for hand transplantation. It is however, a viable option for a young bilateral amputee who is relatively healthy. Although in the rare case of a twin born with a limb deformity, whose sibling dies, limb transplantation is an attractive option since the complications with immunosuppression are no longer present. Future studies with larger samples are required to assess long-term outcomes, complications, and psychological issues that have not yet been adequately addressed.[37]

2.2 Current Status

Besides hand transplantation, there are other areas of CTA which have developed clinically over the last 50 years. Since 1963, surgeons have made various attempts at transplanting tracheal allografts (1979), nonvascularized nerve allografts (1988), flexor tendon apparatus (1967), knee allografts (1996), laryngeal allografts (1969), abdominal wall allografts (1999), and most recently, partial face allografts (2005). Full facial/scalp allograft transplantation has received much recent attention and clinical application seems to be close on the horizon.[38–40]

2.2.1 Trachea

Tracheal allograft transplantation has been investigated since the 1970s, with three documented attempts. A distinct obstacle in trachea allograft transplantation is its small network of nutrient vessels, eliminating the possibility of a vascularized pedicle. To overcome this surgeons have attempted to achieve neoangiogenesis using the sternocleidomastoid muscle and greater omentum. In 1979, Rose reported the first allogeneic human trachea transplant.[41] The trachea was first implanted heterotopically into the recipient's sternocleidomastoid muscle for 3 weeks, and then transferred into its anatomical position completing a two-stage operation. Although the surgeon did not use any additional immunosuppression, initial reports at 9 weeks were satisfactory. No further follow-up has been documented.

Levashov accomplished the second human trachea transplant in 1993, describing a one-stage operation entailing an omentum-wrapped tracheal allograft on a 24-year-old female suffering from idiopathic fibrosing mediastinitis. Postoperatively, the patient received CsA immunosuppression and had "good" results at 2-month follow-up. At 4 months the patient required a stent for tracheal stenosis. Long-term viability and function data for this patient are also not available.[42]

In 2003, Klepetko reported the third attempt at heterotopic tracheal allograft transplantation. Their patient, a 57-year-old man with terminal chronic obstructive pulmonary disease was referred for bilateral lung transplantation. It was decided that because of this patient's anatomy, a single-stage operation using both tracheal allograft reconstruction with bilateral lung transplantation was indicated. Placement of the tracheal allograft was accomplished intra-abdominally, wrapped within the distal portion of the greater omentum, and attached to the anterior abdominal wall similar to a stoma, allowing daily inspection, secretion clearance, and observational biopsies. The patient received triple immunosuppression therapy consisting of CsA, MMF, and steroids, a regimen indicated primarily for his coinciding bilateral lung transplant. Although the heterotopic tracheal allograft was not needed for reconstructive purposes at the second operation 8 months later, the graft was explanted, demonstrating mechanically stability and acceptable vascularization.[43]

2.2.2 Peripheral Nerve

Although peripheral nerve, by definition, does not qualify as true CTA, its development has grown in accordance with and has a tremendous presence in the area of reconstructive surgery. Mackinnon has attempted the largest series of peripheral nerve allograft transplants, providing sole treatment for large peripheral defects ($n=2$) or in combination with autografts ($n=5$). Their immunosuppressive regimen included FK506 or CsA, azathioprine and prednisone; with the addition of cold preservation of the allografts at 5 °C for 7 days prior to transplantation. All immunosuppression was stopped once there was distal neuronal regeneration (between 12 and 26 months). Results from this series were mixed in reference to functional recovery, but successfully demonstrated an undefined role for nerve allograft transplantation.[44–48]

2.2.3 Flexor Tendon Apparatus

Peacock (1967) was the first to report successful human composite flexor tendon allotransplantation. Within a 10-year period (1957–1967), 11 cadaveric transplants were performed involving ten patients. Indications included failure of conventional autografting and/or when surrounding tissues (i.e., infection) made autografting unfeasible. Results in terms of active motion were "successful" in 7/10 patients. More impressively, no immunosuppression was used. The author reported that flexor allograft recipients displayed no clinical evidence of rejection other than self-limiting epitrochlear adenopathy. He concluded that insoluble collagen, specific to this type of CTA, is "relatively nonantigenic."[49,50]

In 1988, Guimberteau (France) successfully transplanted a vascularized flexor tendon apparatus dependent on an ulnar vessel pedicle in two patients. One allograft was cadaveric and the other was a nonrelated living donor (who underwent elective resection of their fifth digit). Immunosuppression included only CsA for 6 months and follow-up results at 1 year were acceptable in terms of functional range of motion.[51,52]

2.2.4 Vascularized Knee

The first reported human knee joint transplant was by Lexer in 1908. Since success was minimal, it took almost a century of immunological research and animal experimentation until the first vascularized knee joint program was started in Germany by Hofmann in 1996. They have since completed six vascularized knee transplants for soft-tissue defects in patients' status posttrauma or infectious destruction. Their immunosuppressive regimens include CsA, azathioprine, methylprednisolone, and antithymocyte globulin. The first five knee allografts were quite problematic, resulting in three amputations and two arthrodeses. In 2002, the sixth knee transplant was executed differently and included a new regimen of immunosuppressive therapy. In addition, Hofmann used a "sentinel skin graft" implanted into the transplant recipient's skin to simultaneously monitor for early signs of graft rejection. This new modified technique seems more efficacious and recent reports include a "well-perfused knee graft on angiography with acceptable mobile function" over 3 years later.[53–55]

2.2.5 Lower Extremity

In May 2006, surgeons from Canada reported the successful transplantation of a normal appearing lower extremity limb from an ischiopagus twin (conjoined twins sharing the lower-half) to her otherwise healthy sister into the appropriate pelvic position. At 3-month follow-up, the surgeons documented "encouraging return of muscle function with intact neurological sensation." Additionally, there was evidence of cortical motor function. There was, however, no immunosuppression indicated because of the twin's immune capability which drastically favored the risk–benefit ratio of the operation. Although this is a syngeneic limb transplant by definition, it displays the potential feasibility of future lower limb transplantation.[56]

2.2.6 Larynx

One of the most impressive areas of CTA to develop since hand transplantation was the first successful laryngeal allograft transplant by Strome in 1980. The first actual attempt at treating laryngeal carcinoma with allograft transplantation was reported by Kluyskens in 1969. This operation entailed subtotal resection, preserving perichondrium to revascularize the allograft, thus eliminating microvascular and neural anastomoses. Obvious rapid reoccurrence of tumor impinged progression for over a decade.[57]

Eleven years later, Strome revisited this operation on a 40-year-old male who had suffered severe laryngeal trauma in a motor vehicle collision at the age of 21. Despite multiple attempts at reconstruction, the patient remained aphonic and laryngeal transplantation seemed to be his last option. The entire pharyngolaryngeal complex, which included six tracheal rings, the thyroid, and the parathyroid glands, was transplanted to the superior thyroid arteries bilaterally, the right internal jugular vein, and the left middle thyroid vein, respectively. Both superior laryngeal nerves and the right recurrent laryngeal nerve were anastomosed, respectively. Initial immunosuppressive therapy consisted of anti-CD3 monoclonal antibodies, CsA, methylprednisone, and MMF. At 2 years, his maintenance regimen included tacrolimus, MMF, and prednisone.

At 8 years posttransplant, the patient has regained a normal sounding voice, possessing acceptable force and intonation. Postoperative complications include one episode of graft rejection requiring steroids and one case of pneumonia requiring antibiotics. As per the patient, his quality of life has increased "immeasurably." He was previously unemployed prior to his transplant and now has become a motivational speaker.[58]

2.2.7 Abdominal Wall

One of the unfortunate obstacles in abdominal organ transplantation is the closure of the abdominal wall, thus leading CTA surgeons to the inevitable birth of abdominal wall allotransplantation. Since 1999, there have been ten successful abdominal wall allotransplants by Tzakis, nine of them with accompanying intestinal autotransplantations. The cadaveric graft is a full-thickness, vascularized, myocutaneous free flap. Either one or both rectus abdominus muscles are included with its overlying fascia, subcutaneous tissue and skin. Harvest is based upon the inferior epigastric vessels left in continuity with the donor's femoral/iliac vessels and then anastomosed to the recipient's common iliac arteries (except for one particular child whose graft was anastomosed to the infrarenal aorta and inferior vena cava).

Induction immunosuppression includes an anti-CD52 monoclonal antibody (alemtuzumab) and tacrolimus for maintenance. In the particular case of abdominal wall allotransplantation, skin biopsies for suspected rejection are obviously quite feasible. Vessel patency is monitored using Doppler ultrasound. Several episodes of acute graft rejection have been reported and all of which have responded to corticosteroids. There has been no documentation of GVHD.[59]

A recent report published in 2004 by the senior author states that nearly half of the abdominal wall graft recipients are alive and that none of the postoperative fatalities were related to graft complications. In addition, two of the abdominal grafts were removed due to venous thrombosis. In conclusion, Tzakis has successfully demonstrated abdominal wall allotransplantation feasibility and its undefined role in complex abdominal wound closure.[60]

2.2.8 Partial Face

On November 27th, 2005, a team of French surgeons led by Duvauchelle and Dubernard transplanted a triangular allograft consisting of a distal nose, lips, and chin to a 38-year-old female recipient in Amiens, France. The world's first partial face allograft, entailing skin, mucosa, fat, and some muscle, was used to restore a defect resulting from a disfiguring dog-bite. The 5 h transplant operation (after an allograft ischemia time = 4 h) included revascularization via the facial arteries and veins bilaterally. Two infusions of donor bone-marrow cells were given in addition to a standard immunosuppressive regimen. At 4-month follow-up, the surgeons report complications limited to mild signs of clinical graft rejection at day 20 that were alleviated by intravenous steroids.[61]

The second partial face transplant took place in April 2006 at the Xijing Hospital in Xi'an, China. The male recipient, whose face had been badly disfigured by a black bear attack 2 years prior, received a composite tissue transplant consisting of a cheek, upper lip, nose, and an eyebrow.[62]

2.2.9 Complete Face/Scalp

Full facial transplantation has become the newest and most controversial CTA topic in recent years. Current plastic surgical technique fails to achieve total surface coverage of the face in a monoblock fashion, as well as, overcoming the difficult match of quality, texture, and color of the patient's facial skin. Recent attempts include skin grafts, local advancement flaps, prefabricated flaps, expanded adjacent flaps, and free tissue flaps; all of which have been less than satisfactory in both aesthetics and function. Part of the reason for aesthetic failure is due to the need for approximately 1,200 cm^2 of skin, enough to cover an entire face, scalp, front of neck, and ears.[63,64]

The success of CTA over the last few decades has provided surgeons with the vision of a complete facial-scalp allotransplant. This option would provide a feasible alternative to hundreds of individuals suffering facial disfigurement secondary to burns, traumatic avulsions, cancer, and congenital defects. It goes without saying that facial disfigurement would be detrimental to anyone and that this potential answer would be invaluable. Although quite appealing, it comes with an unprecedented amount of psychosocial issues.[65]

To date successful facial/scalp allotransplantation has been limited to animal and cadaveric studies. At present there is an established full facial-scalp allograft model in rats which includes a bilateral external ear component.[66] The flap is elevated from the facial muscles and then divided based on its vascular pedicle, the common carotid arteries, and external jugular veins. Siemionow has recently shown in rats that acceptance of facial allografts can be drastically increased (up to 100% at 200 days posttransplant) when modifying the arterial anastomoses to include only a unilateral common carotid artery anastomosis. Immunosuppressive therapy is both inducted and maintained using CsA.[67]

In 2004, the Cleveland Clinic Hospital (Cleveland, OH) led by Siemionow, became the first within the United States to have an IRB-approved protocol for facial transplantation. In addition, London's Royal Free Hospital's research committee gave Butler and colleagues permission to begin evaluating potential recipients as well.

Later in 2004, a report was published by England's Royal College of Surgeons estimating that a facial allograft recipient would have a 10% chance of graft loss due to acute rejection in their first postoperative year, and a 30–50% risk of graft loss due to chronic rejection in their first 2–5 years. While the English remain pessimistic, the United States' ASRM (American Society for Reconstructive Microsurgery) and ASPS (American Society of Plastic Surgeons) have jointly issued a set of guidelines recommending facial transplantation to be performed by only IRB-approved institutions in patients whose reconstructive options have been exhausted.[68]

Needless to say further investigation is warranted prior to the vision of clinical face allotransplantation becoming reality, but similar skepticism existed toward rat hindlimb allotransplantation in the 1980s.

References

1. K. S. Black, C. W. Hewitt, L. A. Fraser, et al., Cosmas and Damian in the laboratory, N Engl J Med 306(6), 368–369 (1982).
2. J. Parra, J. A. Torres, F. Alvarez, et al., Kidney homografts: induction of specific tolerance through the lymphoid tissues, Ann NY Acad Sci 30(120), 524–534 (1964).

3. E. M. Billaud, Clinical pharmacology of immunosuppressive drugs: year 2000-time for alternatives, Therapie 55(1), 177–183 (2000).
4. W. A. Morrison, B. M. O'Brien, A. M. MacLeod, A. Gilbert, Neurovascular free flaps from the foot for innervation of the hand, J Hand Surg 3(3), 235–242 (1978).
5. R. M. Merion, D. J. White, S. Thiru, et al., CsA: five years' experience in cadaveric renal transplantation, N Engl J Med 19(310), 148–154 (1984).
6. R. Y. Calne, CsA and liver transplantation, Mt Sinai J Med 54(6), 465–466 (1987).
7. I. G. Brons, R. Y. Calne, Pancreas transplantation at Cambridge: more than 10 years experience at the CsA era, Transplant Proc 23(4), 2215–2216 (1991).
8. C. W. Hewitt, K. S. Black, L. A. Fraser, et al., Composite tissue (limb) allografts in rats. I. Dose-dependent increase in survival with CsA, Transplantation 39(4), 360–364 (1985).
9. K. S. Black, C. W. Hewitt, L. A. Fraser, et al., Composite tissue (limb) allografts in rats. II. Indefinite survival using low-dose CsA, Transplantation 39(4), 365–368 (1985).
10. C. W. Hewitt, K. S. Black, S. F. Dowdy, et al., Composite tissue (limb) allografts in rats. III. Development of donor-host lymphoid chimeras in long-term survivors, Transplantation 41(1), 39–43 (1986).
11. C. W. Hewitt, K. S. Black, L. E. Henson, et al., Lymphocyte chimerism in a full allogeneic composite tissue (rat-limb) allograft model prolonged with CsA, Transplant Proc 20(2 Suppl 2), 272–278 (1988).
12. C. W. Hewitt, K. S. Black, A. M. Aguinaldo, et al., CsA and skin allografts for the treatment of thermal injury. I. Extensive graft survival with low-level long-term administration and prolongation in a rat burn model, Transplantation 45(1), 8–12 (1988).
13. C. W. Hewitt, K. S. Black, J. A. Stenger, et al., Comparison of kidney, composite tissue, and skin allograft survival in rats prolonged by donor blood and concomitant limited CsA, Transplant Proc 20 (3 Suppl 3), 1110–1113 (1988).
14. L. M. Ferreira, J. P. Anthony, S. Mathes, et al., Complications of allogeneic microsurgical transplantation of a limb (composite tissue), in rats, Rev Assoc Med Bras 41(3), 213–218 (1995).
15. B. M. Achauer, K. S. Black, C. W. Hewitt, et al., Immunosurgery, Clin Plast Surg 12(2), 293–307 (1985).
16. G. Guzman-Stein, A. R. Shons, Functional recovery in the rat limb transplant model: a preliminary study, Transplant Proc 19(1 Pt2), 1115–1117 (1987).
17. J. Randzio, H. Kniha, M. E. Gold, et al., Growth of vascularized composite mandibular allografts in young rabbits, Ann Plast Surg 26(2), 140–148 (1991).
18. M. E. Gold, J. Randzio, H. Kniha, et al., Transplantation of vascularized composite mandibular allografts in young cynomolgus monkeys, Ann Plast Surg 26(2), 125–132 (1991).
19. P. Benhaim, J. P. Anthony, L. Y. Lin, et al., A long-term study of allogeneic rat hindlimb transplants immunosuppressed with RS-61443, Transplantation 56(4), 911–917 (1993).
20. P. Benhaim, J. P. Anthony, L. Ferreira, et al., Use of combination of low-dose CsA and RS-61443 in a rat hindlimb model of composite tissue allotransplantation, Transplantation 61(4), 527–532 (1996).
21. M. Z. Siemionow, D. M. Izycki, M. Zielinski, Donor-specific tolerance in fully major histocompatibility complex-mismatched limb allograft transplants under an anti-alpha/beta T-cell receptor monoclonal antibody and cyclosporine A protocol, Transplantation 76(12), 1662–1668 (2003).
22. M. Siemionow, T. Ortak, D. Izycki, et al., Induction of tolerance in composite-tissue allografts, Transplantation 74(9), 1211–1217 (2002).
23. M. Siemionow, D. Izycki, K. Ozer, et al., Role of thymus in operational tolerance induction in limb allograft transplant model, Transplantation 81(11), 1568–1576 (2006).
24. C. Tai, M. Goldenberg, K. M. Schuster, et al., Composite tissue allotransplantation, J Invest Surg 16(4), 193–201 (2003).
25. J. H. Barker, W. C. Breidenbach, C. W. Hewitt, Second international symposium on composite tissue allotransplantation. introduction, Microsurgery 20(8), 359 (2000).
26. B. Kann, C. W. Hewitt, Composite tissue (hand) allotransplantation: Are we ready? Plast Reconstr Surg 107(4), 1060–1065 (2001).

27. E. T. Ustuner, M. Zdichavsky, X. Ren, et al., Long-term composite tissue allograft survival in a porcine model with cyclosporine/mycophenolate mofetil therapy, Transplantation 66(12), 1581–1587 (1998).
28. J. M. Dubernard, E. Owen, N. Lefrancois, et al., First human hand transplantation. Case report, Transpl Int 13(Suppl 1), S521–514 (2000).
29. J. W. Jones, S. A. Gruber, J. H. Barker, et al., Successful hand transplantation. One-year follow-up. Louisville Hand Transplant Team, N Engl J Med 343(7), 468–473 (2000).
30. J. M. Dubernard, P. Henry, H. Parmentier, et al., First transplantation of two hands: results after 18 months, Ann Chir 127(1), 19–25 (2002).
31. C. G. Francois, W. C. Breidenbach, C. Maldonado, et al., Hand transplantation: comparisons and observations of the first four clinical cases, Microsurgery 20(8), 360–371 (2000).
32. J. M. Dubernard, P. Petruzzo, M. Lanzetta, et al., Functional results of the first human double-hand transplantation, Ann Surg 238(1), 128–136 (2000).
33. S. Schneeberger, M. Ninkovic, H. Piza-Katzer, et al., Status 5 years after bilateral hand transplantation, Am J Transplant 6(4), 834–841 (2006).
34. P. Petruzzo, J. P. Revillard, J. Kanitakis, et al., First human double hand transplantation: efficacy of a conventional immunosuppressive protocol, Clin Transplant 17(5), 455–460 (2003).
35. M. Lanzetta, P. Petruzzo, G. Vitale, et al., Human hand transplantation: what have we learned? Transplant Proc 36(3), 664–668 (2004).
36. F. Schuind, C. Van Holder, D. Mouraux, et al., The first Belgian hand transplantation-37 month term results, J Hand Surg 31(4), 371–376 (2006).
37. M. Lanzetta, P. Petruzzo, R. Margreiter, et al., The international registry on hand and composite tissue transplantation, Transplantation 79(9), 1210–1214 (2005).
38. F. Petit, L. Lantieri, M. A. Randolph, W. P. Lee, Future research in immunology for composite tissue allotransplantation, Ann Chir Plast Esthet 51(1), 11–17 (2006).
39. J. M. Dubernard, Composite tissue allografts: a challenge for transplantologists, Am J Transplant 5(6), 1580–1581 (2005).
40. S. Hettiaratchy, M. A. Randolph, F. Petit, et al., Composite tissue allotransplantation—a new era in plastic surgery? Br J Plast Surg 57(5): 381–391 (2004).
41. K. G. Rose, K. Sesterhenn, F. Wustrow, Tracheal allotransplantation in man, Lancet 1(8113), 433 (1979).
42. Yu. N. Levashov, P. K. Yablonsky, S. M. Cherny, et al., One-stage allotransplantation of thoracic segment of the trachea in a patient with idiopathic fibrosing medistinitis and marked tracheal stenosis, Eur J Cardiothorac Surg 7(7), 383–386 (1993).
43. W. Klepetko, G. M. Marta, W. Wisser, et al., Heterotopic tracheal transplantation with omentum wrapping in the abdominal position preserves functional and structural integrity of a human tracheal allograft, J Thorac Cardiovasc Surg 127(3), 862–867 (2004).
44. M. J. Brenner, J. N. Jensen, J. B. Lowe 3rd, et al., Anti-CD40 ligand antibody permits regeneration through peripheral nerve allografts in a nonhuman primate model, Plast Reconstr Surg 114(7), 1802–1814 (2004).
45. R. V. Weber, S. E. Mackinnon, Bridging the neural gap, Clin Plast Surg 32(4), 605–616 (2005).
46. M. J. Brenner, J. B. Lowe 3rd, I. K. Fox, et al., Effects of Schwann cells and donor antigen on long-nerve allograft regeneration, Microsurgery 25(1), 61–70 (2005).
47. I. K. Fox, A. Jaramillo, D. A. Hunter, et al., Prolonged cold-preservation of nerve allografts, Muscle Nerve 31(1), 59–69 (2005).
48. S. K. Sen, J. B. Lowe 3rd, M. J. Brenner, et al., Assessment of the immune response to dose of nerve allografts, Plast Reconstr Surg 115(3), 823–830 (2005).
49. E. Peacock, J. W. Madden, Human composite flexor tendon allografts, Ann Surg 166(4), 624–629 (1967).
50. E. Peacock, W. Van Winkle, Surgery and biology of wound repair. Philadelphia: Saunders; (1970) pp. 398–404.
51. J. C. Guimberteau, B. Panconi, R. Boileau, Simple and composite ulnar transplants in reconstructive surgery of the hand, Ann Chir Plast Esthet 39(3), 301–317 (1994).

52. J. C. Guimberteau, J. Baudet, B. Panconi, et al., Human allotransplant of a digital flexion system vascularized on the ulnar pedicle: a preliminary report and 1-year follow-up of two cases, Plast Reconstr Surg 89(6), 1135–1147 (1992).
53. G. O. Hofmann, M. H. Kirschner, F. D. Wagner, et al., Allogeneic vascularized transplantation of human femoral diaphyses and total knee joints-first clinical experiences, Transplant Proc 30(6), 2754–2761 (1998).
54. G. O. Hofmann, M. H. Kirschner, F. D. Wagner, et al., Allogeneic vascularized grafting of human knee joints under postoperative immunosuppression of the recipient, World J Surg 22(8), 818–823 (1998).
55. G. O. Hofmann, M. H. Kirschner, Clinical experience in allogeneic vascularized bone and joint allografting, Microsurgery 20(8), 375–383 (2000).
56. R. M. Zuker, R. Redett, B. Alman, et al., First successful lower-extremity transplantation: technique and functional result, J Reconstr Microsurg 22(4), 239–244 (2006).
57. P. Kluyskens, S. Ringoir, Follow-up of a human larynx transplantation, Laryngoscope 80(8), 1244–1250 (1970).
58. M. A. Birchall, R. R. Lorenz, G. S. Berke, et al., Laryngeal transplantation in 2005: a Review, Am J Transplant 6(1), 20–26 (2006).
59. P. A. Bejarano, D. Levi, M. Nassiri, et al., The pathology of full-thickness cadaver skin transplant for large abdominal defects: a proposed grading system for skin allograft acute rejection, Am J Surg Pathol 28(5), 670–675 (2004).
60. G. Selvaggi, D. M. Levi, T. Kato, et al., Expanded use of transplantation techniques: abdominal wall transplantation and intestinal autotransplantation, Transplant Proc 36(5), 1561–1563 (2004).
61. B. Devauchelle, L. Badet, B. Lengele, et al., First human face allograft: early report, Lancet 368(9531), 203–209 (2006).
62. R. Khamsi, World's second face transplant performed in China, New Sci 14, 29 (2006).
63. M. Siemionow, S. Unal, G. Agaoglu, A. Sari, A cadaver study in preparation for facial allograft transplantation in humans: part I. What are alternative sources for total facial defect coverage, Plast Reconstr Surg 117(3), 864–875 (2006).
64. M. Siemionow, G. Agaoglu, S. Unal, A cadaver study in preparation for facial allograft transplantation in humans: part II. Mock facial transplantation, Plast Reconstr Surg 117(3), 876–878 (2006).
65. O. Wiggins, J. Barker, S. Martinez, et al., On the ethics of facial transplantation research, Am J of Bioethics 4(3), 1–12 (2004).
66. Y. Demir, S. Ozmen, A. Klimczak, et al., Tolerance induction in composite facial allograft transplantation in the rat model, Plastic Reconstr Surg 114(7), 1790–1801 (2004).
67. S. Unal, G. Agaoglu, J. Zins, M. Siemionow, New surgical approach in facial transplantation extends survival of allograft recipients, Ann Plast Surg 55(3), 297–303 (2005).
68. S. Okie, Brave new face, N Engl J Med 354(9), 889–894 (2006).

Chapter 3
The Impact of the Discovery of Cyclosporine on Transplantation of Composite Tissue Allografts

Zsolt T. Csapo, Bence Forgacs, and Barry D. Kahan

3.1 Introduction

Over the past 30 years, progress in basic science, immunopharmacology, and clinical practice has engendered exciting improvements in the field of transplantation that have resulted in longer patient and graft survivals and a better quality of life for recipients. Composite tissue transplantation has benefited from developments in organ transplantation: harvest of tissue from deceased donors and improved immunosuppression. The goal of organ transplantation – an efficient yet nontoxic immunosuppressive regimen – is particularly necessary for composite transplants because these grafts are not vital to host survival.

The first generation of chemical immunosuppressants in clinical use – azathioprine, cyclophosphamide, methotrexate – as well as the more recent agent mycophenolate mofetil, all exert an indiscriminate blockade of cell division, which prevents expansion of the number of immunocompetent elements. The next development in this therapeutic area was the introduction of lymphoid depleting modalities – antilymphocyte sera, total lymphoid irradiation, and thoracic duct drainage. The most recent stage utilizes compounds that display greater selectivity for immunocompetent than nonspecific host resistance elements. Cyclosporine (CsA), as the first drug to fulfill this goal, had an important impact on the biology and practice of immunosuppression.

3.2 History of Composite Transplantation

Some authors trace the history of transplantation to 400 BC when the Indian physician Sushruta used skin grafts from the cheek to reconstruct noses and ear lobes. Transplantation of skin or other body parts from animals or later from humans were utilized by surgeons. In 1668, the Dutchman Job van Meeneren claimed to have performed a successful bone graft from a dog's skull to repair a defect in the human cranium. In 1682, a canine bone was reportedly used to repair the skull of an injured Russian aristocrat who was later said to have had the bone removed because of threats of excommunication from the church.

A major step was the first temporary skin transplant from a deceased donor in 1881. The surgeon used skin from a deceased person as a temporary graft for a seriously burned patient. Following the possibilities of finer surgical techniques in 1906, the first successful human corneal allograft transplant was reported by Eduard Zirm in Olmutz (Moravia). The graft maintained some degree of transparency. Few other surgeons matched Zirm's success until after the Second World War, when fine needles and suture material became available.

The first unsuccessful knee-joint transplant from a deceased donor was performed by Erich Lexer in Germany in 1908. A few years later, in 1911, Yamanouchi performed the first homologous vein transplant for arterial reconstruction. The increasing number of reported transplants encouraged surgeons to transplant various tissues and organs. In 1920, the first monkey testes were transplanted into humans in France by Serge Voronoff. By the early 1930s, more than 500 men were reported to have received transplanted testes, but the fallacy of this approach was evident shortly thereafter. In 1964, an attempt at a hand transplant was undertaken in Ecuador, but the graft was rejected within 2 weeks. A partial larynx transplant was done in Belgium in 1969, but the patient died without speaking.

3.3 Immunosuppression

Although the surgical techniques have been successful in composite transplantation, graft survival or function has been poor, showing that control of rejection was the most important issue. In humans, total body irradiation had proved useful in achieving successful bone marrow homografts. Unfortunately, in the settings of other organ transplants, including kidney grafts, irradiation treatment alone generally led to dismal outcomes because of the profound bone marrow depression, which impaired nonspecific host resistance.

A major advance in the control of rejection of transplanted organs was achieved with the introduction of chemical immunosuppressants. Schwartz and Dameshek observed that treatment with 6-mercaptopurine prevented rabbits from producing antibodies toward foreign proteins such as human albumen. Subsequent experiments showed that the drug prolonged canine renal allograft survival. In 1961, Joseph Murray prescribed 6-mercaptopurine for a recipient of a human kidney transplant; however, the patient unfortunately died from drug toxicity. After a disappointing experience with total body irradiation, Roy Calne's experimented with azathioprine, an imidazole analog of 6-mercaptopurine that showed superior oral absorption. However, when used alone, azathioprine was not effective in suppressing human responses to allotransplants. Cortisone, which had been discovered to be an immunosuppressant in 1936, was combined with azathioprine by French investigators initially and later by Starzl. In 1964, Hume noted that regular doses of prednisone were not only useful to prevent graft failure, but in larger doses also reversed renal allograft rejection episodes. However, this combination, which remained the standard of care throughout the 1970s, severely impaired nonspecific host resistance, thereby enhancing the risk of serious infections.

3.4 Cyclosporine: Discovery and Structure

The CsA story began in 1969 when the Microbiology Department of Sandoz (Basle Switzerland) tested two new strains of fungi imperfecti that had been isolated from soil samples obtained in Hardanger Vidda, a high treeless plain in Southern Norway. Although it synthesized CsA, *Cylindrocarpon lucidum* Booth only grew in surface culture, making it less suitable for fermentation cultures than the other strain, *Tolypocladium inflatum* Gams. Antibiotic testing revealed that the only marginal fungistatic activity in vivo was primarily directly against clinically irrelevant organisms. In 1973, Ruegger et al. reported the purification of the active compound of CsA from the fermentation mixture (24–556). Subsequently, the culture conditions needed to produce compounds were substantially improved to optimize yields.[14]

Chemical degradation and X-ray analysis were used to elucidate the structure of an iodo-derivative of CsA.[36,42] CsA is a neutral, hydrophobic cyclic peptide composed of eleven amino acid residues, having the configuration of the natural L-amino acids except a D-alanine in position 8. Seven N-methylated amino acid residues occupy positions 1, 3, 4, 6, 9, 10, and 11. Ten amino acids are aliphatic, namely, alpha-aminobutyric acid in position 2, sarcosine in position 3, *N*-methyl-leucine in positions 4, 6, 9, and 10, valine in position 5, alanine in position 7, D-alanine in position 8, and *N*-methylvaline in position 11. One novel N-methylated amino acid in position 1, the C-9-amino acid, is composed of nine carbon atoms with a double bond, which was found for the first time in nature in CsA and had never before been isolated or known in free form (Fig. 3.1). Finally, the complete molecule was successfully synthesized by Wenger in 1980. However, the compound designated 24–556 showed unusually low toxicity.

In 1972, Jean F. Borel discovered the marked immunosuppressive effects of 24–556 (Cyclosporine A) in mouse and rat models of autoimmunity and alloimmunity. In his experiments, fitted pinch grafts of skin from male DBA/2 donors were transplanted to male BALB/c recipients with rejection determined by daily observations of epithelial survival. The group receiving 100–300 mg/kg daily oral administration of compound displayed significantly prolonged skin allograft survival. BDF/1 female mice showed graft-versus-host reactions following male spleen cells reconstitution after a sublethal dose of cyclophosphamide. CsA delayed the onset of death due to a graft-versus-host reaction. Experimental allergic encephalomyelitis, which was induced in Lewis rats with inoculation of *Mycobacterium phlei* into both hind foot pads, was evidenced by paralysis. CsA considerably reduced the incidence of paralysis at doses of 50 or 100 mg/kg/day. Freund's adjuvant arthritis was induced in female OFA rats with intradermal injection of heat-killed *Mycobacterium smegmae* into one hind paw. The vertical and horizontal diameters of noninjected

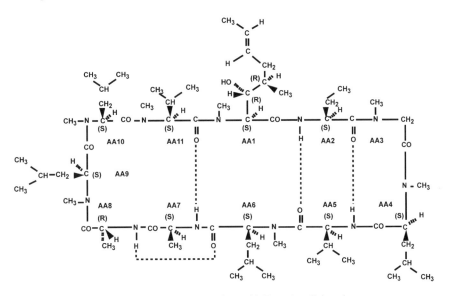

Fig. 3.1 The structure of cyclosporine. AA, amino acid; R, active, S, inactive

paws were recorded on days 0 and 19. Total suppression of paw swelling was obtained with 30 mg/kg/day CsA dose with a pronounced inhibition observed following a prolonged therapeutic schedule.[5] Further experiments with pure CsA supported the concept of a selective action of CsA on lymphoid cells.[5–7,18]

Because of its selectivity, this drug was the prototype of a new generation of immunosuppressants that selectively act on adaptive resistance while sparing nonspecific host resistance. At the 1976 Spring meeting of the British Society for Immunology, Borel first communicated his experimental animal results with CsA: (1) It showed selectivity for lymphocytes; mainly for T helper cells; (2) It suppressed humoral and cell-mediated immune reactions; (3) It inhibited the induction phase of lymphoid cell proliferation by affecting early mitogenic triggering but not mitosis; (4) It was not lymphocytotoxic because the effect was reversible; (5) It was effective in all species tested: the mouse, rat, guinea pig, rabbit, and monkey.

These properties interested D.J.G. White of Cambridge, UK, who initiated the first experimental animal studies performed outside Sandoz, starting with heterotopic heart allografts in rats.[9,31] Impressive results were obtained by the Cambridge group in many transplantation models.

Thereafter, these findings were duplicated with lung allografts in dogs[35] as well as small bowel transplants in pigs[10,11,41] and dogs.[13] Grafted skeletal muscle[47], composite tissue allografts[4] and nerve and Schwann cells[50] were shown to recover their normal function. Prolonged survival was observed for concordant xenografts of kidney[28] and heart.[24]

The first recipients of mismatched cadaver kidney transplants were treated by Calne and colleagues,[11,12] and a cohort of bone marrow transplants reported by Powles et al.[37] These experiences revealed that CsA also displays strong immunosuppressive effects in man. Corneal transplantation was reported in three groups during a similar time period,[1,43,44] with topical application alone proving sufficient to ensure graft survival.[25] Since this time, thousands of reports have been delivered at scientific congresses and in the medical literature, leading to the general acceptance of CsA by the health authorities and registration as an approved drug in 1983.[27,34,48]

The major practical field of interest for CsA has been organ transplantation as described in a volume celebrating the 20th anniversary (Transplantation Proceedings 2004)[52].

3.5 Cyclosporine: Mechanism of Action

CsA is a prodrug. To gain pharmacologic activity it must bind to cytoplasmic components termed immunophilins. After binding to the *cis–trans* prolyl-petidyl isomerase, namely, cyclophilin (CyP), the drug undergoes a structural change that everts the hydrophilic region of amino cids 1, 2, 3 from the inside to the outside of the ring. The CsA–CyP complexes bind near the junction of the heterodimeric calcineurin A and B chains, which are complexed with Ca++ and calmodulin. The inhibitory pentameric association prevents dephosphorylation, transport, and release in the nucleus of transcriptional promoters – the nuclear factor of activated T-cells (NF-AT) as well as NF-Kappa-KB and other factors.[20,26] Inhibition of calcineurin action prevents generation of nuclear promoters and blocks the expression of several cytokine genes that promote T-cell activation, including IL-2, IL-4, and IFN-gamma[15] (Fig. 3.2).

3.6 Biologic Effects of Cyclosporine

The discovery of CsA, with its marked immunosuppressant effects to produce successful transplantation of tissues of varying immunogenicity and, particularly, its good tolerability, allowed exploration of composite tissue allografts. Unlike solid organ allografts, composite allografts, such as a hand or an entire limb, are histologically heterogeneous being composed of tissues that show varying degrees of antigenicity. Among these tissues are the highly antigenic skin and muscle, as well as immunocompetent components, such as bone marrow and lymph nodes, which may participate in the immunological reaction leading to a challenging treatment of surgical and immunological aspects. Table 3.1 lists some composite allograft studies performed using CsA.

In the 1980s, Hewitt and associates reported numerous studies on the use of CsA to significantly prolong the survival of limb allografts in rats.[4,21,22,23] After subcutaneous delivery of CsA daily for 20 days postoperatively, three of five rats receiving

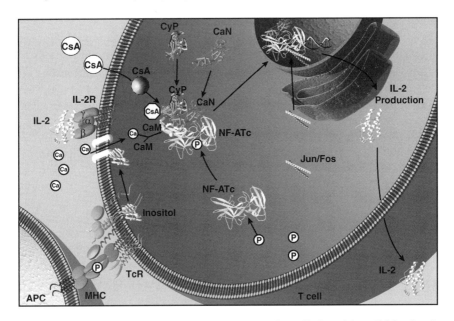

Fig. 3.2 The action of cyclosporine. APC, antigen presenting cell; Ca, calcium; CaM, calmodulin; CaN, calcineurin; CsA, cyclosporine; CyP, cyclophilin; IL-2, Interleukin-2; Jun/Fos, Jun/Fos proteins; MHC, major histocompatibility complex; NF-ATc, nuclear factor of activated T cells; TcR, T-cell receptor

Table 3.1 Studies with cyclosporine

Date	Researcher	Surgery	Immunosuppression
1982	Siliski[45]	Whole-knee-joint	Alone CsA
1983	Press[38]	Rat limb	CsA + Prednisone
1984	Kim[29]	Rat hindlimb	AZA + Steroid
1984	Fritz[16]	Rat hindlimb	CsA
1987	Guzman-Stein[19]	Rat hindlimb	High-dose CsA
1989	Kniha[30]	Rabbit forelimb	CsA
1991	Randzio[40]	Rabbit hemi-mandible	High-dose CsA
1991	Gold[17]	Monkey hemi-mandible	CsA
1993	Benhaim[2]	Rat hindlimb	Alone CsA
1996	Benhaim[3]	Rat hindlimb	CsA + MMF
1995	Lee[33]	Rat distal femur	Alone CsA
1998	Ustuner[46]	Swine radial forelimb	Alone CsA

twice weekly maintenance therapy displayed more than 400-day allograft survivals. Survivals in treated versus untreated animals were 101 versus 18 days, respectively. In 1982, Siliski et al.[45] described prolonged survival of whole-knee-joint allografts in rabbits using CsA as the only immunosuppressant. Although in 1983, Press et al.[38,39] were unable to prolong rat limb allograft survival with intraperitoneal CsA plus prednisone therapy, 3 years later when they repeated the study using a lower CsA dose they noted prolonged survival of the limb grafts despite rejection of the corresponding skin.

In 1984, Kim et al.[29] observed early rejection of hindlimb transplants among rats that were treated with azathioprine and steroids, but prolonged survival with CsA. In the same year, Fritz et al.[16] reported prolonged hindlimb graft survival among rats receiving continuous CsA treatment.

Using immature rats, Guzman-Stein et al.[19] demonstrated good functional recovery of hindlimb transplants, which showed normal bone healing, bone growth, and reinnervation of skin and muscle. Rejection episodes were reversed by increasing the dose of CsA. In 1989, Kniha et al.[30] observed 75–80% growth of immature forelimb transplants in rabbits using CsA. In 1991, Randzio et al.[40] reported a successful hemi-mandible transplant in rabbits treated with CsA. Although the allografts functioned well, the toxic effects of high doses of CsA prevented long-term survival. In the same year, Gold et al.[17] reported hemi-mandible transplants in monkeys using CsA. Two of the four animals chewed, ate normal diets, and gained weight. These animals displayed graft survivals of more than 60 days. Using CsA, Lee et al.[33] reported transplantation of the distal femur and surrounding musculature in rats. The rats showed weight bearing and bone healing.

The introduction of mycophenolate mofetil at the beginning of the 1990s provided another tool for composite tissue allotransplants. In 1993, Benhaim et al.[2] reported rejection of transplanted hindlimbs in rats using CsA alone, but 3 years later the animals survived with functioning grafts for more than 32 weeks when the authors used CsA in combination with mycophenolate mofetil. In 1998, Ustuner et al.[46] employed similar immunosuppression in a swine radial forelimb osteomyocutaneous flap model. Among the eight surviving animals, two had severe rejection, three mild to moderate responses, and three no reactions after 90 days.

After numerous successful composite tissue allografts in small animals, primate transplantation studies had only limited success. Although hand transplantation was performed with restoration of acceptable neuromuscular function, rejection was observed often, and attempts to reverse rejection had only limited success.[32]

Although CsA has an appropriate safety profile for the success of complex tissue transplants, a more potent degree of immunosuppression is necessary, such as that provided by the second-generation calcineurin antagonist tacrolimus. However, CsA has played a critical role in launching successful composite tissue allotransplantation.

References

1. Bell, T. A., Easty, D. L., and McCullagh, K. G., 1982, A placebo-controlled blind trial of cyclosporin-A in prevention of corneal graft rejection in rabbits, *Br J Ophthalmol.* **66**:303.
2. Benhaim, P., Anthony, J. P., Lin, L. Y.-T., McCalmont, T. H., and Mathes, S. J., 1993, A long-term study of allogeneic rat hindlimb transplants immunosuppressed with RS-61443, *Transplantation.* **56**:911.

3. Benhaim, P., Anthony, J. P., Ferreira, L., Borsanyi, J-P., and Mathes, S. J., 1996, Use of combination of low-dose cyclosporine and RS-61443 in a rat hindlimb model of composite tissue allotransplantation, *Transplantation.* **61**:527.
4. Black, K. S., Hewitt, C. W., Fraser, L. A., Howard, E. B., Martin, D. C., Achauer, B. M., and Furnas, D. W., 1985, Composite tissue (limb) allografts in rats. II. Indefinite survival using low-dose cyclosporine, *Transplantation.* **39**:365.
5. Borel, J. F., Feurer, C., Gubler, H. U., and Stahelin, H., 1976, Biological effects of cyclosporin A: a new antilymphocytic agent, *Agents Action.* **6**:468.
6. Borel, J. F., Feurer, C., Magnee, C., and Stahelin, H., 1977, Effects of the new anti-lymphocytic peptide cyclosporin A in animals, *Immunology.* **32**:1017.
7. Burckhardt, J. J., and Guggenheim, B., 1979, Cyclosporin A: in vivo and in vitro suppression of rat T-lymphocyte function, *Immunology.* **36**:753.
8. Calne, R. Y., 1960, The rejection of renal homografts: inhibition in dogs by using 6-mercaptopurine. Lancet **1**:417.
9. Calne, R. Y., and White, D. J. G., 1977, Cyclosporin A—a powerful immunosuppressant in dogs with renal allografts, *Surg Transplant.* **5**:595.
10. Calne, R. Y., Sells, R. A., Pena, J. R., Davis, D. R., Millard, P. R., Herbertson, B. M., Binns, R. M., and Davies, D. A., 1969, Induction of immunological tolerance by porcine liver allografts, *Nature.* **223**:472.
11. Calne, R. Y., White, D. J., Rolles, K., Smith, D. P., and Herbertson, B. M., 1978, Prolonged survival of pig orthotopic heart grafts treated with cyclosporin A, *Lancet.* **1**:1183.
12. Calne, R. Y., Rolles, K., White, D. J., Thiru, S., Evans, D. B., McMaster, P., Dunn, D. C., Craddock, G. N., Henderson, R. G., Aziz, S., and Lewis, P., 1979, Cyclosporin A initially as the only immunosuppressant in 34 recipients of cadaveric organs: 32 kidneys, 2 pancreases, and 2 livers, *Lancet.* **2**:1033.
13. Craddock, G. N., Nordgren, S. R., Reznick, R. K., Gilas, T., Lossing, A. G., Cohen, Z., Stiller, C. R., Cullen, J. B., and Langer, B., 1983, Small bowel transplantation in the dog using cyclosporine, *Transplantation.* **35**:284.
14. Dreyfuss, M., Harri, E., Hofmann, H., Kobel, H., Pache, W., and Tscherter, H., 1976, Cyclosporine A and C – new metabolites from Trichoderma polysporum (Link ex pers) Rifai, *Eur J Appl Microbiol.* **3**:125.
15. Danovitch, G. M., 2001, *Handbook of Kidney Transplantation*, Lippincott Williams and Willkins, Philadelphia, USA
16. Fritz, W. D., Swartz, W. M., Rose, S., Futrell, J. W., and Klein, E., 1984, Limb allografts in rats immunosuppressed with cyclosporine A, *Ann Surg.* **199**:211.
17. Gold, M. E., Randzio, J., Kniha, H., Kim, B. S., Park, H. H., Stein, J. P., Booth, K., Gruber, H. E., and Furnas, D. W., 1991, Transplantation of vascularized composite mandibular allografts in young cynomolgus monkeys, *Ann Plast Surg.* **26**:125.
18. Gordon, M. Y., and Singer, J. W., 1979, Selective effects of cyclosporin A on colony-forming lymphoid and myeloid cells in man, *Nature.* **31**;279:433.
19. Guzman-Stein, G., and Shons, A. R., 1987, Functional recovery in the rat limb transplant model: a preliminary study. *Transplant Proc.* **9**:1115.
20. Henderson, D. J., Naya, I., Bundick, R. V., Smith, G. M., and Schmidt, J. A., 1991, Comparison of the effects of FK-506, cyclosporin A and rapamycin on IL-2 production, *Immunology.* **73**:316.
21. Hewitt, C. W., Black, K. S., Fraser, L. A., Howard, E. B., Martin, D. C., Achauer, B. M., and Furnas, D. W., 1983, Cyclosporine A is superior to prior donor-specific blood transfusion for the extensive prolongation of rat limb allograft survival, *Transplant Proc.* **15**:514.
22. Hewitt, C. W., Black, K. S., Fraser, L. A., Howard, E. B., Martin, D. C., Achauer, B. M., and Furnas, D. W., 1985, Composite tissue (limb) allografts in rats. I. Dose-dependent increase in survival with cyclosporine, *Transplantation.* **39**:360.
23. Hewitt, C. W., Black, K. S., Dowdy, S. F., Gonzalez, G. A., Achauer, B. M., Martin, D. C., Furnas, D. W., and Howard, E. B., 1986, Composite tissue (limb) allografts in rats. III. Development of donor-host lymphoid chimeras in long-term survivors, *Transplantation.* **41**:39.

24. Homan, W. P., Williams, K. A., Fabre, J. W., Millard, P. R., and Morris, P. J., 1981, Prolongation of cardiac xenograft survival in rats receiving cyclosporin A, *Transplantation.* **31**:164.
25. Hunter, P. A., Wilhelmus, K. R., Rice, N. S. C., and Jones, B. R., 1981, Cyclosporine A applied topically to the recipient eye inhibits corneal graft rejection. *Clin Exp Immunol.* **45**:173.
26. Johansson, A., and Moller, E., 1990, Evidence that the immunosuppressive effects of FK506 and cyclosporine are identical, *Transplantation.* **50**:1001.
27. Kahan, B. D., and Ponticelli, C., 2000, *Principles and Practice of Renal Transplantation*, Martin Dunitz Ltd, London, UK.
28. Dieperink H., and Starklint H., 1983, Effect of cyclosproin A on ischaemically damaged rabbit kidneys. Dan Med Bull. **30**(4):278–80.
29. Kim, S. K., Aziz, S., Oyer, P., and Hentz, V. R., 1984, Use of cyclosporine in allotransplantation of rat limbs, *Ann Plast Surg.* **12**:249.
30. Kniha, H., Randzio, J., Gold, M. E., Fudem, G. M., Cruz, H. G., Park, H. H., and Furnas, D. W., 1989, Growth of forelimb allografts in young rabbits immunosuppressed with cyclosporine, *Ann Plast Surg.* **22**:135.
31. Kostakis, A. J., White, D. J. G., and Calne, R. Y., 1977, Prolongation of the rat heart allograft survival by cyclosporin A, *IRCS Med Sci.* **5**:280.
32. Lanzetta, M., Pozzo, M., Bottin, A., Merletti, R., and Farina, D., 2005, Reinnervation of motor units in intrinsic muscles of a transplanted hand, *Neurosci Lett.* **10**;373:138.
33. Lee, W. P., Pan, Y. C., Kesmarky, S., Randolph, M. A., Fiala, T. S., Amarante, M. T., Weiland, A. J., and Yaremchuk, M. J., 1995, Experimental orthotopic transplantation of vascularized skeletal allografts: functional assessment and long-term survival, *Plast Reconstr Surg.* **95**:336; discussion 350.
34. Morris, P. J., 1981, Cyclosporin A, *Transplantation.* **32**:349.
35. Norin, A. J., Veith, F. J., Emeson, E. E., Montefusco, C. M., Pinsker, K. L., and Kamholz, S. L., 1981, Improved survival of transplanted lungs in mongrel dogs treated with cyclosporin A, *Transplantation.* **32**:259.
36. Petcher, T. J., Weber, H. P., and Ruegger, A., 1976, Crystal and molecular structure of an iodo-derivative of the cyclic undecapeptide cyclosporine A, *Helv Chim Acta.* **59**:1480.
37. Powles, R. L., Barrett, A. J., Clink, H., Kay, H. E., Sloane, J., and McElwain, T. J., 1978, Cyclosporin A for the treatment of graft-versus-host disease in man, *Lancet.* **2**:1327.
38. Press, B. H., Sibley, R. K., and Shons, A. R., 1983, Modification of experimental limb allograft rejection with cyclosporin and prednisone: a preliminary report, *Transplant Proc.* **5**:3057.
39. Press, B. H., Sibley, R. K., and Shons, A. R., 1986, Limb allotransplantation in the rat: extended survival and return of nerve function with continuous cyclosporine/prednisone immunosuppression, *Ann Plast Surg.* **16**:313.
40. Randzio, J., Kniha, H., Gold, M. E., Chang, T. T., Su, L. D., Park, H. H., Cho, J. S., Booth, K., and Furnas, D. W., 1991, Growth of vascularized composite mandibular allografts in young rabbits, *Ann Plast Surg.* **26**:140.
41. Ricour, C., Revillon, Y., Laufenberger, A., et al., 1981, Effect of cyclosporin A on the survival of piglet small intestine allografts, *Eur Soc Paediat Gastroentrol Nutr.* (Abstract).
42. Ruegger, A., Kuhn, M., Lichti, H., Loosli, H. R., Huguenin, R., Quiquerez, C., and von Wartburg, A., 1976, Cyclosporin A, ein immunosuppressiv wirksamer Peptidmetabolit aus Trichoderma polysporum Rifai, *Helv Chim Acta.* **59**:1075–1092.
43. Gebhardt, B. M., 1981, Suppression of corneal allograft rejection by cyclosporin A, *Arch Ophthalmol.* **99**:1640–1643
44. Shepherd, W. F., Coster, D. J., Chin Fook, T., Rice, N. S. C., and Jones, B. R., 1980, Effect of Cyclosporin A on the survival of corneal grafts in rabbits, *Br J Ophthal.* **64**:148.
45. Siliski, J. M., Simkin, S., Green, C. J., 1984, Vascularized whole knee joint allografts in rabbits immunosuppressed by cyclosporin A, *Arch Orthop Trauma Surg.* **103**:26.

46. Ustuner, E. T., Zdichavsky, M., Ren, X., Edelstein, J., Maldonado, C., Ray, M., Jevans, A. W., Breidenbach, W. C., Gruber, S. A., Barker, J. H., and Jones, J. W., Long-term composite tissue allograft survival in a porcine model with cyclosporine/mycophenolate mofetil therapy, *Transplantation*. **66**:1581.
47. Watt, D. J., Partridge, T. A., and Sloper, J. C., 1981, Cyclosporine A as a means of preventing rejection of skeletal muscle allografts in mice, *Transplantation*. **31**:266.
48. White, D. J. G., Plumb, A. M., Pawelec, G., and Brons, G., 1979, Cyclosporine A: an immunosuppressive agent preferentially active against proliferating T cells, *Transplantation*. **27**:55.
49. Zalewski, A. A., and Gulati, A. K., 1981, Rejection of nerve allografts after cessation immunosuppression with Cyclosporin A, *Transplantation*. **31**:88.
50. Zalewski, A. A., and Silvers, W. K., 1980, An evaluation of nerve repair with nerve allografts in normal and immunologically tolerant rats, *J Neurosurg*. **52**:557.
51. Zirm, E., 1906, Eine erfolgreiche totale Keratoplastik Graefes, *Arch Ophthalmol*, **64**:580.
52. Kahan, B. D., The era of cyclosporine: twenty years forward and twenty years back. Transplantation Proceedings, Volume **36**:5S-6S.

Chapter 4
The First Limb Transplants with Cyclosporine

Christopher J. Salgado, Samir Mardini, and Charles W. Hewitt

4.1 Introduction

Cyclosporine was first described in 1976 as a fungal metabolite and found to have remarkable immunosuppressive properties both experimentally and clinically.[1] It was several years later that at the University of California, Irvine, College of Medicine, Drs. Kirby Black (Research Director for the Plastic Surgery Division within the Department of Surgery) and Charles W. Hewitt (Director of Research for the Division of Urology within the Department of Surgery) found themselves next door to one another, each directing the research efforts of their respective divisions. Dr. Black's interests at the time were in developing models of ischemia reperfusion injury and flap studies in the field of Plastic Surgery and Dr. Hewitt's primary interests were in studying transplant rejection and mechanisms of tolerance induction, as the Division of Urology was the division that was primarily responsible for kidney transplantation at the University of California, Irvine.

Dr. Black's ischemia-reperfusion model involved amputation and replantation of a rat hindlimb, and the mechanisms of ischemia-reperfusion injury by reattachment of these preserved amputated limbs under various conditions. In specific, the effects of temperature on tissue survival were evaluated with the use of a refrigerated environmental chamber located in Dr. Hewitt's lab. A discussion concerning these experiments ensued between Hewitt and Black and ultimately an investigative partnership was formed, along with a very meaningful friendship. Each investigator became interested in the other investigator's research, and further discussions ensued.

4.2 The Questions

From the model developed for replantation of the amputated limbs and the results of organ graft prolongation came a mutual realization that it would be very interesting to test additional mechanisms related to transplantation using the hindlimb model. Thus, the two investigators eventually decided to investigate the answer for a fairly unique question, namely, could this model be used to study limb transplantation and some of the developments found successful in prolonging organ transplantation? It was hypothesized that these new and unique types of transplants, integumentary musculoskeletal transplants, would have particular usefulness in plastic and reconstructive surgery applications and indications. In specific, these composite tissue allografts or substructures thereof would be useful for reconstructing full-thickness soft tissue defects such as those encountered in victims of severe burn injury or other traumas or after tumor extirpation, in addition to possible restoration of muscle function for recessive myopathies. Therefore, a bond was formed, initially as an alliance between a transplantation immunology laboratory and a plastic surgery microvascular surgical laboratory, which later blended and integrated the two investigator's interests into one focus of pursuit over the next 20 years, and which represented the pioneering efforts for these investigators in the field of composite tissue transplantation.

4.3 Materials and Methods

All were not successful in the early years. For a year and a half, these investigators used every proven technique that was successfully developed in the kidney transplant model and applied it to the rat hindlimb composite tissue transplant model. There were only minor successes, with perhaps a few days here and there of prolonged graft survival.[2,3] Although cyclosporine-induced prolongation of skin graft survival in mice was obtained for about 20 days in earlier years[4] and muscle allograft transplantation in rats was feasible with cyclosporine,[5] it became readily apparent that this particular allograft entire limb transplantation model was indeed a difficult one in which to achieve graft prolongation and success. The failures became frustrating and several discussions resulted concerning dropping the whole idea of composite tissue transplantation, as it just did not seem feasible in view of the results that were obtained. It was during this time that this new immunosuppressive compound came onto the scene; however, its reputation was rather uncertain. Cyclosporine's promise was in debate, due to concerns of its reported toxicities.[6,7] In regard to wound healing, however, no detrimental effects specifically related to cyclosporine administration had been observed. Indeed the considerable problems in wound healing were undoubtedly related to the continuous use of steroids. Thus cyclosporine, a steroid sparing drug, gave an advantage.

In Dr. Black and Hewitt's laboratory it was a drug that was initially viewed as not very promising. However, once the two investigators realized that failures were common with respect to prolonging limb transplant survival, the attitude changed and the two were willing to try new and promising interventions and drug therapies to improve their results.

4.4 Cyclosporine and Limb Transplants

After a story put forth in the *Los Angeles Times*, a student who was working on the limb transplant project, approached Drs. Black and Hewitt about a remarkable and miraculous immunosuppressant agent. Although Kirby Black and Charles Hewitt were both quite aware of the new drug in development, it was decided after this student's urging to try cyclosporine in the limb transplant model. It was decided that the student would write to the company that was developing the drug (Sandoz), to see if an experimental quantity could be obtained to study whether this "miracle drug" would prolong limb transplant survival. A wonderful scientist and gentleman, David Winter, who was then the Director of Immunology at Sandoz, became intrigued with the prospects of these proposed limb transplantation experiments and sent a large quantity of cyclosporine to try in these rather unique experiments. Shortly after the drug arrived, it was mixed according to Sandoz directions and the laboratory initiated testing of this compound for its ability to extend limb transplant survival. Within the first week of experimentation, it was noted that there were dramatic differences between these experiments and any previous ones that had been undertaken in the laboratory. By days 5 and 6 there was notable stubble of hair growth forming on the limb, something which had not been achieved before. Two weeks after transplantation, luxuriant black hair growth occurred over the entire transplanted limb. The animals did quite well and soon they were actually walking on these new transplanted limbs. It was truly amazing and the investigators in the laboratory became cyclosporine converts. They were so impressed with the ability of this compound to prolong tissue transplant survival compared to any former drug therapy or treatment tried previously to manipulate the immune system that they were convinced this was a true twentieth century miracle drug. The first experiments with cyclosporine were then detailed in the literature.[8–10]

4.5 The Return of Cosmas and Damian

In 1981, a compelling editorial was written in the *New England Journal of Medicine* regarding analogies between the legend of Cosmas and Damian and whether cyclosporine would usher in the twentieth century equivalent of Cosmas and Damian.[11] The title of the article was "Cosmas and Damian in the 20th Century". The legend of Cosmas and Damian, twin saints, a physician and a surgeon, are well known to the transplant community and have served as a symbol for the desired successes of transplantation. It was in AD 348 that, according to Jacopo de Varagine's thirteenth century "Legenda aurea", Saints Cosmas and Damian had performed a miraculous transplantation and the coincidence was that the type of tissue they actually transplanted was reported to be a limb transplant. The limb was taken from a recently deceased Ethiopian moor and transplanted to a Roman church custodian of one of their shrines. As famous paintings depict, the black leg was successfully transplanted on this white individual due to miraculous healing powers of the sainted twins. The real miracle, however, was that the sainted brothers had performed this procedure posthumously, since they were beheaded early in the third century AD, as Christian martyrs.[12] Due to the analogies drawn between the miraculous feats of Cosmas and Damian and the new compound cyclosporine, to in effect achieve the twentieth century equivalent, some poetic license was granted in a short report published in the *New England Journal of Medicine*, in response to Dr. Kahan's editorial appearing in a previous issue.[6]

The first reported results with limb transplants and cyclosporine were made with the initial quantities of cyclosporine that was granted by David Winter from Sandoz. The results were used to answer Dr. Kahan's editorial in a most affirmative manner, again drawing the important analogies of the miraculous features of the drug to prolong limb transplant survival, similar to what Cosmas and Damian had done. There were no winged angels flying around the microsurgery operating table at Irvine and the real miracle was in this immunosuppressive compound. The other serendipitous analogy involved the genetic model that the investigators had chosen in Irvine due to the immunology and transplant barrier of the rat strains utilized: a black donor and white recipient were used. Thus, the analogies to the original Cosmas and Damian's legend were emphasized.

References

1. J. F. Borel, C. Feurer, H. U. Gubler, et al., Biological effects of cyclosporine A: A new anti-lymphocytic agent, *Agents Actions* **468** (1976).
2. K. S. Black, C. W. Hewitt, T. L. Woodard, et al., Efforts to enhance survival of limb allografts by prior administration of whole blood in rats using a new survival end-point, *J Microsurg* **3**, 162–167 (1982).
3. C. W. Hewitt, K. S. Black, L. A. Fraser, et al., Cyclosporin A (CyA) is superior to prior donor-specific blood (DSB) transfusion for the extensive prolongation of rat limb allograft survival, *Transplant Proc* **15**, 514–517 (1983).
4. J. F. Borel, C. Feurer, H. U. Gubler, et al., Biological effects of cyclosporine A: A new anit-lymphocytic agent, *Agents Actions* **6**, 468 (1976).
5. A. K. Gulati, A. A. Zalewski, Muscle allograft survival after cyclosporin A immuno-suppression, *Exp Neurol* **77**, 378 (1982).
6. A. W. Thomson, I. D. Cameron, Immune suppression with cyclosporin A-optimism and caution, *Scott Med J* **26**(2), 139–144 (1981).
7. B. D. Kahan, Cyclosporine: the agent and its actions, *Transplant Proc* **17**(4), 5–18 (1985).
8. K. S. Black, C. W. Hewitt, L. A. Fraser, et al., Cosmas and Damian in the laboratory, *N Engl J Med* **306**, 368–369 (1982).
9. C. W. Hewitt, K. S. Black, L. A. Fraser, et al., Composite tissue (limb) allografts in rats: I. Dose-dependent increase in survival with cyclosporine, *Transplantation* **39**, 360–364 (1985).
10. K. S. Black, C. W. Hewitt, L. A. Fraser, et al., Composite tissue (limb) allografts in rats: II. Indefinite survival using low dose cyclosporine, *Transplantation* **39**, 365–368 (1985).
11. B. D. Kahan, Cosmas and Damian in the 20th Century, *N Engl J Med* **305**(5), 280–281 (1981).
12. B. D. Kahan, Cosmas and Damian revisited, *Transplant Proc* **4**(Suppl 1), 2211 (1983).

Section II

Chapter 5
Translational Research in Composite Tissue Allotransplantation

Linda C. Cendales, David E. Kleiner, and Allan D. Kirk

5.1 Introduction

Patients suffering from severe tissue loss secondary to burns, traumatic injuries, or tumor resections have limited options for reconstruction when autologous tissue for reconstruction is scarce. Composite tissue allotransplantation (CTA) has recently been introduced as a potential clinical treatment for functionally significant tissue loss. CTA has emerged as an amalgamation of advanced microsurgical techniques for limb and flap autotransplantation, and improved immunosuppressive agents to prevent rejection. However, as a developing field, it is yet to have its unique immunological properties established.

To date, the International Registry for Hand and Composite Tissue Transplantation has reported 24 hand transplant recipients[1] and 39 CTA patients worldwide.[2] A more comprehensive analysis of the clinical cases is considered elsewhere in this book. Although graft and patient outcomes have steadily improved in solid organ transplants due to the use of potent immunosuppressive agents preventing rejection and the use of antibiotic prophylaxis and diagnostic tools, transplantation continues to require that patients trade their condition for life-long immunosuppression. As such, two critical goals of this emerging field are an improved understanding of the biology of rejection as it relates specifically to CTA, and the optimization of immunosuppressive drug regimens for application in early clinical trials. Several practical advancements are necessary to meet these goals.

Most CTA recipients have experienced reversible episodes of acute rejection,[1,3-6] but given the infrequent application of CTA to date, no single group has accumulated sufficient experience to determine histological patterns of rejection. As such, a grading scheme for ranking the pathological severity of rejection, specifically one based on the most accessible component of the graft, the skin, has not been established. This is a basic requirement for international communication related to allograft biology.

Moreover, although CTA rejection has been presumed to be mediated by mechanisms similar to solid organ transplantation, it is under investigation whether CTA tissues differ in their propensity to attract an allospecific infiltrate, or if some elements are spared rejection. Important studies have been performed in small animal models to study the intricacies of the different tissues. These data are presented elsewhere in this book. Questions of pathway and mechanisms are appropriate for small animals whereas large animal models answer questions of practicality, toxicity, and more generalized efficacy. In transplantation in particular, the histology and cadence of unmodified allograft rejection in nonhuman primates is essentially identical to that of humans. Although there are differences between animals and humans, experiments in large animal models have been and continue to be the paramount way to acquire adequate experience to commence ethically designed human trials.[7]

It is therefore the purpose of this chapter to present some ongoing work in the initiation of a standardization process for CTA reporting as well as in the development of a preclinical model in nonhuman primates (NHPs) for the study of CTA.

5.2 Classification of Human Skin Rejection in CTA

Vascularized skin, a common component included in many composite tissue allografts, is a highly immunogenic tissue that introduces the possibility of a more vigorous rejection response. However, the visibility of the skin also provides an advantage in detecting rejection early in the process. Unlike more homogeneous solid organ allografts, the tempo of the alloimmune response toward the varying tissues in CTA continues to require study. At present, the aggregate pace of rejection in CTA appears to be similar to solid organ transplantation. It remains to be seen whether individual components present different susceptibilities and rates of demise.

The fundamental aspects of CTA allograft biology seem generally similar to other forms of transplantation. Specifically, each recipient holds a distinctive immune history shaped by genetic predispositions and environmental exposures occurring throughout their lives which condition their immune responses (e.g., vaccines, transfusions, infections, pregnancy). This influences each individual's precursor frequencies and the threshold to respond to any immune event. At the time of transplantation, reperfusion injury and endothelial trauma lead to platelet activation which in turn, interacts with antigen presenting cells (APCs) and endothelial cells. APCs likely rally to the regional lymph nodes, although the disruption of lymphatics may alter this in CTA as it does in other vascularized grafts. The aggregate response evokes an alloreactive cytotoxic effector reaction.

Cytotoxic T cells, arising from the afferent immune response, travel to the graft through a combination of adhesion receptor upregulation, endothelial damage, and chemotactic cytokine and chemokine release. In addition to each individual's multifaceted immune system, each graft has its own intrinsic susceptibility adding complexity to the rejection process.[8] Indeed, one of our focuses is to better understand rejection as well as to continue to improve drug efficiency to ideally transplant tissues amidst differences. We devised a classification scheme for human CTA rejection that allows pathologic changes to be grouped by severity.[9] This system is reproducible by independent pathologists and represents the largest and first multicenter collective experience in the world to date.[10]

The initial classification experience consisted of 29 samples collected from specimens from hand and abdominal wall transplantation from international centers. The cases were previously procured from 1 month to 3 years after transplantation and showed a range of changes from mild to severe rejection causing graft loss. All patients underwent immunosuppressive protocols according to their respective center and for this study, no correlation was used. Eleven biopsies were ranked by severity based on the intensity of the overall infiltration, and the degree of involvement of adnexa and the epidermis. Reproducibility of the system was tested using the second set of 18 biopsies. Three independent pathologists from three different institutions categorized blindly the tissue slides according to the newly described system. The nonparametric Kendall coefficient of concordance (W) was used to assess the amount of agreement among the three pathologists in their classification grades.[11] This tool is useful to statistically test whether there is significant agreement and to offer an easily interpreted nonparametric Spearman correlation among pairs of examiners. The computed value of Kendall's W (corrected for ties) was 0.9375 and the p value was highly significant ($p = < 0.0001$). The corresponding average Spearman correlation among pairs of assessors was 0.906.

Clinically, rejection was characterized by patchy or generalized erythematous rash localized solely to the allograft that ranged from a mild rash to, in one case, erythematous-scaly papules, superficial erosion, and necrosis requiring revision amputation of the limb due to rejection.[12] All samples displayed at least some degree of perivascular infiltrate suggesting that this is one of the earliest findings in skin rejection. Adnexal structures were involved with increasing severity. In the case of graft loss, confluent necrosis of the epidermis and other structures was seen and although perineural inflammation was also present, frank neuritis was not observed. Myositis was observed in two muscle samples, but, since muscle was not obtained in all cases, it was not apparent how the severity or the tempo of myositis related to the dermal changes or clinical appearance of rejection. In mild cases, the infiltrate was mainly of CD4+ T cells while in cases with more severe infiltrate it was predominantly CD8+ T cells (Fig 5.1).

On the basis of our initial observations, we proposed the following preliminary classification system to standardize reporting of CTA rejection (Fig. 5.2). Grade 0; nonspecific changes: No or only mild lymphocytic infiltration without involvement of the superficial dermal structures or epidermis. Grade 1; mild rejection: superficial perivascular inflammation with involvement of superficial vessels and without involvement of overlying epidermis. Grade 2; moderate rejection: Features of Grade 1 with involvement of the epithelium of adnexal structures. Grade 3; severe rejection: Bandlike superficial dermal infiltrate with more continuous involvement of the epidermis and middle and deep perivascular infiltrate. Grade 4; necrotizing rejection (not shown): Includes features of Grade 3 along with frank necrosis of the epidermis or other tissues.[10]

Other clinical scoring systems with similar observations have been put forward. These include studies in full-thickness cadaver skin transplants for large abdominal defects,[13] the evaluation of allograft rejection in human hands,[14] and observations based on a case report.[15] Although these studies provide valuable information,

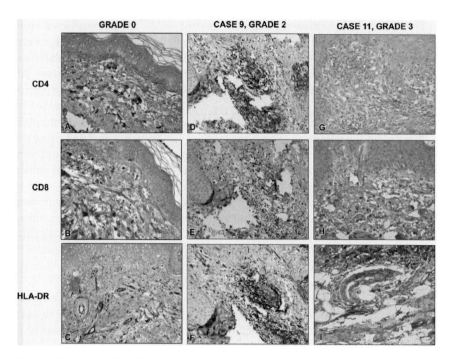

Fig. 5.1 Immunostaining of three cases from CTA. Panels (**a–c**) CTA biopsy that showed no evidence of inflammation or epidermal injury (Grade 0). Panels (**d–f**) A case of moderate acute rejection (Case 9, Grade 2). Panels (**g–i**) A case of severe acute rejection (Case11, Grade 3). Only rare inflammatory cells were seen on the immunostains, and HLA-DR was positive only on capillary endothelial cells and the mature, keratinized epithelial cells. Note that in the case of mild rejection, most of the T cells are CD4+ (panel **d**) and that only scattered CD8+ cells are seen (panel **e**), whereas in the severe rejection case about equal numbers of CD4 and CD8+ cells were seen (panels **g** and **h**, respectively). HLA-DR staining of these cases show essentially no staining of keratinocytes in the mild case (panel **f**), whereas in the severe rejection there was staining of some adnexal structures (panel **i**). In both cases of rejection the inflammatory infiltrate was strongly positive for HLA-DR. (All at ×400 magnification). Reproduced with permission. From [10]

currently no single center has extensive experience in prospective analysis of graft rejection. Standardization of a scoring system will require a consensus forum such as that provided by the Banff congresses held for other solid allografts.[16]

5.3 Development of a Nonhuman Primate Model for the Study of CTA

The current ethical environment of large animal experimentation is similar to that of humans; NHPs are intelligent social beings with physical and emotional needs.[17] As such, we have established a technically feasible NHP model for the study of

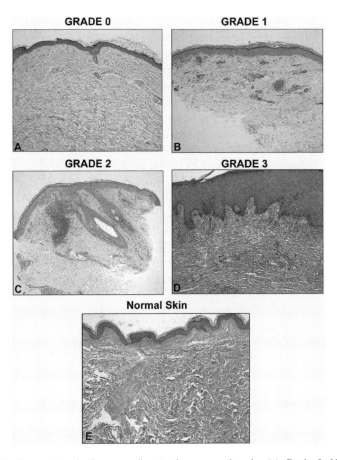

Fig. 5.2 Grading acute rejection according to the proposed scale. (**a**) Grade 0. Nonspecific changes – there is some epidermal atrophy, but essentially no inflammatory infiltrate is seen. (**b**) Grade 1. Mild rejection – there is a mild, superficial perivascular infiltrate in this biopsy. There is no infiltration of inflammatory cells into the epidermis, but a few lymphocytes were seen infiltrating into the adnexal glands. (**c**) Grade 2. Moderate rejection. – the inflammatory infiltrate is more intense than in the Grade 1 example, but is still predominantly perivascular. There is also clear infiltration of lymphocytes into the epidermis and the hair shaft. Very little keratinocyte necrosis is seen. Grade 3. Severe rejection – in addition to prominent perivascular inflammation, there is now a band-like infiltrate just beneath the dermal–epidermal junction. Infiltration of the epidermis and adnexal glands is present. Normal skin is shown for comparison in panel **e**. (All H&E, ×100) Reproduced with permission. From [10]

CTA that is particularly sensitive to the evolving ethical requirements of primate testing. Nonhuman primate models are essential for transitioning many experimental theories to clinical therapies in organ transplantation.[17–19] Although some aspects of NHPs make them a rigorous testing ground many avenues are only approachable through NHPs systems. As noted previously, the general physiology, anatomy, and the histology and pace of unmodified rejection are comparable to that of humans.

NHPs allow for the testing of human-specific immunosuppressants and furthermore, the noteworthy similarities between the human and the NHP major histocompatibility complex provide important implications for T-cell responses which are like that of human beings. Experimentation in NHPs however, should only be considered after the experimental rationale has been tested in vitro and in lower animals.[17]

Old world monkeys are phylogenetically closer to humans. Three species in particular are generally used in transplantation research; *Macaca mulatta* (rhesus monkey), *Macaca fascicularis* (cynomolgus monkey), and *Papio cynocephalus* (baboon). NHP studies in CTA include the transplantation of hands and neurovascular free flaps in baboons, partial hands in rhesus monkeys, and mandibular allograft in cynomolgus monkeys.[20–26] We sought to establish our model with outbred *Macaca fascicularis* to facilitate the systematic study of the progression and resolution of CTA rejection, and to serve as a suitable preclinical testing ground for novel antirejection strategies. Limb manipulations in NHPs could impair their social development, thus, our model incorporates all elements of a limb CTA, yet leaves no functional deficit despite graft rejection or excision.[27]

Our model is based on a sensate osteomyocutaneous forearm flap.[28] Each animal included in the protocol serves both as a donor and recipient and pairs are based on MHC nonidentity and high responsiveness status in mixed lymphocyte reactions. Allograft procurement is performed as previously described.[27] Briefly, under general anesthesia and intraoperative antibiotic prophylaxis, surgery is performed using standard microsurgical techniques. The flaps are dissected from the ulnar to the radial aspects and include a unicortical segment of the radius, the palmaris longus tendon, medial and lateral antebrachial cutaneous nerves, brachioradialis muscle, radial artery, cephalic vein, and the overlying skin (Fig. 5.3a,d,e).

The donor flap is perfused with cold (4 °C) Euro-Collins solution or University of Wisconsin solution (UWS), and stored in perfusate at 4 °C. Transplantation begins with the osteosynthesis with typically two self-tapping screws (Fig. 5.3b). An end-to-end anastomosis between the donor and recipient's radial artery is performed and systemic heparin (100 units/kg) is administered. Vasospasm is treated as needed with topical papaverine over the anastomosis. Repair of the brachioradialis muscle follows. A flow-through anastomosis of the cephalic vein and the neurorrhaphy of the lateral antebrachial cutaneous nerve and the medial antebrachial cutaneous nerve are performed. The skin is closed in one layer after the repair of the palmaris longus tendon (Fig. 5.3c). An X-ray of the forearm and wrist is taken after skin closure. Animals are transported without a splint to the intensive care unit cage. Autografts are performed using this technique replanted orthotopically.

5.3.1 Postoperative Management

All animals undergo close monitoring. We continue anticoagulation for 1 week followed by aspirin for 2 weeks. Routine pain and antibiotic prophylaxis are administered. The transplant is evaluated daily and changes suggestive of rejection

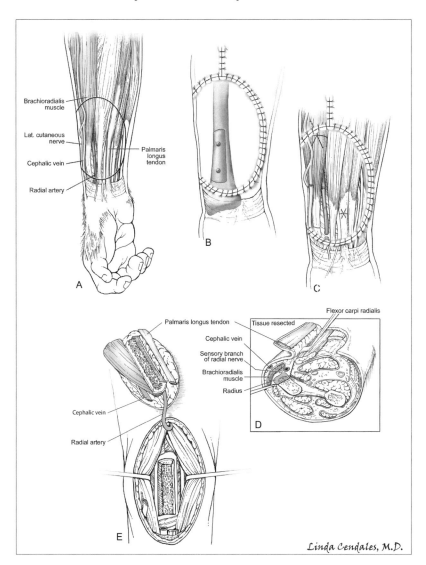

Fig. 5.3 Sensate osteomyocutaneous radial forearm flap with palmaris longus tendon. (**a**) Anatomy. (**b**) The osteosynthesis of the radius is performed with screws. (**c**) The palmaris longus tendon, brachioradialis muscle, cephalic vein, sensory branch of the radial nerve, and the proximal end of the radial artery are repaired anatomically after transplantation. (**d**) Cross-section view. The flap dissection begins ulnarward to include the deep fascia and the palmaris longus tendon. (**e**) The flap is isolated on the proximal vascular pedicle. Reproduced with permission. From [27]

(e.g., vesiculation, erythema, and epidermolysis) prompt a full skin biopsy for histological evaluation.

In our initial experience, the primary objective of the protocol was the establishment of the model. Thus, rejection episodes were not rescued. Excisional biopsies were indicated when the graft showed gross signs of severe rejection (erythema, with partial necrosis or epidermolysis) and they were performed at the operating room under general anesthesia. Histological and immunohistochemical evaluation included fixation with hematoxylin and eosin, identification of T cells with antihuman CD3 (Dakicytomation, 1:150), and antihuman CD68 (Dako, 1:50) for macrophages.

Our initial experience included an autograft group ($n = 5$) and an untreated allograft group ($n=7$). Other animals received a calcineurin inhibitor (tacrolimus 1 mg/kg every 12 h orally with a targeted level from 15 to 20 ng/ml), an antiproliferative agent (mycophenolate mofetil 20 mg/kg every 12 h orally), and methylprednisolone at 15 mg/kg intramuscular for 3 days followed by 7.5 mg/kg for 2 days and a 50% reduction every 2 days until the dose was 1 mg/kg in seven animals.

5.3.2 Results

All the animals included in this study achieved full range of motion immediately after surgery. Two technical failures were experienced in the first group; a vascular occlusion due to the absence of anticoagulation and a hematoma formation secondary to excessive anticoagulation. An incidental radius fracture was observed in a follow-up X-ray which was treated with open reduction and internal fixation without complications. During the first three postoperative days, all animals undergoing surgery without immunosuppression revealed a generalized severe purple discoloration limited to the allograft (Fig. 5.4a). Histologically, perivenular inflammation and a mild perivascular CD3 positive infiltrate in the superficial dermis were observed (Fig. 5.4b,c). In the group treated with immunosuppression, a pink rash, slower in progression, developed (Fig. 5.5a). Some animals demonstrated a patchy discoloration but – similar to the animals without treatment – this observation was limited to the transplant. In one animal, vesiculation was the presenting sign of rejection. We completed the excisional biopsies of the flaps at days 5, 8, 15, 17, 24, 73, and 76 after surgery.

Histological examination of the treated animals revealed a dermal lymphocytic infiltrate similar in magnitude and distribution to the clinical rejection viewed in hand transplant recipients[10] (Fig 5.2). Dermal mononuclear cell infiltrates were mainly of lymphocytes (Fig. 5.5b,c). Moderate multifocal perivascular lymphocytic dermal infiltrates, with mild lymphocytic infiltrates at the dermal–epidermal junction were seen. These lymphoid infiltrates were strongly CD3 positive on immunostaining (Figs. 5.4d). Staining with anti-C4d was positive in native, autograft and allograft capillaries. Further studies are needed to draw conclusions regarding the role of complement in CTA rejection.

We have initiated histological analysis of bone, tendon, muscle, nerve, artery, vein, and skin. While the speed of rejection is too fast in unmodified grafts to evaluate nonvascular tissues, as stated previously, animals treated with immunosuppression provided histological samples that are indistinguishable from reported human

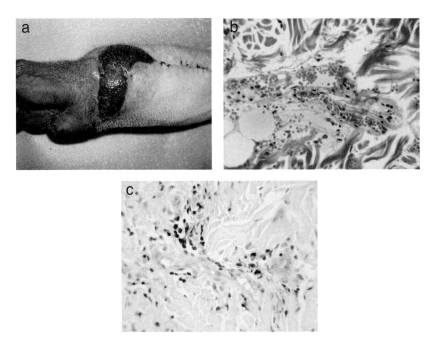

Fig. 5.4 Appearance of animals without immunosuppression. (**a**) Skin discoloration in nonhuman primate composite tissue allografts (**b**) Hemorrhage adjacent to venules in the allografted skin dermis. (Hematoxylin and eosin, ×400). (**c**) Nonhuman primate skin transplant without immunosuppression 3 days post surgery. Mild infiltration of CD3 positive lymphocytes adjacent to venules in superficial dermis (anti-CD3 immunostain, ×400). Reproduced with permission. From [27]

cases. In addition to histological findings, this model permits transcriptional analysis of all tissues. We have preliminarily established relevant NHP primer sets for polymerase chain reaction-based analysis. This too, is a novel aspect of this model that we are using in ongoing studies.

5.4 Conclusions

Interest in CTA is growing rapidly and the field stands poised at the brink of a critical growth period. That growth can be frenetic or methodical. As we favor the latter, we have proposed a scoring system for clinical histopathological reporting in CTA based on the largest and first multicenter collective experience to date. We have also established an NHP model allowing for the systematic evaluation of primate-specific questions to facilitate a rational progression from the bench to bedside. These logistical necessities will, we hope, be added to the experience of others to set the tone for the future of CTA.

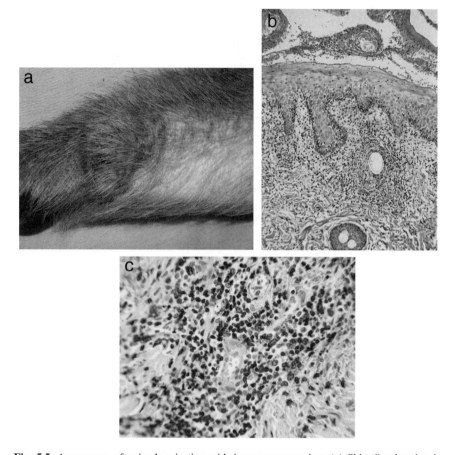

Fig. 5.5 Appearance of animals rejecting with immunosuppression. (**a**) Skin discoloration in nonhuman primate composite tissue allografts. Note the hair growth in the transplant. (**b**) Allogeneic skin transplant 14 days post transplantation. Parakeratotic hyperkeratosis with a serocellular crust is evident. A moderate dermal, perifollicular, and perivascular mononuclear cell infiltrate is present. (Hematoxylin and eosin, ×100). (**c**) Lymphocytic infiltrates are strongly positive for CD3 on immunostaining (anti-CD3 immunostain ×400). Reproduced with permission. From [27]

As the evolution of surgery is incremental, much work lies ahead. We have "Promises to keep, and miles to go before we sleep" (R. Frost, 1874–1963). But a greater understanding of CTA will be achieved through the collaborative application of the scientific method toward our ultimate goal: the improvement of our patients' health.

Acknowledgments The authors are beholden with the coauthors of the manuscripts generated from these data; John Bacher, Michael Eckhaus, Margaret Moresi, Phillip Ruiz, and He Xu. The authors gratefully acknowledge the selfless contributions to the clinical study through the generous gifts of allografted tissue received from Darla Granger, Warren Breidenbach, Carolyn Burns, Carrie Marcell, Jean-Michel Dubernard, Nadey Hakim, Raimund Margreiter, Deborah Weppler,

Andreas Tzakis, Frederic Schund, and Carlo Van Holder. The authors would like to thank Bob Wesley for his expert statistical support. The authors thankfully acknowledge the expert technical assistance of the Veterinary Surgical Service staff and of Mr. Frank Leopardi in the development of the preclinical model.

References

1. Lanzetta M, Petruzzo, Dubernard JM, et al., Second report (1998–2006) of the International Registry on Hand and Composite Tissue Transplantation, *Transpl Immunol* **18**(1): 1–6, 2007 Jul.
2. International Registry on Hand and Composite Tissue Transplantation; http://www.hand registry.com. (accessed on 09-27-2007) September 27, (2007).
3. D. M. Levi, A. G. Tzakis, T. Kato, J. Madariaga, N. K. Mittal, J. Nery, S. Nishida, P. Ruiz, Transplantation of the abdominal wall, *Lancet* **361**(9376), 173–176 (2003).
4. L. Cendales, W. Breidenbach, Hand Transplantation. *Hand Clinics North Am* **17**(3), 499–510 (2001).
5. R. Margreiter, G. Brandacher, M. Ninkovic, et al., A Double-hand transplant can be worth the effort, *Transplantation* **74**(1), 85–90 (2002).
6. J. Kanitakis, D. Jullien, P. Petruzzo, N. Hakim, A. Claudy, J. Revillard, E. Owen, J. Dubernard, Clinicopathologic features of graft rejection of the first human hand allograft, *Transplantation* **76**, 688–693 (2003).
7. A. Kirk, Crossing the bridge: large animal models in translational transplantation research, *Immunol Rev* **196**, 176–196 (2003).
8. A. D. Kirk, Induction Immunosuppression, *Transplantation* **82**(5), 593–602 (2006).
9. L. Cendales, D. Kleiner, Proposed classification of human composite tissue allograft acute rejection, *Am J Transplant* **3**(Suppl 5), S154 (2003).
10. L. Cendales, A. Kirk, M. Moresi, P. Ruiz, D. Kleiner, Composite tissue allotransplantation: classification of clinical acute skin rejection, *Transplantation* **81**(3), 418–422 (2006).
11. Siegel, Sidney, Castelan, Nonparametric Statistics for the Behavioral Sciences, 2nd edition. McGraw Hill, New York, 1988, pp. 262–272.
12. J. Kanitakis, D. Jullien, P. Petruzzo, N. Hakim, A. Claudy, J. Revillard, E. Owen, J. Dubernard, Clinicopathologic features of graft rejection of the first human hand allograft, *Transplantation* **76**, 688–693 (2003).
13. P. A. Bejarano, D. Levi, M. Nassiri, V. Vincek, et al., The pathology of full-thickness cadaver skin transplant for large abdominal defects, *Am J Surg Pathol* **28**(5), 67–75 (2004)
14. J. Kanitakis, P. Petruzzo, D. Jullien, et al., Pathological score for the evaluation of allograft rejection in human hand (composite tissue) allotransplantation, *Eur J Dermatol* **(4)**, 235–238 (2005).
15. S. Schneeberger, A. Kreczy, G. Brandacher, et al., Steroid and ATG-resistant rejection after double forearm transplantation responds to Campath 1-H, *Am J Transplant* **4**(8), 1372–1374 (2004).
16. L. Racusen, K. Solez, R. Colvin, The Banff 97 working classification of renal allograft pathology, *Kidney Int* **2**, 713–723 (1999).
17. A. D. Kirk, Transplantation tolerance: a look at the nonhuman primate literature in the light of modern tolerance theories, *Crit Rev Immunol* **19**(5–6), 349–388 (1999).
18. World Medical Association Statement Declaration of Helsinki on Animal Use in Biomedical Research. Adopted by the 41st World Medical Assembly Hong Kong, 1989.
19. S. M. Rose, N. Blustein, and D. Rotrosen, Recommendations of the expert panel on ethical issues in clinical trials of transplant tolerance, *Transplantation* **66**, 1123–1125 (1998).
20. E. P. Egerszegi, D. D. Samulack, R. K. Daniel, Experimental models in primates for reconstructive surgery utilizing tissue transplants, *Ann Plast Surg* **13**, 423–430 (1984).
21. R. K. Daniel, E. P. Egerszegi, D. D. Samulack, S. E. Skanes, R. W. Dykes, W. R. Rennie, Tissue transplants in primates for upper extremity reconstruction: a preliminary report, *J Hand Surg* [Am] **11**, 1–8 (1986).

22. G. B. Stark, W. M. Swartz, K. Narayanan, A. R. Moller, Hand transplantation in baboons, *Transplant Proc* **19**, 3968–3971 (1987).
23. E. R. Hovius, H. Stevens, P. van Nierop, W. Rating, R. van Strik, J. van der Meulen, Allogeneic transplantation of the radial side of the hand in the rhesus monkey; technical aspects, *Plastic Reconstr Surg* **89**(4), 700–709 (1992).
24. H. Stevens, S. Hovius, J. Heeney, et al., Immunologic aspects and complications of composite tissue allografting for upper extremity reconstruction: a study in the rhesus monkey, *Transpl Proc* **23**(1), 623–625 (1991).
25. P. Egerszegi, D. Samulack, R. Daniel, Experimental models in primates for reconstructive surgery utilizing tissue transplants, *Ann Plastic Surg* **13**(5), 423–430 (1994).
26. M. Gold, J. Randzio, H. Kniha, et al., Transplantation of vascularized composite mandibular allografts in young cynomolgus monkeys, *Ann Plastic Surg* **26**(2), 125–132 (1991).
27. L. Cendales, H. Xu, J. Bacher, M. Eckhaus, D. Kleiner, A. Kirk, Composite tissue allotransplantation: development of a preclinical model in nonhuman primates, *Transplantation* **80**(10), 1447–1454 (2005).
28. L. R. Scheker, The radial forearm flap. In *Atlas of Microsurgical Composite Tissue Transplantation*, Edited by Donald Serafin. WB Saunders Co., Boston, Massachusetts, pp. 389–400.

Chapter 6
Relative Antigenicity of Allograft Components and Differential Rejection

Jignesh Unadkat, Justin M. Sacks, Stefan Schneeberger, and W. P. Andrew Lee

Abstract A composite tissue comprises tissues derived from all three germ layers: ectoderm, mesoderm, and endoderm. Following transplantation, each component induces an immune response, which differs in character and intensity.

Skin has been shown to be the most antigenic tissue and is the first tissue to be rejected in animal models and human transplants. The heightened antigenicity of skin has been attributed to Langerhans' dendritic cells and skin-specific antigens. Muscle, bone, cartilage, and nerve predictably induce a relatively lower immune response in that order. However, rejection of even one component of a composite tissue renders the entire allograft vulnerable to dysfunction.

The knowledge of relative antigenicity can lead to the development of strategies intended to decrease the antigenicity of a specific component. In addition, a better understanding of this relative antigenicity of allograft components enables the concept of tailored immunosuppression targeting only specific cellular and humoral components of rejection. This would limit the amount of immunosuppression used and the consequent related complications of opportunistic infections and malignancies.

6.1 Introduction

The origins of modern transplantation immunology are commonly dated to experiments performed by Medawar in 1953.[1,2] In these experiments, skin allograft rejection was shown to be primarily a host versus graft response. As further cellular, humoral, and complement constituents of the immune response were discovered over the last century, the mechanisms leading to allograft rejection became elucidated. Immunosuppressive modalities have been formulated to target these mechanisms of rejection and to suppress physiological immune responses.[3]

Surgical technique and immunosuppressive therapy have evolved over the following decades and were successfully introduced into organ transplantation. The remarkable results in solid organ transplantation have expanded the boundaries of transplantation into the transplantation of more complex tissue constructs such as the abdominal wall, face, hand, larynx, and trachea.[4]

The first human hand transplantation took place in Ecuador in 1964 using systemic steroids and azathioprine (AZA), a purine antimetabolite as immunosuppressive therapy. However, this immunosuppression, though occasionally successful in promoting long-term survival in solid organ transplantation, was inadequate in preventing hand allograft rejection. As a consequence, the first hand allograft was rejected within fourteen days.[5] The first hand transplant of the modern era of immunosuppressive therapy was performed in Lyon, France, in 1998.[6] Successive hand transplants have been performed in Austria, China, Belgium, Italy, Malaysia, and the United States.[4]

Transplantation of the human hand differs from solid organ transplantation in varied ways.[7] A composite tissue allograft (CTA) consists of tissues derived from ectoderm, endoderm, and mesoderm.[4] These germ layers give rise to skin, adipose tissue, muscle, cartilage, bone, nerve, and vessels. A hand allograft represents a CTA largely consisting of ectoderm and mesoderm. An immunosuppressive regimen designed to prevent rejection of a hand transplant must be capable of preventing rejection of the individual tissue components of the CTA.[4,8] Additionally, it has been shown that the various components of CTAs interact with the host immune system in a complex but predictable pattern with differing timing and intensity.[8]

Experimental models for the transplantation of individual vascularized components of CTAs have been developed.[8] Skin, subcutaneous tissue, muscle, bone, nerve, and blood vessels have been individually assessed for their relative antigenicities.[8] The aim of this discussion will be to elucidate and quantify the antigenicity of these allograft components both individually and collectively.

6.2 Components of Vascularized Tissue Allograft

A vascularized CTA, unlike an organ allograft, challenges the host immunity with a myriad of antigens derived from all three germ layers – ectoderm, mesoderm, and endoderm.[9] The immune system has been shown to differentially reject components of a CTA.[10] This selective rejection process leads to dysfunction of individual components potentially leading to failure of the entire CTA. For example, in a hand transplant, failure of the skin component would render the host exposed to various infections. Nerve rejection would render the hand allograft insensate and prone to unconscious injuries as seen in diabetic neuropathy.

Skin derived from the ectoderm is considered an exquisitely antigenic tissue.[11-13] Subcutaneous tissue produces a similar pattern as observed in the skin.[8] Muscle predictably produces a low cellular and humoral response.[14] Bone induces a medium to strong immune response.[15] Blood vessels are considered to have a lower antigenicity requiring minimal or no immunosuppression.[16] However, both rejection and deterioration of the cellular elements may contribute to the relatively high failure rates when used solely as by-pass grafting material.[16] Nerve allograft has shown variability in its antigenicity initially being composed of donor allogeneic cells and then being replaced by host tissue. This suggests the possible role of finite immunosuppression.[17,18]

6.2.1 Skin

Skin is the largest organ in the body. It functions as both a physical and immunological barrier between an organism and its environment. This function necessitates the need for a robust and effective immunoregulatory system at the local level to survey the entry of pathogens into the body. Similar patterns of antigenicity have also been found in the small intestine and lungs in mice,[19] which are barriers to ingested and inhaled pathogens, respectively. Extremely efficient in its intrinsic immune function, the skin lends itself as a primary target of rejection when transplanted.

Skin is highly antigenic.[11] Several studies by different investigators have demonstrated this unique property.[8,20] Skin allografts from a chimeric donor are rejected in spite of stable hemopoietic chimerism in the host.[21] This correlates with the clinical finding in a CTA that the skin initially shows the first signs of rejection[22] and is also associated with maximal cellular infiltrate in a situation of established rejection.[23]

The heightened antigenicity of skin may be explained in part to several factors. These include possible expression of potent antigens specific to skin such as Skn and Epa-1.[24] Keratinocytes, which constitute the major epidermal component of skin, play an important role in skin antigenicity. In addition, the presence of highly efficient dendritic cells leads to the direct presentation of these antigens to the host immune system.

6.2.1.1 Antigens

Embryonic pre-albumin 1 (Epa-1) is a tissue restricted, loss mutation, and target-cell determinant in the murine skin. It is present on epidermal cells, fibroblasts, and macrophages inducing formation of anti-Epa-1 cytotoxic T lymphocytes (CTL). These CTLs besides causing direct lysis of Epa-1 expressing cells also cause extensive damage of "innocent bystander" tissue by chemokine expression that recruits other inflammatory cells.[25] Skn and Epa-1 act as major antigenic determinants and also as targets in graft versus host disease. Similar skin specific alloantigens have been suggested in miniature swine.[26] Human skin may similarly possess as yet unidentified skin-specific antigens.

6.2.1.2 Keratinocytes

The keratinocyte (KC) is an important component of the skin immune system. It constitutively expresses MHC I but no MHC II. However, on activation by interferon gamma or inflammation, KC have been shown to upregulate the MHC I expression as well as express MHC II.[27] Intercellular adhesion molecule-1 (ICAM-1) is expressed at a very low level or is absent from KC. On activation, KC express

ICAM-1, which plays an important role in trafficking of T cells through the epidermis.[28] Activated KC has also been shown to express CD36 that is involved in cell adhesion.[29] In addition, KC secretes many pro-inflammatory cytokines such as interleukin-1 (IL-1)[30], interleukin 12 (IL-12),[31] interleukin 6 (IL-6),[32] and chemokines such as IL-1 and interleukin 8 (IL-8).[33]

6.2.1.3 Skin Dendritic Cells

Dendritic cells (DCs) are derived from hematopoietic bone marrow (BM) stem cells and migrate via circulation to sites bordering the external environment particularly the skin.[24] These APCs, because of their migratory property, carry antigenic information from skin into secondary lymphoid organs and present it to lymphocytes for priming and stimulation. Several skin DC types have been described including the epidermal Langerhans' cells and the phenotypically different, dermal dentrilic cells.

Langerhans cells (LCs) are immature DCs that are specific to skin and are extremely efficient at presenting antigens and activating naïve T cells.[34] They are present in the epidermis and selectively express c-type lectin Langerin (CD207) and high amount of CD1a as markers, which enable their identification and characterization.[35] LCs are dependent on transforming growth factor-β1 (TGF-β1) for their development and localization. The antigenicity of skin directly correlates with the LC density. Thus, mice tail skin has fewer LCs and is weakly antigenic when compared to flank or ear skin, which is highly antigenic and has 5–10 times the LC density.[36,37] In the epidermis, they are found in the immature state, but become mature on application of inflammatory stimuli such as tumor necrosis factor-alpha (TNF-α). Contact between neighboring immature LCs is rarely observed; however, following maturation, the dendritic processes abut each other communicating signals that lead to their mobilization out of the epidermis toward the draining lymph nodes.[35] Dermal DCs migrate to lymph nodes. These cells (DDC) express CD1a at a lower level, and function similar to LCs, although at a lower efficiency. On activation, like LC, these cells migrate to specific regions, distinct from LCs, in regional lymphoid organs to prime T cells.[38]

6.2.1.4 Pathogenesis of Skin Rejection

CTA transplants introduce potent donor LCs bearing the donor MHC as well as skin-specific antigens into the recipient. Following transplantation, LCs are activated and migrate via lymphatics to recipient secondary lymphoid organs where they present the host antigen to naïve T cells. This strong direct presentation of donor antigen by LC strongly activates donor-specific CD4$^+$ cytotoxic T cells toward the skin component.[39] In fact, Barker and Billingham have shown that severing graft lymphatics abrogated skin rejection, thereby demonstrating the significance of LC migration in skin rejection.[40] In addition, recipient APCs circulate through the allograft phagocytosing donor antigen and presenting it on self-MHC to CD8+ T cells. This indirect presentation augments the alloreactive-stimulus. On activation, allospecific T cells migrate into the allograft, initially in the dermal perivascular space. Following this, the infiltrate spreads to the interphase between dermis and epidermis, sequentially progressing toward the outermost layers of the skin. This is followed by necrosis of single layer of KCs and then necrosis and loss of the epidermis.[51] Thus, a primed recipient immune system eventually leads to graft destruction.[41]

Animal studies in the rat have shown that without cyclosporine, skin allografts induce a potent cell mediated response to vascularized as well as nonvascularized grafts. In addition, a potent humoral response is detected two weeks following a vascularized allograft as shown in Fig. 6.1.[8]

6.2.1.5 Pathology of Skin Rejection

Skin rejection is graded on the relative amount and stage of mononuclear cell infiltrate[42] (Table 6.1).

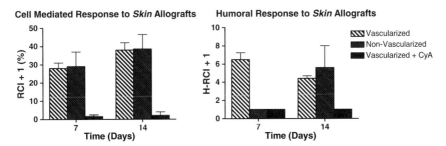

Fig. 6.1 (*Left*) Cell-mediated responses in rats with various skin allografts: vascularized, non-vascularized, and vascularized with cyclosporine treatment. (*Right*) Humoral response in rats with various skin allografts

Table 1 Skin is graded based on mononuclear cell infiltration and histological status of the skin

Description	Grade	Histology
Minimal rejection	Grade I	Perivascular lymphocytic and eosinophilic infiltrates
Mild rejection	Grade II	Additional interphase reaction in epidermis and/or adnexal structures
Moderate rejection	Grade III	Diffuse lymphocytic infiltration of epidermis and dermis
Severe rejection	Grade IVa	Necrosis of single keratinocytes and focal dermal–epidermal separation
	Grade IVb	Necrosis and loss of the epidermis

6.2.2 Muscle

Muscle tissue derived from the mesoderm germ layer forms an integral part of a CTA. All myocytes uniformly express self-antigen.[43] Striated muscles being devoid of specific resident APC fail to induce allorecognition via the direct presentation pathway. In fact studies have demonstrated a lack of MHC I or MHC II expression on normal mature muscle fibers.[52]

During the inflammatory state, sarcolemmal class I antigens are expressed.[43] The trauma of allotransplantation possibly leads to low grade ischemia reperfusion damage and may induce inflammation and subsequent expression of MHC. The immune response to the muscle component of CTA is predictably delayed and lower than skin.

Various investigators have demonstrated a lower antigenic potential for muscle compared to skin in various animal models. In rat heterotopic hind-limb allografts, a high cellular infiltrate but a medium to low humoral response to allografted muscle was observed.[8] Subsequent studies involving the cytokine profile in host rats allografted with muscle have demonstrated lower Th1 cytokine interferon-gamma (IFN-γ) and a Th2 deviant cytokine milieu (IL-4, IL-10)[20] This profile suggests a favorable immunological recognition by the host.

Differential rejection pattern of muscle has been observed. Long term acceptance to the musculoskeletal component of a CTA, but not the skin, has been shown using a hemopoietic BM transplant and transient low dose immunosuppression in miniature swine models.[44] Clinically, this correlates with findings in human hand transplants of only a moderate lymphocytic infiltrate in the muscle in the presence of established skin rejection.[22]

Being highly vascular, muscle tissue has a greater amount of circulating recipient APC rendering its rejection process to be primarily affected via the indirect pathway. Muscle tissue rejects beginning with a mononuclear cell infiltrate, progressing to mixed infiltrate, damage to myocytes, and finally total necrosis.[14]

6.2.3 Tendon

Similar to muscle tissue, tendons express antigenicity lower than the skin. However, due to reduced vascularity compared to muscle, tendons are associated with lower mononuclear cell infiltrate in rejection of the CTA. Studies in animals have shown that tendon allografts undergo a similar process of revascularization, repair, and ligamentization compared with that seen in autografts.[45] Shino et al. found no evidence of immune reaction in patients who received allogenic tendon grafts procured by fresh frozen tissue preservation.[46]

Low antigenicity of tendons has been exploited in using tendon allografts for reconstruction of various tendon deficits[47] including hand flexor tendons,[48] anterior cruciate ligament reconstruction and chronic Achilles tendon rupture reconstruction.[49] In addition, the report on the first human vascularized flexor tendon allograft reported acceptance and good function after one year.[50]

6.2.4 Cartilage

Cartilage in the CTA is encountered in varied locations. It is found in tracheal rings in tracheal allotransplants, in articular cartilage in the joints of a hand transplant and in laryngeal allotransplants. Histologically, the cartilage is hyaline consisting of chondrocyte filled lacunae that are surrounded by composite matrix (type II collagen and proteoglycan molecules) enclosed in the perichondrium. The articular cartilage however lacks perichondrium.[51]

The distribution of major histocompatibility antigens (MHC) on individual components of a cartilage graft determines its overall antigenicity. The perichondrium variably expresses MHC class I and II antigens. This is distributed on cellular elements such as fibroblasts, APCs, and DCs. However, these cells are extremely few in number and as such the perichondrium carries relatively less immunogenicity.[52] Cartilage matrix does not express either MHC class I or II molecules and as such is nonantigenic. Chondrocytes uniformly express MHC I antigen and variable amounts of MHC II.[53] These cells predictably induce a strong antigenic response by themselves. However, in normal circumstances, these antigenic cells are enclosed within lacunae surrounded by nonantigenic matrix and hence protected from immune recognition and/or destruction.[54] Indeed, preventing the chondrocytes from exposure leads to cartilage survival as evidenced in transplanted articular[55] and corneal cartilage grafts.[56] The epithelium covering the cartilage however is highly antigenic and influences the overall rejection process.[57] Thus, it appears that chondrocytes in a CTA potentially remain immunologically protected. Animal studies demonstrate a low immune response to transplanted cartilage.[58] In addition, biopsies taken following amputation of the first rejected human hand transplant reveal minimal to no cellular infiltrate or architectural destruction.[22] Allorecognition in a nonvascularized cartilage graft is initiated by the perichondrium. Pathologically, cartilage rejection is characterized by a multifocal lymphocytic infiltrate accompanied by a roughened articular surface and periosteal and fibrovascular proliferation.[10]

6.2.5 Bone

Bone allografts are exposed to exactly the same immunologic processes as other tissue grafts and may be rejected by the host's immune system. Bone allograft antigens are the proteins or glycoproteins on cell surfaces. The rejection of a bone allograft is considered a cellular rather than a humoral response, although the humoral component may contribute.[59] Studies in the rat have demonstrated a prominent cellular response to vascularized and nonvascularized bone allografts and a low humoral response[8] (Fig. 6.2).

Immune responses directed against osteochondral allografts have been demonstrated in animal models.[15,60] Antigenicity of bone allografts from histocompatibility

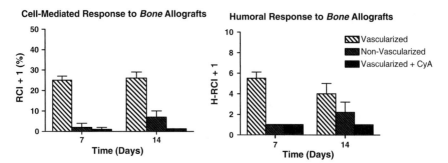

Fig. 6.2 (*Left*) Cell-mediated responses in rats with various bone allografts: vascularized, non-vascularized, and vascularized with cyclosporine treatment. (*Right*) Humoral responses in rats with various bone allografts

complexes is reduced by deep-freezing the allograft prior to transplantation. These respsonses are further reduced when allograft tissues are freeze-dried.[61] The antigenicity of frozen cortical and corticocancellous bone allografts placed orthotopically in rabbits was investigated. It was observed that bone allografts and frozen corticocancellous bone evoked humoral and cell-mediated immunity. In contrast, freeze-dried cortical bone allografts were minimally antigenic.[62] In a similar study, dog leukocyte antigen (DLA)-matched and mismatched, fresh and frozen osteochondral allografts were implanted orthotopically. Fresh allografts stimulated the formation of donor specific antibody against cell-surface antigens, while DLA-matched grafts did not. Antibody titers were significantly reduced when the allograft was frozen.[63]

Bone allograft antigenicity is dependent upon histocompatibility barriers. In a rat vascularized knee allograft model, cyclosporine was administered continuously and in short term as host treatment. Across a strong histocompatibility barrier, continuous cyclosporine was required for long-term graft survival, whereas short-term therapy delayed rejection for 4–6 weeks. Across a weak histocompatibility barrier, short-term therapy was just as effective as continuous therapy in achieving long-term survival.[15] Bone antigencity can be tempered with appropriate MHC antigen matching.

Relative antigenicity of vascularized bone in a canine model has been found to be dependent upon MHC antigen matching. Vascularized bone allografts in matched or immunosuppressed recipients paralleled functional results of vascularized autografts.[64] The vascularized orthotopically placed fibular bone grafts were analyzed quantitatively. Preservation of blood flow and repair patterns were delayed but were not clinically different from vascularized autografts.

In an orthotopic transplant model of the rat distal femur and a surrounding muscular cuff, long-term graft function in fracture healing and weight bearing was assessed. Weak- and strong-barrier MHC mismatches were transplanted. Graft viability and function was prolonged with continuous immunosuppression using cyclosporine. As the graft barrier increased, viability and function of the allograft deteriorated if immunosuppression was not administered in a continuous mode.[65]

Relative antigenicity of bone appears to be related to MHC matching of donor and host in animal models. Results of animal studies will provide valuable information as further vascularized human CTA transplants involving bone are performed. The utility of MHC matching based on animal data for correlation into human practice is supported by these studies.

6.2.6 Nerve

With advent of modern immunosuppressants and knowledge of nerve allo-immunity and refined microsurgical techniques, isolated nerve allografts have become clinically possible with limited immunosuppression.[18] Human hand transplantation has allowed the transfer of intact neural constructs.

Various animal studies have delineated the antigenic status of nerves. Schwann cells have been shown to express both MHC I and MHC II as well as inter cellular adhesion molecule-1 (ICAM-1).[66] In addition, following orthotopic transplantation in rats, MHC II has been shown to become upregulated.[67] Other structures proposed as antigenic include myelin, perineural cells, and fibroblasts, but this data is limited.[68] Schwann cells, because of the expression of ICAM-1 and MHC II, act as APC and trigger a prompt immune response following transplantation. Subsequently, the nerve undergoes a chimeric state, which is progressively replaced by host tissue. This phenomenon suggests the need for only finite host immunosuppression.[66]

Due to replacement of donor Schwann cells by host tissue, nerves are accepted following a period of immune reaction and thus induce a lower cellular infiltrate. In addition, nerves have been shown to induce a low to medium Th1 cytokine profile.[20] This lowered antigenicity is supported by evidence from human hand transplantation studies. Biopsies from clinically rejected hand allografts show perineural inflammation but no frank neuritis even in the most severe cases of rejection.[23]

The low antigenicity of peripheral nerves along with limited low dose immunosuppression helps in reconstructing short and long gap nerve deficits where autologous nerve reconstruction is not possible.

6.2.7 Vessels

Blood vessels including arteries and veins are essential components of CTA transplantation. These vessels are the first donor tissues to come into direct contact with the recipient blood. Endothelial cells (EC) lining the lumen play a sentinel role in allograft rejection.

Human EC have been shown to express MHC I and on activation MHC II. In addition, they have been shown to express co-stimulatory markers such as CD80, CD86,[69] and CD40.[70] This enables the EC to act like APC and stimulate proliferation of allogeneic $CD4^+$ and $CD8^+$ T cells.[71] Human ECs can also constitutively and inducibly express various adhesion molecules and proinflammatory cytokines that serve to recruit circulating leukocytes to local sites of antigenic challenge.[72] Blood vessel media, composed of smooth muscle cells, and adventia express variable levels of MHC antigens.

Endothelial cells have been found to have a relatively high antigenicity in the rat model. However, the blood vessels induced a low cellular infiltrate and low humoral response compared to other constituents of a CTA.[8] This seemingly contrasting result can be explained by the fact that following allo-transplantation, donor EC are progressively replaced by recipient EC, thus leading to decreased allogeneic stimulus toward the blood vessel. This has been demonstrated in various experimental allograft rejections,[73] and clinical transplantations involving kidneys[74] and hearts.[75]

Pathology data from human hand transplants have demonstrated low antigenicity. Human hand transplant tissue biopsies show arteritis in medium and large vessels in sub cutis only in established rejection, further demonstrating the low antigenicity of blood vessels. However, the presence of intimal fibrosis, vascular smooth muscle hyperplasia, and luminal narrowing in chronically rejected allografts suggest an important role of blood vessel antigenicity in chronic rejection.[76]

6.3 Discussion

Composite tissue allotransplantation has evolved to a critical stage where the knowledge gained from first clinical experiments needs to be translated into a sound concept for future immunosuppressive protocols. Novel regimes are required to prevent severe acute rejection while avoiding the profound systemic toxicity associated with conventional high dose maintenance immunosuppression. The key step to achieve such a goal is to understand the relative immunogenicity of the various components of a CTA and to adjust the treatment accordingly.

Herein, we describe and conceptualize the immune response toward different tissues with particular regard to the driving force for rejection in the situation of composite tissue allotransplantation. Components of a vascularized CTA demonstrate an established role with regard to the strength of the immune response induced, the amount of immunosuppression required for allograft survival, and the impact and consequence of rejection. In this context, composite tissue allotransplantation represents a situation different from and more challenging than solid organ transplantation but also provides the opportunity to target tissue components individually.

Studies on relative antigenicity of various components of a vascularized CTA have established the hierarchy of antigenicity as skin > muscle > bone > cartilage > nerves. Also, it has been demonstrated that the immunogenicity of a CTA such as the limb is lower than its individual components. Mechanisms that might promote this phenomenon are "antigen consumption," antigen competition, the induction of enhancing antibodies, and activation of T-suppressor cells[8] (Fig. 6.3). Although the difference in

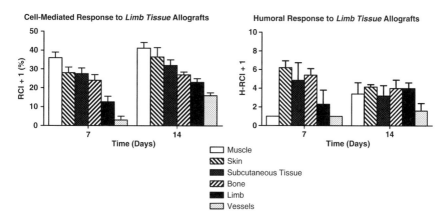

Fig. 6.3 (*Left*) A systematic comparison of cell-mediated responses in rats with various vascularized limb-tissue allografts: muscle, skin, subcutaneous tissue, bone, whole limb, and blood vessels. (*Right*) A systematic comparison of humoral responses in animals with various vascularized limb-tissue allografts

the severity of the immune response toward the various components of a CTA has been elucidated and confirmed in experimental models as well as in the first clinical cases, the significance of the combination of various components has not been understood in its full complexity.

The severity of the immune activation invoked by the individual composition of a vascularized CTA cannot be adequately predicted.[48] The impact of the individual constitution of a CTA with regard to the type and mass of each single component remains thus to be investigated. Therefore, caution is recommended when proceeding with different types of CTAs such as a partial face, full face, or any other parts of the body as the severity of the immune response might not be equal in different types of transplants. We feel that it is important to consider these issues instead of proceeding from hand to any type of skin transplantation because the presence or absence and the amount of components such as bone or muscle can influence the pattern of the response to the allograft as a whole. In this context, the implication of factors such as direct versus indirect antigen presentation, cellular versus humoral immune response, or Th1 versus Th2 response to various components of a vascularized CTA remain to be determined.

In the context of hand transplantation under conventional immunosuppression, experimental as well as clinical data confirm that the skin represent the major – if not the only – target for rejection. Although not fully understood in its complexity and details, various mechanisms such as expression of skin-specific antigens such as Skn and Epa-1, MHC class II expression on keratinocytes,[25] and the presence of a high proportion of supreme antigen presenting cells within the skin have been shown to induce the movement of allospecific activated T-cells toward the epidermis. Accordingly, a higher level of immunosuppression is required to prevent rejection of a CTA carrying a skin component when compared to a CTA without skin.[10] Reducing the antigenicity of a CTA by "selective transplantation" of a graft without the skin component and consecutive replacement of the skin by artificial or autologous tissue has been discussed as an option for minimizing maintenance immunosuppression but does not seem to be clinically feasible. In addition, the "protective effect" of the skin as the major attraction of the immune response over other components has not been adequately investigated[8]. Hence, skin-specific or skin targeted immunosuppression might provide the solution to the dilemma of skin rejection. The unique situation that the skin is accessible to local or topical treatment allows interfering with the mechanisms involved in skin rejection while avoiding exposure of the individual to high levels of systemic immunosuppression. In this context, the mechanisms of lymphocyte adhesion, transmigration, and trafficking toward the epidermis as the ultimate target of the immune response have been outlined in this article and shall be addressed in future experimental as well as clinical trials.

Each distinct tissue component of a CTA serves a particular function, which cumulatively adds to the functionality of the CTA as a whole. This interdependence sets the requirements for a definite acceptance of all components by the recipient, irrespective of the varying antigenic potential. Hence, monitoring of all components of a CTA for signs of rejection would be desirable. Skin can be monitored by inspection and skin biopsy, but muscle, connective tissue, nerve, or bone cannot be routinely monitored in a comparable fashion. Therefore, other non-invasive methods need to be developed in order to individually monitor the different components of a CTA and adequately adjust immunosuppression.

In conclusion, the relative antigenicity of different components of a CTA represent a major hurdle for the application of CTA in a higher number of patients and a key issue for designing adequate immunosuppressive protocols in this field. Although the complexity of the immune response toward a CTA warrants further clarification, current knowledge can be translated into specifically designed immunosuppressive regimes targeting the skin as the most critical component of CTAs.

References

1. Starzl TE. Back to the future. *Transplantation.* 2005;79(9):1009–1014.
2. Billingham RE, Medawar PB. Desensitization to skin homografts by injections of donor skin extracts. *Ann Surg.* 1953;137(4):444–449.
3. Kirk AD. Immunosuppression without immunosuppression? How to be a tolerant individual in a dangerous world. *Transpl Infect Dis.* 1999;1(1):65–75.
4. Siemionow M, Ozer K. Advances in composite tissue allograft transplantation as related to the hand and upper extremity. *J Hand Surg [Am].* 2002;27(4):565–580.
5. Barker JH, Francois CG, Frank JM, Maldonado C. Composite tissue allotransplantation. *Transplantation.* 2002;73(5):832–835.
6. Dubernard JM, Owen E, Herzberg G, et al. Human hand allograft: report on first 6 months. *Lancet.* 1999;353(9161):1315–1320.
7. Lee WP, Mathes DW. Hand transplantation: pertinent data and future outlook. *J Hand Surg [Am].* 1999;24(5):906–913.
8. Lee WP, Yaremchuk MJ, Pan YC, Randolph MA, Tan CM, Weiland AJ. Relative antigenicity of components of a vascularized limb allograft. *Plast Reconstr Surg.* 1991;87(3):401–411.

9. Prabhune KA, Gorantla VS, Maldonado C, Perez-Abadia G, Barker JH, Ildstad ST. Mixed allogeneic chimerism and tolerance to composite tissue allografts. *Microsurgery.* 2000;20(8): 441–447.
10. Buttemeyer R, Jones NF, Min Z, Rao U. Rejection of the component tissues of limb allografts in rats immunosuppressed with FK-506 and cyclosporine. *Plast Reconstr Surg.* 1996;97(1):139–148; discussion 149–151.
11. Murray JE. Organ transplantation (skin, kidney, heart) and the plastic surgeon. *Plast Reconstr Surg.* 1971;47(5):425–431.
12. Moseley RV, Sheil AG, Mitchell RM, Murray JE. Immunologic relationships between skin and kidney homografts in dogs on immunosuppressive therapy. *Transplantation.* 1966;4(6): 678–687.
13. Tanaka S, Sakai A. Stimulation of allogeneic lymphocytes by skin epidermal cells in the rat. *Transplantation.* 1979;27(3):194–199.
14. Tan CM, Yaremchuk MJ, Randolph MA, Lee WP, Burdick J, Weiland AJ. Vascularized muscle allografts and the role of cyclosporine. *Plast Reconstr Surg.* 1991;87(3):412–418.
15. Paskert JP, Yaremchuk MJ, Randolph MA, Weiland AJ. The role of cyclosporin in prolonging survival in vascularized bone allografts. *Plast Reconstr Surg.* 1987;80(2):240–247.
16. Wengerter K, Dardik H. Biological vascular grafts. *Semin Vasc Surg.* 1999;12(1):46–51.
17. Bain JR, Mackinnon SE, Hudson AR, Falk RE, Falk JA, Hunter DA. The peripheral nerve allograft: an assessment of regeneration across nerve allografts in rats immunosuppressed with cyclosporin A. *Plast Reconstr Surg.* 1988;82(6):1052–1066.
18. Mackinnon SE, Doolabh VB, Novak CB, Trulock EP. Clinical outcome following nerve allograft transplantation. *Plast Reconstr Surg.* 2001;107(6):1419–1429.
19. Zhang Z, Zhu L, Quan D, et al. Pattern of liver, kidney, heart, and intestine allograft rejection in different mouse strain combinations. *Transplantation.* 1996;62(9):1267–1272.
20. Tung TH, Mohanakumar T, Mackinnon SE. TH1/TH2 cytokine profile of the immune response in limb component transplantation. *Plast Reconstr Surg.* 2005;116(2):557–566.
21. Boyse EA, Old LJ. Loss of skin allograft tolerance by chimeras. *Transplantation.* 1968;6(4): 619.
22. Kanitakis J, Jullien D, Petruzzo P, et al. Clinicopathologic features of graft rejection of the first human hand allograft. *Transplantation.* 2003;76(4):688–693.
23. Cendales LC, Kirk AD, Moresi JM, Ruiz P, Kleiner DE. Composite tissue allotransplantation: classification of clinical acute skin rejection. *Transplantation.* 2006;81(3):418–422.
24. Steinman RM. The dendritic cell system and its role in immunogenicity. *Annu Rev Immunol.* 1991;9:271–296.
25. Steinmuller D, Wakely E, Landas SK. Evidence that epidermal alloantigen Epa-1 is an immunogen for murine heart as well as skin allograft rejection. *Transplantation.* 1991;51(2): 459–463.
26. Fuchimoto Y, Gleit ZL, Huang CA, et al. Skin-specific alloantigens in miniature swine. *Transplantation.* 2001;72(1):122–126.
27. Volc-Platzer B, Majdic O, Knapp W, et al. Evidence of HLA-DR antigen biosynthesis by human keratinocytes in disease. *J Exp Med.* 1984;159(6):1784–1789.
28. Dustin ML, Singer KH, Tuck DT, Springer TA. Adhesion of T lymphoblasts to epidermal keratinocytes is regulated by interferon gamma and is mediated by intercellular adhesion molecule 1 (ICAM-1). *J Exp Med.* 1988;167(4):1323–1340.
29. Simon M, Jr., Hunyadi J. Expression of OKM5 antigen on human keratinocytes in positive intracutaneous tests for delayed-type hypersensitivity. *Dermatologica.* 1987;175(3):121–125.
30. Luger TA, Stadler BM, Katz SI, Oppenheim JJ. Epidermal cell (keratinocyte)-derived thymocyte-activating factor (ETAF). *J Immunol.* 1981;127(4):1493–1498.
31. Aragane Y, Riemann H, Bhardwaj RS, et al. IL-12 is expressed and released by human keratinocytes and epidermoid carcinoma cell lines. *J Immunol.* 1994;153(12):5366–5372.
32. Partridge M, Chantry D, Turner M, Feldmann M. Production of interleukin-1 and interleukin-6 by human keratinocytes and squamous cell carcinoma cell lines. *J Invest Dermatol.* 1991;96(5): 771–776.

33. Barker JN, Jones ML, Mitra RS, et al. Modulation of keratinocyte-derived interleukin-8 which is chemotactic for neutrophils and T lymphocytes. *Am J Pathol.* 1991;139(4):869–876.
34. Richters CD, van Pelt AM, van Geldrop E, et al. Migration of rat skin dendritic cells. *J Leukoc Biol.* 1996;60(3):317–322.
35. Nishibu A, Ward BR, Jester JV, Ploegh HL, Boes M, Takashima A. Behavioral responses of epidermal Langerhans cells in situ to local pathological stimuli. *J Invest Dermatol.* 2006; 126(4):787–796.
36. Bergstresser PR, Fletcher CR, Streilein JW. Surface densities of Langerhans cells in relation to rodent epidermal sites with special immunologic properties. *J Invest Dermatol.* 1980;74(2): 77–80.
37. Chen HD, Silvers WK. Influence of Langerhans cells on the survival of H-Y incompatible skin grafts in rats. *J Invest Dermatol.* 1983;81(1):20–23.
38. Kissenpfennig A, Henri S, Dubois B, et al. Dynamics and function of Langerhans cells in vivo: dermal dendritic cells colonize lymph node areas distinct from slower migrating Langerhans cells. *Immunity.* 2005;22(5):643–654.
39. Steinmuller D. Passenger leukocytes and the immunogenicity of skin allografts: a critical reevaluation. *Transplant Proc.* 1981;13(1 Pt 2):1094–1098.
40. Barker CF, Billingham RE. The role of afferent lymphatics in the rejection of skin homografts. *J Exp Med.* 1968;128(1):197–221.
41. Tyler JD, Steinmuller D. Evidence of cell-mediated cytotoxicity to skin-specific alloantigens on mouse epidermal cells. *Transplant Proc.* 1981;13(1 Pt 2):1082–1085.
42. Schneeberger S, Kreczy A, Brandacher G, Steurer W, Margreiter R. Steroid- and ATG-resistant rejection after double forearm transplantation responds to Campath-1H. *Am J Transplant.* 2004;4(8):1372–1374.
43. Karpati G, Pouliot Y, Carpenter S. Expression of immunoreactive major histocompatibility complex products in human skeletal muscles. *Ann Neurol.* 1988;23(1):64–72.
44. Hettiaratchy S, Melendy E, Randolph MA, et al. Tolerance to composite tissue allografts across a major histocompatibility barrier in miniature swine. *Transplantation.* 2004;77(4): 514–521.
45. Arnoczky SP, Warren RF, Ashlock MA. Replacement of the anterior cruciate ligament using a patellar tendon allograft. An experimental study. *J Bone Joint Surg Am.* 1986;68(3):376–385.
46. Shino K, Kawasaki T, Hirose H, Gotoh I, Inoue M, Ono K. Replacement of the anterior cruciate ligament by an allogeneic tendon graft. An experimental study in the dog. *J Bone Joint Surg Br.* 1984;66(5):672–681.
47. Deng W, Zhao H, Dong H. [Clinical application of allogeneic tendon]. *Zhongguo Xiu Fu Chong Jian Wai Ke Za Zhi.* 2005;19(8):666–668.
48. Zhang Y, Yang K, Zhu W. [Experimental research and clinical application of allogenic tendon grafting]. *Zhonghua Wai Ke Za Zhi.* 1995;33(9):539–541.
49. Chang Q, Huang X, Guan C. [Treatment of chronic Achilles tendon rupture by use of allogeneic tendon]. *Zhongguo Xiu Fu Chong Jian Wai Ke Za Zhi.* 2004;18(4):336–337.
50. Guimberteau JC, Baudet J, Panconi B, Boileau R, Potaux L. Human allotransplant of a digital flexion system vascularized on the ulnar pedicle: a preliminary report and 1-year follow-up of two cases. *Plast Reconstr Surg.* 1992;89(6):1135–1147.
51. Colnot C. Cellular and molecular interactions regulating skeletogenesis. *J Cell Biochem.* 2005;95(4):688–697.
52. Shaari CM, Farber D, Brandwein MS, Gannon P, Urken ML. Characterizing the antigenic profile of the human trachea: implications for tracheal transplantation. *Head Neck.* 1998;20(6): 522–527.
53. Burmester GR, Menche D, Merryman P, Klein M, Winchester R. Application of monoclonal antibodies to the characterization of cells eluted from human articular cartilage. Expression of Ia antigens in certain diseases and identification of an 85-kD cell surface molecule accumulated in the pericellular matrix. *Arthritis Rheum.* 1983;26(10):1187–1195.
54. Donald PJ. Cartilage grafting in facial reconstruction with special consideration of irradiated grafts. *Laryngoscope.* 1986;96(7):786–807.

55. Langer F, Gross AE. Immunogenicity of allograft articular cartilage. *J Bone Joint Surg Am.* 1974;56(2):297–304.
56. Whitsett CF, Stulting RD. The distribution of HLA antigens on human corneal tissue. *Invest Ophthalmol Vis Sci.* 1984;25(5):519–524.
57. Wang EC, Damrose EJ, Mendelsohn AH, et al. Distribution of class I and II human leukocyte antigens in the larynx. *Otolaryngol Head Neck Surg.* 2006;134(2):280–287.
58. Yang J, Hu J, Wu Z. [Experimental study on the tracheal allografts with decreased antigenicity]. *Zhongguo Xiu Fu Chong Jian Wai Ke Za Zhi.* 2006;20(1):73–76.
59. Burchardt H. The biology of bone graft repair. *Clin Orthop Relat Res.* 1983(174):28–42.
60. Stevenson S, Li XQ, Martin B. The fate of cancellous and cortical bone after transplantation of fresh and frozen tissue-antigen-matched and mismatched osteochondral allografts in dogs. *J Bone Joint Surg Am.* 1991;73(8):1143–1156.
61. Friedlaender GE. Immune responses to osteochondral allografts. Current knowledge and future directions. *Clin Orthop Relat Res.* 1983(174):58–68.
62. Friedlaender GE, Strong DM, Sell KW. Studies on the antigenicity of bone. I. Freeze-dried and deep-frozen bone allografts in rabbits. *J Bone Joint Surg Am.* 1976;58(6):854–858.
63. Stevenson S. The immune response to osteochondral allografts in dogs. *J Bone Joint Surg Am.* 1987;69(4):573–582.
64. Goldberg VM, Powell A, Shaffer JW, Zika J, Bos GD, Heiple KG. Bone grafting: role of histocompatibility in transplantation. *J Orthop Res.* 1985;3(4):389–404.
65. Lee WP, Pan YC, Kesmarky S, et al. Experimental orthotopic transplantation of vascularized skeletal allografts: functional assessment and long-term survival. *Plast Reconstr Surg.* 1995;95(2):336–349; discussion 350–333.
66. Atchabahian A, Mackinnon SE, Hunter DA. Cold preservation of nerve grafts decreases expression of ICAM-1 and class II MHC antigens. *J Reconstr Microsurg.* 1999;15(4): 307–311.
67. Ansselin AD, Pollard JD. Immunopathological factors in peripheral nerve allograft rejection: quantification of lymphocyte invasion and major histocompatibility complex expression. *J Neurol Sci.* 1990;96(1):75–88.
68. Evans PJ, Mackinnon SE, Levi AD, et al. Cold preserved nerve allografts: changes in basement membrane, viability, immunogenicity, and regeneration. *Muscle Nerve.* 1998;21(11):1507–1522.
69. Linsley PS, Greene JL, Brady W, Bajorath J, Ledbetter JA, Peach R. Human B7-1 (CD80) and B7-2 (CD86) bind with similar avidities but distinct kinetics to CD28 and CTLA-4 receptors. *Immunity.* 1994;1(9):793–801.
70. Hollenbaugh D, Mischel-Petty N, Edwards CP, et al. Expression of functional CD40 by vascular endothelial cells. *J Exp Med.* 1995;182(1):33–40.
71. Biedermann BC, Pober JS. Human endothelial cells induce and regulate cytolytic T cell differentiation. *J Immunol.* 1998;161(9):4679–4687.
72. Briscoe DM, Alexander SI, Lichtman AH. Interactions between T lymphocytes and endothelial cells in allograft rejection. *Curr Opin Immunol.* 1998;10(5):525–531.
73. Plissonnier D, Nochy D, Poncet P, et al. Sequential immunological targeting of chronic experimental arterial allograft. *Transplantation.* 1995;60(5):414–424.
74. Lagaaij EL, Cramer-Knijnenburg GF, van Kemenade FJ, van Es LA, Bruijn JA, van Krieken JH. Endothelial cell chimerism after renal transplantation and vascular rejection. *Lancet.* 2001;357(9249):33–37.
75. Quaini F, Urbanek K, Beltrami AP, et al. Chimerism of the transplanted heart. *N Engl J Med.* 2002;346(1):5–15.
76. Cailhier JF, Laplante P, Hebert MJ. Endothelial apoptosis and chronic transplant vasculopathy: recent results, novel mechanisms. *Am J Transplant.* 2006;6(2):247–253.

Chapter 7
On the Road to Tolerance Induction in Composite Tissue Allotransplantation

Mark A. Hardy

7.1 Introduction

In 1954, the first successful kidney transplant between identical twins opened the way for the clinical application of solid organ transplantation. Recognizing that transplantation between identical twins would not be the route to widespread relief of organ failure because of the unique avoidance of rejection, researchers directed attention to widening the donor pool. Allotransplantation was the goal and this implied a search for methods to prevent rejection and destruction of the transplant. Over time it became apparent that the use of immunosuppressive drugs carried associated toxicity along with it. The goal of many transplant clinicians and immunobiologists was to induce tolerance without altering the recipient's response to infection and other antigens.

The transplant literature is replete with review articles on how to achieve immunologic unresponsiveness to allogeneic organ transplants. The following summary will briefly focus on the cells, mechanisms, and clinical possibilities that may impact future successful composite tissue allografts (CTA). The intent of this review is not to be comprehensive, but rather to summarize the existing evidence on the importance of various cells in the immune process and how signaling between cells can be manipulated. By summarizing and interpreting sometimes conflicting experimental results in this field, I hope to show how to utilize existing information to achieve clinical success with CTA.

CTA as a source of antigen comes with its own professional and nonprofessional antigen presenting cells (donor APCs), its own stem cells in the bone marrow, and various organ-specific antigens, including bone, skin, muscle, nerves, arteries, and veins. This is unique to transplant immunity and will be discussed extensively in other chapters in this book.

Currently, the major goal of transplantation immunology is to induce donor-specific tolerance in such a manner that the extended suppression of immune responses is specific for the allograft and leaves the rest of the immune system competent to fight infections and malignancies. Although it is intuitive that the immune system did not evolve for the purpose of rejection of transplanted tissues, it is these immune responses against tissues from nongenetically identical individuals that lead to rejection of such tissues. While new immunosuppressive drugs have decreased the incidence and severity of acute rejection, chronic rejection remains a major problem. Induction of tolerance promises to increase allograft survival while reducing the risks of chronic immunosuppression, which are associated with major morbidity and excess mortality. The establishment of immune tolerance to organ transplants remains a major goal in clinical organ transplantation, and this is particularly true in composite tissue transplantation where alternatives, although generally unsatisfactory, exist, and where the transplant is not a life saving procedure.

The first descriptions of actively acquired transplant tolerance were by Owen[1] and by Billingham, Brent, and Medawar.[2] They showed that fetal exposure to major histocompatibility complex (MHC) mismatched donor antigen in utero in Freemantle cattle[1] or neonatal exposure in the mouse[2] led to acceptance of donor strain skin grafts during adulthood without need for any immunosuppression or manipulation. Transplantation tolerance has been defined in many different ways but the most accurate description is that of the state in which a recipient is unresponsive to an allograft but retains immunity to other third-party antigens, especially pathogens. It also implies that a second-set, donor-type allograft is accepted without rejection while a third-party allograft is rejected in the normal fashion.

Because of the great difficulty in achieving transplantation tolerance, the term "operative tolerance" has been used to describe the state in which unresponsiveness to an allograft is maintained with minimal or intermittent chronic immunosuppression. Although initially it was thought that neonatal tolerance depended primarily on thymic education that distinguished self and nonself, it has become apparent that neonatal tolerance occurs by multiple mechanisms, including clonal deletion, anergy, and immunoregulation. While it is still debated whether the neonatal immune system has intrinsic defects that favor tolerance induction, induction of neonatal tolerance remains one of the best models of central tolerance induction that we have. Evidence exists that tolerance is the result of the dose and nature of the donor antigen. Although it is plausible that the neonatal immune system is easier to fool to achieve tolerance, the mechanisms involved remain unclear.

As we proceed with this review we must remember that the immune reaction to CTA involves an extremely diverse alloreactive repertoire. Many cell types are involved in the initiation and the ultimate destruction of the allograft where the alloantigens are presented to the immunocompetent host, both by direct and indirect methods and where the large mass of alloreactive clones (as many as one in ten T cells can be alloreactive) creates an important barrier to tolerance induction. Despite tremendous progress in the field of organ transplantation over the past 40 years, primarily due to development of new immunosuppressive agents and greater experience in using them, our current immunosuppressive strategies are clearly not tolerogenic. Drugs which are very effective in prolonging graft survival, such as cyclosporine or tacrolimus may disrupt the normal mechanisms of self-tolerance induction in the thymus[3] and can blunt the ability of costimulation blockade to induce both cardiac allograft tolerance and mixed chimerism in mice.[4] Since active immunologic mechanisms are required to induce transplantation tolerance, several commonly used immunosuppressive agents may actually be counterproductive by the effect of such agents on cosignaling and particularly by the effects on activation, proliferation, and suppressive function of regulatory T cells (Tregs).

Successful induction of tolerance, primarily to immediately vascularized allografts such as CTA, has been achieved in rodent models, but only rarely in large animal models or in clinical situations. Most experimental efforts have been based on one or more of the following techniques:

(1) maximal T-cell depletion without endangering the life of the host using total lymphoid irradiation, total body irradiation, and/or various monoclonal or polyclonal antibodies along with other immunologic manipulations, such as costimulatory blockade
(2) donor antigen infusion and alteration of allogeneic signaling so as to induce a population of donor-specific suppressor and regulatory T cells
(3) donor hematopoietic stem cell infusions following T-cell depletion using various cytoreductive regimens sufficient to allow donor bone marrow engraftment and creation of a transient chimera without causing graft versus host disease
(4) direct infusion or augmentation of T regulatory cells.

Experiments in large animals and humans have relied primarily on the third approach, as summarized by Fehr and Sykes[5] based on existence of transient macrochimerism in nonhuman primates and humans. Interestingly, it is effective for kidney transplantation and not for cardiac transplantation. Little data are available for CTA, which includes donor bone marrow and therefore should be favored, as emphasized elsewhere in this book by Gordon and his colleagues.

To assess various approaches to tolerance induction that may become practical for CTA transplantation, we first need to describe and evaluate the various immunologic mechanisms that have been hypothesized to be important in establishing immunological unresponsiveness. In this chapter I favor concepts that imply an active process (turning switch on) rather than a deletional process (turning switch off).

7.2 T-Cell Tolerance

T-cell tolerance to self-antigens and the regulation of immune responses to environmental antigens are an intrinsic part of the immune system. Immune tolerance is initially achieved during thymic development by negative selection of T cells with high affinity for self-peptides. Additional regulation is required in the periphery to control the responses of autoreactive T cells that have escaped negative selection in the thymus and to control responses to foreign antigens. Several peripheral mechanisms of T-cell regulation have been identified including the induction of anergy, activation induced cell death (AICD), and Tregs.

7.3 Regulatory T Cells

T cells are essential for allograft rejection and are the ultimate targets of peripheral tolerance. Mechanisms contributing to "tolerance" include deletion, anergy, ignorance, immune deviation, and immunoregulation.[6–8] These are not mutually exclusive, but their relative contribution depends in part on immunogenicity of the donor–recipient pair and graft type (e.g., skin versus heart).[9–12] Natural regulatory T cells (natural Tregs) comprise 5–10% of CD4 cells in mice and humans and exhibit potent regulatory activity. Natural Tregs are selected in the thymus and emerge expressing a CD45RBLo CD25+ phenotype. A high proportion also expresses glucocorticoid-induced TNF receptor (GITR) and CTLA-4. These markers, and CD25 in particular, have been extremely useful for identification of natural Tregs. Generally, T-cell tolerance is induced in two main sites: (1) in the thymus during early T-cell differentiation (central tolerance); and (2) in the secondary lymphoid tissue after export of mature T cells from the thymus (peripheral tolerance). Lymphocyte precursors in the thymus, whose T-cell receptors (TCRs) bind with high affinity to peptide–MHC complexes on thymic Ag presenting cells, undergo apoptosis in a process of negative selection (central tolerance). Two types of regulatory T cells have been reported in association with tolerance: CD4+CD25+[13] and CD4+CD45RBlow.[14] The thymic CD4+CD25+ T cells migrate from the thymus to the periphery.[15] There are also polyclonal immunoregulatory CD4+CD25+ T cells induced by specific Ag and which originate in the periphery rather than the thymus.[16]

An important advance in the understanding of the biology of Treg was discovery of Foxp3, a forkhead/winged helix transcription factor expressed by Treg that regulate their thymic development.[17] CD25-Foxp3+ cells exhibit Treg activity, and are in equilibrium with CD25+ cells.[18] By following Foxp3 as a specific marker, the in vivo behavior of natural Treg can now be more accurately assessed. Tregs are anergic in vitro, however, they proliferate in vivo in response to endogenous or exogenous antigens.[19–21] Natural Tregs are found in unmanipulated animals, derived in the thymus, and express Foxp3. Somewhat distinct Treg can be generated from peripheral CD4 cells by antigen (Ag) exposure such as repetitive stimulation in vitro in the presence of IL-10, or Vitamin D3 + dexamethasone which gives rise to IL-10 secreting T regulatory cells.[22–24]

The study of Tregs in transplant setting has been complicated by the potential effects of therapeutic agents and the focus on the importance of other mechanisms of tolerance (e.g., chimerism, costimulatory blockade). We now know that CD4+ Tregs are present in tolerant allograft recipients and can adoptively transfer donor-specific graft survival to naive hosts.[25–27] The balance between natural CD25+ Treg and effector cells may play an important role in establishing a tolerant state. Natural Treg can proliferate in vivo in response to an allograft and then exhibit increased potency and Ag-specificity, presumably due to expansion of the appropriate Ag-reactive/cross-reactive clones.[21] In this regard, any strategy that blocks effector cells may allow outgrowth and tip the balance in favor of allograft acceptance.

The importance of Tregs in transplantation tolerance has been shown in a variety of experimental models using nondepletional T-cell antibodies or costimulatory blockade. Tregs could build up over time by homeostasis when the effector response is inhibited, hence the possible importance of "induction" therapy with polyclonal or monoclonal antibodies. This may lead to specifically induced proliferation of natural Treg by de novo conversion of non-Treg, hence the importance of manipulating the dendritic cells (DCs) and initial antigen presentation.

A therapeutically applicable approach that can directly initiate a shift in the immune response from immunity to tolerance by converting T effector cells to Treg in the periphery would be exciting. Another possibility recently described by several groups,[28] and extended to human renal transplants (personal communication – Kiel University Nephrology group) is to proliferate the Tregs in vitro and infuse them back into patients receiving a renal allograft.

A minimal requirement for tolerance is the depletion of alloaggressive T-cell clones. However, unless complete central (thymic) deletion is achieved via creation of mixed chimerism, the long-term maintenance of the tolerant state is also dependent on self-perpetuating immunoregulatory mechanisms that actively constrain the remaining alloaggressive T cells. In the absence of effective therapy, the more rapid expansion of alloaggressive T cells overcomes the protective effects of regulatory lymphocytes. Hence, the allograft outcome, rejection or tolerance, depends on the balance between cytotoxic and regulatory T cells. The decrease of the pool size of alloreactive T cells by transient pharmacologic ablation (e.g., antilymphocyte serum) would be therefore required to allow regulatory T cells to proliferate and exert their suppressive effects before tolerance can be achieved.

7.4 T Suppressor Cells

Research on T suppressor cells has reemerged in the late 1990s when several subsets of T cells were shown to inhibit the proliferation of other T cells. While natural Treg cells play a major role in regulating self-reactive T cells and preventing autoimmune diseases another set of regulatory T cells, the CD8+CD28+ Ts cells are characterized by their antigen-specific activity.[29] It has been shown that CD8+CD28+ Ts specific for alloantigens could be generated in vitro by repeated antigenic stimulation.[30–38] In vivo, such cells can act as antigen-specific suppressors in patients with heart, kidney, or liver allografts.[39–48] These antigen-specific CD8+CD28+ Ts express Foxp3, are MHC class I restricted, have no killing capacity, and do not produce cytokines.[30,42,43] Instead they act on professional DCs and non-professional (endothelial cells) antigen-presenting cells (APC) directly, i.e., by cell-to-cell contact, inducing qualitative changes characteristic of an alternative pathway of maturation toward a tolerogenic rather than immunogenic phenotype. It has been suggested by Suciu Foca (personal communication) that T-cell-mediated suppression may result from the sequential interactions first between T suppressor cell and APC and next between "tolerized" APC and T helper cell (Th) (first stage of effector cell). In turn, anergic Th acquire regulatory capacity, in conjunction with Foxp3 expression, and further perpetuate tolerance.[29,43]

7.5 Pharmacologic Induction Strategies

To develop tolerance induction strategies, new agents must be introduced that affect the central role of T cells in transplant rejection by mechanisms other than deletion alone. Studies on the generation and characterization of antigen-specific Ts, Treg cells, and tolerogenic APC may pave the way to development of such new agents and thereby the induction of immunologic tolerance.

While the immunosuppressive drugs used in current practice focus on T-cell deletion which is effective in preventing rejection, some of the newer agents are addressing the costimulation issue and therefore increasing the specificity of that modality of treatment and shifting the host's cellular repertoire toward donor-specific tolerogenic responses.

7.6 Costimulation Blockade

Prevention of full T-cell activation by means of blockade of costimulation through B7:CD28 or CD40:CD40L pathways[44] or IL2 activity,[45] or alloantigen presentation by immature (iDC) or plasmacytoid dendritic cells (pDC)[46] are among the strategies that may induce Ag-specific T-cell anergy or clonal deletion. More recently, many transplant models have shown the correlation between tolerance and the induction of CD4+ Tregs, that express CD25, CTLA-4, and FoxP3,[47] and are capable of preventing or blocking T-cell alloreactivity.[48] The evidence that the tolerogenic effect of Tregs occurs prior to the development of complete peripheral tolerance[49] suggests that these cells are critical, particularly in the early phases after transplant, and may not be required for maintenance of long-term tolerance.

The two-signal model of T-cell activation has been a dominant concept in immunology for the past two decades. To generate an effective response in vivo, T cells must not only receive signal one delivered via the T-cell receptor (TCR), but they also require costimulatory signals (signal two).[44] Several families of costimulatory molecules have been identified. Among the best studied are members of the immunoglobulin (in particular CD28) and the tumor necrosis factor receptor (TNF: TNFR) super families.[45,46] The concept of blocking costimulatory pathways to prevent rejection or promote tolerance has focused on two of the originally discovered, and probably most important, pathways, CD28 and CD40. Short-term blockade of the CD28 pathway with the CTLA-4-Ig fusion protein proved to be a potent inhibitor of rejection in many rodent transplant models.[47–50] Although initial clinical results using CTLA-4-Ig were disappointing, LEA29Y (now known as Belatacept©) proved to be more promising in nonhuman primate transplant experiments.[51–53] A large Phase II study of Belatacept© in human recipients of de novo renal allografts demonstrated that Belatacept© was as effective as cyclosporine without evidence of nephrotoxicity.[54] Phase III studies are underway and studies using Belatacept© in calcineurin-inhibitor free and steroid-free protocols in renal and islet transplantation have begun in 2007.

Many transplantation therapies have been developed to target other costimulatory molecules to inhibit graft-specific T cells when they are undergoing active stimulation.[55] Another costimulatory molecule that has been targeted most extensively experimentally is CD154 (CD40L). The CD40 receptor is expressed on APCs, epithelial cells, and activated T cells. CD40 binds CD154 (CD40L). Anti-CD154 therapy has successfully induced tolerance to cardiac allografts in mice, along with long-term survival of allografts in nonhuman primates.[56] Many mechanisms have been identified that may explain the tolerogenic effects of anti-CD154 mAb. Most studies have suggested that suppression by Tregs is the most important basis for tolerance induced by anti-CD154 mAb.[57–59] Anti-CDI54 can also prevent the costimulatory effects downstream of CD154 engagement on activated T cells thereby limiting the expansion of alloreactive T cells.[59] Although clinical trials with anti-CD154 mAb have been halted because of life-threatening thromboembolic side effects,[60] targeting of the CD40/CD154 pathway is again being considered for clinical use. Insight into the expression of CD154 on platelets and how it functions to stabilize thrombi in a CD40-independent manner suggested that targeting this pathway via CD40 rather than CD154 might allow interruption or inhibition of the CD154/CD40-dependent interactions critical for T-cell responses while leaving unaltered the CD154-integrin interactions. Anti-CD40 mAbs have now been shown to prolong allograft survival successfully in nonhuman primates without triggering thromboembolism.[61,62]

It is clear that we need better understanding of the effects of the new blockers of costimulation on T-cell responses and the mechanisms by which T cells can escape blockade of these pathways as CD28 blockers progress in clinical trials, and the success of alternative approaches to target CD40 show promise in nonhuman primate models. In recent years, additional costimulatory pathways, including ICOS, OX40, CD70, and 4-1BB have been described. It seems likely that continued investigation of these and other as yet not known pathways will provide insights and additional therapeutic opportunities to overcome the redundancy of the immune system.

It is clear that blockade of any given pathway is less effective than blocking multiple pathways (i.e., CD40 and CD28 pathways) as has been previously shown.[51,63,64] Highly immunogenic allografts, such as those of intestine and skin, require more effective tolerogenic therapies as will probably CTA. Among these, the combination of costimulatory blockade with immunosuppressive drugs (Rapamycin© (RAPA) with a CD154 mAb and CTLA-4-Ig) has been shown to result in long-term graft acceptance.[65] Although increased allograft survival can be achieved by targeting independent co-stimulatory pathways, a much greater success may be gained when several pathways are targeted simultaneously, and in some cases, when alloreactive T cells are sufficiently initially eliminated. Since the highest inflammatory reaction in the host results from surgery and healing of a highly immunogenic allograft, the early treatment or "induction" immediately after transplantation is not an ideal time in which to induce a state of immunologic tolerance. Ideally, costimulation blockade or any other induction treatment should be used in a preemptive fashion along with a donor-specific transplant antigen surrogate such as donor bone marrow or other cells, modified to be nonimmunogenic by chemical or physical means. The immune system is most effective at inducing peripheral tolerance when the environment is quiescent. On the basis of this belief, tolerance may be achieved by exposing the recipient to donor antigens concomitantly with costimulation blockade prior to transplantation, in an effort to facilitate preemptive tolerance induction.

7.7 Donor-Specific Transfusions

The goal of donor-specific transfusions (DST) is to modify the host immune response to alloantigens prior to the immunogenic introduction of an allograft. Historically, although the infusion of whole blood from the donor into graft recipients was effective in rodents, it only modestly prolonged the longevity of allografts in humans.[66–71] In mice, the prolonged allograft survival following DST can be substantially lengthened or rendered permanent if the DST is combined with blocking of CD154.[72] The finding that DST predominantly, if not exclusively, induces tolerance via indirect presentation provided the first clues that DST and anti-CD154 collaborated in induction of peripheral allotolerance. It is thought that the infused DST cells rapidly undergo apoptosis and then are presented by host APCs which are impaired in maturation by anti-CD154. This commits the immature APCs to the tolerogenic presentation of DST-derived allopeptides which when deprived of CD40 signal become apoptotic. Delivery of peptides via apoptotic cells appears to be an extremely efficient means to induce peripheral tolerance. Delivery of immunodominant synthetic allopeptides, as we have also done,[73,74] may be equally effective.

7.8 T-Cell Activation

The two signal hypotheses of T-cell activation is an accepted paradigm that describes the early requirements for T-cell activation versus anergy.[75] This paradigm states that the proficient induction of an immune response requires TCR and MHC/peptide interaction (signal one) followed by the interaction between costimulatory molecules, namely CD80/86 and CD28 (signal two). If signal one is generated in absence of signal two, then the outcome is not immunity, but tolerance. Providing signal one and signal two is the responsibility of the APC, which must efficiently engage and trigger multiple T-cell surface molecules. To achieve this, the APCs must first "mature." CD154 is unique in helping the APCs mature by providing a spectrum of signals that trigger the upregulation of costimulatory molecules, cytokines, and chemokines. When this is blocked, the APCs remain immature and tolerance ensues.

In transplantation, T–APC interactions can be direct or indirect. Donor APC rapidly migrate from the allograft to secondary lymphoid organs,[76] and depletion of allograft APC may impair antigen presentation and rejection.[77] Priming of recipient effector T cells by this direct pathway may take place both in secondary lymphoid organs and/or directly in the graft.[78] In CTA, the majority of donor APCs probably reside in the donor bone marrow, although a significant number are also present in the skin. The other components of CTA clearly carry both professional and non-professional APCs and it is still uncertain what the role of organ or tissue-specific transplantation antigens is in provoking rejection or acceptance of the graft. Manipulation of the donor limb with depleting agents prior to transplantation has not been explored and might offer the possibility of significantly modifying the immunogenicity of CTA. Since donor APC are very short lived, a significant contribution to effector T-cell priming and rejection must be through indirect presentation of donor alloantigens by recipient APC to recipient CD4+ T cells. Indeed, many recent investigations demonstrate that indirect presentation is the major pathway of alloantigen presentation, and it occurs extremely early after transplantation.

7.9 Dendritic Cells

The predominant roles of DCs as APCs in direct and indirect pathways and their ability to induce tolerance in the immature state have provided a rational basis for the manipulation of donor and recipient DCs.[79–84] DCs are rare, ubiquitously distributed, migratory leukocytes, derived from CD34+ stem cells. They convey Ag from peripheral sites, such as the skin, or other nonlymphoid tissues, to T cells in secondary lymphoid organs. DC present Ag peptides bound to MHC class II molecules to CD4+ (Th) cells. To generate cytotoxic T lymphocytes (CTL) with the capacity to reject allografts, DC must present Ag peptides complexed with MHC class I to CD8+ T cells. DCs must be mature for the initiation of acquired immune reactivity.

There are three major subsets of DCs – myeloid (M), lymphoid-related, and plasmacytoid DC, which include preplasmacytoid DC (pre-pDC). DC can be generated from CD34+ hematopoietic progenitors whereas monocytes differentiate into MDC in response to GM-CSF and IL-4. In humans, besides classic MDC, a second subset of "preplasmacytoid" DC is found in secondary lymphoid tissue. pDC represent a relatively high proportion of circulating DC in tolerant human organ transplant recipients compared with patients requiring maintenance immunosuppression.[85] It has been strongly suggested that they may play a critical role for therapy of organ transplantation and in tolerance induction.

Tolerance exhibited following intrathymic inoculation of alloAg appears to be dependent on thymic DC.[86] We showed that BM-derived host MDC pulsed with allopeptide and injected intrathymically, can induce organ (heart, intestine) or pancreatic islet transplant tolerance in pre-transplant antilymphocyte serum

(ALS)-conditioned hosts.[87,88] While Sayegh et al.[86] concluded that thymic recognition of immunodominant class II MHC allopeptides leads to peripheral T-cell unresponsiveness, we found that intrathymic injection of immunodominant donor MHC class I peptide or intravenous injection of host MDC primed in vitro with an immunodominant allopeptide also induced cardiac, islet, and even bone marrow allograft survival of > 200 days with full acceptance of second set allografts and rejection of third party allografts.[87–93] Our observations provided the first compelling evidence that the induction of tolerance through the indirect pathway enhanced allograft survival. Furthermore, we highlighted the importance of the indirect pathway of allorecognition in acquired thymic tolerance and that thymic or BM-derived host DCs pulsed with donor MHC class I allopeptide could be effective when delivered intravenously.[87] Although this regimen circumvented the limitations imposed by intrathymic administration, it required depletion of peripheral T cells by transient ALS.

The permanent and specific tolerance to several types of donor organs in the rat appeared to be dependant on CD4+CD25+ FoxP3+ Tregs that could be adoptively transferred to naïve hosts. The resultant tolerance was highly dependant on the relative quantity of the Tregs infused.[89,90] The capacity of DC to downregulate immune reactivity has been extensively reviewed previously.[78] Various agents, including UVB-radiation,[71] corticosteroids,[91] cyclosporine,[92] rapamycin (Rapa©),[93] mycophenolate mofetil,[94] vitamin D3,[95] or the CTLA-4-Ig[96] can confer tolerogenic properties on DC, either in vitro or in vivo. Several reviews have addressed the mechanisms by which DCs can exert their tolerogenic effect.[97–99] It appears that DCs promote the induction of Treg cells, a mechanism that could insure long-term, Ag-specific unresponsiveness.

The concept that interstitial "passenger leukocytes" are the most important immunogenic components of transplanted whole organs has prevailed for many years. Increases in graft survival when thyroid, pancreatic islet, skin, or kidney allografts were depleted of "passenger leukocytes," was consistent with the belief that, at least for certain organs or tissues, donor-derived leukocytes provided the main immunological stimulus for graft rejection.[100–102] Key evidence implicating DC was provided by the "parking" experiments of Lechler and Batchelor.[100] When nonlymphoid tissues of long-surviving, successful human organ allograft recipients were shown by Starzl et al.[103] to contain donor DCs (microchimerism), it was proposed that the ability of an organ to be tolerogenic was dependent on its passenger leukocytes, and not on its parenchymal cell component.[101]

Recently, Kuwana et al.[104] reported that immature pDCs, freshly isolated from human peripheral blood, induced Ag-specific anergy in CD4+ T-cell lines. This suggests that immature pDCs in blood anergize effector CD4+ T cells responsive to foreign- or self-Ags. It is possible that a combination of pDC with specific therapeutic agents can enhance and maintain their inhibitory effect on alloreactive T-cell responses and therefore may lead to tolerance. CTAs, with the bone marrow generously represented in the donor organ, may be an ideal organ to utilize the micro- or preferably mixed-macrochimeric mechanisms for its acceptance.

7.10 Microchimerism

Initially, donor bone marrow cells (DBMC) were used together with the transplanted organ based on the hypothesis that marrow cells would engraft in the recipient. The hope was that the DBMC would result in tolerance of the recipient toward donor HLA antigens, thus facilitating the acceptance of the organ. In clinical trials of liver, kidney, intestine, lung, heart, and pancreas transplantation DBMC did not modify patient or donor organ survival. The DBMC were not selected or modified prior to infusion into patients and only recently has this become a focus of interest, particularly in relation to selection of CD34 cells (stem cells). The CTA carries it own supply of DBMC and this may partially account for a relatively high success found in CTA transplantation in its initial trials plagued primarily by noncompliance, rather than a high rate of severe immunologic rejection. The question of microchimerism in CTA clinical transplantation has not yet been answered. It is not clear if unmanipulated or nonselected DBMC can lead to the induction of partial peripheral tolerance through a partial chimerism or microchimerism in the lymphoid organs, or through the development of T suppressor/regulatory cells in the recipient. Although no significant objective advantage has been yet found in the use of donor BM along with an allograft, this possibility cannot be readily excluded in CTA transplants where the donor BM is constantly available while the donor organ is in place.

7.11 Mixed Chimerism

The clinical application of donor BMT for induction of tolerance has largely been avoided until recently because of the formidable problems of graft-versus-host disease (GVHD) and by the toxicity of the host conditioning thought to be necessary to allow bone marrow (BM) to engraft. In an effort to avoid such problems the concept of mixed chimerism was developed by Ildstad and Sachs[105] and is addressed thoroughly in another chapter in this book. Mixed chimerism is the condition in which hematopoietic populations of both the recipient and the donor coexist in the recipient. Mixed chimerism can be achieved by milder treatments that do not ablate host hematopoietic cells.[106] In the case of CTA hematopoietic stem cells contained in the donor BM inoculum need to "home" to the BM compartment of the recipient and this is facilitated by treatment with anti-T cell mAbs or with costimulatory blockade[107,108] without treating the hosts with TBI or chemotherapy. High doses of DBMC, present in CTA, can also help to overcome other barriers to mixed chimerism as summarized by Fehr and Sykes.[5]

The mechanisms by which stable mixed chimerism results in tolerance to organ grafts have been studied extensively in laboratory animals.[105] This approach is currently being applied to clinical protocols in which the overall goal is to withdraw immunosuppressive drugs completely.[106–110] The main mechanism of donor-specific tolerance in mixed chimerism relies on central deletion by seeding of the thymus by donor hematopoietic progenitor cells giving rise to DCs which mediate clonal deletion in the thymus through the physiologic process of negative selection.[111] The result is a T-cell repertoire that is tolerant toward the donor and the host.

Tolerance to kidney allografts has been achieved with transient chimerism after HLA-matched bone marrow and kidney transplantation in five patients with multiple myeloma using a nonmyeloablative regimen.[109] Even with only transient chimerism in four of the five patients, they all retained their kidney grafts for several years after the complete withdrawal of immunosuppressive drugs.[109] Long-term graft acceptance has also been achieved in haplotype-matched patients without myeloma.[107,109,110] The mechanism of graft acceptance is unclear in the absence of stable chimerism in the clinical trials but appears to be at least partially related to a shift in the balance toward T regulatory cells in the periphery.

7.12 Conclusion

Taking account of the available experimental and clinical data that I have briefly summarized and that have been recently extensively discussed and presented at the World Transplant Congress (WCT) held in Boston in June 2006, and which are included in the Supplement to *American Journal of Transplantation*, 2006, pp. 1–1145, the progress along the road toward clinical tolerance induction is rapid and extensive. It incorporates developments of (1) new, highly targeted immunosuppressive agents, such as Belatacept© and anti-CD40 MoAb; (2) in vivo production of donor targeted Tregs that can be expanded in vitro, and reinfused into recipients prior to and after an allograft; (3) induction of mixed chimerism in allograft recipients without major myeloablative treatments; (4) trials of induction of microchimerism with donor bone marrow infusions to achieve unresponsiveness to an allograft ("operative" tolerance); and even (5) return to major deletional treatment during induction, using Compath 1H (anti-CD52) followed by gradual withdrawal, initially of Tacrolimus (2 months) and then of Rapamycin (at 1 year) prior to withdrawal of all immunosuppression. The reader interested in further details of the various issues raised in this chapter would do well to review the abstracts and papers recently presented which are both provocative and instructive.

Tolerance has been the goal of all transplant surgeons, clinicians, and immunobiologists ever since the first identical twin left Peter Bent Brigham Hospital with his brother, and did not require any immunosuppressive medications. Despite many experiments in rodents that predicted success, the induction of tolerance in nonhuman primates and in humans has been extraordinarily difficult to achieve in a predictable fashion. When it is achieved, it is at either no cost in morbidity because it is found unexpectedly in an occasional noncompliant patient who stops all his/her medications while continuing to maintain normal transplant organ function, or at a significant cost in initial potential morbidity when it is induced with either deletional or nonmyeloablative regimens. In either case it appears that the Holy Grail[112] has been seen, that the directions to it are known, and that it can be approached from various paths, but that it can be drunk from carefully for fear that it may fall and break. It is not yet ready for mass consumption, but it can be imported, perhaps best wrapped in a CTA.

References

1. R. D. Owen, Immunogenetic consequences of vascular anastomoses between bovine twins, *Science* **102**, 400–401 (1945).
2. R. E. Billingham, L. Brent, P. B. Medawar, "Actively acquired tolerance" of foreign cells, *Nature* **172**, 603–606 (1953).
3. A. D. Hess, A. C. Fischer, Immune mechanisms in cyclosporine-induced syngeneic graft versus host disease, *Transplantation* **48**, 895–900 (1989).
4. P. Blaha, et al., The influence of immunosuppressive drugs on tolerance induction through bone marrow transplantation with co stimulation blockade, *Blood* **101**, 2886–2893 (2003).
5. T. Fehr, M. Sykes, Tolerance induction in clinical transplantation, *Transpl Immunol* **13**, 117–130 (2004).
6. R. Lechler, J. Bluestone, Transplantation tolerance: putting the pieces together, *Cur Opin Immunol* **9**, 631–633 (1997).
7. A. D. Wells, X. C. Li, Y. Li, M. C. Walsh, X. X. Zheng, Z. Wu, G. Nunez, A. Tang, M. Sayegh, W. W., Hancock, T. B. Strom, L A. Turka. Requirement for T-cell apoptosis in the induction of peripheral transplantation tolerance, *Nat Med* **5**, 1303–1307 (1999).
8. K. Kishimoto, S. Sandner, J. Imitola, M. Sho, Y. Li, P. B. Langmuir, D. M. Rothstein, T. B. Strom, L. A. Turka, M. H. Sayegh, Th1 cytokines, programmed cell death, and alloreactive T cell clone size in transplant tolerance, *J Clin Invest* **109**, 1471–1479 (2002).
9. M. Sho, A. Yamada, N. Najafian, A. D. Salama, H. Harada, S. E. Sandner, A. Sanchez-Fueyo, X. X. Zheng, T. B. Strom, M. H. Sayegh, Physiological mechanisms of regulating alloimmunity: cytokines, CTLA-4, CD25+ cells, and the alloreactive T cell clone size, *J Immunol* **169**, 3744–3751 (2002).
10. N. E. Phillips, T. G. Markees, J. P. Mordes, D. L. Greiner, A. A. Rossini, Blockade of CD40-mediated signaling is sufficient for inducing islet but not skin transplantation tolerance, *J Immunol* **170**, 3015–3023 (2003).
11. M. A. Williams, J. Trambley, J. Ha, A. B. Adams, M. M. Durham, P. Rees, S. R. Cowan, T. C. Pearson, C. P. Larsen, Genetic characterization of strain differences in the ability to mediate CD40/CD28-independent rejection of skin allografts, *J Immunol* **165**, 6849–6857 (2000).
12. A. van Maurik, K. J. Wood, N. D. Jones, Impact of both donor and recipient strains on cardiac allograft survival after blockade of the CD40-CD154 costimulatory pathway, *Transplantation* **74**, 740–743 (2002).
13. E. Suri-Payer, A. Z. Amar, A. M. Thornton, E. M. Shevach, CD4+CD25+ T cells inhibit both the induction and effector function of autoreactive T cells and represent a unique lineage of immunoregulatory cells, *J Immunol* **160**, 1212–1218 (1998).
14. F. Powrie, R. Correa-Oliveira, S. Mauze, R. L. Coffman, Regulatory interactions between CD45RBhigh and CD45RBlow CD4+ T cells are important for the balance between protective and pathogenic cell-mediated immunity, *J Exp Med* **179**, 589–600 (1994).
15. M. Papiernik, M. L. de Moraes, C. Pontoux, F. Vasseur, C. Penit, Regulatory CD4 T cells: expression of IL-2R alpha chain, resistance to clonal deletion and IL-2 dependency, *Int Immunol*, **10**, 371–378 (1998).
16. K. M. Thorstenson, A. Khoruts, Generation of anergic and potentially immunoregulatory CD25+CD4 T cells in vivo after induction of peripheral tolerance with intravenous or oral antigen, *J Immunol* **167**, 188–195 (2001).
17. J. D. Fontenot, M. A. Gavin, A. Y. Rudensky, FoxpS programs the development and function of CD4+CD25+ regulatory T cells, *Nat Immunol* **4**, 330–336 (2003).

18. J. D. Fontenot, J. P. Rasmussen, L. M. Williams, J. L. Dooley, A. G. Farr, A. Y. Rudensky, Regulatory T cell lineage specification by the forkhead transcription factor foxpS, *Immunity* **22**, 329–341 (2005).
19. L. S. Walker, A. Chodos, M. Eggena, H. Dooms, A. K. Abbas, Antigen-dependent proliferation of CD4+CD25+ regulatory T cells in vivo, *J Exp Med* **198**, 249–258 (2003).
20. L. Klein, K. Khazaie, H. von Boehmer, In vivo dynamics of antigen-specific regulatory T cells not predicted from behavior in vitro, *Proc Natl Acad Sci USA* **100**, 8886–8891 (2003).
21. E. Nishimura, T. Sakihama, R. Setoguchi, K. Tanaka, S. Sakaguchi, Induction of antigenspecific immunologic tolerance by in vivo and in vitro antigen-specific expansion of naturally arising Foxp3+CD25+CD4+ regulatory T cells, *Int Immunol* **16**, 1189–1201 (2004).
22. H. Groux, A. O'Garra, M. Bigler, M. Rouleau, S. Antonenko, J. E. de Vries, M. G. Roncarolo, A CD4+ T-cell subset inhibits antigen-specific T-cell responses and prevents colitis, *Nature* **389**, 737–742 (1997).
23. F. J. Barrat, D. J. Cua, A. Boonstra, D. F. Richards, C. Grain, H. F. Savelkoul, R. de Waal-Malefyt, R. L. Coffman, C. M. Hawrylowicz, A. O'Garra, In vitro generation of interleukin 10-producing regulatory CD4(+) T cells is induced by immunosuppressive drugs and inhibited by T helper type 1 (Th1)- and Th2-inducing cytokines, *J Exp Med* **195**, 603–616 (2002).
24. P. L. Vieira, J. R. Christensen, S. Minaee, E. J. O'Neill, F. J. Barrat, A. Boonstra, T. Barthlott, B. Stockinger, D. C. Wraith, A. O'Garra, IL-10-secreting regulatory T cells do not express FoxpS but have comparable regulatory function to naturally occurring CD4+CD25+ regulatory T cells, *J Immunol* **172**, 5986–5993 (2004).
25. K. J. Wood, S. Sakaguchi, Regulatory T cells in transplantation tolerance, *Nat Rev Immunol* **3**, 199–210 (2003).
26. S. Sakaguchi, Naturally arising CD4+ regulatory T Cells for immunologic self-tolerance and negative control of immune responses, *Annu Rev Immunol* **22**, 531–562 (2004).
27. H. Waldmann, L. Graca, S. Cobbold, E. Adams, M. Tone, Y. Tone, Regulatory T cells and organ transplantation. *Semin Immunol* **16**, 119–126 (2004).
28. A. Proneth, B. G. Exner, J. H. Fechner, E. K. Geissler, F. Fandrich, S. J. Knechtle, Monocyte-dervided cells from monkeys induce regulatory cells in vitro: a potential new cell therapy approach for transplant tolerance, *Am J Transpl Transplant* (supplement WCT Congress Abstracts) **1621**, 608 (2006).
29. N. Suciu-Foca, J. S. Manavalan, R. Cortesini, Generation and function of antigen-specificsuppressor and regulatory T cells, *Transpl Immunol* **11**, 235 (2003).
30. Z. Liu, S. Tugulea, R. Cortesini, N. Suciu-Foca, Specific suppression of T helper alloreactivity by allo-MHC class I-restricted CD8+CD28- T cells, *Int Immunol* **10**, 775 (1998).
31. R. Ciubotariu, A. I. Colovai, G. Pennesi, Z. Liu, D. Smith, P. Berlocco, R. Cortesini, N. Suciu-Foca, Specific suppression of human CD4+ Th cell responses to pig MHC antigens by CD8+CD28- regulatory T cells, *J Immunol* **161**, 5193 (1998).
32. S. Jiang, S. Tugulea, G. Pennesi, Z. Liu, A. Mulder, S. Lederman, P. Harris, R. Cortesini, N. Suciu-Foca, Induction of MHC-class I restricted human suppressor T cells by peptide priming in vitro, *Hum Immunol* **59**, 690 (1998).
33. A. I. Colovai, Z. Liu, R. Ciubotariu, S. Lederman, R. Cortesini, N. Suciu-Foca, Induction of xenoreactive CD4+ T-cell anergy by suppressor CD8+CD28- T cells, *Transplantation* **69**, 1304 (2000).
34. Z. Liu, S. Tugulea, R. Cortesini, S. Lederman, N. Suciu-Foca, Inhibition of CD40 signaling pathway in antigen presenting cells by T suppressor cells, *Hum Immunol* **60**, 568 (1999).
35. J. Li, Z. Liu, S. Jiang, R. Cortesini, S. Lederman, N. Suciu-Foca, T suppressor lymphocytes inhibit NF-kappa B-mediated transcription of CD86 gene in APC, *J Immunol* **163**, 6386 (1999).
36. C. C. Chang, R. Ciubotariu, J. S. Manavalan, J. Yuan, A. I. Colovai, F. Piazza, S. Lederman, M. Colonna, R. Cortesini, R. Dalla-Favera, N. Suciu-Foca, Tolerization of dendritic cells by T(S) cells: the crucial role of inhibitory receptors ILT3 and ILT4, *Nat Immunol* **3**, 237 (2002).
37. N. Suciu-Foca Cortesini, F. Piazza, E. Ho, R. Ciubotariu, J. LeMaoult, R. Dalla-Favera, R. Cortesini, Distinct mRNA microarray profiles of tolerogenic dendritic cells, *Hum Immunol* **62**, 1065 (2001).

38. R. Cortesini, J. LeMaoult, R. Ciubotariu, N. S. Cortesini, CD8+CD28- T suppressor cells and the induction of antigen-specific, antigen-presenting cell-mediated suppression of Th reactivity, *Immunol Rev* **182**, 201 (2001).
39. A. I. Colovai, M. Mirza, G. Vlad, S. Wang, E. Ho, R. Cortesini, N. Suciu-Foca, Regulatory CD8+CD28- T cells in heart transplant recipients, *Hum Immunol* **64**, 31 (2003).
40. R. Ciubotariu, R. Vasilescu, E. Ho, P. Cinti, C. Cancedda, L. Poli, C. Late, Z. Liu, P. Berloco, R. Cortesini, N. Suciu-Foca Cortesini, Detection of T suppressor cells in patients with organ allografts, *Hum Immunol* **62**, 15 (2001).
41. R. Cortesini, E. Renna-Molajoni, P. Cinti, R. Pretagostini, E. Ho, P. Rossi, N. Suciu-Foca Cortesini, Tailoring of immunosuppression in renal and liver allograft recipients displaying donor specific T suppressor cells, *Hum Immunol* **63**, 1010 (2002).
42. J. S. Manavalan, P. C. Rossi, G. Vlad, F. Piazza, A. Yarilina, R. Cortesini, D. Mancini, N. Suciu-Foca, High expression of ILT3 and ILT4 is a general feature of tolerogenic dendritic cells, *Transpl Immunol* **11**, 245 (2003).
43. J. S. Manavalan, S. Kim-Schulze, L. Scotto, A. J. Naiyer, G. Vlad, P. C. Colombo, C. Marboe, D. Mancini, R. Cortesini, N. Suciu-Foca, Alloantigen specific CD8+CD28- FOXP3+ T suppressor cells induce ILT3+ILT4+ tolerogenic endothelial cells, inhibiting alloreactivity, *Int Immunol* **16**, 1055 (2004).
44. M. K. Jenkins, The ups and downs of T cell costimulation, *Immunity* **1**, 443–446 (1994).
45. R. J. Greenwald, G. J. Freeman, A. M. Sharpe, The B7 family revisited, *Ann Rev Immunol* **23**, 515–548 (2005).
46. S. A. Quezada, L. Z. Jarvinen, E. F. Lind, R. J. Noelle, CD40/CD154 interactions at the interface of tolerance and immunity, *Ann Rev Immunol* **22**, 307–328 (2004).
47. T. C. Pearson, D. Z. Alexander, M. Corbascio, R. Hendrix, S. C. Ritchie, P. S. Linsley, D. Faherty, C. P. Larsen, Analysis of the B7 costimulatory pathway in allograft rejection, *Transplantation* **63**, 1463–1469 (1997).
48. T. C. Pearson, D. Z. Alexander, K. J. Winn, P. S. Linsley, R. P. Lowry, C. P. Larsen, Transplantation tolerance induced by CTLA4-Ig, *Transplantation* **57**, 1701–1706 (1994).
49. M. H. Sayegh, E. Akalin, W. W. Hancock, M. E. Russell, C. B. Carpenter, P. S. Linsley, L. A. Turka, CD28-B7 blockade after alloantigenic challenge in vivo inhibits Th1 cytokines but spares Th2, *J Exp Med* **181**, 1869–1874 (1995).
50. D. Lenschow, Y. Zeng, J. Thistlethwaite, A. Montag, W. Brady, M. Gibson, P. Linsley, J. Bluestone, Long-term survival of xenogeneic pancreatic islet grafts induced by CTLA4Ig, *Science* **257**, 789–792 (1992).
51. A. D. Kirk, D. M. Harlan, N. N. Armstrong, T. A. Davis, Y. Dong, G. S. Gray, X. Hong, D. Thomas, J. H. Fechner, S. J. Knechtle, CTLA4-Ig and anti-CD40L prevent renal allograft rejection in primates, *Proc Natl Acad Sci USA* **94**, 8789–8794 (1997).
52. M. G. Levisetti, P. A. Padrid, G. L. Szot, N. Mittal, S. M. Meehan, C. L. Wardrip, G. S. Gray, D. S. Bruce, J. R. Thistlethwaite, Jr., J. A. Bluestone, Immunosuppressive effects of human CTLA4Ig in a non-human primate model of allogeneic pancreatic islet transplantation, *J Immunol* **159**, 5187–5191 (1997).
53. C. P. Larsen, T. C. Pearson, A. B. Adams, P. Tso, N. Shirasugi, E. Strobertm, D. Anderson, S. Cowan, K. Price, J. Naemura, J. Emswiler, J. Greene, L. A. Turk, J. Bajorath, R. Townsend, D. Hagerty, P. S. Linsley, R. J. Peach, Rational development of LEA29Y (Belatacept©), a high-affinity variant of CTLA4-Ig with potent immunosuppressive properties, *Am J Transplant* **5**, 443–453 (2005).
54. F. Vincenti, C. Larsen, A. Durrbach, T. Wekerle, B. Nashan, G. Blanche, P. Lang, J. Grinyo, P. P. Halloran, K. Solez, D. Hagerty, E. Levy, W. Zhou, K. Natarajan, B. Charpentier, Costimulation blockade with belatacept in renal transplantation, *N Engl J Med* **353**, 770–781 (2005).
55. T. Wekerle, J. Kurtz, S. Bigenzahn, Y. Takeuchi, M. Sykes, Mechanisms of transplant tolerance induction using costimulatory blockade, *Curr Opin Immunol* **14**, 592 (2002).
56. M. R. Clarkson, M. H. Sayegh, T-cell costimulatory pathways in allograft rejection and tolerance, *Transplantation* **80**, 555 (2002).

57. K. Honey, S. P. Cobbold, H. Waldmann, CD40 ligand blockade induces CD4+ T cell tolerance and linked suppression, *J Immunol* **163**, 4805 (1999).
58. L. Graca, K. Honey, E. Adams, S. P. Cobbold, H. Waldmann, Cutting edge: anti-GDI 54 therapeutic antibodies induce infectious transplantation tolerance, *J Immunol* **165**, 4783 (2000).
59. S. A. Quezada, K. Bennett, B. R. Blazar, A. Y. Rudensky, S. Sakaguchi, R. J. Noelle, Analysis of the underlying cellular mechanisms of anti-GDI 54-induced graft tolerance: the interplay of clonal anergy and immune regulation, *J Immunol* **175**, 771 (2005).
60. P. I. Sidiropoulos, D. T. Boumpas, Lessons learned from anti-CD40L treatment in systemic lupus erythematosus patients, *Lupus* **13**, 391 (2004).
61. K. G. Haanstra, E. A. Sick, J. Ringers, J. A. Wubben, E. M. Kuhn, L. Boon, M. Jonker, Costimulation blockade followed by a 12-week period of cyclosporine A facilitates prolonged drug-free survival of rhesus monkey kidney allografts, *Transplantation* **79**, 1623 (2005).
62. A. B. Adams, N. Shirasugi, T. R. Jones, M. M. Durham, E. A. Strobert, S. Cowan, P. Rees, R. Hendrix, K. Price, N. S. Kenyon, D. Hagerty, R. Townsend, D. Hollenbaugh, T. C. Pearson, C. P. Larsen, Development of a chimeric anti-CD40 monoclonal antibody that synergizes with LEA29Y to prolong islet allograft survival, *J Immunol* **174**, 542 (2005).
63. C. P. Larsen, et al., CD40-gp39 interactions play a critical role during allograft rejection. Suppression of allograft rejection by blockade of the CD40-gp39 pathway, *Transplantation* **61**, 4–9 (1996).
64. C. P. Larsen, et al., Long-term acceptance of skin and cardiac allografts after blocking CD40 and CD28 pathways, *Nature* **381**, 434–438 (1996).
65. Y. Li, X. X. Zheng, X. C. Li, M. S. Zand, T. B. Strom, Combined costimulation blockade plus rapamycin but not cyclosporine produces permanent engraftment, *Transplantation* **66**, 1387–1388 (1998).
66. C. B. Anderson, et al., Beneficial effects of donor-specific transfusions on long-term renal allograft function, *Transplant Proc* **27**, 991–994 (1995).
67. M. L. Wood, R. Gottschalk, A. P. Monaco, Comparison of immune responsiveness in mice after single or multiple donor-specific transfusions, *J Immunol* **132**, 651–655 (1984).
68. S. F. Oluwole, C. Iga, H. Lau, M. A. Hardy, Prolongation of rat heart allografts by donor-specific blood transfusion treated with ultraviolet irradiation, *Heart Transplantation* **4**, 385–389 (1985).
69. S. F. Oluwole, J. Chabot, P. Pepino, K. Reemtsma, M. A. Hardy, Mechanisms of immunologic unresponsiveness induced by UV-irradiated donor-specific blood transfusions and peritransplant cyclosporine, *Transplantation* **46**, 352–358 (1988).
70. S. F. Oluwole, K. Reemtsma, M. A. Hardy, Characteristics and function of suppressor T-lymphocytes in immunologically unresponsive rats following pretreatment with UV-B-irradiated donor leukocytes and peritransplant Cyclosporine, *Transplantation* **47**, 1001–1007 (1989).
71. M. A. Hardy, S. F. Oluwole, Effect of ultraviolet radiation on immunogenicity of tissues and organ allografts, *Transplant Rev* **5**, 46–62 (1991).
72. D. C. Parker, et al., Survival of mouse pancreatic islet allografts in recipients treated with allogeneic small lymphocytes and antibody to CD40 ligand, *Proc Natl Acad Sci USA* **92**, 9560–9564 (1995).
73. H. A. DePaz, O. O. Oluwole, A. O. Adeveri, P. Witkowski, M. X. Jin, M. A. Hardy, S. F. Oluwole, Immature rat myeloid dendritic cells generated in low dose granulocyte macrophage–colony stimulating factor prolong donor-specific rat cardiac allograft survival, *Transplantation* **75**, 521–528 (2003).
74. O. O. Oluwole, H. A. DePaz, A. Adeyeri, M. X. Jin, M. A. Hardy, S. F. Oluwole, Role of CD4+CD25+ regulatory T cells from naïve host thymus in the induction of acquired transplant tolerance by immunization with allo-major histocompatibility complex peptide, *Transplantation* **75**, 1136–1142 (2003).
75. A. Mondino, A. Khoruts, M. K. Jenkins, The anatomy of T-cell activation and tolerance, *Proc Natl Acad Sci USA* **93**, 2245–2252 (1996).
76. C. P. O'Larsen, P. J. Morris, J. M. Austyn, Migration of dendritic leukocytes from cardiac allografts into host spleens, *J. Exp. Med.* **171**, 307–314 (1990).
77. Z. Wang, A. Castellaneta, A. D. Creus, W. J. Shufesky, A. E. Morelli, A. W. Thomson, Heart, but not skin allografts from donors lacking Flt3 ligand exhibit markedly prolonged survival time, *J Immunol* **172**, 5924–5930 (2004).

78. M. Baratin, K. Bonin, C. Daniel, Frontline: peripheral priming of alloreactive T cells by the direct pathway of allorecognition, *Eur J Immunol* **34**, 3305–3314 (2004).
79. R. M. Steinman, D. Hawiger, M. C. Nussenzweig, Tolerogenic dendritic cells, *Annu Rev Immunol* **21**, 685–711 (2003).
80. M. V. Dhodapkar, R. M. Steinman, J. Krasovsky, C. Munz, N. Bhardwaj, Antigenspecific inhibition of effector T cell function in humans after injection of immature dendritic cells, *J Exp Med* **193**, 233–238 (2001).
81. Z. X. Lian, T. Okada, X. S. He, H. Kita, Y. J. Liu, A. A. Ansari, K. Kikuchi, S. Ikehara, M. E. Gershwin, Heterogeneity of dendritic cells in the mouse liver: identification and characterization of four distinct populations, *J Immunol* **170**, 2323–2330 (2003).
82. Y. J. Liu, H. Kanzler, V. Soumelis, M. Gilliet, Dendritic cell lineage, plasticity and cross-regulation, *Nat Immunol* **2**, 585–589 (2001).
83. L. Lu, A. W. Thomson, Dendritic cell tolerogenicity and prospects for dendritic cell-based therapy of allograft rejection and autoimmune disease. In *Dendritic Cells*, Second Edition. M. T. Lotze, A. W. Thomson, editors. Academic Press, San Diego, pp. 587–607 (2001).
84. R. I. Lechler, W. F. Ng, R. M. Steinman, Dendritic cells in transplantation – friend or foe, *Immunity* **14**, 357–368 (2001).
85. A. W. Thomson, L. Lu, Dendritic cells as regulators of immune reactivity: implications for transplantation, *Transplantation* **68**, 1–8 (1999).
86. M. H. Sayegh, N. Perico, L. Gallon, O. Imberti, W. W. Hancock, G. Remuzzi, C. B. Carpenter, Mechanisms of acquired thymic unresponsiveness to renal allografts. Thymic recognition of immunodominant allo-MHC peptides induces peripheral T cell anergy, *Transplantation* **58**, 125–132 (1994).
87. M. Garrovillo, A. Ali, H. A. Depaz, R. Gopinathan, O. O. Oluwole, M. A. Hardy, S. F. Oluwole, Induction of transplant tolerance with immunodominant allopeptide-pulsed host lymphoid and myeloid dendritic cells, *Am J Transplant* **1**, 129–137 (2001).
88. M. Garrovillo, A. Ali, S. F. Oluwole, M. A. Hardy, Indirect allorecognition in acquired thymic tolerance: induction of donor-specific tolerance to rat cardiac allografts by allopeptide-pulsed host dendritic cells, *Transplantation* **68**, 1827–1834 (1999).
89. A. Ali, M. Garrovillo, M. X. Jin, M. A. Hardy, S. F. Oluwole, Major histocompatibility complex class I peptide-pulsed host dendritic cells induce antigen-specific acquired thymic tolerance to islet cells, *Transplantation* **69**, 221–226 (2000).
90. S. F. Oluwole, O. O. Oluwole, H. A. DePaz, A. O. Adeyeri, P. Witkowski, M. A. Hardy, CD4+CD25+ regulatory T cells mediate acquired transplant tolerance, *Transpl Immunol* **11**, 287–293 (2003).
91. P. Kalinski, C. M. Hilkens, E. A. Wierenga, M. L. Kapsenberg, T-cell priming by type-1 and type-2 polarized dendritic cells: the concept of a third signal, *Immunol Today* **20**, 561–567 (1999).
92. J. I. Lee, R. W. Ganster, D. A. Geller, G. J. Burckart, A. W. Thomson, L. Lu, Cyclosporine A inhibits the expression of costimulatory molecules on in vitro-generated dendritic cells: association with reduced nuclear translocation of nuclear factor kappa B, *Transplantation* **68**, 1255–1263 (1999).
93. T. Hackstein, T. Taner, A. F. Zahorchak, A. E. Morelli, A. J. Logar, A. Gessner, A. W. Thomson, Rapamycin inhibits IL-4-induced dendritic cell maturation in vitro and dendritic cell mobilization and function in vivo, *Blood* **101**, 4457–4463 (2003).
94. A. Mehling, S. Grabbe, M. Voskort, T. Schwarz, T. A. Luger, S. Beissert, Mycophenolate mofetil impairs the maturation and function of murine dendritic cells, *J Immunol* **165**, 2374–2381 (2000).
95. G. Penna, L. Adorini, 1 Alpha,25-dihydroxyvitamin D3 inhibits differentiation, maturation, activation, and survival of dendritic cells leading to impaired alloreactive T cell activation, *J Immunol* **164**, 2405–2411 (2000).
96. A. W. Thomson, L. Lu, Are dendritic cells the key to liver transplant tolerance? *Immunol Today* **20**, 27–32 (1999).
97. J. Banchereau, F. Briere, C. Caux, J. Davoust, S. Lebecque, Y. J. Liu, B. Pulendran, K. Palucka, Immunobiology of dendritic cells, *Ann Rev Immunol* **18**, 767–811 (2000).

98. P. T. Coates, A. W. Thomson, Dendritic cells, tolerance induction and transplant outcome, *Am J Transplant* **2**, 299–307 (2002).
99. R. J. Steptoe, A. W. Thomson, Dendritic cells and tolerance induction, *Clin Exp Immunol* **105**, 397–402 (1996).
100. R. I. Lechler, J. R. Batchelor, Restoration of immunogenicity to passenger cell-depleted kidney allografts by the addition of donor strain dendritic cells, *J Exp Med* **155**, 31–41 (1992).
101. D. Talmage, G. Dart, J. Radovich, K. Lafferty, Activation of transplant immunity: effect of donor leucocytes on thyroid allograft rejection, *Science* **191**, 385–388 (1976).
102. M. Rouabhia, L. Germain, F. Belanger, F. A. Auger, Cultured epithelium allografts: Langerhans cell and Thy-1+ dendritic epidermal cell depletion effects on allograft rejection, *Transplantation* **56**, 259–264 (1993).
103. T. E. Starzl, A. J. Demetris, N. Murase, S. Ildstad, C. Ricordi, M. Trucco, Cell migration, chimerism, and graft acceptance, *Lancet* **339**, 1579–1582 (1992).
104. M. J. Kuwana, J. Kaburaki, T. M. Wright, Y. Kawakami, Y. Ikeda, Induction of antigen-specific human CD4(+) T cell anergy by peripheral blood DC2 precursors, *Eur J Immunol* **31**, 2547–2557 (2001).
105. S. T. Ildstad, D. H. Sachs, Reconstitution with syngeneic plus allogeneic or xenogeneic bone marrow leads to specific acceptance of allografts or xenografts, *Nature* **307**, 168–170 (1984).
106. M. Sykes, D. H. Sachs, Mixed chimerism, *Philos Trans R Soc Lond B Biol Sci* **356**, 707–726 (2001).
107. E. H. Field, S. Strober, Tolerance, mixed chimerism and protection against GVHD after TLI, *Philos Trans R Soc Lond Biol Sci* **356**, 1–10 (2001).
108. S. Strober, R. J. Lowsky, J. A. Shizuru, J. D. Scandling, M. T. Millan, Approaches to transplantation tolerance in humans, *Transplantation* **77**, 932–936 (2004).
109. L. H. Buhler, T. R. Spitzer, M. Sykes, D. H. Sachs, F. L. Delmonico, N. Tolkoff-Rubin, S. L. Saidman, R. Sackstein, S. McAfee, B. Dey, C. Colby, A. B. Cosimi, Induction of kidney allograft tolerance after transient lymphohematopoietic chimerism in patients with multiple myeloma and end-stage renal disease, *Transplantation* **74**, 1405–1409 (2002).
110. A. B. Cosimi, D. H. Sachs, Mixed chimerism and transplantation tolerance, *Transplantation* **77**, 943–946 (2004).
111. J. W. Kappler, N. Roehm, P. Marrack, T cell tolerance by clonal elimination in the thymus, *Cell* **49**, 273–276 (1987).
112. P. Nickerson, W. Streurer, J. Steiger, T. B. Strom, In pursuit of the "Holy Grail": Allograft tolerance, *Kidney Intl* **45**, 840–49 (1994).

Chapter 8
Donor-Specific Tolerance

Au H. Bui, Gerald Lipshutz, and Jerzy Kupiec-Weglinski

8.1 Introduction

The widespread use of immunosuppressive drugs within the last several decades has without doubt contributed to the effectiveness and overall success of solid organ transplantation. In 1965, the first immune suppressive drugs consisted of treatment with azathioprine and corticosteroids.[1] Since then, more efficacious drugs (e.g., calcineurin inhibitors, mycophenolate mofetil, rapamycin, monoclonal antibodies against CD3, and CD25) have emerged such that the problems associated with acute rejection have been mainly overcome. Chronic rejection though still remains a serious problem and limitation to organ transplantation. In fact, only 50% of kidney transplants that survive the first 12 months are still functioning 7.5–9.5 years later.[2] Long-term immune suppression has not provided the benefits observed in short-term graft survival.

The clinical efficacy of solid organ transplantation has allowed the field of composite tissue allotransplantation (CTA) to become a clinical reality. The technical and ethical issues of CTA were overcome and introduced into the modern era with the first successfully described hand transplant performed in Lyon, France.[3] Since then, teams from Louisville, KY[4] and Guangzhou, China[5] have also reported successful hand allograft transplants. Using a combination of tacrolimus, mycophenalate, and corticosteroids effective immunosuppression was achieved with adequate clinical outcomes in at least 18 individuals (6 double-hand transplants and 12 single hand transplants). The immunologic challenges of solid organ transplantation parallel that of CTA. Most notably, the skin is a highly immunogenic organ that often requires higher immunosuppressive regimen to achieve adequate clinical efficacy. As such, acute rejection appears to be a more significant problem with the current immunosuppressive medications in CTA than solid organ transplantation.

The practice of immunosuppressive administration can currently be divided into three phases: induction, maintenance, and rescue therapies.[6] Induction immunotherapy is used as a means to overcome the ischemic injury and surgical trauma an allograft undergoes during the transplant process. The injury thus sustained by transplanted allografts creates an immunogenic organ that is more susceptible to immunologic attacks. The purpose of induction therapy therefore is to sufficiently suppress recipient immune responses. Maintenance therapy is defined as immune suppression that is typically much lower in dose than induction therapy and therefore applicable in a chronic setting. Rescue therapy is similar to induction therapy in that it employs high-dose immune suppression and is usually instigated in response to a rejection episode.

The use of chronic medications is not without significant health risks. Most notably, drug toxicity and their multiple side effects, an increased susceptibility to opportunistic infection, and the high occurrence of spontaneous neoplasms are all risks associated with long-term immune suppression.[7] Additionally, use of many drugs such as calcineurin-inhibitors is associated with direct nephrotoxicity often leading to chronic allograft or native kidney dysfunction. In the hand transplants thus far described, the primary complication observed was infection. Complications commonly observed in solid organ transplantation such as malignancies, cardiovascular-related disease, nephrotoxicity, gastrointestinal adverse effects, and diabetes have not yet been reported.[8] As such, one of the key tenets in the future success of solid organ and composite tissue transplantation is the development of immunologic tolerance. Research has thus focused on two guiding principles; the first to develop immunologic strategies that will improve organ tolerance while reducing the use of immunosuppressive drugs, and secondly to prevent chronic rejection and late allograft dysfunction. This has lead to an active field of research by which alternative immune tolerance specific to donor antigen is achieved with a reduction in standard immune suppression.

A number of tolerant induction protocols have been successfully employed in various animal models. In this chapter, we attempt to address the critical issues and factors that are currently relevant in donor-specific tolerance. In particular, the emphasis will be work performed in animal systems as they have proven invaluable as tools to explore the immunological mechanisms by which to achieve donor-specific tolerance. Animal systems are not without their drawbacks, and it is important to be aware of the significant limitations of using animal models as we strive to understand the immune response triggered by organ transplantation. Kidney transplantation in rhesus monkeys demonstrated long-term graft survival with anti-CD154 antibody for 6-month treatment.[9] Careful examination of the allografts though demonstrated mononuclear cell infiltration and nephropathy in kidney grafts thus providing a false impression of graft tolerance. True induction tolerance therefore must include in its definition an absence of donor-specific alloantibodies and no evidence of destructive lymphocyte infiltration in allografts.

8.2 Physiologic Mechanisms of Induction Therapy

8.2.1 T Cells

T cells have emerged as a major role in the regulation of transplant tolerance. One important issue is the high donor-specific T-cell precursor frequency often seen in many pretransplant patients. Due to the exponential nature of the immune response, even modest increases in the T-cell precursor frequency can have profound alterations in the early immunologic environment.[10] Though precursor frequency may vary greatly among patients due to secondary factors such as prior immune history and MHC mismatch, the T-cell activation threshold requirements may also be considerably different. In general, primed T cells have less stringent activation requirements than naïve T cells. Thus, the transplantation response creates an immunogenic organ susceptible to attack from the recipient immune system.[11] More specifically, endothelial damage injury, ischemic reperfusion damage, and surgical trauma are all factors that contribute to the immunogenicity of the transplanted organ. To counteract these opposing forces, higher induction pharmacologic doses are required to suppress recipient immune responses.

There are two known pathways in which T cells recognize donor antigens present in transplanted tissue. In the first, known simply as the direct pathway, the responding T cells recognize intact allogeneic MHC molecules on the surface of donor-derived antigen presenting cells (APCs). This is believed to be the pathway responsible for rejection during the early period following transplantation.[12] The indirect pathway involves recipient APCs which process donor-derived allo-MHC molecules into peptides and subsequently present these peptides to T cells on self-MHC molecules.[13] Donor-derived APCs are short lived which suggests that the indirect pathway is the dominant pathway through which chronic alloresponse progresses.

Additionally, experimental transplant tolerance methods have been divided into two categories: central and peripheral tolerance. Central tolerance generally refers to the use of bone marrow transplantation to create a mixed chimerism within the recipient.[14] This creates a coexistence of recipient and donor lymphoid and myeloid cell lines within the host. As a result of this process, developing T cells that are donor reactive will be subsequently deleted before they can exit the thymus, in the same manner as self-reactive T cells.[15] Peripheral tolerance refers to the use of antibodies or pharmacologic agents that block or modulate T-cell activation or growth factor receptor pathways in mature T cells.[16] This usually has the effect of inducing apoptosis among the T cells that are responding to donor alloantigens. The degree of resistance to tolerance is dependent upon several factors, most importantly the allograft employed, the allogenic disparity between donor and recipient, and other genetic factors not yet fully defined.

8.3 Generation of T Regulatory Cells

The induction and maintenance of graft tolerance is a complex process that requires multiple coordinated systems to work cooperatively to prevent allograft rejection. The immune system consists of a series of systems that may regulate its effector functions. One component that has gained prominence due to its ability to suppress effector functions and its role in maintaining immune tolerance is the T regulatory cell (Treg). The role of T regulatory cells (Tregs) has expanded in recent years with identification of a population of cells containing different cell-surface phenotypes and, to some extent, with different mechanisms of action.[17] One of the initial limitations of recognizing this population of T cells was the lack of a consistent identifying marker. Prior to the identification of CD25 as a marker for Tregs, the existence of such a T-cell population was often questioned. It was not until Sakaguchi et al. described a naturally occurring subset of CD4+ T cells that arose during T-cell development in the thymus and was defined by constitutive expression of the α chain of the IL-2 receptor, CD25, that the existence of such a population gained prominence.[18] The molecular marker CD25 was initially thought to be found only on activated T cells, but their discovery on a subset of CD4+ T cells that had regulatory functions now allowed researchers a means to identify this T-cell subset.[19]

One of the inherent characteristics of naturally occurring Tregs is the ability to suppress other cells. In naïve animals, this subset of CD4 T cells has the ability to control autoreactive T cells in vivo. These cells were found not only to be hyporesponsive to antigenic stimulation but demonstrated the ability to suppress reactive T cells via a contact–contact mechanism. Moreover, it was soon discovered that animals deficient in Tregs developed severe autoimmune disease. These observations allowed researchers to conclude that Tregs play a crucial role in preventing various forms of autoimmune disease and that they function to regulate key elements in maintaining self-tolerance.

There appears to be two distinct Treg populations involved in immune control. The first is a naturally occurring subset that originates during T-cell development in the thymus and defined by constitutive express of the α chain of the IL-2 receptor. A second population believed to play an important role is derived from a T-cell population that proliferates following a pathogen response. These Tregs suppress the immune response following antigen stimulation in order to prevent secondary autoimmunity. Current research is directed towards these peripheral Tregs as they are believed to play an important role in transplant tolerance. The Treg population is not limited to the CD4+ compartment as investigators have learned that CD8+ and NK cells may have differing roles in transplant tolerance. CD8+ Tregs, TCR+CD4–CD8– T cells, and NK Tregs have all been reported to play a role in different transplantation tolerance models.[20]

The identification of Treg markers other than CD25 and their different mechanisms of action has established that multiple Tregs may exist.[17] CD45RB, CTLA-4, glucocorticoid-induced TNF receptor family–related receptor (GITR or TNFRSF18), CD122, CD103 (αEβ7 integrin), CD134 (OX40), and CD62L (L-selectin) are all markers whose relative expression levels have been used to define and isolate CD4+CD25+ Tregs.[21] One of the limitations soon discovered was that none of these markers alone are definitive to the naturally occurring Treg population. Instead, they are found on many T-cell populations, most notably activated T cells. Recently, the helical transcription FoxP3 was found to be uniquely expressed by naturally occurring CD4+CD25 Treg cells and act as a regulatory mechanism for Treg differentiation. Unfortunately, even though markers exist for identifying FoxP3, the intracellular location of the transcription factor limits the viability of the cell following staining.[22]

There are currently two inducible Treg populations believed to play an important role in transplant tolerance: Th3 and Tr1 cells. Th3 cells were first identified due to their influence primarily through TGF-β secretion produced through ingestion of oral antigens, a term also known as oral tolerance.[23] Tr1 cells were first characterized in studies involving the regulation of autoimmune colitis. Though functionally similar to Th3 cells, they are characterized by the ability to secrete large amounts of the cytokine IL-10.[24] There are certain characteristics that differentiate the naturally occurring T cells and the ones induced in the periphery. Recent evidence suggests that peripheral T cells are able to acquire this immunosuppressive characteristic through peripheral interactions while naturally occurring Tregs develop in the thymus. There appears to be no evidence to suggest that peripheral Tregs require thymic stimulus for differentiation. Secondly, in vitro studies have demonstrated that CD4+CD25 Tregs suppress T-cell effectors via cell–cell interactions. While it thus appears that naturally occurring Tregs influence cells via a cell contact dependent mechanism and cytokine-independent mechanism, Tr1 and Tr3 regulatory cells suppress cellular activity through secretion of particular cytokines (e.g., TGFβ and IL-10) that influence the immune response.[25]

The induction of a regulatory T-cell population in an otherwise alloreactive T-cell population following allotransplantation has been proposed as one of the key factors in creation of a tolerant environment in multiple animal systems.[26] One tolerant strategy reports differentiation of a Treg population by repeated exposure of naïve allogeneic dendritic cells (DCs).[27] In fact, the maturation and phenotypic characteristics of allograft DCs appear to play a critical role in T-cell characterization. Immature and naïve DCs have poor costimulatory and cytokine profiles that can produce a poor T-cell alloreactive response and in some cases a suppressive regulatory T-cell population.

The success in the development of Treg populations in animal models has not translated into clinical success. One of the current obstacles postulated to be a deterrent is the large number of alloreactive T cells initially present that prevent the induction of tolerance by Treg populations. By thus reducing the high numbers of graft destructive T cells, this would facilitate the suppressive characteristics of the Treg population to develop a tolerant state. Costimulatory blockade has emerged as a tolerant strategy that may generate and spare the necessary regulatory T-cell population while reducing the numbers of alloreactive T cells. With this idea in mind, Strom et al. demonstrated that selective deletion of nonregulatory CD25+ alloreactive T cells and persistence of Treg cells could be achieved through administration of an agonistic IL-2–Fc receptor fusion protein. In fact, administration of this fusion protein in combination with selective blockade of IL-15 signaling, which is important for effector T-cell proliferation and memory generation, resulted in graft acceptance in a stringent transplantation model.[28] Thus a paradigm has emerged that supports the idea that a balance between deletion and regulation plays a critical role in the development of transplantation tolerance.

8.4 T-Cell Costimulatory Blockade

T cells require two distinct signals for activation. The first signal involves binding the T-cell receptor (TCR/CD3) to the appropriate MHC peptide bound class molecule found on an APC.[29] The second signal is an antigen-independent signal that serves to augment the T response following TCR binding. The binding of a nonspecific surface costimulatory molecule found on T cells and APCs acts to provide the necessary second signal for T-cell activation. Indeed, TCR binding without costimulatory engagement results in T-cell anergy and/or apoptosis.[30] In addition, costimulation molecule expression levels were found to be increased in response to ischemic reperfusion injury that contributed to T-cell activation.[31]

One of the first costimulatory molecule identified was the CD28 receptor found on T cells. CD28 is constitutively expressed by CD4 cells while CD8 expression is dependent on the its activated state. The binding of the CD28 molecule to either of its respective ligands, B7-1 or B7-2 expressed on APCs results in the delivery of a "positive" costimulatory signal to the T cell. The resulting antigen-specific T-cell expansion is characterized by IL-2 production, expression of characteristic cell surface markers (CD44, CD62L), and a memory/effector phenotype.[32] CD28 blockade can be achieved by monoclonal antibodies directed against B7-1 and B7-2 by the recombinant fusion protein CTLA4Ig.[33] The efficacy of this molecule is based upon the observation that CTLA4 has a significantly higher binding affinity to the B7 molecules than CD28. Binding to the B7 molecules thus acts as a competitive agonist to CD28. Various experiences have been described in which interruption of CD28 signaling creates a tolerogenic effect in animal transplantation models.[34]

The "negative" costimulatory molecules CTLA4, programmed cell death 1 (PD-1), and its respective ligands PDL-1 and PDL-2 have recently generated great interest. PD-1, a member of the CD28 family, was originally isolated using subtractive hybridization in a thymic T-cell line undergoing apoptosis.[35] The role of PD-1 as a negative costimulator was first observed in PD-1 knockout mice. These knockout mice developed spontaneous autoimmune diseases such as lupus-like glomerulonephritis and arthritis with deposition of IgG3 and C3 in the glomeruli.[36] Unlike CTLA4, which is found exclusively on T cells, PD-1 is also expressed on B and myeloid cells, suggesting possibly a greater role in immune regulation than that seen with CTLA4. PDL-1 is constitutively expressed in many different immunologic cell types including T cells, B cells, macrophages, and DCs.[37] The PDL-1 has also been found in a variety of nonlymphoid cell types including endothelial cells in the heart, glial cells in the inflamed brain, and β cells of the pancreas. PDL-2 expression is more limited, largely confined to activated macrophages and DCs. PD-1 may play a role in inhibiting the immune response as recent evidence demonstrates that during chronic viral infections, PD-1 expression is abnormally high in exhausted T cells.[37]

The role of costimulatory molecules expanded considerably with the discovery of a class of costimulatory molecules that may act a "negative" signal following T-cells binding. The emergence of this second class of costimulatory molecule creates an intriguing model by which T-cell regulation is possibly modulated by the differential expression of both "positive" versus "negative" signaling molecules. The engagement of both TCR and costimulatory molecules following antigenic stimulation may thus reflect a summation of both positive and negative signals which direct the T cell toward activation or anergy T-cell activation.

Clinical agents designed to target costimulatory work mechanistically by reducing the efficiency of antigen presentation and increasing the threshold for activation of naïve T lymphocytes. The focus of experimental work continues to be concentrated in tolerance induction with the elimination of maintenance therapy. The clinical focus, however, has been on the pairing of costimulatory blockade with minimization of maintenance medications particularly calcineurin sparing approaches. Recently, work using humanized monoclonal Abs directed towards CD154, hu5c8, and IDEC-131 in nonhuman primates demonstrated promise by preventing acute rejection for years without additional immunosuppression.[38] Unfortunately, the favorable effects observed in the animal studies have not translated to successful clinical effects in humans. Early trials were aborted due to inadequate efficacy and a predilection toward thromboembolism.[39] Some progress in the clinical development of medications targeting costimulatory molecules has made progress with the advent of two agents specific for the B7 molecules. The first consists of humanized antibodies specific for CD80 and CD86, and the other is a high-affinity B7-specific fusion protein combining an engineered version of CD152 with the constant region of human IgG1, Belatacept. Both have shown to be beneficial in studies with nonhuman primates in calcineurin and steroid sparing maintenance immunosuppression.[40,41] Promising results were seen with belatacept in the treatment of patients receiving kidney transplants.[42]

8.5 Donor-Specific Transfusion

Numerous studies have demonstrated that pretransplantation infusion of allogeneic donor cells, especially when there is no major histocompatibility complex antigens mismatch, has the potential to induce tolerance to a specific allograft.[43–47] Prior to the introduction of cyclosporine to transplantation and during the azathioprine–prednisone era, patients were routinely given preoperative blood transfusions.[48–52] Data comparing transfused and nontransfused kidney transplant recipients demonstrated that patients who received blood transfusions had significantly longer graft survival.[53–56] Several studies showed that those patients who received random third-party blood transfusion prior to transplantation had dramatically improved 1-year graft survival rates. Opelz et al. demonstrated that patients who received greater than 10 units of blood before undergoing transplantation had 66% graft survival whereas those who did not receive a transfusion had 29% graft survival. Another study demonstrated that DST provided long-term graft survival in recipients with greater than 20 transfusions (71.5% at 1-year and 65.5% at 4 years) as compared to those who received no transfusion (42.2 and 30.3%, respectively).[57] This was further expanded to include the pediatric population. In one study, 37 pediatric living-related renal transplants demonstrated a 6-year 93% graft survival.[58] Until the 1980s, the concept of pretransplant blood transfusion was well accepted as beneficial and resulted in improved allograft survival.

The molecular mechanism responsible for donor-specific transfusion (DST) immune suppression is poorly characterized. Postulated immunomodulatory mechanisms include clonal deletion,[59] induction of anergy (Takeuchi T), generation of regulatory cells (Vignes), (Quigley) regulation of cytokine production (Yang), (Takeuchi), (Liang) promotion of microchimerism (Liang), and provision of soluble MHC antigens (Masroor).[60] It is generally believed that the priming with donor antigens ultimately blocks the recipient immune response. This occurs when a graft that shares MHC antigens with the blood transfusion is performed. The degree of HLA sharing between donor blood and recipient is crucial in the modulation of the recipient immune system. Sharing of one HLA-DR antigen is associated with induction of tolerance, whereas HLA-DR mismatched transfusions lead to rejection. Possible explanation for this may be due to the increased donor-specific IFN-γ production with no detectable IL-10 in mismatched blood transfusions, whereas matched transfusion decreased IFN-γ production and increased IL-10 production.

After the introduction of cyclosporine, the beneficial effects of DST became controversial and were often not detectable.[61,62] One of the reasons DST has fallen out of favor is that the fear of sensitization is of paramount concern.[63,64] In a highly mismatched histocompatible mouse cardiac graft model, pretreatment of donor recipients with DST without immunosuppression resulted in hyperacute graft rejection. However, concomitant use of cyclophosphamide immunosuppression and DST resulted in prolongation of cardiac graft survival. Human protocols with three DSTs without simultaneous azathioprine resulted in the development of antibodies against donor HLA antigens, which unfortunately prevented subsequent kidney transplantation in almost one-third of donor-recipient pairs.[65,66] While azathioprine reduced sensitization to 8–14% if administered at the time of transfusion,[67,68] cyclosporine further decreased sensitization to 4%.[69] Improvements in pharmacologic immune suppression demonstrated that transfusions did not improve cadaveric renal survival in patients receiving optimal cyclosporine therapy and that equally good living-related donor graft survival could be achieved with DST and conventional immunosuppression or no DST and cyclosporine.[70] Furthermore, the fear of sensitization or transmission of hepatitis and HIV has further contributed to the disappearance of DST strategies.

8.6 Gene Therapy for Tolerance Induction

Gene therapy offers the promise of novel interventions for a variety of both inherited and acquired conditions. In organ transplantation, gene therapy is being investigated in the prevention of acute and chronic rejection through down-regulation of adhesion molecules involved in rejection, production of noninflammatory cytokines, and in inducing donor-specific unresponsiveness in the recipient. The ultimate goal is to induce transplantation tolerance to alloantigens while allowing normal responses to viruses, bacteria, and malignant cells.[71] The induction of donor-specific tolerance has been sought by mechanisms involving the normal tolerance induction pathways including both central and peripheral routes.[72] This would allow for the removal of pharmacological immunosuppression and its unintended side effects (e.g., risk of malignancy, coronary vascular disease, infections) in transplant recipients. However, their use is not without risks. All viruses induce an immunological response and have inherent risks such as insertional mutagenesis and toxicity. Viral genetic capacity is also limited and large scale production may often prove difficult.

8.6.1 Gene Therapy Vectors

Gene therapy agents are generally classified into (1) viral vectors and (2) nonviral methods of DNA transfer. Viral vectors include oncoretroviruses, lentiviruses, adenoviruses, and adeno-associated viruses (AAVs). Retroviruses are a class of enveloped single-stranded RNA viruses. Following infection, the viral genome is reverse transcribed into double-stranded DNA which integrates into the host genome. The viral genome is approximately 10kb and it contains at least three genes: gag (core proteins), polymerase (reverse transcriptase), and env (envelope protein). At the terminal end of the genome are long terminal repeats (LTRs) which include promoter/enhancer sequences involved in integration. A packaging sequence (psi) is also present. The tropism of viruses differ and replacing the env gene with that of the vesicular stomatitis virus G protein has extended the host range in a technique known as pseudotyping. This has generally been used with the Maloney murine leukemia virus (Mo-MLV)-derived vectors. A requirement for retroviral integration and expression is that the target cells must be proliferating and this limits gene therapy to dividing cells in vivo or in vitro. Though transgene expression is usually adequate in vitro and initially in vivo, prolonged expression in vivo can be difficult to maintain as retroviruses are inactivated by c1 complement protein present in human sera.

Lentiviruses are a subclass of retroviruses which are able to infect both proliferating and nonproliferating cells. Human immunodeficiency virus is an example. They are considerably more complicated than simple retroviruses, containing an additional six proteins: tat, rev, vpr, vpu, nef, and vif. Current packaging cell lines have separate plasmids for a pseudotype envelope gene, a transgene construct, and a packaging plasmid supplying the structural and regulatory genes in trans. This leads to improved safety with less risk of the development of infectious virus. Studies demonstrate prolonged in vivo expression in muscle, liver, and nervous tissue without the requirement for cellular proliferation.

Adenoviruses are a class of viruses with double-stranded DNA genomes that cause respiratory, intestinal, and eye infections in humans. They are nonenveloped viruses containing a linear double-stranded DNA genome. Serotypes 2 or 5 are predominantly used as vectors. The life cycle does not normally involve integration into the host genome; they remain as episomal elements in the nucleus of the host cell and provide no risk of insertional mutagenesis. Adenoviral vectors are efficient at transducing target cells proliferating or not, and can be generated at high titers ($>10^{11}$ plaque forming units/mL). Transgene expression in vivo tends to be short-lived with 90% of the administered vector degraded in the liver by a nonimmune-mediated mechanism following intravenous injection. Following this, cytotoxic T-cells activation results in the elimination of virus-infected cells while humoral responses develop with antiadenoviral antibody and antitransgene antibody.

Persisting antibody prevents subsequent administration of the vector thereby limiting its use in gene therapy.

AAVs are nonpathogenic human parvoviruses. They are dependent on a helper virus to proliferate and are capable of infecting both dividing and nondividing cells. The wild-type genome is a single-stranded DNA molecule, consisting of two genes: rep (coding for replication proteins) and cap (coding for capsid structural proteins). At either end of the genome is a 145 bp inverted terminal repeat. In the absence of rep genes in the recombinant vector used for gene therapy, the AAV vector will only integrate at random, as a single provirus or head-to-tail concatamer resulting in prolonged transgene expression (years in some cases).

Nonviral methods of DNA transfer require only a small number of proteins, have a virtually infinite capacity, and have no infectious or mutagenic capability. Nonviral methods include liposomes, naked DNA, and molecular conjugates. The simplest method is the direct introduction of DNA into target cells. This approach is limited in its application because it can be used only with certain tissues and requires large amounts of DNA. Though not very efficient, this can result in prolonged low-level expression in vivo. It has been used in vivo with intravascular pressure in small animal models resulting in hepatic gene expression.

Another nonviral approach involves the creation of an artificial lipid sphere. DNA spontaneously associates to the external surface of cationic liposomes by virtue of its positive charge. These complexes can then interact with the cell membranes allowing DNA to pass through the target cell's membrane resulting in cellular transfection. In vitro up to 90% of certain cell lines may be transfected by this method. Molecular conjugates consist of protein or synthetic ligands to which a DNA binding agent has been attached.

Four areas to consider for gene therapy in tolerance induction in organ transplantation are (1) chemokine antagonists, (2) major histocompatibility complex molecules, (3) immunosuppressive cytokines, and (4) blockage of costimulatory signals. Examples have demonstrated some success in donor-specific unresponsiveness.

8.6.2 Chemokine Antagonists

Allografts express immunomodulatory proteins and these are critical in allograft rejection in the recruitment of host inflammatory cells. Cells enter transplant allografts within hours by binding to adhesion molecules on the endothelial cells. Inflammatory cells then infiltrate the allograft and result in cellular injury and the release of inflammatory cytokines.[73]

Reports have demonstrated the importance of chemokine receptors CCR1 and CCR5 and their ligands (RANTES, MIP-1α, and MIP-1β) in promoting heart allograft rejection. Alteration of these pathways utilizing inhibitors or performing studies in knock-out mice has been shown to prolong organ survival.[74–76] RANTES 9–68 is a truncated form of the native human RANTES molecule; the first eight amino acids of the amino-terminal end have been deleted. RANTES 9–68 can compete with the wild-type RANTES chemokine for both receptor binding and occupancy.[77] Lentiviral gene transfer of RANTES 9–68 has been performed in a rat cardiac transplantation model by ex vivo gene transfer. Graft survival was prolonged with reduced cellular infiltration and intragraft expression of IFN-γ, RANTES, TGF-β, and TNF-α.[78]

8.6.3 MHC Molecules

Multiple groups have demonstrated the induction of long-term tolerance following gene transfer of MHC class I or class II molecules.[79–82] These were generally performed to create matching MHC between donor organs and recipients in transplantation in murine models.

Autologous bone marrow hematopoietic stem cells have been transduced with retroviruses carrying donor-type MHC antigens. Modified cells are used to reconstitute conditioned hosts resulting in molecular chimerism.[83] In murine studies, prolonged disparate skin graft survival occurred after reconstitution of lethally irradiated mice with autologous bone marrow cells transduced with retroviral vectors carrying the allogeneic MHC class I gene of the skin graft. In some studies, where retrovirally expressed MHC was low on the surface of bone marrow-derived cells, the mechanism responsible for this does not appear to be the induction of central tolerance as cytotoxic T-cell precursors capable of lysing the skin graft were detectable. Lack of immune unresponsiveness could be lost after providing sufficient T-cell help. This suggests that a peripheral mechanism was involved[83,84] in this state.

However, in other studies where more vigorous expression of MHC class I on the surface of transduced bone marrow was performed, survival of congenic skin grafts (for MHC class I antigen K^b) was long term (>100 days). Such murine experiments suggest that efficient expression of retrovirally transduced alloantigens on BM-derived cells is sufficient to induce specific immunologic tolerance.[82] This approach or the introduction of donor MHC into recipient thymus with a conditioning regimen is a plausible therapy that continues to be investigated to obtain donor-specific tolerance induction.

8.6.4 Immunosuppressive Cytokines

Interleukin-10 (IL-10) is a potent immunomodulatory cytokine that interacts with APCs. It inhibits production of cytokines such as IL-1, -6, -8, and tumor necrosis factor-α.[85,86] Gene transfer and gene therapy leading to IL-10 expression in allogeneic transplants may therefore be a promising therapy to impair effective antigen presentation, reduce graft immunogenicity, and inhibit inflammation.

Lipid-mediated gene transfer of viral IL-10 resulted in prolonged survival of cardiac allografts in a mouse model of heterotopic heart transplantation.[87] Grafts demonstrated fewer donor-specific cytotoxic T lymphocytes (CTLs) compared with control allografts. In addition, activated splenic CTLs were rare in the IL-10 treated group. Allografts also demonstrated fewer infiltrating helper T cells. Donor-specific IgM alloantibody was not detected in animals with prolonged cardiac allograft survival. Allografts did demonstrate a histology characterized by a moderate mononuclear infiltrate composed of unactivated cells. However, cardiac allograft survival was not indefinite; this was likely due to the transient expression of IL-10 by lipid-mediated transfection. Other investigations in pancreatic islets did not show the same results; however, cellular IL-1o was utilized which enhancing immunostimulatory activities and induces T-cell differentiation; these are not properties of viral IL-10.[88]

8.6.5 Blockage of Costimulatory Signals

Another approach is to use gene therapy vectors encoding immunomodulatory molecules to develop a state of immune unresponsiveness. In a high-responding liver transplant model, this approach has been applied.[89,90] Adenoviral vectors encoding CTLA4Ig, blocking the costimulatory pathway of CD80/86-CD28 resulted in liver allograft acceptance for more than 300 days. Similarly an adenoviral vector blocking the CD40-CD154 costimulatory pathway (CD40Ig) had similar results of long-term liver allograft survival.

Simultaneous blockage of both pathways with recombinant adenoviral vectors has led to long-term acceptance of full MHC-mismatched cardiac grafts in a rat model.[91] However, tolerance was not induced in this cardiac model. Secondary skin grafts derived from both donor and third-party strains were ultimately rejected in recipients that had accepted the cardiac allograft. Certainly the mechanism of allograft rejection is not identical among different organs, cells, and tissues. It is possible that in some conditions of tolerance that secondary skin grafts can be rejected while other vascularized organs may survive.[92] Costimulatory blockade remains an active area of investigation in both animal models and humans.

	Plasmid	Oncoretrovirus	Lentivirus	Foamy	Herpes	Adenovirus	AAV
Genetic material	DNA	RNA	RNA	RNA	DNA	DNA	DNA
Genetic material packaging capacity	No limitation	9 kb	10 kb	12 kb	> 30 kb	30 kb	4.7 kb
Duration of expression	Transient	Long	Long	Long	Transient	Transient	Long in post-mitotic tissues
Genome integration	Yes	Yes	Yes	No	No	Rarely	Rarely
Transduction of postmitotic cells	No	Low	Low	High	High	Moderate	Moderate

Modified from [93]. *kb* kilobase; *AAV* adeno-associated virus

8.7 Conclusion

Although considerable progress has been made in the understanding of immunologic tolerance, there are a number of active issues that remain to be solved. Animal models have proven invaluable in our understanding of donor-specific tolerance but the many successes observed in these experimental models has not yet translated to clinical efficacy. Development of clinical tolerance in humans and nonhuman primates has proven more difficult than observed in rodent models. There are several possible reasons for this, one of which may be due to heterologous immunity.[94] This refers to the exposure of viral and bacterial infections that triggers a cross-reactive immune response to the transplanted allograft. This was made due to the observation that rodent models are generally bred in clean, pathogen-free environments that do not mimic the infectious environment humans, and nonhuman primates are regularly exposed. Thus a strategy involving T-cell depletion may be a more appropriate clinical approach than producing regulatory cells as further infections may overcome the regulatory response.

On the basis of existing rodent and nonhuman primate evidence, new protocols must be established that will limit the degree of toxicity of newer treatments while reducing the administration of broad immunosuppressive medications. The broad immunosuppressive medications employed in solid organ transplantation have nonetheless helped shape the success of CTA. One caveat to realize is the clinical experience thus far observed in CTA may well be different from that of solid organ transplantation. As the complications from CTA are revealed and collected, the immunologic therapy may need to be tailored to suit the appropriate organ transplanted. This may require several concomitant approaches to produce a true tolerant state. Nevertheless, selective immunosuppressive therapy will reduce the complications associated with broad immunosuppression and is the future to continued success in organ transplantation.

References

1. R. Y. Calne, B. A. Hurn, Combined immunosuppressive action of phytohaemagglutinin and azathioprine (Imuran) on dogs with renal homotransplants, *Br Med J* **5454**, 154–155 (1965).
2. J. Cecka, *Clinical Transplants*, UCLA Tissue Typing Laboratory, pp. 1–14 (1996).
3. J. M. Dubernard, G. Herzberg, et al., Human hand allograft: report on first 6 months, *Lancet* **353**, 1315 (1999).
4. J. W. Jones, J. H. Barker, W. C. Breidenbach, Successful hand transplantation. One-year follow-up. Louisville Hand Transplant Team, *N Engl J Med* **343**, 468 (2000).
5. C. G. Francois, C. Maldonado, et al., Hand transplantation: comparisons and observations of the first four clinical cases, *Microsurgery* **20**, 360 (2000).
6. A. Kirk, Induction Immunosuppression, *Transplantation* **82**, 593–602 (2006).
7. M. Pascual, T. Kawai, N. Tolkoff-Rubin, A. B. Cosimi, Strategies to improve long-term outcomes after renal transplantation, *N Engl J Med* **346**(8), 580–590 (2002).
8. M. Lanzetta, R. Margreiter, et al., The international registry on hand and composite tissue transplantation, *Transplantation* **79**, 1210 (2005).

9. A. D. Kirk, D. S. Batty, R. E. Baumgartner, J. D. Berning, K. Buchanan, Treatment with humanized monoclonal antibody against CD154 prevents acute renal allograft rejection in nonhuman primates, *Nat Med* **5**(6), 686–693 (1999).
10. R. Germain, The art of the probable: system control in the adaptive immune system, *Science* **293**, 240 (2001).
11. P. Matzinger, The danger model: a renewed sense of self, *Science* **296**, 301 (2002).
12. M. H. Sayegh, C. B. Carpenter, Mechanisms of T cell recognition of alloantigen: the role of peptides, *Transplantation* **57**, 1295–1302 (1994).
13. R. I. Ciubotariu, J. R. Batchelor, et al., Persistent allopeptide reactivity and epitope spreading in chronic rejection of organ allografts, *J Clin Invest* **101**, 398–405 (1998).
14. Nikolic B, Skyes M. Mixed hematopoietic chimerism and transplantation tolerance, *Immunol Res* **16**(3), 217–228 (1997).
15. J. O. Manilay, K. G. Swenson, M. Sykes, Intrathymic deletion of alloreative T cells in mixed bone marrow chimeras prepared with a nonmyeloablative conditioning regiment, *Transplantation* **66**(1), 96–102 (1998).
16. X. C. Li, T. B. Strom, L. A. Turka, A. D. Wells, T cell death and transplantation tolerance, *Immunity* **14**, 407–416 (2001).
17. H. Jonuleit, E. Schmitt, The regulatory T cell family: distinct subsets and their interrelations, *J Immunol* **171**, 6323–6327 (2003).
18. S. Sakaguchi, M. Asano, et al., Immunologic self-tolerance maintained by activated T cells expressing IL-2 receptor alpha-chains (CD 25). Breakdown of a single meechanism of self tolerance causes varius autoimmune diseases, *J. Immunol* **155**, 1151–1164 (1995).
19. C. Baecher-Allan, G. Freeman, et al., CD4+Cd25+ high regulatory cells in human peripheral blood, *J Immunol* **167**, 1245 (2001).
20. M. Gilliet, Generation of human Cd8 T regulatory cells by CD40 ligand-activated plasmacytoide dendritic cells, *J Exp Med* **195**, 695–704 (2002).
21. K. J. Wood, Regulatory T cells in transplantation tolerance, *Nat Rev Immunol* **3**, 199–210 (2003).
22. S. Hori, S. Sakaguchi, Control of regulatory T cell development by the transcription factor Foxp3, *Science* **299**, 1057–1061 (2003).
23. Y. Chen, V. K. Kuchroo, J. Inobe, et al., Regulatory T cell clones induced by oral tolerance: suppression of autoimmune encephalomyelitis, *Science* **265**, 1237–1240 (1994).
24. H. Groux, et al., A CD4+ T cell subset inhibits antigen specific T cell responses and prevents colitis, *Nature* **389**, 737–742 (1997).
25. M. Stassen, E. Schmitt, H. Jonuleit, Human CD(4+)CD(25+) regulatory T cells and infectious tolerance, *Transplantation* **77** (1 Suppl), S23–S25 (2004).
26. H. Waldmann, S. Cobbold, Regulating the immune response to transplants: a role for CD4+ regulatory cells? *Immunity* **14**, 399–406 (2001).
27. H. Jonuleit, E. Schmitt, G. Schuler, J. Knop, A. H. Enk, Induction of interleukin 10-producing, nonproliferating CD4(+) T cells with regulatory properties by repetitive stimulation with allogeneic immature human dendritic cells, *J Exp Med* **192**, 1213–1222 (1992).
28. X. X. Zheng, et al., Favorably tipping the balance between cytopathic and regulatory T cells to create transplantation tolerance, *Immunity* **19**, 503–514 (2003).
29. D. M. Rothstein, et al., T cell costimulatory pathways in allograft rejection and tolerance, *Immunol Rev* **196**, 85 (2003).
30. R. Schwartz, A cell culture model for T lymphocyte clonal anergy, *Science* **248**(4961), 1349 (1990).
31. M. Takada, K. C. Nadeau, et al., The role of the B7 costimulatory pathway in experimental cold ischemia/reperfusion injury, *J Clin Invest* **100**, 1199 (1997).
32. M. K. Jenkins, S. D. Norton, K. B. Urdahl, CD28 delivers a costimulatory signal involved in antigen specific IL-2 production by human T cells, *J Immunol* **147**(8), 2461 (1991).
33. P. S. Linsley, J. Johnson, et al., Immunosuppression in vivo by a soluble form of the CTLA-4 T cell activation molecule, *Science* **257**, 789–792 (1992).
34. R. I. Lechler, L. A. Turka, The complementary roles of deletion and regulation in transplantation tolerance, *Nat Rev Immunol* **3**(2), 147–158 (2003).

35. Y. Ishida, K. Shibahara, T. Honjo, Induced expression of PD-1, a novel member of the immunoglobulin gene superfamily, upon programmed cell death, *EMBO J* **11**, 3887–3895 (1992).
36. H. Nishimura II, et al., Development of lupus-like autoimmune diseases by disruption of the PD-1 gene encoding an ITIM motif-carrying immunoreceptor, *Immunity* **11**, 141–151 (1992).
37. G. J. Freeman, R. Ahmed, A. H. Sharpe, Reinvigorating exhausted HIV-specific T cells via PD-1PD-1 ligand blockade, *J Exp Med* **203**(10), 2223–2227 (2006).
38. A. D. Kirk, N. N. Armstrong, et al., CTLA4Ig and anti-CD40 ligand prevent renal allograft rejection in primates, *Proc Natl Acad Sci USA* **94**, 8789 (1997).
39. A. D. Kirk, H. Sollinger, et al., Preliminary results of the use of humanized anti-CD154 in human renal allotransplantation, *Am J Transplant* **1**, S191 (2001).
40. A. D. Kirk, A. Celniker, et al., Induction therapy with monoclonal antibodies specific for CD80 and CD86 delays the onset of acute renal allograft rejection in non-human primates, *Transplantation* **72**, 377 (2001).
41. C. P. Larsen, A. B. Adams, et al., Rational development of LEA29Y (belatacept), a high affinity variant of CTLA4-Ig with potent immunosuppressive properties, *Am J Transplant* **5**, 443 (2005).
42. F. Vincenti, A. Durrbach, et al., Costimulation Blockade with belatacept in renal transplantation, *N Engl J Med* **353**, 770–781 (2005).
43. Y. Sharabi, D.H. Sachs, Mixed chimerism and permanent specific transplantation tolerance induced by a nonlethal preparative regimen, *J Exp Med* **169**(2), 493–502 (1989).
44. E. L. Lagaaij, et al., Effect of one-HLA-DR-antigen-matched and completely HLA-DR-mismatched blood transfusions on survival of heart and kidney allografts, *N Engl J Med* **321**(11), 701–705 (1989).
45. D. Middleton, et al., Transfusion of one HLA-DR antigen-matched blood to potential recipients of a renal allograft, *Transplantation* **58**(7), 845–848 (1994).
46. W. Wong, P. J. Morris, K. J. Wood, Syngeneic bone marrow expressing a single donor class I MHC molecule permits acceptance of a fully allogeneic cardiac allograft. *Transplantation* **62**(10), 1462–1468 (1996).
47. A. de Vries-van der Zwan, et al., Specific tolerance induction and transplantation: a single-day protocol, *Blood* **89**(7), 2596–2601 (1997).
48. O. Salvatierra Jr., et al., Pretreatment with donor-specific blood transfusions in related recipients with high MLC, *Transplant Proc* **13**(1 Pt 1), 142–149 (1981).
49. G. Opelz, B. Graver, P. I. Terasaki, Induction of high kidney graft survival rate by multiple transfusion, *Lancet* **1**(8232), 1223–1225 (1981).
50. C. B. Carpenter, Deliberate transfusion of potential renal transplant recipients with specific donor blood, *Am J Kidney Dis* **1**(2), 116–118 (1981).
51. T. Leivestad, et al., Effect of pretransplant donor-specific transfusions in renal transplantation, *Transplant Proc* **14**(2), 370–373 (1982).
52. C. B. Anderson, G. A. Sicard, E. E. Etheredge, Pretreatment of renal allograft recipients with azathioprine and donor-specific blood products, *Surgery* **92**(2), 315–321 (1982).
53. G. Opelz, et al., Effect of blood transfusions on subsequent kidney transplants, *Transplant Proc* **5**(1), 253–259 (1973).
54. N. Akiyama, et al., Effects of donor-specific blood transfusion on the survival of living related renal grafts, *Jpn J Exp Med* **54**(5), 225–227 (1984).
55. W. J. Burlingham, et al., Improved renal allograft survival following donor-specific transfusions. I. Induction of antibodies that inhibit primary antidonor MLC response, *Transplantation* **39**(1), 12–17 (1985).
56. W. W. Pfaff, et al., Planned random donor blood transfusion in preparation for transplantation. Sensitization and graft survival, *Transplantation* **38**(6), 701–703 (1984).
57. G. Opelz, P. I. Terasaki, Improvement of kidney-graft survival with increased numbers of blood transfusions, *N Engl J Med* **299**(15), 799–803 (1978).
58. D. Potter, et al., Effect of donor-specific transfusions on renal transplantation in children, *Pediatrics* **76**(3), 402–405 (1985).

59. L. Yang, et al., Mechanisms of long-term donor-specific allograft survival induced by pretransplant infusion of lymphocytes, *Blood* **91**(1), 324–330 (1998).
60. D. C. Brennan, T. Mohanakumar, M. W. Flye, Donor-specific transfusion and donor bone marrow infusion in renal transplantation tolerance: a review of efficacy and mechanisms, *Am J Kidney Dis* **26**(5), 701–715 (1995).
61. W. H. Barber, Donor-specific transfusions in renal transplantation, *Clin Transplant* **8**(2 Pt 2), 204–206 (1994).
62. M. Otsuka, et al., Long-term graft survival of living-related kidneys after donor-specific transfusion, *Transplant Proc* **32**(7), 1741–1742 (2000).
63. E. van Twuyver, et al., Pretransplantation blood transfusion revisited, *N Engl J Med* **325**(17), 1210–1213 (1991).
64. E. van Twuyver, et al., High-affinity cytotoxic T lymphocytes after non-HLA-sharing blood transfusion-the other side of the coin, *Transplantation* **57**(8), 1246–1251 (1994).
65. O. Salvatierra Jr., et al., Deliberate donor-specific blood transfusions prior to living related renal transplantation. A new approach, *Ann Surg* **192**(4), 543–552 (1980).
66. B. W. Colombe, et al., Two patterns of sensitization demonstrated by recipients of donor-specific transfusion. Limitations to control by Imuran, *Transplantation* **44**(4), 509–515 (1987).
67. C. B. Anderson, et al., Pretreatment of renal allograft recipients with immunosuppression and donor-specific blood, *Transplantation* **38**(6), 664–668 (1984).
68. R. M. Radvany, K.M. Patel, Donor-specific transfusions. Donor-recipient HLA compatibility, recipient HLA haplotype, and antibody production, *Transfusion* **28**(2), 137–141 (1988).
69. J. S. Cheigh, et al., Minimal sensitization and excellent renal allograft outcome following donor-specific blood transfusion with a short course of cyclosporine, *Transplantation* **51**(2), 378–381 (1991).
70. D. E. Potter, et al., Are blood transfusions beneficial in the cyclosporine era? *Pediatr Nephrol* **5**(1), 168–172 (1991).
71. K. J. Wood, J. Fry, Gene therapy: potential applications in clinical transplantation. *Expert Rev Mol Med* **1999**, 1–20 (1999).
72. D. J. Moore, J. F. Markmann, S. Deng, Avenues for immunomodulation and graft protection by gene therapy in transplantation, *Transpl Int* **19**(6), 435–445 (2006).
73. W. W. Hancock, Chemokine receptor-dependent alloresponses, *Immunol Rev* **196**, 37–50 (2003).
74. R. Horuk, et al., A non-peptide functional antagonist of the CCR1 chemokine receptor is effective in rat heart transplant rejection, *J Biol Chem* **276**(6), 4199–4204 (2001).
75. W. Gao, et al., Targeting of the chemokine receptor CCR1 suppresses development of acute and chronic cardiac allograft rejection, *J Clin Invest* **105**(1), 35–44 (2000).
76. W. Gao, et al., Beneficial effects of targeting CCR5 in allograft recipients, *Transplantation* **72**(7), 1199–1205 (2001).
77. J. H. Gong, et al., RANTES and MCP-3 antagonists bind multiple chemokine receptors, *J Biol Chem* **271**(18), 10521–10527 (1996).
78. G. Vassalli, et al., Lentiviral gene transfer of the chemokine antagonist RANTES 9–68 prolongs heart graft survival, *Transplantation* **81**(2), 240–246 (2006).
79. D. Forman, C. Tian, J. Iacomini, Induction of donor-specific tolerance in sublethally irradiated recipients by gene therapy, *Mol Ther* **12**(2), 353–359 (2005).
80. N. Emmanouilidis, C. P. Larsen, Induction of chimerism and tolerance using freshly purified or cultured hematopoietic stem cells in nonmyeloablated mice, *Methods Mol Med* **109**, 459–468 (2005).
81. H. Hayashi, et al., Role of the thymus in donor specific hyporesponsiveness induced by retroviral transduction of bone marrow using an MHC class I gene, *Transplant Proc* **29**(1–2), 1133 (1997).
82. J. Bagley, et al., Induction of T-cell tolerance to an MHC class I alloantigen by gene therapy, *Blood* **99**(12), 4394–4399 (2002).
83. J. Bagley, J. Iacomini, Gene therapy progress and prospects: gene therapy in organ transplantation, *Gene Ther* **10**(8), 605–611 (2003).
84. R. S. Mayfield, et al., The mechanism of specific prolongation of class I-mismatched skin grafts induced by retroviral gene therapy, *Eur J Immunol* **27**(5), 1177–1181 (1997).

85. R. de Waal Malefyt, et al., Interleukin 10(IL-10) inhibits cytokine synthesis by human monocytes: an autoregulatory role of IL-10 produced by monocytes, *J Exp Med* **174**(5), 1209–1220 (1991).
86. P. Ralph, et al., IL-10, T lymphocyte inhibitor of human blood cell production of IL-1 and tumor necrosis factor, *J Immunol* **148**(3), 808–814 (1992).
87. L. A. DeBruyne, et al., Lipid-mediated gene transfer of viral IL-10 prolongs vascularized cardiac allograft survival by inhibiting donor-specific cellular and humoral immune responses, *Gene Ther* **5**(8), 1079–1087 (1998).
88. M. S. Lee, et al., Pancreatic islet production of murine interleukin-10 does not inhibit immune-mediated tissue destruction, *J Clin Invest* **93**(3), 1332–1338 (1994).
89. N. Yanagida, et al., Tolerance induction by a single donor pretreatment with the adenovirus vector encoding CTLA4Ig gene in rat orthotopic liver transplantation, *Transplant Proc* **33**(1–2), 573–574 (2001).
90. M. Nomura, et al., Induction of donor-specific tolerance by adenovirus-mediated CD40Ig gene therapy in rat liver transplantation, *Transplantation* **73**(9), 1403–1410 (2002).
91. K. Yamashita, et al., Long-term acceptance of rat cardiac allografts on the basis of adenovirus mediated CD40Ig plus CTLA4Ig gene therapies, *Transplantation* **76**(7), 1089–1096 (2003).
92. L. J. West, K. Tao, Acceptance of third-party cardiac but not skin allografts induced by neonatal exposure to semi-allogeneic lymphohematopoietic cells, *Am J Transplant* **2**(8), 733–744 (2002).
93. A. C. Nathwani, A.M. Davidoff, D.C. Linch, A review of gene therapy for haematological disorders, *Br J Haematol* **128**(1), 3–17 (2005).
94. A. B. Adams, C. P. Larsen, Heterologous immunity: an overlooked barrier to tolerance, *Immunol Rev* **196**, 147–160 (2003).

Chapter 9
Immune Tolerance Induction: Basic Concepts for Composite Tissue Allotransplantation

Patricio Andrades, Clement Asiedu, and Judith M. Thomas

9.1 The Clinical Problem and Possible Solution

Despite remarkable progress in contemporary transplantation there are still major unresolved problems in the field.[1] First, although immunosuppressive drugs have dramatically improved the life of transplant recipients over the past 30 years, they are associated with significant toxicities. This includes both the toxicities of immunosuppression itself (enhanced risk of opportunistic infections and selected malignancies), and side effects unrelated to immunosuppression (nephrotoxicity of calcineurin inhibitors, hypertension and cardiovascular disease from corticosteroids, etc.). Second, these agents have proven very successful in the prevention and treatment of acute rejection, but similar success has not been achieved in preventing chronic rejection and extending graft survival for decades. Even though various promising new agents are currently being developed and investigated, the undeniable conclusion is that chronic immunosuppressive drug therapy in its present status is not a satisfactory solution to the unremitting problem of host alloaggressiveness. This is a major obstacle to widespread application of composite tissue transplantation that can potentially be eliminated by induction of transplantation tolerance.

Half a century ago, the concept of transplantation tolerance emerged from a set of elegantly simple experiments. Medawar, seeking to understand skin graft rejection, observed that rabbits reject foreign skin grafts more quickly if the animals were retransplanted with a graft from the same donor.[2] At the same time, Owen noted that nonidentical cattle that share a common placenta fail to reject skin grafts from littermates but not from other cattle.[3] These findings demonstrated that the immune system could respond to transplantation by rejection or by induction of tolerance. In 1953, Billingham, Brent, and Medawar, in what is probably one of the most famous papers in transplantation immunology, described acquired immunological tolerance to alloantigens in mice.[4] The possibility of harnessing the immune system to produce antigen-specific immunological unresponsiveness to major histocompatibility complex (MHC) nonidentical allogeneic donor grafts in mature transplant recipients, without lifelong dependence on immunosuppressive drugs, has been and remains the goal of transplant research scientists. With current technology this goal is tantalizingly close, yet intangible.

Tolerance is sought as a potential solution for all these problems because it would enable indefinite allograft acceptance without the harmful side effects and economic burden of lifelong immunosuppression. Hundreds of tolerance strategies have emerged in experimental transplantation, but it is not a simple matter to transfer inbred rodent transplant tolerance protocols to the clinical setting. Thus, studies of transplant tolerance in outbred large animals, including nonhuman primates (NHPs), become necessary to identify and optimize the most promising clinical approaches. With better understanding of the mechanisms favoring successful induction and maintenance of tolerance in preclinical models that have close immunological homology to humans, the prospect of safe and effective induction of antigen-specific regulation in human organ transplantation may become tangible.[5]

9.2 Immune Tolerance Definition

A strategic perspective of tolerance induction demands a workable definition of the concept at the onset. Over the years, the strict definition of tolerance has transformed with the introduction of different therapeutic strategies and with the better understanding of the molecular mechanisms related to its induction and maintenance.[6] One thing is clear that the once-simple definition of tolerance as "specific absence of an immune response to an antigen" is no longer sufficient to describe the available phenomena. From the immunologic standpoint, a definition of tolerance requires the following essential elements:

Antigen-specific unresponsiveness state that determines a prolonged (indefinite) allograft acceptance and survival, with normal function and histology devoid of encroaching or attacking mononuclear cells (allogeneic nonaggressiveness)

Preservation of an otherwise normal recipient immune response, maintaining the capacity to reject third-party allograft and to accept a second donor-specific allograft

Absence of a requirement for continuing nonspecific immunosuppressive therapy, thus avoiding immunosuppression-related infection, neoplasia, or other side effects

Such a tolerant state, if complete, would imply normal graft survival with normal function and graft histology without any requirement of immunosuppression. On the other hand, the state of tolerance in the recipient might be incomplete and less clear-cut, requiring reduced amount of maintenance immunosuppression and acceptable but not normal allograft function. Calne introduced this concept of *almost tolerance* with donor-specific hyporesponsiveness under lower dosage of immunosuppressive drugs and named it *prope tolerance*.[7] He suggests that tolerance can be lost by low-grade, ill-understood chronic rejection process or acute rejection following generalized immune stimulus as encountered in viral infections, or allergic responses. Conceivably, a minimal nontoxic dose of maintenance immunosuppression could guard against these hazards, although acute intervention might be useful to dampen activated innate immunity to reduce the downstream production of proinflammatory cytokines and chemokines that can confound the regulatory mechanisms that sustain the tolerance state.

From the clinical point of view, a strict mechanistic definition of tolerance is unhelpful, since an "operationally tolerant state" is all that is needed for the welfare of a patient. A useful working definition for operational or clinical tolerance would be the long-term functional graft survival in a patient not requiring maintenance immunosuppression.[8] Sachs introduced an updated definition, stating that tolerance is not merely the absence of a response, but may involve an active down-regulatory response induced through a variety of mechanisms.[9] At the present time, identification of a complete or partial donor-specific tolerance state can only be confirmed by elimination/withdrawal or reduction/minimization of maintenance immunosuppression.[7] No reliable in vitro, in vivo, or intragraft monitoring assays for tolerance are currently available.

9.3 Immune Mechanisms Implicated in Tolerance

Recent insights into the requirements for T-cell activation and normal mechanisms of immunologic homeostasis and self-tolerance suggest several new approaches to achieve transplantation tolerance.[10] In general, three distinct immune mechanisms exist by which operational transplantation tolerance can be achieved. One involves deleting or inactivating alloreactive clones in the thymus at the time of antigen exposure (central tolerance). Another involves deleting, inactivating, or regulating the activation of alloreactive precursor cells in the peripheral circulation and lymphoid tissues (peripheral tolerance).[11] The third involves immune ignorance, which is less well understood. Here the lymph node milieu is disorganized, usually by impairment of one or both NF-κB signal pathways, such that host alloreactive precursor cells cannot successfully undergo the precise, regimented sequence of events – ranging from lymph node homing, specific antigen presentation, costimulation, and activation to become mature immune effectors and exit to the periphery.[12]

9.3.1 Central Tolerance

The original clonal selection theory of antigen-specific tolerance proposed a physical absence of self-antigen-reactive clones due to a deletional process during ontogeny.[13] During intrathymic development, immature T cells that are potentially reactive to autoantigens are either physically deleted (clonal deletion) or functionally inactivated (clonal anergy). Tolerance induced by myeloablative conditioning regimen followed by immune system reconstitution with donor bone marrow takes advantage of this process.[14] After this procedure the recipients harbor a mixture of self and donor hematopoietic cells in a state called mixed chimerism. The presence of donor antigen presenting cells (APC) in the thymus leads to the deletion of donor reactive T cells, which is a principal mechanism of tolerance in this system. As a result, donor and recipient lymphocyte combatants achieve a truce and coexist for an indeterminate period of time.

However, the need for chemotherapy or irradiation to ablate the recipient immune system as a preconditioning regimen has largely prevented the widespread adoption of this model. It has also been demonstrated that the clonal deletion of host immune cells in chimeric models of tolerance is only relevant in mixed chimeras in which host immune cells persist. It is also clear that chimerism is not a necessary and sufficient condition for organ graft acceptance, because in some animal models of combined bone marrow and organ transplantation, the organ graft is rejected despite the acceptance of the donor marrow cells and sustained multilineage chimerism.[15] Chimeric models of transplantation tolerance pose the risk of graft-versus-host disease (GVHD), particularly chronic GVHD following infusion of donor hematopoietic cells, because small numbers of mature donor T cells in the inoculum can become activated by donor cells.[16] Therefore, chimerism-based tolerance models need to provide a resolute means of preventing GVHD.[17]

An important consideration is that every graft is to some degree also a lympho-hematopoietic graft because of the substantial numbers of passenger lymphoid cells (sessile and bloodborne) either within the graft or from attached lymph nodes. These donor leukocyte populations contain not only differentiated lymphoid and myeloid cells, but also self-renewing hematopoietic stem cells. Long-term follow-up studies have shown that patients treated with grafts, excluding specific transfusion and marrow infusion, can exhibit significant levels of chimerism for decades, even after immunosuppressive drugs have been discontinued.[18] Thus, organ grafts have the capacity to function as marrow grafts of sorts, with the differences being fundamentally quantitative.[19]

9.3.2 Peripheral Tolerance

Tolerance can also occur via mechanisms operating outside the thymus. Hence the term "peripheral tolerance" is applied to suppression, deletion, or anergy of alloreactive T cells that takes place in the periphery as opposed to the thymus in central tolerance. It should be noted that these mechanisms are not mutually exclusive, so that following the induction of peripheral tolerance, graft-derived donor cells may migrate and take up residence in the host thymus and facilitate tolerance. Thus, peripheral and central tolerance can and do operate in concert to promote long-term graft acceptance. A number of strategies for achieving peripheral tolerance are detailed in the following paragraphs.

9.3.2.1 T-Cell Depletion

Activated T helper cells play a major role in the immune response to the allograft by releasing cytokines, which regulate the proliferation and function of B cells, macrophages, and other immune reactive cells. Cytotoxic T cells also attack and destroy graft cells directly. Hence, depletion of T cells is a prominent component of tolerance-inducing protocols and can be accomplished by means of irradiation, antibodies, and immunosuppressive drugs. Problems associated with T-cell depletion include nonspecific targeting of non-T cells, failure to deplete lymph node T cells efficiently, especially in lymphoid tissues, and increased morbidity from infection.[20,21] Recipient APC in germinal centers of the lymph nodes can process donor antigens for presentation to residual recipient T helper cells in the microenvironment, leaving open a potential path of immune escape T-cell activation to bring about rejection of the allograft. Since T-cell depletion protocols have been most successful in inducing tolerance in NHP transplantation, they are likely candidates for tolerance translation to clinical transplantation.

Our group has used peritransplant T-cell depletion plus 15-deoxyspergualin (DSG) therapy to induce long-term tolerance to pancreatic islet allografts in NHP.[22,23] Profound depletion of circulating and noncirculating T cells was achieved with a specific anti-CD3 monoclonal antibody conjugated to a modified diphtheria toxin. The immunosuppressive drug DSG transiently arrests dendritic cell maturation, ostensibly by preventing the nuclear translocation of NF-κB family members RelB and p52, upon which dendritic cell maturation depends[24] (and unpublished data). In our studies we noticed a striking switch of cytokine expression toward an immunoregulatory pattern, with sustained high-level production of circulating IL-10 in the absence of proinflammatory cytokines.[25] Other T-cell depletion protocols, e.g., antilymphocyte serum or the anti-CD52-specific monoclonal antibody Campath-1H in combination with donor bone marrow or tacrolimus and rapamycin, are currently underway in preclinical and clinical models.[26]

9.3.2.2 Costimulatory Blockade

The need for specific T cell/APC interactions stems from the fact that T cells require two signals to generate a productive immune response. The first signal is provided by APC-borne MHC-peptide complexes through the T-cell receptor (TCR), and the second is a costimulatory signal that is provided by a ligand (on APC) and receptor (on T cell) interaction, necessary for the T cell to respond optimally to the antigen. By their nature costimulatory signals are not antigen-specific but, rather, amplify and synergize with the TCR ligation to provide crucial signals to the activated T cells.[27] Consequently, antibodies that interfere with costimulatory pathways are promising candidates for tolerance induction. Experimental transplantation models have demonstrated that a state of anergy and apoptosis of donor-reactive T cells ensues when antigen stimulation occurs in the absence of a costimulatory signal.[28,29]

The best-understood costimulatory signal is provided through the T-cell surface molecule CD28, that has two ligands, the homologous molecules CD80 (B7–1) and CD86 (B7–2); both of which are members of the Ig superfamily and are expressed on activated APC and some other cell types. Ligation of CD28 optimizes T-cell responses and without its costimulation, T-cell reaction is weak and transient.[27] Blocking CD28-B7 costimulation using either monoclonal antibodies or CTLA4Ig (receptor immunoglobulin fusion protein that binds CD80 and CD86 with higher affinity than CD28) prolonged allograft survival in rodent models.[30] Similar results were observed when anti-CD154 antibodies were used to block the CD154–CD40 costimulatory pathway.[31] Unfortunately, neither blockade of either one of the above costimulatory pathways nor both has been shown to induce stable drug-free tolerance in NHPs and humans.[32] Of note, CD154-specific monoclonal antibody therapy has been associated with increased incidence of thromboembolic events in clinical trials.[33] In contrast, CTLA4Ig has been used in many clinical trials without limiting toxicities,[34,35] and a second-generation agent LEA29Y, which has higher affinity for CD80 and CD86 than CTLA4Ig, seems to be more effective and is currently undergoing regulatory revisions.[36] In addition to CD28 and CD154, other costimulatory pathways like ICOS and CD134 have been identified recently and suggested as potential targets for therapeutic interventions.[37] Other strategies designed to promote tolerance by direct stimulation of negative pathways like CTLA-4 and PD-1 are theoretically attractive and worth pursuing further.[38]

9.3.2.3 Regulatory T Cells

Successful strategies to induce transplantation tolerance should mimic normal mechanisms of self and nonself discrimination of the immune system. Regulatory T cells (Tregs, also known as suppressor T cells) are a specialized subpopulation of T cells in charge of maintaining immune system homeostasis and tolerance to self. Interest in regulatory T cells has been heightened by evidence from experimental mouse models that the immunosuppressive potential of these cells can be harnessed therapeutically to treat autoimmune diseases and facilitate transplantation tolerance.[39] The observation that T cells from a tolerant host can be adoptively transferred to another otherwise unmanipulated naive animal to induce tolerance has clearly established the power of Tregs. These observations have prompted the development of strategies to promote the deletion of alloreactive effectors T cells while sparing Tregs.

One potential strategy is in vitro expansion of Tregs using a mixture of antibodies to CD3 plus CD28 in combination with IL-2. Although not yet tested in clinical transplantation ex vivo expansion has generated large numbers of regulatory T cells that have proven capable of preventing autoimmunity or inducing allograft tolerance.[40] Strategies to promote induction of Tregs in vivo are under investigation as well. One such approach is the combination therapy with IL-15 (to inhibit effector cell proliferation), long acting agonistic IL-2Fc (which promotes apoptosis of effector but not regulatory T cells) plus rapamycin that has been tested in rodent and NHP models with promising results.[41]

9.3.2.4 Cytokines Modulation

Although cytokines have long been thought to be a potential target for immune intervention the relevance of the Th1/Th2 paradigm to allograft tolerance is controversial.[42] According to this paradigm, Th2 cells that produce IL-4 and IL-10 favor tolerance, whereas INF-γ producing Th1 cells favor rejection. There is some evidence that Th2 cytokine deviation is pivotal for tolerance induction by costimulatory blockade and T-cell depletion strategies.[5,22,43] Credibility for the Th1/Th2 paradigm is bolstered by findings in which tolerance is blocked by neutralizing antibodies to IL-4.[44] Recent studies suggest that targeting IL-15, a proinflammatory cytokine which inhibits T-cell apoptosis may promote tolerance,[45] especially in combination with IL-2 sparing, the latter promoting activation-induced cell death.[46]

9.4 Composite Tissue Allograft Rejection

The primary basis for allograft rejection is the ability of T cells to recognize through their TCR, a variety of proteins referred to as alloantigens. The most important alloantigens are those encoded within the major MHC. MHC genes are among the most polymorphic known, with hundreds of different alleles so far identified at five major human MHC loci (HLA-A, HLA-B, HLA-C, HLA-DR, and HLA-DQ). Consequently, finding a completely matched, unrelated organ graft donor is minimal. However, since HLA matching is advantageous with respect to long-term graft survival, most organ distribution algorithms favor transplantation of well-matched grafts.[47]

Composite tissue allotransplantation (CTA) involves the transplantation of various tissues derived from ectoderm and mesoderm typically containing skin, fat, muscle, nerves, lymph nodes, bone, cartilage, ligaments, bone marrow, etc., as opposed to a single organ in solid organ transplantation (SOT). The function and immunologic properties of composite tissue grafts are more difficult to define, because each individual component tissue possesses its own unique characteristics that ultimately affect the successful outcome of the transplant. Cartilage, ligaments and fat present low antigenicity while bone, muscles, nerves, and vessels exhibit moderate antigenicity. In contrast, skin is the most antigenic component that elicits the most severe rejection because of the abundance of dendritic cells within the epidermis and dermis.[48] Another big difference is that SOT is designed to restore the physiologic function of the particular organ, preserve life, and improve quality of life. But CTA predominantly improves the quality of life for nonlife-threatening conditions and aims to restore anatomic, functional, and cosmetic integrity. Hence, the benefits of performing CTA should be balanced against the morbidity of the surgical procedure and the long-term immunosuppression therapy necessary to prevent graft rejection.[49]

The most important factor retarding progress in widespread clinical application of the CTAs is the high immunogenicity of the skin component.[48] This increased immune reactivity of CTA requires higher doses of immunosuppressive therapy to control the frequent rejection episodes, with consequent risk of toxicity and overimmunosuppression. For this reason, it was thought that clinical CTA might be prohibited based on the toxicity and morbidity of immunosuppression in the experimental models.[50] The development of new and more effective drugs and successful preclinical animal trials paved the way for the first clinical CTA. Definition of effective tolerance induction strategies will eliminate the last hurdle preventing widespread application of clinical CTA. There are positive aspects of CTA in that direct visualization of the graft allows early detection of complications, and local therapies for rejection control are possible. Transfer of immunocompetent donor cells from the bone marrow and lymph node components of CTA has resulted in GVHD and chimerism in rodent models.[49,51] That GVHD and chimerism have not been demonstrated in human hand transplantation cases yet may be due to the relatively small amount of donor bone marrow in the graft or the type of immunosuppressive therapy that was used.[52]

9.5 Strategies for Tolerance Induction in CTA

While transplantation tolerance has been achieved using numerous experimental approaches in rodents, very few strategies have been successfully translated to large animal models such as NHP. Human transplantation tolerance has been only reported in rare circumstances, but this will hopefully be on the rise as better assays become available to define a tolerant state and safely allow discontinuation of immunosuppressive therapies. Although the current clinical experience provides insight into the immune response to composite tissue allografts, widespread application will be facilitated by the development of modalities that can reduce or even eliminate the need for long-term immunosuppression.[53] Because of their genetic similarities to humans,[54] NHP are the best model for preclinical testing of immune tolerance. Unfortunately, only a few studies on CTA transplants have been performed in NHP due to prohibitive costs and the difficulties in obtaining the appropriate permission and infrastructure.[55]

The first communications of CTA transplants in NHP were published in the 1980s.[56,57] In those studies, hand allotransplants were performed under the cover of cyclosporine A (CsA) plus prednisone. The results were poor because the majority of the CTA were rejected during the first 15 days with only a few long-term survivals. Stevens et al.[58,59] obtained an improved survival time by the addition of monoclonal antibodies and blood transfusions, but all the recipients had severe complications and died from sepsis or lymphoid tumors. With CsA monotherapy resulting in prolonged survival Gold et al.[60] demonstrated the feasibility of mandibular CTA transplantation. To surpass the problems encountered by the pioneering studies, more selective immunosuppressive regimens and modalities need to be incorporated into the concept of CTA transplantation in NHP.[55]

The application of genetic matching could allow for the reduction of long-term immunosuppression in CTA. Lee et al.[61] have been successful in inducing tolerance to vascularized musculoskeletal allografts in major MHC-matched, minor antigen-mismatched swine receiving only a 12-day course of cyclosporine immediately after transplant. Although this model did not contain a cutaneous component, graft viability was assessed by histologic criteria after 260–360 days, and donor-specific tolerance was demonstrated by host acceptance of donor skin grafts and rejection of third-party skin grafts.[62] These findings suggest a potentially important role for major MHC matching in future hand transplants to reduce or eliminate the immunosuppression needed.

Another approach has been the creation of stable chimeras in rodents, large animals, and primates. These protocols required recipient preconditioning for ablation of the hematopoietic system with whole body irradiation and then reconstitution with a mixture of syngeneic and allogeneic bone marrow to obtain specific tolerance to skin allografts.[63] However, these preconditioning regimens are not clinically practical due to possible host toxicity, graft failure, GVHD, and the requirement of waiting for chimerism to develop prior to transplantation. The approach has since been rendered less toxic by using specific nonmyeloablative conditioning involving T-cell depleting antibody treatment with promising results.[64–67] This technique has been extended to pilot clinical trials in which tolerance has been achieved in patients with multiple myeloma and end stage renal disease by a nonmyeloablative regimen followed by HLA-matched donor bone marrow and renal allotransplantation.[68,69] Active research is going on in this area to bring tolerance induction closer to CTA.

As mentioned before, by blocking the secondary costimulatory signals using monoclonal antibodies, a long-lasting immune downregulation occurs with specificity to the bound antigen.[49] On the basis of these principles, nonlymphoablative and nonmyeloablative conditioning regimens based on costimulatory blockade have been demonstrated to induce tolerance to skin allografts in rodents.[70,71] Elster et al.[72] have shown prolonged acceptance of allogeneic skin graft in primates, utilizing anti-CD154 monoclonal antibodies. This approach holds much promise in the context of CTA, although the potential risk of hypercoagulability remains to be clarified.[33] In our laboratory, we have tested our protocol of T-cell depletion plus deoxyspergualin in a murine skin allograft model and observed that IL-10 was critical for prolonged allograft survival,[73] and we have also applied it to NHP models showing a 40% long-term skin graft tolerance (nonpublished data).

Finally, although tolerance continues to be a highly desirable goal, there are still many difficulties in conducting clinical tolerance trials. One of those difficulties is the risk of compromising short-term success rates as many of these trials call for new or reduced immunosuppressive approaches. The other problem is that acute rejection and short-term graft survival should not be used as end points in trials. In this context, tolerance markers are urgently needed to determine the safety of drug withdrawal to demonstrate achieved tolerance. The advances in the last few years have increased our understanding of the underlying mechanisms by which tolerance can be achieved and should allow for clinical application in the near future.

References

1. R. I. Lechler, M. Sykes, A. W. Thomson, L. A. Turka, Organ transplantation-how much of the promise has been realized? Nat Med 11(6), 605–613 (2005).
2. P. B. Medawar, The behavior and fate of skin autografts and skin homografts in rabbits, J Anat 78, 176–178 (1944).
3. R. D. Owen, Immunogenetic consequences of vascular anastomoses between bovine twins, Science 102, 400–401 (1945).
4. R. E. Billingham, L. Brent, P. B. Medawar, Actively acquired tolerance of foreign cells, Nature 172, 603–606 (1953).
5. J. M. Thomas, K. M. Verbanac, Transplant tolerance induction: basic concepts and therapeutic approaches, Lieberman R, Mukherjee A, editors. New York: R. G. Landes Compony; 1996.
6. A. P. Monaco, P. J. Morris, Clinical tolerance: the end of the beginning, Transplantation 77(6), 921–925 (2004).
7. R. Y. Calne, Prope tolerance – the future of organ transplantation from the laboratory to the clinic, Int Immunopharmacol 5(1), 163–167 (2005).
8. A. P. Monaco, Prospects and strategies for clinical tolerance, Transplant Proc 36(1), 227–231 (2004).
9. D. H. Sachs, Tolerance: of mice and men, J Clin Invest 111(12), 1819–1821 (2003).
10. L. A. Turka, What's new in transplant immunology: problems and prospects, Ann Intern Med 128(11), 946–948 (1998).
11. S. H. Adler, L. A. Turka, Immunotherapy as a means to induce transplantation tolerance, Curr Opin Immunol 14(5), 660–665 (2002).
12. F. G. Lakkis, A. Arakelov, B. T. Konieczny, Y. Inoue, Immunologic 'ignorance' of vascularized organ transplants in the absence of secondary lymphoid tissue, Nat Med 6(6), 686–688 (2002).
13. F. M. Burnet, The clonal selection theory of acquired immunity, New York: Cambridge University Press; 1959.
14. M. Sykes, D. H. Sachs, Bone marrow transplantation as a means of inducing tolerance, Semin Immunol 2(6), 401–417 (1990).
15. J. Miller, J. M. Mathew, V. Esquenazi, Toward tolerance to human organ transplants: a few additional corollaries and questions, Transplantation 77(6), 940–942 (2004).
16. A. L. Lobashevsky, X. L. Jiang, J. M. Thomas, Allele-specific in situ analysis of microchimerism by fluorescence resonance energy transfer (FRET) in nonhuman primate tissues, Hum Immunol 63(2), 108–120 (2002).
17. S. Strober, R. J. Lowsky, J. A. Shizuru, J. D. Scandling, M. T. Millan, Approaches to transplantation tolerance in humans, Transplantation 77(6), 932–936 (2004).
18. A. S. Rao, T. E. Starzl, A. J. Demetris, M. Trucco, A. Thomson, S. Qian, N. Murase, J. J. Fung, The two-way paradigm of transplantation immunology, Clin Immunol Immunopathol 80(3 Pt 2), S46–S51 (1996).
19. W. J. Hubbard, J. M. Thomas, Cytoablation and cytoreduction strategies in transplant tolerance, Curr Opin Immunol 2, 36–46 (1997).
20. R. D. Moses, J. T. Sundeen, K. S. Orr, R. R. Roberts, R. E. Gress, Cardiac allograft survival across major histocompatibility complex barriers in the rhesus monkey following T lymphocyte-depleted autologous marrow transplantation. III. Late allograft rejection, Transplantation 48(5), 769–773 (1989).
21. R. I. Lechler, M. Sykes, A. W. Thomson, L. A. Turka, Organ transplantation – how much of the promise has been realized? Nat Med 11(6), 605–613 (2005).

22. J. M. Thomas, J. L. Contreras, C. A. Smyth, A. Lobashevsky, S. Jenkins, W. J. Hubbard, D. E. Eckhoff, S. Stavrou, D. M. Neville Jr., F. T. Thomas, Successful reversal of streptozotocin-induced diabetes with stable allogeneic islet function in a preclinical model of type 1 diabetes, Diabetes 50(6), 1227–1236 (2001).
23. G. Meng, Y. Jiang, W. Hubbard, J. M. Thomas, The effect of anti-CD3-immunotoxin on T lymphocyte function in vitro, Transpl Immunol 6(1), 53–59 (1998).
24. W. J. Hubbard, J. L. Contreras, D. E. Eckhoff, F. T. Thomas, J. M. Thomas, Immunotoxins and tolerance induction in primates, Curr Opin Immunol 5, 29–34 (2000).
25. A. Hutchings, J. M. Thomas, Transplantation: tolerance, Curr Opin Investig Drugs 4(5), 530–535 (2003).
26. T. E. Starzl, N. Murase, K. Abu-Elmagd, E. A. Gray, R., et al, Tolerogenic immunosuppression for organ transplantation, Lancet 361(9368), 1502–1510 (2003).
27. H. Gudmundsdottir, L. A. Turka, T cell costimulatory blockade: new therapies for transplant rejection, J Am Soc Nephrol 10(6), 1356–1365 (1999).
28. Y. Li, X. C. Li, X. X. Zheng, A. D. Wells, L. A. Turka, T. B. Strom, Blocking both signal 1 and signal 2 of T-cell activation prevents apoptosis of alloreactive T cells and induction of peripheral allograft tolerance, Nat Med 5(11), 1298–1302 (1999).
29. Z. Dai, B. T. Konieczny, F. K. Baddoura, F. G. Lakkis, Impaired alloantigen-mediated T cell apoptosis and failure to induce long-term allograft survival in IL-2-deficient mice, J Immunol 161(4), 1659–1663 (1998).
30. H. Lin, S. F. Bolling, P. S. Linsley, R. Q. Wei, D. Gordon, C. B. Thompson, L. A. Turka, Long-term acceptance of major histocompatibility complex mismatched cardiac allografts induced by CTLA4Ig plus donor-specific transfusion, J Exp Med 178(5), 1801–1806 (1993).
31. C. P. Larsen, D. Z. Alexander, D. Hollenbaugh, E. T. Elwood, S. C. Ritchie, A. Aruffo, R. Hendrix, T. C. Pearson, CD40-gp39 interactions play a critical role during allograft rejection. Suppression of allograft rejection by blockade of the CD40-gp39 pathway, Transplantation 61(1), 4–9 (1996).
32. S. P. Montgomery, H. Xu, D. K. Tadaki, A. Celniker, L. C. Burkly, J. D. Berning, F. Cruzata, E. A. Elster, G. Gray, R. L. Kampen, S. J. Swanson, D. M. Harlan, A. D. Kirk, Combination induction therapy with monoclonal antibodies specific for CD80, CD86, and CD154 in non-human primate renal transplantation, Transplantation 74(10), 1365–1369 (2002).
33. B. D. Elzey, J. Tian, R. J. Jensen, A. K. Swanson, J. R. Lees, S. R. Lentz, C. S. Stein, B. Nieswandt, Y. Wang, B. L. Davidson, T. L. Ratliff, Platelet-mediated modulation of adaptive immunity. A communication link between innate and adaptive immune compartments, Immunity 19(1), 9–19 (2003).
34. J. R. Abrams, M. G. Lebwohl, C. A. Guzzo, B. V. Jegasothy, M. T. Golddfarb, et al., CTLA4Ig-mediated blockade of T-cell costimulation in patients with psoriasis vulgaris, J Clin Invest 103(9), 1243–1252 (1999).
35. J. M. Kremer, R. Westhovens, M. Leon, E. Di Giorgio, R. Alten, S. Steinfeld, et al., Treatment of rheumatoid arthritis by selective inhibition of T-cell activation with fusion protein CTLA4Ig, N Engl J Med 349(20), 1907–1915 (2003).
36. C. P. Larsen, T. C. Pearson, A. B. Adams, P. Tso, N. Shirasugi, E. Strobertm, et al., Rational development of LEA29Y (belatacept), a high-affinity variant of CTLA4-Ig with potent immunosuppressive properties, Am J Transplant 5(3), 443–453 (2005).
37. D. M. Rothstein, M. H. Sayegh, T-cell costimulatory pathways in allograft rejection and tolerance, Immunol Rev 196, 85–108 (2003).
38. E. Ozkaynak, L. Wang, A. Goodearl, K. McDonald, S. Qin, et al., Programmed death-1 targeting can promote allograft survival, J Immunol 169(11), 6546–6553 (2002).
39. S. Sakaguchi, Naturally arising CD4+ regulatory t cells for immunologic self-tolerance and negative control of immune responses, Annu Rev Immunol 22, 531–562 (2004).
40. Q. Tang, K. J. Henriksen, M. Bi, E. B. Finger, G. Szot, et al., In vitro-expanded antigen-specific regulatory T cells suppress autoimmune diabetes, J Exp Med 199(11), 1455–1465 (2004).

41. X. X. Zheng, A. Sanchez-Fueyo, C. Domenig, T. B. Strom, The balance of deletion and regulation in allograft tolerance, Immunol Rev 196, 75–84 (2003).
42. K. Kishimoto, V. M. Dong, S. Issazadeh, E. V. Fedoseyeva, et al., The role of CD154-CD40 versus CD28-B7 costimulatory pathways in regulating allogeneic Th1 and Th2 responses in vivo, J Clin Invest 106(1), 63–72 (2000).
43. I. C. Rulifson, A. I. Sperling, P. E. Fields, F. W. Fitch, J. A. Bluestone, CD28 costimulation promotes the production of Th2 cytokines, J Immunol 158(2), 658–665 (1997).
44. Z. Dai, F. G. Lakkis, The role of cytokines, CTLA-4 and costimulation in transplant tolerance and rejection, Curr Opin Immunol 11(5), 504–508 (1999).
45. X. C. Li, G. Demirci, S. Ferrari-Lacraz, C. Groves, A. Coyle, T. R. Malek, T. B. Strom, IL-15 and IL-2: a matter of life and death for T cells in vivo, Nat Med 7(1), 114–118 (2001).
46. Y. Li, X. C. Li, X. X. Zheng, A. D. Wells, L. A. Turka, T. B. Strom, Blocking both signal 1 and signal 2 of T-cell activation prevents apoptosis of alloreactive T cells and induction of peripheral allograft tolerance, Nat Med 5(11), 1298–1302 (1999).
47. G. Opelz, Correlation of HLA matching with kidney graft survival in patients with or without cyclosporine treatment, Transplantation 40(3), 240–243 (1985).
48. W. P. Lee, M. J. Yaremchuk, Y. C. Pan, M. A. Randolph, C. M. Tan, A. J. Weiland, Relative antigenicity of components of a vascularized limb allograft, Plast Reconstr Surg 87(3), 401–411 (1991).
49. C. Tai, M. Goldenberg, K. M. Schuster, B. R. Kann, C. W. Hewitt, Composite tissue allotransplantation, J Invest Surg 16(4), 193–201 (2003).
50. S. E. Hovius, H. P. Stevens, P. W. van Nierop, W. Rating, R. van Strik, J. C. van der Meulen, Allogeneic transplantation of the radial side of the hand in the rhesus monkey: I. Technical aspects, Plast Reconstr Surg 89(4), 700–709 (1992).
51. B. Yazdi, M. P. Patel, R. Ramsamooj, R. Llull, B. M. Achauer, K. S. Black, C. W. Hewitt, Vascularized bone marrow transplantation (VBMT): induction of stable mixed T-cell chimerism and transplantation tolerance in unmodified recipients, Transplant Proc 23(1 Pt 1), 739–740 (1991).
52. C. G. Francois, W. C. Breidenbach, C. Maldonado, T. P. Kakoulidis, et al., Hand transplantation: comparisons and observations of the first four clinical cases, Microsurgery 20(8), 360–371 (2000).
53. W. P. Lee, J. P. Rubin, J. L. Bourget, S. R. Cober, M. A. Randolph, G. P. Nielsen, F. L. Ierino, D. H. Sachs, Tolerance to limb tissue allografts between swine matched for major histocompatibility complex antigens, Plast Reconstr Surg 107(6), 1482–1490; discussion 1491–1482 (2001).
54. A. Geluk, D. G. Elferink, B. L. Slierendregt, K. E. van Meijgaarden, R. R. de Vries, T. H. Ottenhoff, R. E. Bontrop, Evolutionary conservation of major histocompatibility complex-DR/peptide/T cell interactions in primates, J Exp Med 177(4), 979–987 (1993).
55. M. Siemionow, S. Unal, Strategies for tolerance induction in nonhuman primates, Ann Plast Surg 55(5), 545–553 (2005).
56. R. K. Daniel, E. P. Egerszegi, D. D. Samulack, S. E. Skanes, R. W. Dykes, W. R. Rennie, Tissue transplants in primates for upper extremity reconstruction: a preliminary report, J Hand Surg [Am] 11(1), 1–8 (1986).
57. G. B. Stark, W. M. Swartz, K. Narayanan, A. R. Moller, Hand transplantation in baboons, Transplant Proc 19(5), 3968–3971 (1987).
58. H. P. Stevens, S. E. Hovius, V. D. Vuzevski, P. W. van Nierop, M. Gotte, N. A. Roche, M. Jonker, Immunological aspects of allogeneic partial hand transplantation in the rhesus monkey, Transplant Proc 22(4), 2006–2008 (1990).
59. H. P. Stevens, S. E. Hovius, J. L. Heeney, P. W. van Nierop, M. Jonker, Immunologic aspects and complications of composite tissue allografting for upper extremity reconstruction: a study in the rhesus monkey, Transplant Proc 23(1 Pt 1), 623–625 (1991).
60. M. E. Gold, J. Randzio, H. Kniha, B. S. Kim, H. H. Park, J. P. Stein, K. Booth, H. E. Gruber, D. W. Furnas, Transplantation of vascularized composite mandibular allografts in young cynomolgus monkeys, Ann Plast Surg 26(2), 125–132 (1991).

61. W. P. Lee, J. P. Rubin, J. L. Bourget, S. R. Cober, M. A. Randolph, G. P. Nielsen, F. L. Ierino, D. H. Sachs, Tolerance to limb tissue allografts between swine matched for major histocompatibility complex antigens, Plast Reconstr Surg 107(6), 1482–1490; discussion 1491–1482 (2001).
62. J. L. Bourget, D. W. Mathes, G. P. Nielsen, M. A. Randolph, et al., Tolerance to musculoskeletal allografts with transient lymphocyte chimerism in miniature swine, Transplantation 71(7), 851–856 (2001).
63. S. T. Ildstad, D. H. Sachs, Reconstitution with syngeneic plus allogeneic or xenogeneic bone marrow leads to specific acceptance of allografts or xenografts, Nature 307(5947), 168–170 (1984).
64. Y. Sharabi, D. H. Sachs, Engraftment of allogeneic bone marrow following administration of anti-T cell monoclonal antibodies and low-dose irradiation, Transplant Proc 21(1 Pt 1), 233–235 (1989).
65. Y. Sharabi, D. H. Sachs, Mixed chimerism and permanent specific transplantation tolerance induced by a nonlethal preparative regimen, J Exp Med 169(2),493–502 (1989).
66. T. Kawai, A. B. Cosimi, R. B. Colvin, J. Powelson, et al., Mixed allogeneic chimerism and renal allograft tolerance in cynomolgus monkeys, Transplantation 59(2), 256–262 (1995).
67. R. D. Foster, L. Fan, M. Neipp, C. Kaufman, et al., Donor-specific tolerance induction in composite tissue allografts, Am J Surg 176(5), 418–421 (1998).
68. L. H. Buhler, T. R. Spitzer, M. Sykes, D. H. Sachs, et al., Induction of kidney allograft tolerance after transient lymphohematopoietic chimerism in patients with multiple myeloma and end-stage renal disease, Transplantation 74(10), 1405–1409 (2002).
69. T. R. Spitzer, F. Delmonico, N. Tolkoff-Rubin, S. McAfee, et al., Combined histocompatibility leukocyte antigen-matched donor bone marrow and renal transplantation for multiple myeloma with end stage renal disease: the induction of allograft tolerance through mixed lymphohematopoietic chimerism, Transplantation 68(4), 480–484 (1999).
70. M. M. Durham, A. W. Bingaman, A. B. Adams, J. Ha, S. Y. Waitze, T. C. Pearson, C. P. Larsen, Cutting edge: administration of anti-CD40 ligand and donor bone marrow leads to hemopoietic chimerism and donor-specific tolerance without cytoreductive conditioning, J Immunol 165(1), 1–4 (2000).
71. T. Wekerle, J. Kurtz, H. Ito, J. V. Ronquillo, et al., Allogeneic bone marrow transplantation with co-stimulatory blockade induces macrochimerism and tolerance without cytoreductive host treatment, Nat Med 6(4), 464–469 (2000).
72. E. A. Elster, P. J. Blair, A. D. Kirk, Potential of costimulation-based therapies for composite tissue allotransplantation, Microsurgery 20(8), 430–434 (2000).

Section III

Chapter 10
Allograft Survival with Calcineurin Inhibitors

Neil F. Jones and Esther Voegelin

10.1 Introduction

The immunosuppressive drugs cyclosporine A (CsA) and tacrolimus (FK506), also called calcineurin inhibitors, have truly revolutionized allograft transplantation.[1] The introduction of CsA in 1976[2] was the first major advance in transplantation since the introduction of prednisone and azathioprine made allograft transplantation possible in the early 1950s and 1960s. FK506 was approved in 1994 and led to dramatic improvements in solid organ transplantation,[3-5] allowing highly antigenic lymph node bearing allografts, such as the small bowel, to be transplanted.[6] Recently, FK506 monotherapy has successfully allowed combined small bowel and partial abdominal wall transplantation in humans.[7] The success of FK506 and CsA has made them key drugs in the modern era of transplantation. The purine synthesis inhibitor mycophenolate mofetil (MMF)[8] was approved in 1995, and the drug Sirolimus (rapamycin)[9] was introduced in 1999. Combining these drugs with calcineurin inhibitors has significantly reduced the incidence of acute rejection and improved solid organ allograft survival, with a reduction in adverse effects.[10-12]

10.2 Molecular Action of Calcineurin Inhibitors

Cyclosporine A is a neutral lipophilic cyclic undecapeptide isolated from the fungus *Tolypocladium inflatum*,[2] whereas FK506, also known as tacrolimus, is a macrolide lactone produced from the fermentation broth of *Streptomyces tsukubaensis*.[13] Calcineurin inhibitors exert their effects by regulation of cytokine production. Cytokine production in T cells is regulated by a series of steps involving phosphorylation and dephosphorylation of specific proteins. Both CsA and FK506 are prodrugs, because they must first form a complex with cellular proteins called "immunophilins" before exerting their effects. There are two classes of immunophilins, the FK506 binding proteins (FKBP) which bind tacrolimus and sirolimus, and the cyclophilins (CyP) which bind CsA. Calcineurin is a phosphatase that is crucial for intracellular events leading to interleukin-2 (IL-2) gene transcription and release by T cells. Once the drugs bind to their respective immunophilin, the drug-immunophilin complex inhibits the activity of calcineurin, thereby reducing the production of IL-2 and other cytokines. Both CsA and FK506 block T-cell proliferation by mechanisms that involve the inhibition of the key signaling phosphatase calcineurin, hence their name calcineurin inhibitors. Inhibition of calcineurin activation by CsA and FK506 blocks T-cell receptor (TCR)-mediated production of interleukin-2 (IL-2), a growth factor critical for T-cell proliferation.[14] Blocking T-cell proliferation prevents the immune system from effectively reacting against alloantigens. Recent studies suggest that the effects of these drugs are not limited to blocking calcineurin activation and IL-2 production. Both CsA and FK506 have been shown to modulate the production of various cytokines and growth factors, including transforming growth factor-β (TGF-β), interferon γ, TNF-α, IL-2, IL-4, IL-5, and IL-13. By potentiating the expression of the potent immunosuppressive cytokine TGF-β, TGF-β has been implicated in mediating at least some of the effects and toxicities of CsA and FK506. Another calcineurin-independent mechanism has been shown to be the blockade of epidermal growth factor receptor induced cell growth.[15,16]

FK506 has been shown to be 100 times more potent than CsA.[17] There are four intracellular binding proteins (immunophilins) for FK506 – FKBP–12, –13, –25, and –52, the first being the most important protein crucial for T-cell activation. Binding of FK506 to FKBP-12 receptor protein prevents activation of T cells and is also a potent suppressor of B-cell activation.[18]

Both FK506 and CsA have similar renal and hepatic toxicities but differ in their other toxic side effects, presumably because of differences in the biological actions of their binding proteins. Neurotoxicity and diabetes can complicate the use of FK506.[19] CsA can cause hypercholesterolemia, increasing the risk of cardiovascular complications in recipients receiving maintenance immunosuppression.[20] FK506 possesses other positive effects and has been shown to promote nerve regeneration in small animal and large animal models[21] and in humans[22] after nerve injury.

10.2.1 Immunosuppression with Calcineurin Inhibitors and Survival of Composite Tissue Allografts in Small Animals

Hewitt et al.[23,24] were the first to show that rejection could be prolonged in a rat hindlimb transplantation model by using a short-term course of CsA 25 mg/kg for 20 days with one animal probably developing tolerance showing no signs of rejection for 701 days after transplantation. Long-term intermittent immunosuppression with CsA 8 mg/kg twice weekly produced long-term survival for more than 400 days in three animals, and long-term continuous immunosuppression with CsA 8 mg/kg/day produced four animals in which rejection could be prevented for greater than 200 days. Interestingly, 19.7% of the lymphocytes in the peripheral blood and spleen of these long-term survivors were donor derived, indicating that mixed chimerism may have contributed to their long-term survival.[25] This successful prevention of rejection using CsA immunosuppression has not been replicated by other investigators. Even though Hotokebuchi et al.[26] were able to prevent rejection in the skin component of a limb transplant across a minor histocompatibility barrier for longer than 1 year by using long-term intermittent immunosuppression with CsA 25 mg/kg twice weekly for 14 weeks, they were unable to prevent skin rejection across a major histocompatibility barrier. However, the articular cartilage component of these limb allografts did not show any signs of rejection up to 1 year after surgery.

Therefore there are probably only 18 rat limb transplants in the literature in which the skin component has shown no signs of rejection for longer than 200 days, the obvious conclusion being that long-term intermittent or even continuous immunosuppression with CsA alone is unable to prevent rejection of the skin component of a limb transplant.

FK506 appears to be superior to CsA in preventing the rejection of rat hindlimb allografts. Arai et al.[27] were able to achieve long-term survival for more than 200 days across a major histocompatibility barrier in eight animals by using intermittent immunosuppression with FK506 3 mg/kg weekly. Of concern, 75% of these long-term survivors developed *Pneumocystis carinii* pneumonia, possibly indicative of the development of graft-versus-host disease (GVHD). By using a short-term course of FK506 6 mg/kg/day for 90 days, Fealy et al.[28] were able to prolong rejection in one animal for 345 days. We reported long-term survival for more than 200 days in ten limb allografts across a major histocompatibility barrier using intermittent immunosuppression with FK506 either 1 or 2 mg/kg twice weekly.[29] All these animals lost weight and died of bacterial pneumonia without signs of skin rejection between 273 and 334 days after transplantation, again suggestive of the development of GVHD. Llull et al.[30] demonstrated chimeric expansion throughout 100 days of FK506 administration (1 mg/kg/day for 14 days, then weekly). After discontinuation of FK506, transient nonlethal GVHD occurred in 9 of 13 animals. Their recovery correlated with a slow reduction in cytometrically detectable chimeric leukocytes in the peripheral blood, repopulation of the donor bone marrow with recipient elements, and chronic allograft rejection.

Consequently, there are only 21 animals in the literature in which rejection of the skin component of a limb transplant could be prevented for more than 200 days by using immunosuppression with FK506, but those animals that survived rejection free for more than 300 days died of pneumonias, which may represent either toxic effects of long-term immunosuppression or the development of GVHD.

A comparison of immunosuppression using CsA, FK506, or MMF showed that only long-term FK506 and not CsA or MMF was capable of preventing rejection of the skin component of a composite tissue allograft (CTA). However, FK506 monotherapy did not achieve this without inevitable drug toxicity. Eight of nine animals died of bacterial pneumonia between 273 and 334 days after transplantation without showing signs of rejection.[31,32] In a study of microsurgical whole joint transplantation in rats, long-term intermittent immunosuppression with FK506 (2 mg/kg/day intramuscularly for 14 days, then biweekly) was significantly superior to rapamycin and MMF in preventing rejection of the transplanted articular cartilage of the vascularized knee joint allograft at 6 weeks, 3 and 6 months, and 1 year after surgery. In addition, side effects including wound healing problems and bone marrow suppression resulting in weight loss and death were less frequent using FK506. However, 5 of 19 rats under FK506 immunosuppression died or had to be killed because of pneumonia between 5 and 7 months after transplantation[33] (Table 10.1).

Combination immunosuppressive therapy may improve graft and host survival, while simultaneously decreasing the occurrence of toxic side effects in CTA models. In a study of microsurgical joint transplantation[33] immunosuppressed with a combination of FK506 (1 mg/kg/day intramuscularly for 14 days, then biweekly) and rapamycin (1.25 mg/kg/day orally), three knee joints remained viable at 6 months but animals had to be killed because of severe drug side effects. In the first study of combination immunosuppression, subtherapeutic doses of CsA 1.5 mg/kg/day combined with mycophenolate mofetil (MMF) 15 mg/kg/day prevented rejection in 89% of limb allografts for 231–254 days.[34] Several other studies have investigated combination immunosuppression therapy in rat limb transplantation using CsA and leflunomide (LEF),[35] or FK506 and 15-deoxyspergualin (DOS),[36] or FK506 and MMF,[37] but failed to achieve long-term survival for more than 200 days. Combination of low-dose MMF (15 mg/kg/day) with FK506 (1 mg/kg/day) produced long-term limb survival and minimal toxic side effects, but sporadic rejection episodes were observed in seven of ten animals that completed this 5-month study. All rejection episodes were effectively controlled by administration of FK506 for seven consecutive days and then return to the biweekly regimen without the dose of MMF being changed. However three of the seven animals killed at 5 months demonstrated signs of rejection. Despite the presence of over 1% of donor chimerism in surviving animals, there was no correlation between the presence of donor chimerism and allograft survival[38] (Table 10.2). Prolongation of skin allograft survival has been achieved by using the synergistic effect of CsA combined with a novel immunosuppressive agent such as FTY-720.[39]

The combination of calcineurin inhibitors with new drugs that target signaling pathways such as rapamycin, or macrophage-dependent T-cell function such as DOS, or other mechanisms such as Janus kinase inhibitor,[40] or FTY720[39] may potentially be an effective method of providing corticosteroid-free antirejection therapy in CTAs. Another combination therapy may involve FK506 and rapamycin. Like FK506, rapamycin is an immunosuppressant which binds FKBP-12, but unlike FK506, it does not bind calcineurin. Rapamycin affects the G1 phase of the cell cycle by acting on a unique cellular target, called mammalian target of rapamycin (mTOR) and blocks the late events in the immune cascade compared with the calcineurin inhibitors. In addition, rapamycin has demonstrated a neuroenhancing effect in vitro but not in vivo.[41] In our studies on nerve allograft transplantation in a rat model, the combination of rapamycin 1.25 mg/kg/day orally and FK506 1 mg/kg/day intramuscularly for 14 days then biweekly for 3 months or for 6 months resulted in significantly better somato-sensory evoked potentials (SSEPs) than in

Table 10.1 Immunosuppression with calcineurin inhibitors and survival of composite tissue allografts in small animals

Authors	Animals/model	Drug	Dosage (mg/kg/day)	Duration (days)	No. of rats	Survival (days)	Complications/others
Hewitt 1985[23]	LBN-LEW	CsA	25 s.c.	20	1	701	
Black 1985[24]	Rat hindlimb		8 s.c.	20, then	3	404–451	Epidermal alterations
			8 s.c.	twice weekly			
					4	206–303	
Hotokebuchi 1989[26]	LEW-F344 Rat hindlimb	CsA	8 s.c.		10	365	Elective sacrifice, GVHD
			25 s.c.	16			
			25 s.c.	16, then twice weekly, 14 weeks	10	365	
	BN-F344		25 s.c.	16	10	44.9 ± 11.1	
	Rat hindlimb		25 s.c.	16, then twice weekly, 14 weeks	10	56.4 ± 18.6	
Arai et al. 1989[27]	BN-F344 Rat hindlimb	FK506	10 i.m.	1x postop day 7	6	56.7 ± 20.4	Reversal of rejection
			10 i.m.	1x postop day 10	6	46 ± 4.2 in 3/6 animals	
			10 i.m.	1x postop day 0, then weekly	8	>214, 2/8>300	75% Pneumocystis carinii pneumonia
			3 i.m.				
Fealy et al. 1994[28]	BN-LEW Rat hindlimb	FK506	6 p.o.	90	3	345 (1/3)	

(continued)

Table 10.1 (continued)

Authors	Animals/model	Drug	Dosage (mg/kg/day)	Duration (days)	No. of rats	Survival (days)	Complications/others
Zhao and Jones 1995[29]	ACI-LEW Rat hindlimb	FK506	1 i.m. 1 i.m. 2 i.m. 2 i.m.	Postop days 3–16, then twice weekly	9	149 ± 83.71	
				Postop days 1–14, then twice weekly	10	296 ± 29.78	Weight loss, pneumonia, GVHD
Llull et al. 1997[30]	LEW-BN Rat hindlimb	FK506	1 i.m. 1 i.m.	Postop days 1–14, then weekly	Not specified	176	Transient GVHD 9/13 animals, CAR
Jones et al. 2001[31,32]	ACI-LEW Rat hindlimb	FK506	2 i.m. 2 i.m.	Postop days 1–14, then twice weekly	10	296.1 ± 29.8	8/9 animals died without signs of rejection between 273 and 334 days posttransplantation
		CsA	25 s.c. 25 s.c.	Postop days 1–14, then twice weekly	9	184 (1/9); 61.5 ± 48.2 43.6 ± 15.8	
		MMF	30 p.o. 30 p.o.	Postop days 1–14, then twice weekly	10		
Vögelin et al. 2002[33]	ACI-LEW Vascularized knee joint transplants without skin	FK506	2 i.m. 2 i.m.	Postop days 1–14, then twice weekly	22	18/19 reached endpoints, 5/6, at 365 1/6 rejection at 372	Postop deaths or premat. killing: 5/22 animals between 5 and 7 months (pneumonia) 7/26 animals between 4 and 24 weeks (+ wound healing problems)

	Rapa	2.5 p.o.	26	18/21 rejected between 42 and 90
	MMF	30 p.o.	31	17/22 rejected between 42 and 180
				18/31 animals between 5 and 40 weeks

FK506 tacrolimus; *MMF* mycophenolate mofetil; *CsA* cyclosporine; *Rapa* rapamycin; *CAR* chronic allograft rejection; *s.c.* subcutaneous; *i.v.* intravenous; *p.o.* oral; *i.p.* intraperitoneal.

Table 10.2 Combined immunosuppression with calcineurin inhibitors and survival of composite tissue allografts

Authors	Animals/model	Drug	Dosage	Duration (days)	No. of rats	Survival (days)	Complications/others
Benhaim et al. 1996[34]	BN-F344	CsA	1.5 s.c.		11	20–100	
	Rat hindlimb	MMF	15 p.o.		17	25 to >300	
		CsA + MMF	1.5 s.c. + 15 p.o.		18	231–254 in 16/18 animals	
Yeh et al. 1997[35]	BN-LEW	LEF+	10 p.o.	Days 2–60	6	60	Elective sacrifice
	Rat hindlimb	CsA	5 p.o.				
Muramatsu et al. 1997[36]	DA-LEW	FK506+	1 i.m.	30	9	76 ± 6.3	Skin + bone marrow rejected > 78 days
	Rat hindlimb	DOS	2.5 i.m.	15	10	120 resp. 78	
		FK506+	1 i.m.	30	9	36 ± 1.5	
		DOS	2.5 i.m.	30	3	all dead	
		CsA+	15 i.m.	30			
		DOS	2.5 i.m.	15			
		CsA+	15 i.m.	30			
		DOS	2.5 i.m.	30			
Hebebrand et al. 1998[37]	Hamster-LEW	FK506	2 i.m.	14	13	10.2 ± 7.0	
	Hindlimb xenotransplant	MMF	30 p.o.	14	14	10 ± 2.5	
		FK506+	2 i.m. + 30 p.o.	14	14	<13	
		MMF	1 i.m.	14	12	8.25 ± 1.3	
		FK506+	20 p.o.	14	11	9.2 ± 2.8	
		MMF	2 i.m.+	4–14	10	8.0 ± 1.5	
		FK506+	30 p.o.	4–14			
		MMF	2 i.m.+	14			

Study	Model	Drug	Dose	Schedule	n	Survival (days)	Comments
		FK506 + MMF	30 p.o.				
Vögelin et al. 2002[33]	ACI-LEW Vascularized knee joint transplants without skin	FK506+ Rapa MMF + Rapa	1 i.m.+ 1.25 p.o. 30 p.o.+ 2.5 p.o.	Postop 1–14, then biweekly every second day every second day	4 4	>180 (3/4) 42 (1/4)	Wound break down, bone marrow suppression, premature deaths in all animals
Perez-Abadia et al. 2003[38]	ACI-Wistar Furth (RT1A^u) Rat hindlimb	MMF FK-506	15 p.o. 1 i.p.	Postop 1–14, then twice weekly	10	150, 7/10 reached endpoint	3/7 rejection signs at endpoint, 1–4 rejection episodes, treated with 7 day course of FK506
Cottrell et al. 2006[42]	Wistar Furth (RT1A^b) –(RT1A^u) limb transplant	FK506 MMF	1 i.p. 15 p.o.	Postop 1–14, then twice daily	7	158.2 ± 2.3	4/7 animals single rejection, 2/7 multiple rejections

FK506 tacrolimus; *MMF* mycophenolate mofetil; *CsA* cyclosporine; *Rapa* rapamycin; *LEF* leflunomide; *DOS* 15-Deoxyspergualin; *s.c.* subcutaneous; *i.v.* intravenous; *p.o.* oral; *i.p.* intraperitoneal.

isografts and allografts, or in nerve allografts only receiving FK506 or rapamycin monotherapy. However, the animals only survived between 4 and 5 months due to toxic side effects. The electrophysiological results were even superior at the 6-month evaluation after cessation of combined immunosuppression therapy at 3 months (Vögelin and Jones, unpublished data). In another study, long-term neuroregeneration of revascularized peripheral nerves in a rat limb transplant model using low-dose FK506 (1 mg/kg/day intraperitoneally for 14 days, then biweekly) and MMF (15 mg/kg/day orally) was similar to that of syngeneic transplants. Several acute rejection episodes in the transplanted limbs were successfully treated by increasing the dose of FK506 to a daily regimen for 7 days. After 5 months, neuroregeneration did not seem to be impaired nor improved compared to the controls.[42]

10.2.2 Immunosuppression with Calcineurin Inhibitors and Survival of Composite Tissue Allografts in Large Animals

Limb transplantations have been performed in 12 baboons and 12 rhesus monkeys in three separate studies all using high-dose CsA and steroids. Daniel et al.[43] performed four hand transplants and seven neurovascular free flaps in baboons. Only one hand transplant survived greater than 200 days, until postoperative day 304. Stark et al.[44] performed eight cross-hand transplants in baboons, only one of which survived long term to 296 days. In both these studies, functional results were disappointing despite electrophysiologic evidence of some sensory and motor reinnervation. Finally, Hovius et al.[45] performed partial hand transplants in 12 rhesus monkeys. Ten of the 12 developed rejection and none survived longer than 179 days; three died of opportunistic infections and three of lymphoid tumors. Extrapolating from these three series of limb transplants in baboons and monkeys, rejection was prolonged greater than 200 days in only two animals; the obvious conclusion being that even high-dose CsA and steroids were ineffective in preventing rejection in primate hand transplants.

Two studies have investigated the use of combination immunosuppression in a forelimb osteomyocutaneous flap model in pigs.[46,47] Of ten animals treated with MMF, CsA, and prednisone, two died of anesthetic complications and three developed pneumonia. Of the eight survivors, two developed severe rejection, three developed mild to moderate rejection, and three showed no signs of rejection when the study was terminated only 90 days after transplantation.[46] In a second study using combination immunosuppression with MMF and FK506 in the same model, five of nine animals showed no signs of rejection when the study was terminated at 90 days.[47] Although a combination of oral FK506 and MMF treatment provided a superior antirejection effect, it resulted in more morbidity than CsA and MMF therapy with five animals developing pneumonias, four animals developing septic arthritis, three animals developing toe abscesses, and four animals died (Table 10.3).

Table 10.3 Immunosuppression with calcineurin inhibitors and survival of composite tissue allografts in large animals

Authors	Animals/model	Drug	Dosage mg/kg/day	Duration (days)	No. of animals	Survival (days)	Complications/Others
Daniel et al. 1986[43]	Baboon hand	CsA	14 i.m. dosage adjusted to levels 800–1,000 ng/l + corticosteroids	Day 4 to sacrifice	4	26, 71, 187,[a] 311[a]	[a]Elective sacrifice, rejection in 3/4 animals, followed by infection rejection in 3/7 animals, followed by infection
	Baboon neurovascular free flap	CsA	14 i.m. dosage adjusted to levels 800–1000 ng/l + corticosteroids	Day 4 to sacrifice	7	20, 123,[a] 141,[a] 161, 193,[a] 196,[a] 211[a]	
Stark et al. 1987[44]	Baboon hand	CsA	25 s.c. dosage adjusted to levels > 800 ng/l + corticosteroids	Day 4 to sacrifice	8	2, 5, 7, 13, 13, 15, 296[a]	[a]Elective sacrifice, several rejection episodes, rejection in 5/8 followed by infection
Hovius et al. 1990[45]	Rhesus monkey partial hand	CsA	25 s.c. + corticosteroids	Day 1 to sacrifice	12	21, 22, 29, 30, 33, 33, 79, 85, 97, 121, 144, 179	Rejection in 10/12 animals; reversal of rejection with either steroid or monoclonal antibodies (mAb) Death from sepsis, malignancy in 7/12

(continued)

Table 10.3 (continued)

Authors	Animals/model	Drug	Dosage mg/kg/day	Duration (days)	No. of animals	Survival (days)	Complications/Others
Üstüner et al. 1998[46]	Pig limb (outbred)	CsA + MMF + Prednisone	40 p.o. + 500 p.o. + 2–0.1 p.o.	To sacrifice	10	90 in 6/10	2/10 died postop.,2 severe rejections, 3 mild to moderate rejection; 2 pneumonia, 1 wound infection, 2 septic arthritis
Jones et al. 1999[47]	Pig limb (outbred)	FK506+	1.5 p.o. dosage adjusted to level 3–8 ng/ml	To sacrifice	9	90 in 5/9	4/10 died at 29,30,42, 83 days from pneumonia or gastric rupture; 4/9 temporary rejections: two pneumonias, 4 septic arthritis, 3 toe abscesses
		MMF + Prednisone	500 p.o. 500 i.v. 2.0–0.1 p.o.	Day 0 Days 1–30, 90			

FK506 tacrolimus; *MMF* mycophenolate mofetil; *CsA* cyclosporine; *Rapa* Rapamycin; *s.c.* subcutaneous; *i.v.* intravenous; *p.o.* oral; *i.p.* intraperitoneal.

10.2.3 Clinical Applications of Composite Tissue Transplantation and Immunosuppression with Calcineurin Inhibitors

Several CTA components including nerves,[48] tendons,[49] skin,[50] bone and joints,[51] vessels,[52] and muscle[53] had been transplanted with variable success before the first-hand transplant in 1998.[54–59] According to the hand registry, up until october 2007, 38 hand transplants have been performed in 28 patients worldwide using a triple immunosuppressive regimen. Initial results suggest a high degree of patient satisfaction with minimal morbidity and no mortality so far.[60] The two failures include the first French patient who requested amputation of his transplanted hand at 2 years because of poor functional recovery, several episodes of rejection, and inability to comply with the immunosuppressive protocol. One of the Chinese hand transplants was amputated at 3 years, presumably after suffering from acute rejection.[61,62] It is likely that there are other unrecorded cases of hand transplantation in China.[63] Larynx,[64] abdominal wall,[17] tongue,[65] uterus,[66] and two partial face[67,68] transplantations have also been reported using different combination immunosuppression therapies. Induction immunosuppression usually consists of anti-CD3 or 52 monoclonal antibody, interleukin-2 receptor (IL-2R) inhibitors, or antithymocyte globulin therapy in combination with FK506 or CsA as maintainance therapy combined with purine biosynthesis inhibitors azathioprine or MMF or cytokine gene expression blockers such as prednisone or rapamycin (Target of rapamycin (TOR) inhibitor).

10.2.4 Short-Term Immunosuppression with Calcineurin Inhibitors and Tolerance Induction in Composite Tissue Allografts

The general feasability of CTAs in reconstructive surgery depends on reducing or even eliminating the need for long-term immunosuppression, i.e., inducing host tolerance to the allograft. Numerous ways have been described of achieving tolerance in animal models. All of these diverse protocols aim to manipulate the recipient's immune system so that it recognizes donor tissue as self. When the donor's own immune cells persist with the recipient's cells, mixed chimerism has been achieved. Mixed chimerism seems to be required initially to induce tolerance; however it is not clear whether mixed chimerism is required to maintain tolerance. During the critical period of antigen presentation, a short-term protocol of immunosuppression allows the host's immune system to selectively reprogram to tolerate the transplanted organ. However, prevention of rejection in CTA especially, of the skin component, seems to be more complex than in solid organ transplantation.

One strategy of tolerance induction is to utilize the use of a genetically defined histocompatibility barrier. The efficacy of complete major histocompatibility complex (MCH) matching between donor and recipient on the survival of CTAs was tested using a short course of immunosuppression. Six limb allografts consisting of the distal femur, knee joint, tibia–fibula, and surrounding muscle, from MCH -matched, minor antigen-mismatched donors were immunosuppressed with CsA for only 12 days and showed no histologic evidence of rejection at death between 178 and 372 days after transplantation compared to the mismatched animals that rejected the musculoskeletal allograft at 40 days[69] (Table 10.4). This MHC-match, minor antigen-mismatch transplant barrier is equivalent to that between human siblings sharing the same paternal and maternal haplotypes, which obviously would be too restrictive for application to CTA transplantation. The mechanism of tolerance is postulated to be a relative lack of T-cell help (interruption of the rejection cascade by cyclosporine inhibition of IL-2) during the critical period of antigen presentation.[69] Chimerism was found to be present in the immediate postoperative period, but persistent long-term chimerism did not seem to be necessary for maintainance of the induced tolerance in the histocompatibility complex-matched swine.[70] When these tolerant animals were challenged with donor skin grafts placed after 100 days, survival of the donor skin was prolonged to 48, 90, and 96 days in three of six animals, while the remaining three animals continued to have viable skin grafts at the time of necropsy, indicating that specific tolerance to the musculoskeletal tissues but not the skin had been induced. However, the recipient animals rejected third-party control skin grafts, yet the animals continued to maintain their immunocompetence. Using the same model, six hindlimb allografts were transplanted including a vascularized skin paddle and immunosuppressed with CsA for 12 days. Four of the six animals were tolerant to their musculoskeletal allografts at the time of necropsy between 130 and 190 days but five of the six skin islands showed rejection between 26 and 60 days posttransplant. Frozen donor skin grafts demonstrated accelerated rejection (<10 days) in three animals and led to simultaneous rejection of both the epidermis of the allograft skin island and the skin graft in the long-term tolerant animal. Therefore, a short course of CsA produced tolerance of all but the antigens of the epidermal component of the limb allograft (split tolerance).[71]

Mixed chimerism and tolerance in CTAs can be induced by bone marrow transplantation after pretreatment of the recipient lymphoid system with total body irradiation, antilymphocyte serum (ALS), or antithymocyte globulin or temporary immunosuppression with CsA or FK506.[72,73] Models of mixed chimerism have been developed in rats, miniature swine and monkeys, and long-term tolerance to donor skin grafts and renal allografts has been achieved by such strategies.[74,75] CTAs such as limb allografts contain bone marrow and can be considered as a vascularized bone marrow transplant of donor-derived bone marrow cells to the recipient. Recently, combined use of ALS and CsA over 21 days but not over 7 or 14 days, induced donor specific tolerance in semiallogeneic mismatched hindlimb allografts between Lewis (recipient) and Lewis-Brown Norway (donor) rats. Complete survival of the allograft (>420 days) including the skin was observed in all six animals. The unresponsiveness was donor specific and was confirmed by skin grafting 60 days posttransplantation without any signs of rejection. Under this

Table 10.4 Short-term immunosuppression with calcineurin inhibitors and tolerance induction in composite tissue allografts

Authors	Animals/model	Drug	Dosage mg/kg/day	Duration (days)	No. of animals	Graft (skin)* survival (days)	Complications/others
Lee et al 2001[69]	Miniature swine: MHC match, minor antigen mismatch Heterotopic limb transplant, no skinflap	CsA	10 i.v. adjusted to levels 500–800 ng/ml	Day 0–12	8	>178, >261, >280, >254, >372, >296	Graft rejection in 1 animal (subtherapeutic CsA levels), one animal died from pulmonary embolism on day 110
Bourget et al. 2001[70]	Miniature swine MHC match, minor antigen mismatch	CsA	10–13 i.v. adjusted to levels 500–800 ng/ml	Day 0–12	6	>178 (48),* >261 (96),* >280 (>154),* >254 (>180),* >372 (90),* >296 (>200)*	Donor skin graft survival ( )*. Only 3/6 animals were tolerant at time of necropsy

(continued)

Table 10.4 (continued)

Authors	Animals/model	Drug	Dosage mg/kg/day	Duration (days)	No. of animals	Graft (skin)* survival (days)	Complications/others
	Heterotopic limb transplant, no skin flap						One animal died from pulmonary embolism on day 110 (15)*; donor skin graft viable at time of death
Mathes et al. 2003[71]	Miniature swine MHC match, minor antigen mismatch Heterotopic limb transplant + skin	CsA	13 i.v. adjusted to levels 500–800 ng/ml	Day 0–12	6	>98 (39), >120 (50), >189 (180), >159 (41), >130 (65), >150 (30),	Skin component survival. Donor skin grafts were rejected in 4/4 animals at day 8, 9, 12, and 60. Two animals died on day 98 + 120
Ozer et al. 2003[76]	LBN → LEW	CsA + ALS[a]	16 s.c.	−1 day to 7	7	20, 19, 18, 22, 45, 23, 19	Six long-term survivors (21 day protocol) accepted skin grafts from LBN and LEW

Siemionow et al. 2002[77]	Hindlimb transplantation		0.4 ml i.p.	−1 day to 14	6	21, 22, 25, 22, >360, >360	
				−1 day to 21	6	>420, >420, >425, >422, >426, >427	
Siemionow et al. 2002[78]	LBN→ LEW Hindlimb transplantation	CsA+ Alpha-beta-TCR mAb[b]	16, 8, 4, 2 s.c. tapered every week 250 μg i.p. tapered to 50 μg, every 2 days, every 3 days	−1 day to 35 −1 day to 35 Second Week Third Week	5	>720	All long-term survivors, no signs of rejection, no GVHD, all accepted secondary skin grafts from LBN
Siemionow et al. 2003[79]	LBN→ LEW	CsA+	16 s.c.	Day 0 to 7	6	>350	All long-term survivors, no signs of rejection, no GVHD, all accepted sec. skin grafts from LBN
	Hindlimb transplantation	Alpha-beta-TCR mAb[b]	250 μg i.p.				

(continued)

Table 10.4 (continued)

Authors	Animals/model	Drug	Dosage mg/kg/day	Duration (days)	No. of animals	Graft (skin)* survival (days)	Complications/others
Ozer et al. 2004[80]	LBN → LEW Hindlimb transplantation	CsA + Alpha-beta-TCR mAb[b]	8 s.c. 250 μg i.p. tapered to 50 μg, every 2 days second and third week	−1 day to 5 −1 day to 7 −1 day to 21	5 6 6	370, 367, 368, 371, 378 364, 361, 363, 365, 367, 382 353, 348, 349, 351, 352, 353	All long-term survivors, no signs of rejection, no GVHD, full acceptance of secondary skin grafts from LBN
Prabhune et al. 2003[81]	ACI → WF	+ FK506	1 i.p.	Day 0–14	10	50.7±24 6 −1 day to 35 Second Week Third Week	Five animals died before 60 days, 4 between days 2 and 7, and 1 animal on day 51 post-transplantation. No signs of rejection, no GVHD
	ACI (1,050 cGy) WF (950 cGy) + ACI T-cell deplet. BM cells[c]	+ MMF	followed twice per week 15 p.o.	28 Day 0–28			

| Hettiaratchy et al. 2004[82] | Miniature swine: MHC match, minor antigen mismatch Heterotopic limb transplant + skin HCT[d] source = CM-PBMC[e] or BMC[f] | CM-PBMC (donor) PCD3-CRM9[g] (recipient) +CM-PBMC (recipient from donor) | 100 μg/kg s.c. 0.05 i.v. 150 × 10^8/kg | Day 5 to day 2 −1 day Day 0 to 2 | 7 | 78, 30, 42, >252, >148, >160, 132 | One animal was killed (78 days) and two died with a viable limb (30/42 days). All long-term survivors (five animals) rejected the skin paddle between days 35 and 50 3/4 animals with CM-PBMC developed GVHD, resolved with 10 days CsA. No GVHD with BMC (3 animals) |

(continued)

Table 10.4 (continued)

Authors	Animals/model	Drug	Dosage mg/kg/day	Duration (days)	No. of animals	Graft (skin)* survival (days)	Complications/others
		+CsA	p.o adjusted to levels 700–800 ng/l and	−1 day to 15			
		or BMC	to 400–600 ng/l	16–30	23		
Kanatani et al. 2004[83]	BN→ LEW	+ CsA	7.5×10^6/kg	Day 0			
		FK506	2.0	Day 0–49		365 (6/23 animals), 172–185 (11/23 animals) < 150 (6/23 animals)	Six animals were killed because of ongoing rejection < 150 days, 11 animals between 175 and 185 days. Six animals were tolerant and showed no signs of rejection to the donor skin graft, no GVHD. When FK506 was not tapered but stopped at 24 weeks, rejection of 11/11
	Hindlimb transplantation		1.6	50–56			
			1.2	57–63			
			0.8	64–168			
		+ MMF	15	Day 0–14			
			12	15–21			
			9.0	22–28			
			6.0	29–35			
			3.0	36–42			
			0	>43			
			0.5	Day 0–14			
		+ Prednisolone	0.4	15–21			
			0.3	22–28			
			0.2	29–35			
			0.1	36–42			
			0	>43			

transplanted limbs on 13.8 days postwithdrawal

[a] *ALS* anti-rat lymphocyte serum.
[b] *Alpha-beta-TCR mAb* alpha-beta T-cell-receptor mouse monoclonal antibody.
[c] *ACI T-cell deplet. BM cells* 100 × 10⁶ ACI T-cell-depleted bone marrow cells.
[d] *HCT* source hematopoietic cell transplantation.
[e] *CM-PBMC* cytokine-mobilized-peripheral blood mononuclear cells.
[f] *BMC* bone marrow cells.
[g] *PCD3-CRM9* recombinant porcine CD3-CRM9 immunotoxin for T-cell depletion.
i.v. intravenous; *s.c.* subcutaneous; *p.o.* oral; *i.p.* intraperitoneal; *GVHD* graft versus host disease.

combined regimen, mature T cells from the periphery were successfully eliminated and repopulated in the presence of CTA antigens.[76,77]

To eliminate alpha-beta T cells, responsible for most immune responses including allograft rejection, a monoclonal antibody to specifically eliminate alpha-beta TCR cells has been used in combination with CsA to create a window of immunological incompetence.[78] The T-cell population was depleted by more than 95% between days 21 and 35 and returned to 84% at day 64 when the combined treatment of mouse anti-rat alpha-beta-TCR monoclonal antibodies (mAb) and CsA was discontinued at day 35 in a semiallogeneic CTA model. Tolerance was confirmed when all five animals accepted skin grafts from their donors 100 days after transplantation but third-party grafts from ACI donors were rejected. Indefinite survival of limb allograft recipients over 750 days could be demonstrated including a donor-specific chimerism of 6.7% at 400 days posttransplant.[78] Furthermore, induction and maintenance of tolerance was studied with a short-term (7 days) protocol of alpha-beta-TCR mAb combined CsA therapy in fully mismatched (Lewis recipients, Brown Norway donors) rat hindlimb allograft recipients without need for chronic immunosuppression and recipient conditioning.[79] A 20–25% level of donor-specific chimerism 120 days posttransplantation was associated with unresponsiveness to alloantigens and tolerance maintenance. All six limb allografts survived greater than 350 days without clinical signs of rejection. Standard skin grafting performed 60 days post limb transplantation revealed donor specific tolerance and immuncompetence (rejection of third-party skin grafts). This study showed that treatment with alpha-beta-TCR mAb reduced T-cell numbers in a dose-dependent manner, with a significant reduction even after one dose of antibody. The combination with CsA seemed to deplete the T-cell subpopulation and created a state of unresponsiveness needed for engraftment of the donor-derived bone marrow hematopoietic stem cells delivered with the limb allograft in the form of a vascularized bone marrow transplant even after 7 days of treatment. However, the genetically dependent difference in immunoresponsiveness and the type of chimerism found in this specific rat limb allograft model (Lewis-Brown Norway to Lewis) suggests that several distinct mechanisms may be involved in tolerance induction and maintainance. Whether these mechanisms are applicable to other rat strain combinations or to large animal species with class II antigens need to be answered.[79] In a second study using the same hindlimb transplantation model between Lewis-Brown Norway donors and Lewis recipients, a short protocol of combined alpha-beta TCR mAb along with CsA for 5, 7, or 21 days resulted in graft survival over 350 days, when the therapy was started 12h before surgery. Development of a stable macrochimerism of 12% 120 days posttransplantation and tolerance was demonstrated.[80] In none of these studies, GVHD associated with bone marrow transplantation from the donor limb was observed. Donor specific hematopoietic macrochimerism was found to vary between 12 and 25% indicating that the posttransplant immune response against alloantigens or the histocompatibility barrier could have been unique to this model. The mechanism for unresponsiveness is not well defined nor is the induction of tolerance in different models fully understood. The establishment of tolerance within a chimeric system seems to be dynamic rather than deletional and responds to mutually interacting donor and host-derived elements. The role of chimerism in transplantation tolerance however remains the subject of an extensive ongoing debate.

The degree of host conditioning, the presence of residual host immunocompetent cell populations, and the temporal relationship between host bone marrow reconstitution and allograft transplantation seem to be important host variables. Wistar Furth (WF) hosts conditioned with 950 cGy received irradiated ACI hindlimbs followed by ACI bone marrow infusion and immunotherapy with FK506 1 mg/kg/day for 14 days, followed by 1 mg/kg/day twice per week thereafter for 14 days and MMF 15 mg/kg/day for 28 days,[81] 70% of the animals died before 100 days (50.7±24.6 days) after limb transplantation without evidence of rejection or GVHD. The only animal that survived 150 days post-transplant was negative for rejection of the skin or GVHD. From the ten chimeras prepared using the same protocol (WF conditioned with irradiation receiving irradiated ACI donor hindlimb followed by ACI bone marrow infusion) but no immunosuppression, four animals died between 7 and 42 days without any signs of rejection but mild GVHD was present in one animal. Six animals completed the study (160.5±3.6 days) with no clinical or histologic signs of rejection or GVHD. However, hematopoietic cell transplantation in combination with myeloablative irradiation has been considered too toxic to be acceptable for a tolerance regimen in reconstructive transplantation.

Hettiaratchy et al.[82] investigated whether hematopoietic cell transplantation could generate tolerance to CTAs across a major histocompatibility barrier in miniature swine without the need for irradiation or myelosuppressive drugs. Seven recipient animals were transiently T-cell depleted and a short course of CsA was given for 30 days, followed by a donor hematopoietic cell transplant consisting of cytokine-mobilized peripheral blood mononuclear cells or bone marrow cells in combination with a heterotopic limb transplant. All seven animals accepted the musculoskeletal elements but rejected the skin of the allografts. The animals that received cytokine-mobilized peripheral blood mononuclear cells showed evidence of GVHD. In contrast, none of the animals that received bone marrow cells showed stable chimerism and none developed GVHD.

No additional conditioning of the recipient after the complete withdrawal of immunosuppressive therapy after hindlimb transplantation across the histocompatibility barrier Brown-Norway to Lewis was studied by Kanatani et al.[83] A low-dose combination protocol of FK-506 (2 mg/kg/day for 7 weeks, 1.6 and 1.2 mg/kg/day for 1 week, 0.8 mg/kg/day for 14 weeks); MMF (15 mg/kg/day for 2 weeks, 12 mg/kg/day for 3 weeks, 9, 6, and 3 mg/kg/day for 1 week); and prednisone (0.5, 0.4, 0.3, 0.2, 0.1 mg/kg/day for 1 week) was used. MMF and prednisone were tapered and withdrawn between weeks 2 and 7. When FK-506 was finally stopped after 24 weeks, 6 of 23 limbs were rejected and 11 limbs showed recurrent signs of rejection but six animals still had viable limbs 1 year postoperatively. Tapering of FK-506 over 24 weeks combined with salvage therapy produced donor-specific tolerance in only 6 of 23 animals. Five of six long-term tolerant recipients had experienced rejection episodes during tapering but there was no evidence of graft-versus-host reaction or drug-related side effects. There was no evidence that donor-specific chimerism contributed to tolerance in this model (no donor leukocytes in the recipient thymus by flow cytometry or immunostaining). In a second group of 11 animals, FK506 was stopped without tapering at 24 weeks. All animals rejected their limbs between 9 and 17 days after withdrawal.

10.3 Future Solutions

Side effects associated with immunosuppression, although justifiable for solid organ transplants, may not be acceptable for CTAs. In addition, these regimens may not prevent chronic rejection from compromising long-term graft function. Research focuses on new immunosuppressive or immunomodulatory drugs such as CD-3 immunotoxin[84] or by the use of Campath 1H.[85] The first applications of Campath 1H in human transplantation have successfully prevented rejection using a steroid-free tacrolimus monotherapy protocol.[17] Whether Campath 1H can induce tolerance in composite tissue transplantation with total elimination of the need for immunosuppression remains to be seen. Other novel immunomodulators include FTY720 which inhibits lymphocyte egress from secondary lymphoid tissues and thymus by agonistic activity at sphingosine 1-phosphate receptors showing synergism with CsA and FK-506 which has been shown to be highly effective in experimental allotransplantation and autoimmune disease models.[39,86]

Other research focuses on tolerance induction. To be clinically applicable, a tolerance induction regimen that can be used for reconstructive transplantation must fulfill several criteria. First, the conditioning regimen of the recipient must avoid any unjustifiable morbidity which probably excludes irradiation. Second, the protocol should not rely on genetic matching but should be able to induce tolerance across a complete major histocompatibility barrier. Third, the regimen must be suitable for the scenario of adult cadaveric transplantation, avoiding any prolonged pretreatment of the recipient and conditioning of the donor. Finally the regimen should induce tolerance to all the components of a CTA including the skin.

Currently, the most promising technique to induce tolerance seems to be through hematopoietic chimerism, but there is no guaranteed protocol applicable to CTAs. Short immunodepleting protocols followed by tapered doses of immunosuppressants seem to be a rational strategy, but have failed to show convincing long-term survival in CTAs.

References

1. V.S. Gorantla, J.H. Barker, J.W. Jones, K. Prabhune, C. Maldonado, D.K. Granger, Immunosuppressive agents in transplantation: mechanisms of action and current anti-rejection strategies, Microsurgery 20, 420–429 (2000).
2. J.F. Borel, Cyclosporin A – present experimental status, Transplant Proc 13, 344–348 (1981).
3. J.J. Fung, S. Todo, A. Jain, J. McCauley, M. Alessiani, C. Scotti, T.E. Starzl, Conversion from cyclosporine to FK506 in liver allograft recipients with cyclosporine-related complications, Transplant Proc (Suppl 1) 22(1), 6–12 (1990).

4. S. Todo, J.J. Fung, A.J. Demetris, A. Jain, R. Venkataramanan, T.E. Starzl, Early trials with FK506 as primary treatment in liver transplantation, Transplant Proc (Suppl 1) 22(1), 13–16 (1990).
5. J.M. Armitage, R.L. Kormos, B.P. Griffith, R.L. Hardesty, F.J. Fricker, R.S. Stuart, G.C. Marrone, S. Todo, J. Fung, T.E. Starzl, A clinical trial of FK506 as primary and rescue immunosuppression in cardiac transplantation, Transplant Proc 23(1), 1149–1152 (1991).
6. S. Todo, A.G. Tzakis, K. Abu-Elmagd, J. Reyes, K. Nakamura, A. Casavilla, R. Selby, B.M. Nour, H. Wright, J.J. Fung, A.J. Demetris, D.H. Van Thiel, T.E. Starzl, Intestinal transplantation in composite visceral grafts or alone, Ann Surg 216(3), 223–234 (1992).
7. D.M. Levi, A.G. Tzakis, T. Kato, J. Madariaga, N.K. Mittal, J. Nery, S. Nishida, P. Ruiz, Transplantation of the abdominal wall, Lancet 361(9376), 73–76 (2003).
8. A.C. Allison, E.M. Eugui, Immunosuppression and other effects of mycophenolic acid and an ester prodrug, mycophenolate mofetil, Immunol Rev 136, 5–28 (1993).
9. C. Vézina, A. Kudelski, S.N. Sehgal, Rapamycin (AY-22,989), a new antifungal antibiotic. I. Taxonomy of the producing streptomycete and isolation of the active principle, J Antibiot (Tokyo) 28(10), 721–726 (1975).
10. B.D. Kahan, J. Podbielski, K.L. Napoli, S.M. Katz, H.U. Meier-Kriesche, C.T. Van Buren, Immunosuppressive effects and safety of a sirolimus/cyclosporine combination regimen for renal transplantation, Transplantation 66(8), 1040–1046 (1998).
11. V.C. McAlister, Z. Gao, K. Peltekian, J Domingues, K. Mahalati, A.S. MacDonald, Sirolimus-tacrolimus combination immunosuppression, Lancet 335(9201), 376–377 (2000).
12. A.M.J. Shapiro, J.R.T. Lakey, E.A. Ryan, G.S. Korbutt, E. Toth, G.L. Warnock, N.M. Kneteman, R.V. Rajotte, Islet transplantation in seven patients with type 1 diabetes mellitus using a glucocorticoid-free immunosuppressive regimen, N Engl J Med 343(4), 230–238 (2000).
13. T. Goto, T. Kino, H. Hatanaka, M. Nishiyama, M. Okuhara, M. Kohsaka, H. Aoki, H. Imanaka, Discovery of FK-506, a novel immunosuppressant isolated from Streptomyces Tsukubaensis, Transplant Proc (Suppl 6) 19(5), 4–8 (1987).
14. N.A. Clipstone, G.R. Crabtree, Identification of calcineurin as a key signaling enzyme in T-lymphocyte activation, Nature 357:695–697 (1992).
15. M.M. Hamawy, Molecular actions of calcineurin inhibitors, Drug News Perspect 16(5), 277–82 (2003).
16. M.H. Kapturczak, H.U. Meier-Kriesche, B. Kaplan, Pharmacology of calcineurin antagonists, Transplant Proc 36(Suppl 2S), 25S–32S (2004).
17. S.R. Ghasemian, J.A. Light, C. Currier, T.M. Sasaki, A. Aquino, Tacrolimus vs neoral in renal and renal/pancreas transplantation, Clin Transplant 13, 123–125 (1999).
18. N. Suzuki, T. Sakane, T. Tsunematsu, Effects of a novel immunosuppressive agent, FK506 on human B-cell activation, Clin Exp Immunol 79, 240–245 (1990).
19. M.M. Moxey-Mims, K.K. Kher, J.A. Light, C. Kay, Increased incidence of insulin dependent diabetes mellitus in pediatric renal transplant patients receiving tacrolimus (FK506), Transplantation 65, 617–619 (1998).
20. R. Satterthwaite, S Aswad, V. Sunga, H. Shidban, T. Bogaard, P. Asai, U. Khetan, I. Akra, R.G. Mendez, R. Mendez, Incidence of new-onset hypercholesterolemia in renal transplant patients treated with FK506 or cyclosporine, Transplantation 65, 446–449 (1998).
21. J.N. Jensen, M.J. Brenner, T.H. Tung, D.A. Hunter, S.E. Mackinnon, Effect of FK506 on peripheral nerve regeneration through long grafts in inbred swine, Ann Plast Surg 54, 420–427 (2005).
22. S.E. Mackinnon, V.B. Doolabh, C.B. Novak, E.P. Trulock, Clinical outcome following nerve allograft transplantation, Plast Reconstr Surg 107, 1419–1429 (2001).
23. C.W. Hewitt, K.S. Black, L.A. Fraser, E.B. Howard, D.C. Martin, B.M. Achauer, D.W. Furnas, Composite tissue (limb) allografts in rats: I. Dose-dependent increase in survival with cyclosporine, Transplantation 39, 360–364 (1985).
24. K.S. Black, C.W. Hewitt, L.A. Fraser, E.B. Howard, D.C. Martin, B.M. Achauer, D.W. Furnas, Composite tissue (limb) allografts in rats: II. Indefinite survival using low dose cyclosporine, Transplantation 39, 365–368 (1985).

25. C.W. Hewitt, K.S. Black, S.F. Dowdy, G.A. Gonzalez, B.M. Achauer, D.C. Martin, D.W. urnas, E.B. Howard, Composite tissue (limb) allografts in rats: III. Development of donor-host lymphoid chimeras in long-term survivors, Transplantation 41, 39–43 (1986).
26. T. Hotokebuchi, K. Arai, K. Takagishi, C. Arita, Y. Sugioka, N. Kaibara, Limb allografts in rats immunosuppressed with cyclosporine: as a whole-joint allograft, Plast Reconstr Surg 83, 1027–1036 (1989).
27. K. Arai, T. Hotokebuchi, H. Miyahara, C. Arita, M. Mohtai, Y. Sugioka, N. Kaibara, Limb allografts in rats immunosuppressed with FK506: I reversal of rejection and indefinite survival, Transplantation 48, 782–786 (1989).
28. M.J. Fealy, W.S. Umansky, K.D. Bickel, J.J. Nino, R.E. Morris, B.H.J. Press, Efficacy of rapamycin and FK506 in prolonging rat hindlimb allograft survival, Ann Surg 219, 88–93 (1994).
29. M. Zhao, N.F. Jones, Limb transplantation in rats: immunosuppression with FK506, J Hand Surg 20A:77–87 (1995).
30. R. Llull, N. Marase, Q. Ye, A.J. Demetris, T.E. Starzl, Chimerism, graft vs-host disease, rejection, and their association with reciprocal donor-host immune reactions after cell, organ, and composite tissue transplantation, Transplant Proc 29, 1203–1204 (1997).
31. R. Büttemeyer, N.F. Jones, M. Zhao, U. Rao, Rejection of the component tissues of limb allografts in rats immunosuppressed with FK506 and cyclosporine, Plast Reconstr Surg 97, 139–148 (1996).
32. N.F. Jones, D. Hebebrand, R. Büttemeyer, M. Zhao, P. Benhaim, U. Rao, Comparison of long-term immunosuppression for limb transplantation using cyclosporine, tacrolimus and mycophenolate mofetil: implications for clinical composite tissue transplantation, Plast Reconstr Surg 107, 777–784 (2001).
33. E. Vögelin, N.F. Jones, U. Rao, Long-term viability of articular cartilage after microsurgical whole-joint transplantation and immunosuppression with rapamycin, mycophenolate mofetil, and tacrolimus, J Hand Surg 27A, 307–315 (2002).
34. P. Benhaim, J.P. Anthony, L. Ferreira, J.-P. Borsanyi, S.J. Mathes, Use of a combination of low-dose cyclosporine and RS-61443 in a rat hindlimb model of composite tissue allotransplantation, Transplantation 61, 527–532 (1996).
35. L.S. Yeh, C.R. Gregory, S.M. Griffey, R.A. Lecouter, S.M. Hou, R.E. Morris, Combination leflunomide and cyclosporine prevents rejection of functional whole limb allografts in the rat, Transplantation 64, 919–922 (1997).
36. K. Muramatsu, K. Doi, T. Akino, M. Shigetomi, S. Kawai, Longer survival of rat limb allograft: combined immunosuppression of FK-506 and 15-deoxyspergualin, Acta Orthop Scand 68, 581–585 (1997).
37. D. Hebebrand, N.F. Jones, G. Zohman, U. Rao, N. Soleiman, Limb xenotransplantation using FK506 and RS-61443 immunosuppression, J Reconstr Microsurg 14, 191–194 (1998).
38. G. Perez-Abadia, L. Laurentin-Perez, V.S. Gorantla, C.G. Francois, M. Vossen, P.C.R. Brouha, H.I. Orhun, G.L. Anderson, C. Maldonado, D.J. Pidwell, W.C. Breidenbach III, J.H. Barker, Low-dose immunosuppression in a rat hindlimb transplantation model, Transplant Int 16(12), 835–842 (2003).
39. K. Chiba, Y. Hoshino, C. Suzuki, Y Masabuchi, Y. Yanagawa, M. Ohtsuki, S. Sasaki, T. Fujita, FTY720, a novel immunosuppressant possessing unique mechanisms. I. Prolongation of skin allograft survival and synergistic effect in combination with cyclosporine in rats, Transplant Proc 28, 1056–1059 (1996).
40. L.B. Ivashkiv, Jak-STAT signaling pathways in cells of the immune system, Rev Immunogenet 2, 220–230 (2000).
41. T.M. Myckatyn, R.A. Ellis, A.G. Grand, S.K. Sen, J.B. Lowe, D.A. Hunter, S.E. Mackinnon, The effects of rapamycin in murine peripheral nerve isografts and allografts, Plast Reconstr Surg 109, 2405–2417 (2002).
42. B.L. Cottrell, G. Perez-Abadia, S.M. Onifer, D.S. Magnuson, D.A. Burke, F.V. Grossi, C.G. Francois, J.H. Barker, C. Maldonado, Neuroregeneration in composite tissue allografts: effect

of low-dose FK506 and mycophenolate mofetil immunotherapy, Plast Reconstr Surg 118, 615–623 (2006).
43. R.K. Daniel, E.P. Egerszegi, D.D. Samulack, S.E. Skanes, R.W. Dykes, W.R.J. Rennie, Tissue transplants in primates for upper extremity reconstruction: a preliminary report, J Hand Surg 11A, 1–8 (1986).
44. G.B. Stark, W.M. Swartz, K. Narajanan, A.R. Moller, Hand transplantation in baboons, Transplant Proc 19, 3968–3971 (1987).
45. S.E.R. Hovius, H.P.J.D. Stevens, P.W.M. van Nierop, W. Rating, R. van Strik, J.C. van der Meulen, Allogeneic transplantation of the radial side of the hand in the rhesus monkey: I technical aspects, Plast Reconstr Surg 89, 700–709 (1992).
46. E.T. Üstüner, M. Zdichavsky, X. Ren, J. Edelstein, C. Maldonado, M. Ray, A.W. Jevans, W.C. Breidenbach, S.A. Gruber, J.H. Barker, J.W. Jones, Long-term composite tissue allograft survival in a porcine model with cyclosporine/mycophenolate mofetil therapy, Transplantation 66, 1581–1587 (1998).
47. J.W. Jones, E.T. Üstüner, M. Zdichavsky, J. Edelstein, X. Ren, C. Maldonado, M. Ray, A.W. Jevans, W.C. Breidenbach, S.A. Gruber, J.H. Barker, Long-term survival on an extremity composite tissue allograft with FK506-mycophenolate mofetil therapy, Surgery 126, 384–388 (1999).
48. T.M. Myckatyn, S.E. Mackinnon, A review of research endeavors to optimize peripheral nerve reconstruction, Neurol Res 26, 124–138 (2004).
49. J.C. Guimbertau, J. Baudet, B. Panconi, R. Boileau, L. Potaux, Human allotransplant of a digital flexion system vascularized on the ulnar pedicle: a preliminary report and 1-year follow-up of two cases, Plast Reconstr Surg 89, 1135–1147 (1992).
50. J.R. Wendt, T.R. Ulich, E.P. Ruzics, J.R. Hostetler, Indefinite survival of human skin allografts in patients with long-term immunosuppression, Ann Plast Surg 32, 411–417 (1994).
51. G.O. Hofmann, M.H. Kirschner, F.D. Wagner, L. Brauns, O. Gonschorek, V. Bühren, Allogeneic vascularized grafting of human knee joints under postoperative immunosuppression of the recipient, World J Surg 22, 818–823 (1998).
52. J.P. Carpenter, J.E. Tomaszewski, Immunosuppression for human saphenous vein allograft bypass surgery: a prospective randomized trial, J Vasc Surg 26(1), 39–42 (1997).
53. T.R. Jones, P.A. Humphrey, D.C. Brennan, Transplantation of vascularized allogeneic skeletal muscle for scalp reconstruction in renal transplant patient, Transplant Proc 30(6), 2746–2753 (1998).
54. J.M. Dubernard, E. Owen, G. Herzberg, M. Lanzetta, X. Martin, H. Kapila, M. Dawahra, N.S. Hakim, Human hand allograft: report on the first 6 months, Lancet 353(9161), 1315–1320 (1999).
55. J.W. Jones Jr, S.A. Gruber, J.H. Barker, W.C. Breidenbach III, Successful hand transplantation. One year follow-up, N Engl J Med 343(7), 468–473 (2000).
56. H.D. Kvernmo, V.S. Gorantla, R.N. Gonzalez, W.C. Breidenbach III, Hand transplantation. A future clinical option? Acta Orthop Scand 76(1), 14–27 (2005).
57. G. Pei, L. Zhu, L. Gu, The experience of three cases of human hand allografts in China. In: Composite Tissue Allografts (ed. Dubernard J.-M.). Paris: John Libbey Eurotext, 2001, pp. 69–70.
58. B. Vallet, H. Parmentier, V. Lagouy, N. Dziesmiazkiewiez, Bilateral hand transplant: functional results after 18 months. In: Composite Tissue Allografts (ed. Dubernard J.-M.). Paris: John Libbey Eurotext, 2001, pp. 75–76.
59. M. Lanzetta, Functional results of the Italian hand transplantation program, J Hand Surg (Suppl 1) 28B, 74 (2003).
60. F. Petit, A.B. Minns, J.M. Dubernard, S. Hettiaratchy, W.P.A. Lee, Composite tissue allotransplantation and reconstruction surgery. First clinical applications, Ann Surg 237(1), 19–25 (2003).
61. Petruzzo, J.M. Dubernard, Hand transplantation: Lyon experience. In: Composite Tissue Allografts (ed. Dubernard, J.M.). Paris: John Libbey Eurotext, 2001, pp. 63–67.

62. P. Guoxian, G. Liquiang, Y. Lixin, Long-term follow-up of hand allografts, Abstract, J Reconstr Microsurg 20(1), 111 (2004).
63. F. Schuind, D. Abramowicz, S. Schneeberger, Hand transplantation: the state of the art, J Hand Surg 32(1)B, 2–17 (2007).
64. M. Strome, J. Stein, R. Esclamado, D. Hicks, R.R. Lorenz, W. Braun, R. Yetman, I. Eliachar, J. Mayes, Laryngeal transplantation and 40-month follow-up, N Engl J Med 344(22), 1676–1679 (2001).
65. M. Birchall, Tongue transplantation, Lancet 363(9422), 1663 (2004).
66. A. Altchek, Uterus transplantation, Mt. Sinai J Med 70(3), 154–162 (2003).
67. B. Devauchelle, L. Badet, B. Lengelé, E. Morelon, S. Testelin, M. Michallet, C. D'Hauthuille, J.-M. Dubernard, First human face allograft: early report, Lancet 368, 203–209 (2006).
68. B. Gander, C.S. Brown, D. Vasilic, A. Furr, J.C. Banis Jr., M. Cunningham, O. Wiggins, C. Maldonado, I. Whitaker, G. Perez-Abadia, J.M. Frank, J.H. Barker, Composite tissue allotransplantation of the hand and the face: a new frontier in transplant and reconstructive surgery, Transplant Int 19(11), 868–880 (2006).
69. W.P.A. Lee, J.P. Rubin, J.L. Bourget, S.R. Cober, M.A. Randolph, G.P. Nielsen, F.L. Ierino, D.H. Sachs, Tolerance to limb tissue allografts between swine matched for major histocompatibility complex antigens, Plast Reconstr Surg 107, 1482–1490 (2001).
70. J.L. Bourget, D.W. Mathes, G.P. Nielsen, M.A. Randolph, Y.N. Tanabe, V.R. Ferrara, A. Wu, S. Arn, D.H. Sachs, W.P.A. Lee, Tolerance to musculoskeletal allografts with transient lymphocyte chimerism in miniature swine, Transplantation 71(7), 851–856 (2001).
71. D.W. Mathes, M.A. Randolph, M.G. Solari, J.A. Nazzal, G.P. Nielsen, J.S. Arn, D.H. Sachs, W.P.A. Lee, Split tolerance to a composite tissue allograft in a swine model, Transplantation 75(1), 25–31 (2003).
72. R.D. Foster, L. Fan, M. Neipp, T. McCalmont, N. Ascher, S.T. Ildstad, J.P. Anthony, Donor specific tolerance induction in composite tissue allografts, Am J Surg 176, 418–421 (1998).
73. J.S. Gammie, S. Li, Y.L. Colson, A.J. Demetris, M. Neipp, S.T. Ildstad, S.M. Pham, A partial conditioning strategy for achieving mixed chimerism in rat: tacrolimus and anti-lymphocyte serum substantially reduce the minimum radiation dose for engraftment, Exp Hematol 26, 927–935 (1998).
74. T. Kawai, A.B. Cosimi, R.B. Colvin, J. Powelson, J. Eason, T. Kozlowski, M. Sykus, R. Monrey, M. Tamaka, D.H. Sachs, Mixed allogeneic chimerism and renal allograft tolerance in cynomolgus monkeys, Transplantation 59, 256–262 (1995).
75. Y. Sharabi, D.H. Sachs, Mixed chimerism and permanent specific transplantation tolerance induced by a nonlethal preparative regimen, J Exp Med 169, 493–502 (1999).
76. K. Ozer, R. Oke, R. Gurunluoglu, M. Zielinski, D. Izycki, R. Prajapati, M. Siemionow, Induction of tolerance to hind limb allografts in rats receiving cyclosporine A and antilymphocyte serum: effect of duration of the treatment, Transplantation 75, 31–36 (2003).
77. M. Siemionow, R. Oke, K. Ozer, D. Izycki, R. Prajapati, Induction or donor-specific tolerance in rat hind-limb allografts under antilymphocyte serum and cyclosporine A protocol, J Hand Surg 27A, 1095–1103 (2002).
78. M. Siemionow, T. Ortak, D. Izycki, R. Oke, B. Cunningham, R. Prajapati, J.E. Zins, Induction of tolerance in composite-tissue allografts, Transplantation 74, 1211–1217 (2002).
79. M.Z. Siemionow, D.M. Izycki, M. Zielinski, Donor-specific tolerance in fully major histocompatibility complex-mismatched limb allograft transplants under an anti-aβ T-cell receptor monoclonal antibody and cyclosporine A protocol, Transplantation 76, 1662–1668 (2003).
80. K. Ozer, D. Izycki, M. Zielinski, M. Siemionow, Development of donor-specific chimerism and tolerance in composite tissue allografts under alpha-beta-T-cell receptor monoclonal antibody and cyclosporine A treatment protocols, Microsurgery 24(3), 248–254 (2004).
81. K.A. Prabhune, V.S. Gorantla, G. Perez-Abadia, C.G. Francois, M. Vossen, L.A. Laurentin-Perez, W.C. Breidenbach III, G.G Wang, G.L. Anderson, D.J. Pidwell, J.H. Barker, C. Maldonado, Composite tissue allotransplantation in chimeric hosts part II. A clinically relevant protocol to induce tolerance in a rat model (Experimental transplantation), Transplantation 76(11), 1548–1555 (2003).

82. S. Hettiaratchy, E. Melendy, M.A. Randolph, R.C. Coburn, D.M. Neville Jr., D.H. Sachs, C.A. Huang, W.P.A. Lee, Tolerance to composite tissue allografts across a major histocompatibility barrier in miniature swine, Transplantation 77(4), 514–521 (2004).
83. T. Kanatani, B. Wright, M. Lanzetta, M. Molitor, G.W. McCaughan, G.A. Bishop, Experimental limb transplantation, part III: induction of tolerance in the rigorous strain combination of Brown-Norway donor to Lewis recipient, Transplant Proc 36, 3276–3282 (2004).
84. F. Thomas, P. Ray, J.M. Thomas, Immunological tolerance as an adjunct to allogeneic tissue grafting. Microsurgery 20(8), 435–440 (2000).
85. A.D. Kirk, D.A. Hale, R.B. Mannon, D.E. Kleiner, S.C. Hoffmann, R.L. Kampen, L.K. Cendales, D.K. Tadaki, D.M. Harlan, S.J. Swanson, Results from a human renal allograft tolerance trial evaluating the humanized CD52-specific monoclonal antibody alemtuzumab (Campath-1H), Transplantation 76(1), 120–129 (2003).
86. K. Chiba, FTY720, a new class of immunomodulator, inhibits lymphocyte egress from secondary lymphoid tissues and thymus by agonistic activity at sphingosine 1-phosphate receptors, Pharmacol Ther 108(3), 308–319 (2005).

Chapter 11
Long-Term Prevention of Rejection and Combination Drug Therapy

Thomas H. Tung

11.1 Introduction

This chapter provides an overview of the use of the most current immunosuppressive medications in composite tissue transplantation, and the immunological issues regarding the long-term survival of tissue allografts. Because the clinical application of composite tissue transplantation has been either anecdotal (laryngeal, bone, tendon) or recent (hand transplantation), the risk of late allograft loss is for the most part extrapolated from the organ transplantation literature. Peripheral nerve transplantation is unique because the nerve allograft provides only a temporary scaffold to guide host nerve regeneration; immunosuppressive medication is required for only a couple of years, and long-term allograft survival is not relevant. On the basis of the experience in organ transplantation, chronic rejection remains a significant and unsolved problem despite the use of the most potent immunosuppressive drugs. Since composite tissue transplantation improves quality of life but is nonvital, allograft longevity will continue to be a critical issue in the justification of hand and face transplantation.

11.2 Combination Drug Therapy

The majority of composite tissue transplantation research to date has focused on the use of general immunosuppressive agents to optimize allograft survival. A combination of therapeutic agents is usually used or pharmacologic therapy is combined with other modalities in an attempt to induce chimerism and possibly tolerance. The early literature studied the efficacy of azathioprine, 6-mercaptopurine, prednisolone, and antilymphocyte serum in various combinations and dosages.[1-5] Despite greater success in models of organ transplantation, these agents in general allowed only modest and inconsistent limb allograft survival with significant morbidity and mortality from the well-described effects of systemic immunosuppression (Table 11.1).

Researchers of composite tissue transplantation have studied the most promising drugs and regimens based on the organ transplantation literature. Cyclosporine

Table 11.1 Adverse sequelae of nonspecific immunosuppression

Toxicity
Malignancy
Infection
Nephrotoxicity
Hypertension
Hyperlipidemia
Neurotoxicity
Diabetes
Osteoporosis
Gingival Hyp.
Acne
Hirsutism
Alopecia
GI toxicity
Heme toxicity

A (CsA) was first introduced in the transplantation literature in 1976.[6] Its ability to consistently prolong allograft survival and its antiproliferative effect on lymphocytes was demonstrated in many animal models of organ transplantation.[7–10] In limb transplantation, the introduction of CsA represented a turning point as it permitted for the first time the consistent prolongation of limb allograft survival,[11] and it became the focus of intensive investigation. However, it eventually became evident that CsA alone could not allow long-term limb allograft survival without significant host morbidity and mortality from nonspecific immunosuppression.[12–15]

Tacrolimus (FK506) was discovered in 1987[16] and was demonstrated to be more effective for the survival of composite tissue and limb allografts.[17] It is in the same class of drugs as CsA and both are calcineurin inhibitors. Overall, FK506 therapy produced more consistent and longer survival than CsA[18] and occasionally, long-term survival was seen after only a short postoperative course of treatment.[19] However, ultimately most transplant recipients succumbed to opportunistic infections because of nonspecific immunosuppression.[20,21] Thus, similar to CsA, a level of immunosuppression adequate for consistent and durable limb allograft survival could not be achieved with FK506 alone without significant host toxicity.[22]

Mycophenolate mofetil (MMF) was developed in the late 1980s from mycophenolic acid (MPA) as a result of a search for new agents that could selectively inhibit de novo synthesis of purines.[23,24] Hydrolysis of MMF releases MPA, which blocks the proliferation and clonal expansion of T and B lymphocytes, and prevents antibody production and the generation of effector T cells. It emerged in clinical trials in the early 1990s after encouraging results in animal models of organ transplantation.[25–27] MMF is currently used in combination therapy for the primary prevention of acute rejection of heart and renal allografts, and for rescue treatment of rejection episodes in kidney, heart, and liver transplantation.[28–32] Its introduction has played a significant role in reducing the incidence of acute rejection in organ transplantation.

In animal models of limb transplantation, it has similarly demonstrated the ability to further prolong allograft survival, especially when combined with a calcineurin inhibitor.[33–35] As such, MMF has become an essential component of most induction and maintenance regimens used in hand transplantation.[36]

In clinical transplantation, the combination of multiple nonspecific immunosuppressive drugs with different mechanisms of action remains the key to successful allotransplantation with excellent short-term results. The objective of combination therapy is to minimize the toxic effects of any single agent while maintaining a sufficient level of immunosuppression by interfering with the immune response at multiple levels. Frequently, a synergistic effect is achieved when drugs acting by different mechanisms are combined and this forms the basis of current combination therapy. Many combinations of immunosuppressive drugs have been studied in composite tissue transplantation and generally consist of a calcineurin inhibitor (CsA or FK506) as discussed in the previous chapter, and corticosteroids (Table 11.2).[34,35,37–41] The most promising regimens

Table 11.2 Combination drug therapy and graft survival

Year	Animal model	MHC barrier	n	Immunosuppression	Graft survival (days)
1991[37]	Rat hindlimb	BUF → WF	n/s	CsA 4 mg/kg/d IV X 14 d	58.8 ± 1.8
			n/s	CsA 2 mg/kg/d IV X 14 d	21.2 ± 4.5
				RPM 0.8 mg/kg/d IV X 14 d	59.6 ± 0.9
				RPM 0.08 mg/kg/d IV X 14 d	20.6 ± 4.6
				RPM 0.08 mg/kg/d IV X 14 d + CsA 2 mg/kg/d IV X 14 d	57.8 ± 3.0
1994[38]	Rat hindlimb	LBN → LEW	12	FA 6 mg/cm^2/d TOP	~17^f
			12	CsA 4 mg/kg/d SC	~19^f
			12	CsA 4 mg/kg/d SC + FA 6 mg/cm^2/d TOP cont.	~33^f
1996[34]	Rat hindlimb	BN → F344	11	CsA 1.5 mg/kg/d SC	~20–~100^f
			17	MMF 15 mg/kg/d PO	~25–>300^f
			18	CsA 1.5 mg/kg/d SC + MMF 15 mg/kg/d PO	231–254 in 16/18
1996[39]	Rat neurovascular myocutaneous graft	BN → LEW	6	LEF 10 mg/kg/d PO, day-2 to 60/rejection	24.33 ± 10.48
			6	CsA 5 mg/kg/d PO, day-2 to 60/rejection	28.5 ± 6.12
			7	CsA 5 mg/kg/d PO + LEF 10 mg/kg/d PO day-2 to 60/rejection	60^b in 6/7
1997[40]	Rat hindlimb	DA → LEW	8	CsA 15 mg/kg/d IM X 30 d	37 ± 3.4

(continued)

Table 11.2 (continued)

Year	Animal model	MHC barrier	n	Immunosuppression	Graft survival (days)
			9	DOS 2.5 mg/kg/d IM X 30 d	44 ± 6.2
			12	FK506 1 mg/kg/d IM X 30 d	61 ± 13.3
			9	CsA 15 mg/kg/d IM X 30 d + DOS 2.5 mg/kg/d IM X 15 d	36 ± 1.5
			3	CsA 15 mg/kg/d IM X 30 d + DOS 2.5 mg/kg/d IM X 30 d	All dead
			9	FK506 1 mg/kg/d IM X 30 d + DOS 2.5 mg/kg/d IM X 15 d	76 ± 6.3
			10	FK506 1 mg/kg/d IM X 30 d + DOS 2.5 mg/kg/d IM X 30 d	76 ± 2.6
1997[41]	Rat hindlimb	BN → LEW	6	LEF 10 mg/kg/d PO + CsA 5 mg/kg/d PO day-2 to 60	60[b]
1998[35]	Pig limb	[outbred]	10	CsA 40 mg/kg/d PO (adjusted per trough levels) + MMF 500 mg/d PO + prednisone taper 2–0.1 mg/kg/d PO	90 in 6/10

All animals male or gender unspecified unless otherwise noted; all immunosuppressant drugs administered beginning day of surgery (POD 0) unless otherwise noted. All dosages not otherwise specified represent continuous therapy.

[a] Elective sacrifice.
[b] Estimate based on graphic data; no numeric data provided.

have been tested in a large animal model and are based on the combination of MMF with either CsA or FK506.[42,43] Such data form the basis of the immunosuppressive therapy used in the first clinical applications of composite tissue transplantation.

11.3 First Clinical Applications

The first clinical applications of composite tissue transplantation used allografts consisting of bone and supportive tissues such as tendon and cartilage. In 1988 and 1989, Guimberteau in France reported allotransplantation of a cadaveric vascularized digital flexor tendon unit which was revascularized by the host's ulnar vessels in two cases.[44] Cyclosporine immunosuppression was used at a dose of 7 mg/day for 6 months. Reported follow-up was 1 year at which time the active flexion of the recipient fingers was significantly improved compared to 0° preoperatively. At the proximal interphalangeal joint, active flexion was 75° in one case and 80° in the other, and at the distal interphalangeal joint, flexion improved to 50° and 55°. Active extension at the same time was decreased by 5° in the first case and by 25° in the second case. The results are surprisingly good considering that the use of immunosuppression was only temporary but may be accounted for by the proportion of connective tissue in a tendon allograft with a much lower cellular component compared to soft tissues and organs. It is assumed that donor cells were rejected shortly after cessation of cyclosporine but that the connective tissue framework remained. Therefore, replacement by host scar tissue may allow a tendon allograft to continue its structural function with tendon adhesions minimized by ongoing therapy and use. Long-term allograft survival per se in such cases does not appear to be necessary for successful long-term function.

In 1994, Hofmann and Kirschner in Germany reported a series of vascularized bone allotransplants for the sequelae of chondrosarcoma or osteomyelitis in the lower extremity.[45,46] In three cases, a femoral diaphysis was transplanted from cadaveric donors, and in five cases, the allograft consisted of the entire knee joint and its extensor apparatus. Combination drug therapy was used for immunosuppression and consisted of cyclosporine, azathioprine, ATG, and methyprednisolone for the first three days, and only cyclosporine and azathioprine thereafter. After 6 months, only cyclosporine was continued until there was evidence of complete bony healing. On 2–5 year follow-up, four patients were reported to have bony union and a functional knee joint with satisfactory range of motion.[47,48] But one of three femur allografts and three of five knee allografts were removed because of infection and replaced with autologous bone or a knee prosthesis. Inadequate immunosuppression and monitoring were felt to be important factors. In these cases, the size of the allograft and greater complexity (knee joint) may have played a critical role as compared to a tendon allograft. Possibly 2 or more years of immunosuppression may have allowed sufficient replacement of allograft tissue by host cells, as in a peripheral nerve allograft.

In early 1998, Strome in Cleveland, Ohio transplanted a cadaveric vascularized laryngeal allograft which consisted of the entire pharyngolaryngeal complex in a patient who lost his larynx traumatically 20 years earlier.[49] Induction therapy included monoclonal antibodies OKT3, cyclosporine, MMF, and methyprednisolone, followed by maintenance therapy with FK506, MMF, and prednisone. An episode of rejection 15 months after transplantation was treated successfully with high-dose steroids. Immunosuppressant-related complications have included hypertension treated with antihypertensive medications, three episodes of tracheobronchitis treated with antibiotics, and pneumocystis carinii pneumonia also treated with antibiotics. Efficient deglutition was regained after 3 months, and vocal parameters normalized after 16 months. At the last reported follow-up after 40 months (2001), the patient has a normal sounding voice, and can swallow without aspiration.[50]

These cases demonstrate that except for simple and small allografts with a relatively low cellular component and antigenicity, chronic nonspecific immunosuppression is required for long-term allograft survival and function. The history of composite tissue transplantation in the modern era of current immunosuppressive medications demonstrates impressive acute survival but has been too short for the evaluation of chronic rejection and long-term survival.

11.4 Hand Transplantation

To date, 24 hands have been transplanted onto 18 recipients. The longest surviving hand allograft was transplanted in January 1999 in Louisville, KY.[51] Two failed cases have been reported. In the first case, which is the very first case performed in Lyon, France in September 1998,[52] the patient was noncompliant with immunosuppressive therapy resulting in rejection and the allograft was amputated 861 days after transplantation.[53] In the second case, the patient presented with severe skin inflammation which most likely represented acute rejection and was not responsive to any treatment. Amputation was therefore performed more than 3 years after transplantation and no histologic data regarding this case has been reported.

The most commonly used combination for induction therapy includes antithymocyte globulin (ATG), FK506, MMF, and steroids.[36] ATG was administered for 3–10 days. Initial steroid doses were 500–1,000 mg/day, and were tapered down to 10–20 mg/day by 6–8 weeks following surgery. In some cases, monoclonal antibodies (Basiliximab) were used instead of ATG, and was usually administered in two doses given on postoperative days 1 and 4. In most patients, maintenance therapy consisted of FK506, MMF, and steroids, but in some cases, MMF is not used, and in others, rapamycin is used in place of FK506. Steroid dosage is usually tapered further after 1 year. The majority of patients have experienced at least one episode of acute rejection, and many have had two or more episodes. One patient has presented with an episode of rejection 756 days after transplantation, and another has experienced several episodes starting 510 days after transplantation most likely due to noncompliance with immunosuppressive medication. All episodes were readily reversed except for the second failure described previously. The incidence of immunosuppressive complications has been low, but has most commonly included opportunistic infections (CMV reactivation, cutaneous mycosis), metabolic (hyperglycemia), and surgical complications (skin necrosis, thrombosis).[36]

Allograft dysfunction with eventual progression to late allograft loss is the initial presentation of chronic adverse immunological sequelae. The assessment of long-term functional results should give an indication of the presence of chronic allograft dysfunction. As such, the functional outcomes have been mixed with only the results of the initial procedures having been published.[54,55] Finger flexion and extension have been good based on the recipient's preexisting extrinsic forearm muscles that had remained innervated and functional. Reinnervation of the intrinsic hand muscles, however, has been poor. There has been electromyographic evidence of intrinsic reinnervation and some functional evidence of thenar muscle activity, but overall intrinsic function has been poor, necessitating tendon transfers to improve hand position and function. Sensory reinnervation has also not been as good as predicted, especially considering the neuroenhancing effects of FK506, which has been noted to increase the regeneration rate in recipients of nerve allografts.[56] The first four patients did show clinical and histological evidence of nerve regeneration. However, the only patient to have documented Semmes–Weinstein testing showed diminished protective sensation in his thumb and no protective sensation in the other digits after 3 years.[57] Of 21 hand allografts evaluated by static 2-point discrimination after 2 years, 66% (14/21) displayed recovery of > 15 mm (normal 2–6 mm) or no discriminative sensation. The Carroll test, which integrates mobility, motor function, and sensation to assess global hand function, has also been used on three of the first four patients. The results ranged from a score between 52 and 75, which translates to one good and two fair results.[58,59] At 5-year follow-up, the Carroll test score of the longest-surviving hand allograft had improved to 63 (from 52), but has shown no significant improvement since the 3-year time point.[58,59] On the basis of the most current reports, the mean Carroll test score for the hand allograft recipients by level is 70 for transplantation at the wrist, and 61 at the forearm,[59] versus 81.6 at the wrist and 60.5 at the forearm after replantation.[60] Nevertheless, most of the patients are able to perform activities they previously could not, especially manual activities of daily living, and 15 patients have reported an improvement in their quality of life.[36]

The analysis of hand allograft function is difficult because of the greater complexity of hand function, the lack of standardization of functional tests among the different centers, and the variable of postoperative therapy, the quality and intensity of which can significantly affect overall function. Moreover, changes in overall hand function are noted much more gradually, unlike critical organ allograft function which is monitored more objectively and quickly by blood tests or specific functional parameters. The hand replantation literature provides data to guide realistic expectations of hand function after transplantation. However, definitive conclusions from the direct comparison of nerve regeneration and muscle reinnervation after limb *transplantation* versus *replantation* are difficult because different functional tests are used by different centers, and the hand replantation data spans the last four decades. Postoperative rehabilitation is critical to functional outcome, and therapy protocols vary and have progressed markedly over the years. Replant cases generally include indigent traumatic patients with poor follow-up and compliance who were not carefully screened as the transplant recipients have been. Hand allotransplantation also offers other theoretical advantages over replantation such as an uninjured, intact, and well-preserved limb, and a favorable amputation site. Therefore a significant selection bias likely exists and the return of function after hand replantation would be expected to be even better if patient screening and close postoperative follow-up and therapy were consistently possible. As such, immunological factors are likely to play a role in limiting the ultimate functional recovery of the hand allograft considering the shortcomings of current pharmacologic immunosuppression in the long term as discussed in the next section.

11.5 Chronic Rejection

The main obstacle to long-term allograft survival using current immunosuppressive medication is chronic allograft loss, which can be expected to be as significant a problem in hand transplantation as it is in organ transplantation. Chronic rejection is the prevalent cause of long-term organ allograft failure and its incidence has remained unchanged despite two decades of progress in immunosuppressive therapy and perioperative care.[61] Chronic rejection manifests as bronchiolitis obliterans in lung transplantation, as posttransplant coronary arteriopathy in heart transplantation, and as chronic nephropathy in renal allografts with glomerulopathy, tubular atrophy, fibrosis, and vasculopathy. Chronic rejection with allograft loss is seen in up to 52% of cardiac and lung transplant recipients by 5 years[2,62,63] and in greater than 50% of renal allograft recipients after 7–8 years.[59,64,65] The frequency and timing of episodes of acute rejection remains the single most factor that predicts chronic rejection and allograft failure. On the basis of the renal transplantation literature, the risk of chronic rejection increases threefold with one acute rejection episode, 12-fold with two or more acute episodes, and up to 26-fold with late rejection episodes occurring more than 8 weeks after transplantation.[66] The estimated half-life for cadaveric renal transplants that had an acute rejection episode is 6.6 years, versus 12.5 years for those who did not.[67] In the recent era, the average yearly reduction in the relative risk of chronic graft failure was 4.2% for all recipients, 6.3% for those who did not have acute rejection episodes, and only 0.4% for those who had an acute rejection episode.[68] The 10-year renal allograft survival rates excluding causes of graft loss other than chronic rejection were 94% for patients without an acute rejection episode, 86% with early acute rejection episodes, and only 45% with late acute rejection episodes. In another series, 43% of patients experiencing acute rejection episodes more than 60 days posttransplantation developed biopsy-proven chronic rejection, compared to only 20% with acute rejection 60 days or less, and 0.8% of patients never experiencing a rejection episode.[69]

Experience with hand transplantation so far suggests that averting chronic rejection will be difficult. In the first two patients, acute rejections were noted at 8, 55, and 74 weeks in Lyon, France and 4–6, 18–20, and 77 weeks in Louisville's experience. Of the 18 hand transplants recipients, 12 had at least one episode of acute rejection, eight had two or more, and several had three to five episodes.[36] One patient has presented with an episode of rejection 756 days after transplantation, and another has experienced several episodes starting 510 days after transplantation. These frequent and late acute rejection episodes suggest a substantial risk for chronic rejection. Their impact on nerve regeneration and functional outcome may also be significant. There is evidence to suggest that rejection of skin will also predispose to rejection of a simultaneous nerve allograft, where the nerve allograft alone was previously accepted and supported regeneration.[70] Multiple episodes of acute rejection may thus lead to cumulative inflammation and scarring that altogether significantly impairs nerve regeneration. Thus, episodes of acute rejection in the hand transplant patients represent more than just temporary and reversible setbacks. Even though these episodes have been relatively easily controlled, the very fact that these episodes have been frequent and have occurred late predicts chronic rejection and ultimate failure of the allograft.

Other relevant risk factors for chronic rejection include patient age and donor source. Young patients have been associated with a relatively high state of immune responsiveness to alloantigens,[71] and are more likely to forget to take immunosuppressive medication.[72] In single center studies, young age also appears to be predictive of chronic rejection and graft loss.[73] The mean age of the current hand transplant recipients is 32, whereas in large series of renal transplants, mean recipient age is generally 45–50.[74,75] There is also a higher graft survival rate for living donor kidneys compared to cadaveric kidneys, and the rate of graft loss from chronic rejection for cadaveric donors is double that for living donors.[76] The literature indicates that a living related allograft progresses from acute to chronic rejection at a slower rate than a cadaveric graft, and this has been attributed to the fact that kidneys from living donors are uniformly healthy.[77,78] A hand allograft will always be cadaveric and therefore will remain predisposed to a higher risk for late graft loss.

The current short-term success of organ transplantation is excellent with 1-year allograft survival rates of up to 80–90% or more.[79,80] Average follow-up of all hand transplant recipients reported is currently less than 5 years. To date, no hand allografts have been reported to be lost within the first year after transplantation. However, chronic rejection remains a problem and is the primary cause of long-term allograft failure. Allograft loss in organ transplantation is defined by loss of function rather than overt tissue necrosis since the allograft cannot be directly visualized. The signs of chronic rejection following a hand transplant may possibly include scarring and loss of mobility, axonopathy or small-vessel disease, and ischemia. The onset of chronic rejection in a hand allograft may be signaled by loss of recovered function or cessation of functional progression well in advance of overt tissue necrosis and may not be immediately measurable like organ allograft function. Evidence of chronic rejection may therefore already be present in the earliest recipients and might only become apparent in retrospect. Evaluation methods that may detect early signs of chronic rejection such as immunohistochemistry of tissue specimens for antibody deposition and flow cytometric analysis of recipient serum against donor antigen to determine the presence of donor-specific antibodies have not been performed. Immunohistologic studies of skin biopsy specimens have been performed but have focused on cellular analysis which is more relevant to the acute response.[81] Until such processes can be eliminated, however, the role of nonvital transplantation is likely to remain limited and controversial. Although the timing of chronic rejection in hand transplantation is unknown, based on the organ transplantation literature, it is likely that it will occur in up to 50% or more of hand allograft recipients within 10 years of transplantation despite our most contemporary immunosuppressive drug regimens. There is little doubt that the potential functional recovery after hand replantation or transplantation is superior to a prosthesis, and that a significant improvement in the quality of life both functionally and psychologically is seen in most recipients.[36,55]

However, the long-term sequelae of lifelong nonspecific immunosuppression and the probability of allograft loss in many of the transplant recipients within one decade, considering the young mean age (32) in the current series, may not in the end justify the risks of hand transplantation, especially for unilateral cases. The stakes become much higher for facial transplantation because a hand allograft can be removed much more easily. In the case of face transplantation, loss of the allograft despite optimal compliance will lead to a large facial wound and further skin grafting, which will result in further deformity and scarring both physically and psychologically.

References

1. D. Slome and B. Reeves, Experimental homotransplantation of the knee-joint, Lancet 2, 205 (1966).
2. R. M. Goldwyn, P. M. Beach, D. Feldman, and R. E. Wilson, Canine limb homotransplantations, Plast Reconstr Surg 37, 184 (1966).
3. Doi K, Homotransplantation of limbs in rats, Plast Reconstr Surg 64, 613–621 (1979).
4. E. M. Lance, A. E. Inglis, F. Figarola, and F. J. Veith, Transplantation of the canine hind limb, J Bone Joint Surg 53A, 1137 (1971).
5. V. Goldberg, B. B. Porter, and E. M. Lance, Transplantation of the canine knee joint on vascular pedicles, J Bone Joint Surg 55A, 1314 (1973).
6. J. F. Borel, C. Feurer, H. U. Gubler, and H. Stahelin, Biological effects of cyclosporine A: A new antilymphocytic agent, Agents Actions 6, 468 (1976).
7. R. Y. Calne, D. J. White, K. Rolles, D. P. Smith, and B. M. Herbertson, Prolonged survival of pig orthotopic heart grafts treated with cyclosporin A, Lancet 1, 1183–1185 (1978).
8. A. B. Cosimi, C. F. Shield, C. Peters, R. C. Burton, G. Scott, and P. S. Russell. Prolongation of allograft survival by cyclosporin A, Surg Forum 30, 287–289. 1979.
9. R. Y. Calne, D. J. White, B. D. Pentlow, K. Rolles, T. Syrakos, T. Ohtawa, D. P. Smith, P. McMaster, D. B. Evans, B. M. Herbertson, and S. Thiru, Cyclosporin A: Preliminary observations in dogs with pancreatic duodenal allografts and patients with cadaveric renal transplants, Transplant Proc 11, 860–864 (1979).
10. B. A. Reitz, N. A. Burton, S. W. Jamieson, C. P. Bieber, J. L. Pennock, E. B. Stinson, and N. E. Shumway, Heart and lung transplantation: Autotransplantation and allotransplantation in primates with extended survival, J Thorac Cardiovasc Surg 80, 360–372 (1980).
11. K. S. Black, C. W. Hewitt, L. A. Fraser, J. G. Osborne, B. M. Achauer, D. C. Martin, and D. W. Furnas, Cosmas and Damian in the laboratory, N Eng J Med 306, 368–369 (1982).
12. S. E. Hovius, H. P. Stevens, P. W. van Nierop, W. Rating, R. van Strik, and J. H. van der Meulen, Allogeneic transplantation of the radial side of the hand in the rhesus monkey: I. Technical aspects, Plast Reconstr Surg 89, 700–709 (1992).
13. K. S. Black, C. W. Hewitt, J. S. Hwang, R. W. Borger, and B. M. Achauer, Dose response of cyclosporine-treated composite tissue allografts in a strong histoincompatible rat model, Transplant Proc 20, 266–268 (1988).
14. H. Kuroki, O. Ishida, H. Daisaku, K. Fukuhara, E. Hatano, T. Murakami, Y. Ikuta, A. K. Matsumoto, and M. Akiyama, Morphological and immunological analysis of rats with long-term-surviving limb allografts induced by a short course of FK506 or cyclosporine, Transplant Proc 23, 516–520 (1991).
15. T. Hotokebuchi, K. Arai, K. Takagishi, C. Arita, Y. Sugioka, and N. Karibara, Limb allografts in rats immunosuppressed with cyclosporine: As a whole-joint allograft, Plast Reconstr Surg 83, 1027–1036 (1989).

16. T. Goto, T. Kino, H. Hatanaka, M. Nishiyama, M. Okuhara, M. Kohsaka, H. Aoki, and H. Imanaka, Discovery of FK-506, a novel immunosuppressant isolated from *Streptomyces tsukubaensis*, Transplant Proc 19, 4–8 (1987).
17. H. Kuroki, Y. Ikuta, and M. Akiyama, Experimental studies of vascularized allogeneic limb transplantation in the rat using a new immunosuppressive agent FK-506: Morphological and immunological analysis, Transplant Proc 21, 3187–3190 (1989).
18. Z. Min and N. F. Jones, Limb transplantation in rats: Immunosuppression with FK-506, J Hand Surg 20A, 77–87 (1995).
19. K. Arai, T. Hotokebuchi, H. Miyahara, C. Arita, M. Mohtai, Y. Sugioka, and N. Kaibara, Prolonged limb allograft survival with short-term treatment with FK-506 in rats, Transplant Proc 21, 3191–3193 (1989).
20. K. Arai, T. Hotokebuchi, H. Miyahara, C. Arita, M. Mohtai, Y. Sugioka, and N. Kaibara, Limb allografts in rats immunosuppressed with FK506. I. Reversal of rejection and indefinite survival, Transplantation 48, 782–786 (1989).
21. R. Buttemeyer, N. F. Jones, Z. Min, and U. Rao, Rejection of the component tissues of limb allografts in rats immunosuppressed with FK-506 and cyclosporine, Plast Reconstr Surg 97, 139–148 (1996).
22. W. P. Lee and D. W. Mathes, Hand transplantation: Pertinent data and future outlook, J Hand Surg [Am] 24, 906–913 (1999).
23. T. S. Mele and P. F. Halloran, The use of mycophenolate mofetil in transplant recipients, Immunopharmacology 47, 215–245 (2000).
24. D. B. Kaufman, R. Shapiro, M. R. Lucey, W. S. Cherikh, T. Bustami, and D. B. Dyke, Immunosuppression: Practice and trends, Am J Transplant 4 Suppl 9, 38–53 (2004).
25. R. E. Morris, E. G. Hoyt, E. M. Eugui, and A. C. Allison, Transplantation and its immunology. Prolongation of rat heart allograft survival by RS-61443, Surg Forum 7, 337–338 (1989).
26. R. E. Morris, E. G. Hoyt, M. P. Murphy, E. M. Eugui, and A. C. Allison, Mycophenolic acid morpholinoethylester (RS-61443) is a new immunosuppressant that prevents and halts heart allograft rejection by selective inhibition of T- and B-cell purine synthesis, Transplant Proc 22, 1659–1662 (1990).
27. H. W. Sollinger, E. M. Eugui, and A. S. Allison, RS-61443: Mechanisms of action, experimental and early clinical results, Clin Transplant 5, 523–526 (1991).
28. H. W. Sollinger, F. O. Belzer, M. H. Deierhoi, A. G. Diethelm, T. A. Gonwa, R. S. Kauffman, G. B. Klintmalm, S. V. McDiarmid, J. Roberts, J. T. Rosenthal, et al., RS-61443 (mycophenolate mofetil). A multicenter study for refractory kidney transplant rejection, Ann Surg 216, 513–518 (1992).
29. H. W. Sollinger, M. H. Deierhoi, F. O. Belzer, A. G. Diethelm, and R. S. Kauffman, RS-61443 – a phase I clinical trial and pilot rescue study, Transplantation 53, 428–432 (1992).
30. R. D. Ensley, M. R. Bristow, S. L. Olsen, D. O. Taylor, E. H. Hammond, et al., The use of mycophenolate mofetil (RS-61443) in human heart transplant recipients. Transplantation 56, 75–82 (1993).
31. G. B. Klintmalm, N. L. Ascher, R. W. Busuttil, M. Deierhoi, T. A. Gonwa, R. Kauffman, S. McDiarmid, S. Poplawski, H. Sollinger, and J. Roberts, RS-61443 for treatment-resistant human liver rejection, Transplant Proc 25, 697 (1993).
32. J. K. Kirklin, R. C. Bourge, D. C. Naftel, W. R. Morrow, M. H. Deierhoi, R. S. Kauffman, C. White-Williams, R. I. Nomberg, W. L. Holman, and D. C. Smith, Jr., Treatment of recurrent heart rejection with mycophenolate mofetil (RS-61443): Initial clinical experience, J Heart Lung Transplant 13, 444–450 (1994).
33. P. Benhaim, J. P. Anthony, L. Y. Lin, T. H. McCalmont, and S. J. Mathes, A long-term study of allogeneic rat hindlimb transplants immunosuppressed with RS-61443, Transplantation 56, 911–917 (1993).
34. P. Benhaim, J. P. Anthony, L. Ferreira, J. P. Borsanyi, and S. J. Mathes, Use of combination of low-dose cyclosporine and RS-61443 in a rat hindlimb model of composite tissue allotransplantation, Transplantation 61, 527–532 (1996).

35. E. T. Ustuner, M. Zdichavsky, X. Ren, J. Edelstein, C. Maldonado, M. Ray, A. W. Jevans, W. C. Breidenbach, S. A. Gruber, J. H. Barker, and J. W. Jones, Long-term composite tissue allograft survival in a porcine model with cyclosporine/mycophenolate mofetil therapy, Transplantation 66, 1581–1587 (1998).
36. M. Lanzetta, P. Petruzzo, R. Margreiter, J. M. Dubernard, F. Schuind, W. Breidenbach, S. Lucchina, S. Schneeberger, C. van Holder, D. Granger, G. Pei, J. Zhao, and X. Zhang, The international registry on hand and composite tissue transplantation, Transplantation 79, 1210–1214 (2005).
37. M. Aboujaqude, H. Chen, J. Wu, et al., Efficacy of rapamycin in limb transplantation in the rat, Clin Invest Med 14, A146 (1991).
38. S. Inceoglu, M. Siemionow, L. Chick, C. M. Craven, and G. D. Lister, The effect of combined immunosuppression with systemic low-dose cyclosporin and topical fluocinolone acetonide on the survival of rat hind-limb allografts, Ann Plast Surg 33, 57–65 (1994).
39. L. S. Yeh, C. R. Gregory, S. M. Griffey, R. A. Lecouteur, and R. E. Morris, Effects of leflunomide and cyclosporine on myocutaneous allograft survival in the rat, Transplantation 62, 861–863 (1996).
40. K. Muramatsu, K. Doi, T. Akino, M. Shigetomi, and S. Kawai, Longer survival of rat limb allograft. Combined immunosuppression of FK-506 and 15-deoxyspergualin, Acta Orthop Scand 68, 581–585 (1997).
41. L. S. Yeh, C. R. Gregory, S. M. Griffey, R. A. Lecouter, S. M. Hou, and R. E. Morris, Combination leflunomide and cyclosporine prevents rejection of functional whole limb allografts in the rat, Transplantation 64, 919–922 (1997).
42. M. Vossen, R. K. Majzoub, J. Edelstein, G. Perez-Abadia, M. Voor, C. Maldonado, T. Tecimer, A. W. Jevans, M. Zdichavsky, J. M. Frank, C. Francois, M. Kon, and J. H. Barker, Bone quality in swine composite tissue allografts: Effects of combination immunotherapy, Transplantation 80, 487–493 (2005).
43. M. Vossen, J. Edelstein, R. K. Majzoub, C. Maldonado, G. Perez-Abadia, M. Voor, H. Orhun, T. Tecimer, C. Francois, M. Kon, and J. H. Barker, Bone quality and healing in swine vascularized bone allotransplantation model using cyclosporine-based immunosuppression therapy, Plast Reconstr Surg 115, 529–538 (2005).
44. J. C. Guimberteau, J. Baudet, B. Panconi, R. Boileau, and L. Potaux, Human allotransplant of a digital flexion system vascularized on the ulnar pedicle: A preliminary report and 1-year follow-up of two cases, Plast Reconstr Surg 89, 1135–1147 (1992).
45. G. O. Hofmann, M. H. Kirschner, F. D. Wagner, W. Land, and V. Buhren, Allogeneic vascularized grafting of a human knee joint with postoperative immunosuppression, Arch Orthop Trauma Surg 116, 125–128 (1997).
46. G. O. Hofmann, M. H. Kirschner, F. D. Wagner, L. Brauns, O. Gonschorek, and V. Buhren, Allogeneic vascularized transplantation of human femoral diaphyses and total knee joints–first clinical experiences, Transplant Proc 30, 2754–2761 (1998).
47. M. H. Kirschner, L. Brauns, O. Gonschorek, V. Buhren, and G. O. Hofmann, Vascularised knee joint transplantation in man: The first two years experience, Eur J Surg 166, 320–327 (2000).
48. M. H. Kirschner, F. D. Wagner, A. Nerlich, W. Land, V. Buhren, and G. O. Hofmann, Allogenic grafting of vascularized bone segments under immunosuppression. Clinical results in the transplantation of femoral diaphyses, Transpl Int 11, 195–203 (1998).
49. M. Strome, Human laryngeal transplantation: Considerations and implications, Microsurgery 20, 372–374 (2000).
50. M. Strome, J. Stein, R. Esclamado, D. Hicks, R. R. Lorenz, W. Braun, R. Yetman, I. Eliachar, and J. Mayes, Laryngeal transplantation and 40-month follow-up, N Eng J Med 344, 1676–1679 (2001).
51. Jones JW, Gruber SA, Barker JH, and Breidenbach WC, Successful hand transplantation: One-year follow-up, New Eng J Med 343, 468–473 (2000).
52. J. M. Dubernard, E. Owen, N. Lefrancois, P. Petruzzo, X. Martin, M. Dawahra, D. Jullien, J. Kanitakis, C. Frances, X. Preville, L. Gebuhrer, N. Hakim, M. Lanzetta, H. Kapila,

G. Herzberg, and J. P. Revillard, First human hand transplantation. Case report. Transpl Int 13 Suppl 1, S521–S524 (2000).
53. J. Kanitakis, D. Jullien, P. Petruzzo, N. Hakim, A. Claudy, J. P. Revillard, E. Owen, and J. M. Dubernard, Clinicopathologic features of graft rejection of the first human hand allograft. Transplantation 76, 688–693 (2003).
54. C. G. Francois, W. C. Breidenbach, C. Maldonado, T. P. Kakoulidis, A. Hodges, J. M. Dubernard, E. Owen, G. Pei, X. Ren, and J. H. Barker, Hand transplantation: Comparisons and observations of the first four clinical cases. Microsurgery 20, 360–371 (2000).
55. J. M. Dubernard, P. Petruzzo, M. Lanzetta, H. Parmentier, X. Martin, M. Dawahra, N. S. Hakim, and E. Owen, Functional results of the first human double-hand transplantation, Ann Surg 238, 128–136 (2003).
56. Mackinnon SE, Doolabh VB, Novak CB, and Trulock EP, Clinical outcome following nerve allograft transplantation, Plast Reconstr Surg 107, 1419–1429 (2001).
57. S. Hettiaratchy, M. A. Randolph, F. Petit, W. P. Lee, and P. E. Butler, Composite tissue allotransplantation–a new era in plastic surgery? Br J Plast Surg 57, 381–391 (2004).
58. M. R. Hausman, J. Masters, and A. Panozzo, Hand transplantation: Current status, Mt Sinai J Med 70, 148–153 (2003).
59. H. D. Kvernmo, V. S. Gorantla, R. N. Gonzalez, and W. C. Breidenbach, III, Hand transplantation. A future clinical option? Acta Orthop 76, 14–27 (2005).
60. B. Graham, P. Adkins, T. M. Tsai, J. Firrell, and W. C. Breidenbach, Major replantation versus revision amputation and prosthetic fitting in the upper extremity: A late functional outcomes study, J Hand Surg [Am] 23, 783–791 (1998).
61. K. L. Womer, R. S. Lee, J. G. Madsen, and M. H. Sayegh, Tolerance and chronic rejection, Phil Trans R Soc Lond B 356, 727–738 (2001).
62. J. D. Hosenpud, L. E. Bennett, B. M. Keck, M. M. Boucek, and R. J. Novick, The registry of the international society for heart and lung transplantation: Eighteenth official report-2001, J Heart Lung Transplant 20, 805–815 (2001).
63. S. Z. Gao, J. S. Schroeder, E. L. Alderman, S. A. Hunt, H. A. Valantine, V. Wiederhold, and E. B. Stinson, Prevalence of accelerated coronary artery disease in heart transplant survivors. Comparison of cyclosporine and azathioprine regimens, Circulation 80, III100–III105 (1989).
64. M. S. Orloff, E. M. DeMara, M. L. Coppage, N. Leong, M. A. Fallon, J. Sickel, X. J. Zuo, J. Prehn, and S. C. Jordan, Prevention of chronic rejection and graft arteriosclerosis by tolerance induction, Transplantation 59, 282–288 (1995).
65. Cecka JM and Terasaki PI, The UNOS Scientific Renal Transplant Registry. In *Clinical Transplants 1994*, ed. by Terasaki PI and Cecka JM, pp. 1–18. UCLA Tissue Typing Laboratory, Los Angeles, CA (1994).
66. A. Tejani and E. K. Sullivan, The impact of acute rejection on chronic rejection: A report of the North American Pediatric Renal Transplant Cooperative Study, Pediatric Transplantation 4, 107–111 (2000).
67. A. Lindholm, S. Ohlman, D. Albrechtsen, G. Tufveson, H. Persson, and N. H. Persson, The impact of acute rejection episodes on long-term graft function and outcome in 1347 primary renal transplants treated by 3 cyclosporine regimens, Transplantation 56, 307–315 (1993).
68. S. Hariharan, C. P. Johnson, B. A. Bresnahan, S. E. Taranto, M. J. McIntosh, and D. Stablein, Improved graft survival after renal transplantation in the United States, 1988 to 1996, N Engl J Med 342, 605–612 (2000).
69. G. P. Basadonna, A. J. Matas, K. J. Gillingham, W. D. Payne, D. L. Dunn, D. E. Sutherland, P. F. Gores, R. W. Gruessner, and J. S. Najarian, Early versus late acute renal allograft rejection: Impact on chronic rejection, Transplantation 55, 993–995 (1993).
70. M. J. Brenner, J. N. Jensen, J. B. Lowe, III, T. M. Myckatyn, I. K. Fox, D. A. Hunter, T. Mohanakumar, and S. E. Mackinnon, Anti-CD40 ligand antibody permits regeneration through peripheral nerve allografts in a nonhuman primate model, Plast Reconstr Surg 114, 1802–1814 (2004).

71. B. A. Bradley, Rejection and recipient age, Transpl Immunol 10, 125–132 (2002).
72. L. R. Raiz, K. M. Kilty, M. L. Henry, and R. M. Ferguson, Medication compliance following renal transplantation, Transplantation 68, 51–55 (1999).
73. Z. A. Massy, C. Guijarro, M. R. Wiederkehr, J. Z. Ma, and B. L. Kasiske, Chronic renal allograft rejection: Immunologic and nonimmunologic risk factors, Kidney Int 49, 518–524 (1996).
74. B. Kaplan, J. D. Schold, and H. U. Meier-Kriesche, Long-term graft survival with neoral and tacrolimus: A paired kidney analysis, J Am Soc Nephrol 14, 2980–2984 (2003).
75. R. Mendez, T. Gonwa, H. C. Yang, S. Weinstein, S. Jensik, and S. Steinberg, A prospective, randomized trial of tacrolimus in combination with sirolimus or mycophenolate mofetil in kidney transplantation: Results at 1 year, Transplantation 80, 303–309 (2005).
76. A. Humar, A. Hassoun, R. Kandaswamy, W. D. Payne, D. E. Sutherland, and A. J. Matas, Immunologic factors: The major risk for decreased long-term renal allograft survival, Transplantation 68, 1842–1846 (1999).
77. R. J. Knight, L. Burrows, and C. Bodian, The influence of acute rejection on long-term renal allograft survival: A comparison of living and cadaveric donor transplantation, Transplantation 72, 69–76 (2001).
78. S. A. Joosten, Y. W. Sijpkens, C. van Kooten, and L. C. Paul, Chronic renal allograft rejection: Pathophysiologic considerations, Kidney Int 68, 1–13 (2005).
79. G. Remuzzi, Transplantation tolerance: Facts and future, Transplant Proc 31, 2955–2957 (1999).
80. J. K. Cooper, G. A. Patterson, and E. P. Trulock, Results of single and bilateral lung transplantation in 131 consecutive recipients, J Thorac Cardiovasc Surg 107, 460–471 (1994).
81. J. Kanitakis, D. Jullien, P. Petruzzo, C. Frances, A. Claudy, J. Revillard, and J. Dubernard, Immunohistologic studies of the skin of human hand allografts: Our experience with two patients, Transplant Proc 33, 1722 (2001).

Chapter 12
Locoregional Immunosuppression in Composite Tissue Allografting

Scott A. Gruber

12.1 Introduction

Unlike visceral solid-organ transplants, composite tissue allografts (CTAs) are modules composed of various tissues, each with differing antigenicity, and therefore differing potential for rejection.[1] Skin and muscle (and perhaps synovium) are the most antigenic and appear to be most susceptible to rejection, while bone, tendon, cartilage, and neurovascular tissue appear to be less immunogenic and evoke rejection responses of lower magnitude. Although CTAs have tremendous potential clinical application for functional and structural reconstruction of major congenital and acquired peripheral tissue defects, these transplants have remained one of the last frontiers in clinical organ transplantation because of concerns expressed beginning 15–20 years ago regarding their risk/benefit ratio.[2,3] Even now, with the performance of unilateral hand, bilateral hand, or digit transplantation in a total of 18 patients from 1998 to 2004,[4] there still remains much concern with regard to the risks of long-term immunosuppression and the potential for development of chronic rejection.[5–7] The following two questions address the key issues involved. (1) Can rejection of these highly antigenic tissues be prevented using currently available immunosuppressive regimens with acceptable drug-specific and generalized toxicity? (2) Will function be restored to a significant degree so as to justify the surgical and immunosuppressive risks involved?

Information recently provided on 18 CTA recipients followed for 17–70 months in the aforementioned inaugural report of the International Registry on Hand and Composite Tissue Transplantation has begun to shed some light on the answers to these questions.[4] Virtually all patients received a form of antilymphocyte antibody for induction (Thymoglobulin [ATG] and/or Basiliximab), and tacrolimus (TCL), mycophenolate mofetil, and prednisone therapy for maintenance immunosuppression. Despite this clinically acceptable but nonetheless intensive immunosuppressive regimen, akin to that currently utilized for rejection-prone, nonuremic, insulin-dependent diabetics who receive a pancreas transplant,[8] two of the three patients experienced at least one episode of acute rejection and 50% of patients experienced multiple episodes. In most cases, the episodes were reversed following combination intravenous and/or oral "pulse" steroid and topical TCL-clobetasol cream treatment,

C. W. Hewitt et al. (eds.), *Transplantation of Composite Tissue Allografts*.
© Springer 2008

but in eight instances, ATG ($n=2$), Basiliximab ($n=5$), or Campath 1-H ($n=1$) was required,[9] further significantly increasing the already-elevated immunosuppressive burden in these patients. Along these lines, five recipients developed CMV infection or disease, with the majority of these cases requiring second-line agents more toxic than ganciclovir or valganciclovir to achieve long-term control of viral infection.[10] Metabolic complications from the immunosuppressants included transient hyperglycemia ($n=9$), increased serum creatinine ($n=2$), Cushing's syndrome ($n=1$), and avascular necrosis of the hip ($n=1$). Overall, patient and graft survival were 100% and 89%, respectively, with one of the two graft losses due to noncompliance. All patients achieved protective sensation with 17 achieving discriminative sensation, and extrinsic and intrinsic muscle recovery enabled patients to perform most daily activities. These intermediate-term results suggest that clinical application of CTAs is more likely to gain widespread acceptance if the systemic immunosuppressive burden and its attendant long-term risks of infection, drug-specific side-effects, and although not yet encountered, malignancy, could be reduced while simultaneously preventing rejection and maintaining function.

12.2 Local Immunosuppression

One approach toward reducing the drug-specific and general adverse consequences of systemic immunosuppression in CTA recipients, and thereby improving the clinical feasibility of the procedure, is the utilization of local drug administration systems to establish a more selective presence of currently available nonspecific immunosuppressive agents in the transplanted limb or limb component, with a concomitant reduction in systemic drug exposure.[11] Interestingly, the first report illustrating this concept appeared as early as 1951, in which Billingham et al.[12] found that topical application of cortisone acetate at a dosage that was ineffective when administered systemically prolonged skin allograft survival in a rabbit model. This work was followed by conflicting reports regarding the effectiveness of local treatment of canine and human renal allografts with a variety of antimetabolites and corticosteroids administered via indwelling arterial catheters in the late 1960s.[13–15] With the exception of experimental and clinical studies demonstrating the efficacy of local graft irradiation,[16,17] further examination of local immunosuppression was abandoned for 15 years, awaiting technological advances in drug-delivery systems and a better understanding of both the cellular events within the rejecting allograft and the pharmacokinetics of target-aimed drug delivery.[18]

In 1986, Ruers et al.[19] demonstrated that continuous intra-arterial (IA) infusion of prednisolone in rat renal allograft recipients produced a significant increase in graft survival when compared with same-dose systemic administration. This work was rapidly followed by multiple reports of favorable experiences with local immunosuppressive therapy utilizing a variety of different agents in rat heterotopic cardiac, renal, pancreatic islet cell, and liver allograft models[11,20,21] and in canine renal and liver allografts models.[22–25] In each case, allograft survival was significantly prolonged with IA drug delivery over that achievable with same-dose IV administration. Along these lines, orally administered immunosuppressants with a high first-pass metabolism in either the small intestine or liver, such as the steroid budesonide, have been found to be efficacious either alone or in combination with cyclosporin A (CSA), in preventing rejection of rat liver and intestinal transplants, respectively, with minimal systemic drug exposure.[26,27] Moreover, other targeting systems, such as drug-impregnated polymer rods, controlled-release drug matrices, liposomes, gene transfer, and cellular cotransplantation, have all been effectively used in small-animal models to direct immunosuppressants to the transplanted organ of interest.[28] Finally, the concept of local immunosuppression has already been applied clinically in lung transplantation, with demonstration of the safety and effectiveness of aerosolized CSA in treating allograft recipients with refractory acute[29] and chronic[30] rejection.

Extremity CTAs, such as a hand or limb transplant, are well suited for local drug delivery as a result of two special features. First, unlike a solid-organ transplant which is "hidden" within a body cavity, the skin of a CTA is exposed and continuously available for the use of topically applied immunosuppression. Second, the relatively low blood flow in the upper extremity would theoretically produce a considerable regional pharmacokinetic advantage of IA drug infusion not achievable in other high-flow transplantable organs such as the liver and kidney, as long as tissue blood flow was low relative to drug clearance.[31] The remainder of this report will review the previous pharmacokinetic and pharmacodynamic results of topical and IA infusion therapy in small-animal skin and CTA models.

12.3 Topical Therapy

Following the initial report of Billingham et al.,[12] further examination of the effect of topical treatment on skin allograft survival awaited the introduction of CSA more than 35 years later. Lai and colleagues[32] utilized a topical CSA preparation containing the solvent DMSO in Buffalo-to-Lewis rat skin allograft recipients. Graft survival was dependent upon both dose and interval of administration, with 5-mg CSA producing long-term survival only if administered daily and 10 mg only if applied no less frequently than every other day. Importantly, considerable systemic absorption of CSA occurred in these animals, with mean steady-state whole-blood levels in the 400–1,600 ng/ml range by HPLC near the end of the second week. However, it was difficult to attribute prolongation of graft survival entirely to a systemic effect, since 10-day application of 5 and 10 mg CSA doses to nearby normal recipient skin significantly decreased mean graft survivals from those obtained with direct donor allograft administration of the same doses (16.4–13.9 days and 18.7–16.7 days, respectively), but not down to (untreated) control values (7.4 days). Unfortunately, the authors did not obtain whole-blood drug concentrations in these two groups of animals, nor did they obtain skin tissue CSA levels in any group studied.

In 1988, Black et al.[33] examined the ability of five different formulations of topical CSA to prolong survival of LBN-to-Lewis skin allografts. Although none of the preparations prolonged graft survival when used alone, several formulations were effective when topical treatment was instituted immediately following an initial 10-day course of subcutaneous CSA when compared with controls receiving only systemic treatment. No whole-blood or local tissue CSA concentrations were determined in this study, but the authors hypothesized that systemic therapy was required during a more immunologically challenging "induction phase," before "maintenance-phase" topical therapy could be used effectively.

This hypothesis was further tested by the Irvine group 2 years later using a dual skin allograft model in the same rat strain combination.[34] Following an initial 10-day course of subcutaneous CSA, application of topical CSA significantly enhanced mean graft survival compared with that of vehicle-treated control grafts placed contralaterally on the same animal (45 days versus 28 days, respectively). Importantly, mean whole-blood CSA levels rapidly dropped 16-fold over the 2-week period following cessation of systemic therapy (2,051 ng/ml on day 11 versus 129 ng/ml on day 25), and remained subtherapeutic from this point on (e.g., 69 ng/ml on day 38). This data, when combined with demonstration of (1) 22-fold-higher mean local tissue concentrations of CSA in the drug-treated versus vehicle-treated grafts on day 36; (2) intact or supranormal systemic immune responses on days 31–33; and (3) decreased MHC class I and class II expression and CD4+ lymphocyte infiltration in the allografts during local treatment,[35] strongly suggested that the topical preparation was not significantly absorbed and exerted a locally immunosuppressive effect.

A synergistic effect of oral CSA and fluocinolone acetonide (FA), a topical corticosteroid, on Buffalo-to-Lewis split-thickness skin allograft survival was demonstrated by Zhao and colleagues.[36] Administration of low-dose oral CSA (5.0 mg/kg/d) or topical corticosteroid alone modestly prolonged mean survival time from 10 (untreated controls) to 14 and 24 days, respectively. However, coadministration of the two agents significantly prolonged survival, so that four of seven grafts survived beyond 100 days. The further addition of topical CSA resulted in all (five of five) grafts surviving beyond 100 days. The degree of systemic absorption of the topical steroid was not addressed, since blood levels were not obtained. However, the addition of topical to oral CSA did not significantly increase whole-blood CSA levels, suggesting that topical CSA was exerting its beneficial effect via local mechanisms. These results were extended to the rat hindlimb allograft model by Inceoglu et al.,[37] who subsequently demonstrated that combination of low-dose subcutaneous CSA (4.0 mg/kg/d) and topical FA significantly prolonged overall limb survival rates when compared with either treatment alone. In contrast to single-agent therapy, skin rejection was completely prevented. However, bacterial infiltrates were present in the skin of the majority of animals in this combination therapy group, with uniform findings of progressive weight loss and muscle wasting. These observations, when taken together with the demonstration of FA in the dermis, suggested that systemic absorption of the glucocorticoid contributed to the global immunosuppressive effect produced.

In a follow-up study using the rat dual skin allograft model, Llull et al.[38] examined the effect of combination topical CSA and topical hydrocortisone following a 10-day course of systemic CSA. Coadministration beginning at day 10 was no more effective than topical CSA alone in producing a disparity in survival between experimental and vehicle-treated grafts. However, if topical CSA alone was applied first until initial signs of rejection occurred, and then the combination was begun, a significant disparity in graft survival (synergism) was observed. These results suggest that the timing of corticosteroid addition during immune response induction in combination with CSA may be critical to the efficacy of treatment.

On the basis of the data available from the above studies, one would conclude that topical CSA alone, in the absence of systemic drug absorption or prior systemic drug administration, is not effective in prolonging skin graft/CTA survival. This is in contrast to subsequently reported results in murine and rat skin transplant models using TCL ointment, in which topical application alone significantly prolonged primary skin allograft survival with undetectable systemic drug concentrations.[39,40] Although the relative contribution to rejection reversal made by the systemic and topical (TCL/clobetasol) components of therapy utilized in the hand transplant recipients remains unclear,[4] the clinical use of locally delivered immunosuppression in the management of acute rejection may have obviated the need for antilymphocyte antibody rescue in some of these patients.

12.4 IA Infusion

We developed a vascularly isolated rabbit forelimb model simulating conditions of composite tissue allografting to determine the regional pharmacokinetic advantage achievable in extremity tissue components during IA immunosuppressive drug delivery.[41] In this model, interruption of collateral circulation through the muscle bundles at mid-arm level and ligation of all side branches made the brachial artery the sole source of blood flow to the distal extremity while leaving bone, innervation, and vasculature intact.

In the first study, CSA was infused continuously via osmotic minipump into the right brachial artery at multiple doses ranging from 1.0 to 8.0 mg/kg/d.[42] On day 6, CSA concentrations were measured in aortic whole blood, as well as in skin, muscle, bone, and bone marrow samples from both right and left forelimbs. At 1.0 mg/kg/d, there were no significant differences between right and left mean CSA concentrations for all four tissues examined. However, with a doubling of the IA dose, huge increases in local tissue CSA concentrations were produced with only very modest increases in systemic whole-blood and tissue drug levels, resulting in a fourfold regional advantage (right:left ratio of CSA concentrations) in bone and bone marrow, sevenfold in muscle, and 14-fold in skin. With further dose increases to 8.0 mg/kg/d, the regional advantage decreased to fourfold in skin, increased to ninefold in bone marrow, remained relatively constant in bone, and initially decreased and then increased to ninefold in muscle. These favorable pharmacokinetic results suggested that reduced, local doses of CSA might be useful in preventing extremity CTA rejection with decreased systemic drug exposure.

In contrast, when the above study protocol was repeated using TCL, only a minimal regional advantage of local drug delivery (mean right/left concentration ratios 1.0:1.4) was obtained in all forearm tissues over the 0.05–0.2 mg/kg/d dose range studied.[43] We concluded that TCL was pharmacokinetically inferior to CSA for continuous IA administration to the vascularly isolated rabbit forelimb, and hypothesized that this difference was the result of differences in the distribution of each drug within whole blood. When compared with CSA, TCL is much more strongly bound by red blood cells and presumably is released too slowly to the plasma to get into the tissue as free drug during its first passage through the arterial blood supply of the limb.

12.5 Conclusion

Experimental work in rodent skin and hindlimb allograft models, as well as anecdotal clinical experience from 18 hand transplant patients, suggests that topical formulations of glucocorticoid, CSA, and TCL, individually or in combination, may play a useful adjunctive role together with systemic therapy in the prophylaxis and treatment of acute CTA rejection. While TCL may be more efficacious than CSA when used topically, our results in the vascularly isolated rabbit forelimb model suggest that CSA would be a much more appropriate agent for continuous IA infusion. Finally, the timing of locoregional administration of immunosuppressants relative to each other and to concomitant systemic therapy may be critical to achieving maximal efficacy. It is certainly possible that local administration of immunosuppressive agents via the topical or IA route during the early posttransplant "induction" period may decrease the subsequent requirements for systemic maintenance therapy to prevent rejection.[44]

References

1. W. P. Lee, M. J. Yaremchuk, Y. C. Pan, M. A. Randolph, C. M. Tan, A. J. Weiland, Relative antigenicity of components of a vascularized limb allograft, Plast Reconstr Surg 87, 401–411 (1991).
2. J. P. Paskert, M. J. Yaremchuk, M. A. Randolph, A. J. Weiland, The role of cyclosporin in prolonging survival in vascularized bone allografts, Plast Reconstr Surg 80, 240–247 (1987).
3. Rehabilitation Research and Development Service: Composite Tissue Transplantation Workshop. Department of Veteran Affairs, (1991).
4. M. Lanzetta P. Petruzzo, R. Margreiter, et al., The international registry on hand and composite tissue transplantation, Transplantation 79,1210–1214 (2005).
5. F. Petit, A. B. Minns, J. M. Dubernard, S. Hettiaratchy, W. P. Lee, Composite tissue allotransplantation and reconstructive surgery: first clinical applications, Ann Surg 237,19–25 (2003).

6. P. Petruzzo, L. Badet, M. Lanzetta, J. M. Dubernard, Concerns on clinical application of composite tissue allotransplantation, Acta Chir Belg 104, 266–271 (2004).
7. S. Hettiaratchy, M. A. Randolph, F. Petit, W. P. Lee, P. E. Butler, Composite tissue allotransplantation – a new era in plastic surgery? Br J Plast Surg 57, 381–391 (2004).
8. S. A. Gruber, S. Katz, B. Kaplan, et al., Initial results of solitary pancreas transplants performed without regard to donor/recipient HLA mismatching, Transplantation 70, 388–391 (2000).
9. S. Schneeberger, A. Kreczy, G. Brandacher, W. Steurer, R. Margreiter, Steroid- and ATG-resistant rejection after double forearm transplantation responds to Campath-1H, Am J Transplant 4, 1372–1374 (2004).
10. S. Schneeberger, S. Lucchina, M. Lanzetta, et al., Cytomegalovirus-related complications in human hand transplantation, Transplantation 80, 441–447 (2005).
11. S. A. Gruber, Locoregional immunosuppression of organ transplants, Immunol Rev 129, 5–30 (1992).
12. R. E. Billingham, P. L. Krohn, P. B. Medawar, Effect of locally applied cortisone acetate on survival of skin homografts in rabbits, Br Med J 1, 1049–1053 (1951).
13. A. B. Retik, J. M. Dubernard, W. J. Hester, J. E. Murray, A study of the effects of intra-arterial immunosuppressive drug therapy on canine renal allografts, Surgery 60, 1242–1250 (1966).
14. J. J. Terz, R. Crampton, D. Miller, W. Lawrence, Regional infusion chemotherapy for prolongation of kidney allografts, J Surg Res 9, 13–18 (1969).
15. S. L. Kountz, R. B. Cohn, Initial treatment of renal allografts with large intrarenal doses of immunosuppressive drugs, Lancet 1, 338–340 (1969).
16. N. F. Gergely, J. C. Coles, Prolongation of heterotopic cardiac allografts in dogs by topical radiation, Transplantation 9, 193–202 (1970).
17. E. C. Halperin, F. L. Delmonico, P. W. Nelson, W. U. Shipley, A. B. Cosimi, The use of local allograft irradiation following renal transplantation, J Radiat Oncol Biol Phys 10, 987–990 (1984).
18. W. W. Eckman, C. S. Patlak, J. D. Fenstermacher, A critical evaluation of the principles governing the advantages of intraarterial infusions, J Pharmacokinet Biopharm 2, 257–285 (1974).
19. T. J. M. Ruers, W. A. Buurman, J. F. M. Smits, et al., Local treatment of renal allografts, a promising way to reduce the dosage of immunosuppressive drugs, Transplantation 41, 156–161 (1986).
20. S. A. Gruber, Local immunosuppressive therapy in organ transplantation, Transplant Proc 26, 3214–3216 (1994).
21. K. Yano, Y. Fukuda, R. Sumimoto, K. Sunimoto, H. Ito, K. Dohi, Suppression of liver allograft rejection by administration of 15-deoxyspergualin, Transpl Int 7, 149–156 (1994).
22. S. A. Gruber, W. J. M. Hrushesky, R. J. Cipolle, et al., Local immunosuppression with reduced systemic toxicity in a canine renal allograft model, Transplantation 48, 936–943 (1989).
23. S. A. Gruber, G. R. Erdmann, B. A. Burke, et al., Mizoribine pharmacokinetics and pharmacodynamics in a canine renal allograft model of local immunosuppression, Transplantation 53, 12–19 (1992).
24. S. Ko, Y. Nakajima, H. Kanehiro, et al., The significance of local immunosuppression in canine liver transplantation, Transplantation 57, 1818–1821 (1994).
25. N. Yoshimura, T. Hamashima, Y. Nakamura, Y. Sudo, H. Yura, T. Oka, Effect of local immunosuppressive therapy with FK 506 on renal allograft survival in the mongrel dog, Transplant Proc 30, 3110–3111 (1998).
26. T. Weber, T. Kalbhenn, G. Herrmann, E. Hanisch, Local immunosuppression with budesonide after liver transplantation in the rat: a preliminary histomorphological analysis, Transplantation 64, 705–708 (1997).
27. N. Ozcay, J. Fryer, D. Grant, D. Freeman, B. Garcia, R. Zhong, Budesonide, a locally acting steroid, prevents graft rejection in a rat model of intestinal transplantation, Transplantation 63, 1220–1225 (1997).

28. S. A. Gruber (ed), Local Immunosuppression of Organ Transplants. Austin: R. G. Landes Company (Medical Intelligence Unit Series) (1996).
29. R. J. Keenan, A. Iacono, J. H. Dauber, et al., Treatment of refractory acute allograft rejection with aerosolized cyclosporine in lung transplant recipients, J Thorac Cardiovasc Surg 113, 335–340 (1997).
30. A. T. Iacono, R. J. Keenan, S. R. Duncan, et al., Aerosolized cyclosporine in lung recipients with refractory chronic rejection, Am J Respir Crit Care Med 153, 1451–1455 (1996).
31. J. M. Collins, Pharmacologic rationale for regional drug delivery, J Clin Oncol 2, 498–504 (1984).
32. C.-S. Lai, T. A. Wesseler Jr., J. W. Alexander, G. F. Babcock, Long-term survival of skin allografts in rats treated with topical cyclosporine, Transplantation 44, 83–87 (1987).
33. K. S. Black, C. W. Hewitt, C. L. C. Chau, L. Pizzo, Transdermal application of cyclosporine prolongs skin allograft survival, Transplant Proc 20, 660–662 (1988).
34. K. S. Black, D. K. Nguyen, C. M. Proctor, et al., Site-specific suppression of cell-mediated immunity by cyclosporine, J Invest Dermatol 94, 644–648 (1990).
35. K. S. Black, M. P. Patel, A. P. Patel, et al., Mechanisms of site-specific immunosuppression, Transplant Proc 23, 120–121 (1991).
36. X.-F. Zhao, J. W. Alexander, T. Schroeder, G. F. Babcock, The synergistic effect of low-dose cyclosporine and fluocinolone acetonide on the survival of rat allogeneic skin grafts, Transplantation 46, 490–492 (1988).
37. S. Inceoglu, M. Siemionow, L. Chick, C. M. Craven, G. D. Lister, The effect of combined immunosuppression with systemic low-dose cyclosporin and topical fluocinolone acetonide on the survival of rat hind-limb allografts, Ann Plast Surg 33, 57–65 (1994).
38. R. Llull, T. P. Lee, A. N. Vu, K. S. Black, C. W. Hewitt, Site-specific immune suppression with topical cyclosporine. Synergism with combined topical corticosteroid added during the maintenance phase, Transplantation 59, 1483–1485 (1995).
39. K. Yuzawa, H. Taniguchi, K. Seino, M. Otsuka, K. Fukao, Topical immunosuppression in skin grafting with FK 506 ointment, Transplant Proc 28, 1387–1389 (1996).
40. T. Fujita, S. Takahashi, A. Yagihashi, K. Jimbow, N. Sato, Prolonged survival of rat skin allograft by treatment with FK506 ointment, Transplantation 64, 922–925 (1997).
41. M. V. Shirbacheh, X. Ren, J. W. Jones, et al., Pharmacokinetic advantage of intraarterial cyclosporine delivery to the vascularly-isolated rabbit forelimb. I. Model development, J Pharmacol Exp Ther 289, 1185–1190 (1999).
42. M. V. Shirbacheh, T. A. Harralson, J. W. Jones, et al., Pharmacokinetic advantage of intraarterial cyclosporine delivery to the vascularly-isolated rabbit forelimb. II. Dose-dependence, J Pharmacol Exp Ther 289, 1191–1195 (1999).
43. M. V. Shirbacheh, T. A. Harralson, J. W. Jones, et al, Pharmacokinetics of intraarterial delivery of tacrolimus to the vascularly-isolated rabbit forelimb, J Pharmacol Exp Ther 289, 1196–1201 (1999).
44. S. A. Gruber, The case for local immunosuppression, Transplantation 54, 1–11 (1992).

Chapter 13
New Approaches to Antibody Therapy

Dalibor Vasilic, Moshe Kon, and Cedric G. Francois

13.1 Historical Perspective

The past years have seen the emergence of a new field in plastic surgery: composite tissue allotransplantation (CTA). While it has been used differently depending on context, CTA generally applies to the allotransplantation of vascularized tissues for the purpose of tissue reconstruction. While CTA has been performed for a few decades now (vascularized tendon and bone allotransplants were performed in select experimental settings as early as the 1980s and 1990s), the holy grail of CTA – the transplantation of vascularized tissues that contain a skin component – was achieved only recently (September 23, 1998) with the first human hand transplantation in Lyon (France).

The allotransplantation of a hand, 54 years after the first kidney transplantation, was considered a landmark accomplishment. While the reconstructive aspects of the procedure were – and are – relatively straightforward, the skin is highly susceptible to immune rejection, and no immunosuppressive regimen prior to 1998[1] had been efficacious at preventing the rejection of a transplanted hand.

Hand transplantation, and recently face transplantation,[2] became possible with the advent of new immunosuppressive regimens, an era inaugurated by the introduction of cyclosporine in 1978. Ultimately, the combination regimen of tacrolimus (also called FK506), mycophenolate mofetil (MMF), and steroids fostered the first successful hand transplantation. In recent years, other immunosuppressive agents acting via different mechanisms have been introduced. While these agents are changing the way CTA recipients are induced or desensitized immediately following transplantation, it is important to point out that the maintenance immunosuppressive regimen following CTA is still roughly the same as it was at the time of the first procedures, when it was first established by Ustuner et al.[3]

To understand antibody therapies in CTA, it is important to consider our historical understanding of immune rejection and the difference between immunosuppression and immunomodulation as two different approaches toward preventing it.

13.1.1 Immunosuppression

The history of immunosuppression can be described as a five-decade (successful) attempt to suppress the immune system to the largest extent possible to prevent rejection. It is an approach deeply rooted in the Medawarian principle that the immune system continuously surveys the organism for elements that are "nonself." When such elements are found, they are destroyed. Consequently, by "suppressing" the surveyors (via inactivation or immobilization), rejection can be prevented. The Medawarian understanding of the immune system can actually be compared to Newtonian physics: it is brilliant, easy-to-understand and surprisingly practical. However, while the concept of immunosuppression has revolutionized the field of transplantation surgery, it is far from perfect. Immunosuppression has many undesired secondary effects, including opportunistic infections, end-organ failure, and posttransplant lymphoproliferative disease, all of which are associated with significant morbidity and mortality. Most importantly, the need for immunosuppression is lifelong. Because the "surveyor" cells are contained rather than educated into accepting the transplanted graft as "self," suspension of immunosuppressive therapy makes them immediately available again for graft rejection. The concept of educating the immune system rather than suppressing it is called immunomodulation.

13.1.2 Immunomodulation

Immunomodulation refers to the modulation or coaxing of the immune system into a specific behavior. This can refer to a rejection response against, e.g., neoplasia, or to a dampened response in, e.g., cases of asthma. The holy grail of immunomodulation in the field of transplantation is "tolerance." In "tolerant" recipients, allogeneic organs are accepted by the immune system without the need for lifelong immunosuppression. The goal of immune tolerance has special importance to the field of CTA, where some question whether the benefit of a nonlife saving organ warrants the risks of immunosuppression, a debate that has hampered the acceptance of CTA as a widespread clinical procedure.

Unfortunately, in spite of important recent advances, immune tolerance as a practical alternative to immunosuppression has eluded us for decades and will likely continue to do so for years to come. Like in quantum physics, the intricacies of the immune system are far more complex, impractical, and poorly understood than inferred from the Medawarian principle. In the meantime, however, new, promising immune modulating agents are opening a window into reducing the need for immunosuppression. Especially promising are some of the new antibodies that are finding their way into the clinic.

13.2 Antibodies in CTA

13.2.1 What are Antibodies?

Antibodies are members of the family of biologicals. Biologicals refer to polypeptides and proteins, as opposed to the small chemical molecules that are the hallmark of pharmaceutical agents. On the basis of their mode of action, biologicals can be separated into two categories: biomimetic molecules and antibodies. Biomimetic molecules mimic endogenous proteins. When administered to the human body, they can thus increase the modulating activities of their endogenous counterparts. Because the immune system's functions depend on the carefully crafted balance between endogenous immune modulators, it is a logical approach in which many exciting new avenues are currently being explored in mainly preclinical programs. They will not be the subjects of discussion in this chapter.

Antibodies have a different mode of action. Antibodies are molecules that bind with high specificity and affinity to molecules implicated in pathogenesis. By binding to their target, antibodies can thus successfully prevent or reverse disease processes. While seemingly a perfect model for drug development (they were first explored for their therapeutic potential in the 1970s and were long heralded as the ultimate "cure-for-all-diseases"), antibodies have the disadvantage of being large molecules (a typical IgG antibody is ~150kD in size). Because of their size, they can themselves become targets of immune rejection. This is especially true since most therapeutic antibodies are discovered in nonhuman species such as mice and need to be "humanized" (i.e., changing their amino acid sequence to prevent human immune reactions) for use in patients. The humanization of antibodies is a challenging and expensive operation.

In spite of these difficulties, antibodies have been finding their way to transplantation, and are playing increasingly important roles in the field.

13.2.2 Which Antibodies are Useful in Transplantation?

Virtually all antibodies used in clinical transplantation target a single cell type: T cells. T cells are the principal mediators in acquired immunity[4] and allograft rejection,[5] and silencing, eliminating, or modulating T-cell responses has been the guiding strategic principle of most immunosuppressive and immunomodulatory therapies.

Antibodies have the ability to target T cells and remove them from circulation. They can do so in a nonspecific way or they can target particular T-cell subpopulations to refine the modulatory purpose.

Because of their suitability to one of both purposes, antibodies in the field of transplantation are usually classified into two categories: polyclonal and monoclonal antibodies. A further distinction can be made as to their clinical use in induction, desensitization, antirejection, or antibody-mediated rejection (AMR) therapy.

13.2.3 Monoclonal Versus Polyclonal

Polyclonal antibodies are antibodies that are derived from different B-cell lines. They are a mixture of immunoglobulin molecules directed against a specific antigen, each recognizing a different epitope. Polyclonal antibodies are typically produced by immunization of suitable mammals, such as mice, rabbits, or horses. The antigen in combination with an adjuvant is injected into the mammal according to standard protocols. This induces the B-lymphocytes to produce IgG immunoglobulins specific for the antigen. This IgG can then be isolated and purified from the serum.

The first class of antibodies used to target T cells belonging to the class of polyclonal antilymphocyte agents, i.e., antisera. Antisera quickly became recognized for delaying allograft rejection, prolonging allograft survival,[6] and even inducing tolerance in certain preclinical models.[7] Subsequent studies performed in nonhuman primates,[8] and eventually humans, established antilymphocyte globulins as a basis of induction therapy (see below). Interestingly, the seminal experiments that heralded the importance and efficacy of antibody-based therapies utilized allograft skin transplantation, a highly immunogenic component found in almost any current CTA model.

Monoclonal antibodies (mAb) are antibodies that react against a single well-defined epitope because they were produced by the same B-cell line, all clones of a single parent cell. Monoclonal antibodies are more difficult to produce, but have the important advantage of controllable target binding. Furthermore, the new monoclonal antibody engineering methods confer significantly lower immunogenicity and therefore allow the possibility for repeated courses.

The discovery of monoclonal antibodies represented an important step forward in the field of transplantation, not only for their novel quality to discriminate among lymphocyte subpopulations,[9] but also for their potent lymphocyte depletion/immunomodulatory effect.[10]

13.2.4 Clinical Use of Antibodies

13.2.4.1 Induction Agents

Antibodies used for this purpose can be either monoclonal (daclizumab, basiliximab, muromonab-CD3 or OKT3, and alemtuzumab or CAMPATH-1H) or polyclonal (rabbit or equine antithymocyte globulins) and can be administered shortly before and during the operation and in the postoperative period. Their main purpose is the induction of potent suppression of adverse immunologic activity targeting an allograft at the time of transplantation.

On the basis of the data from The International Registry on Hand and Composite Tissue Transplantation, the majority of hand transplant recipients received ATG (rabbit antithymocyte globulins) and basiliximab (monoclonal anti-IL-2R antibody),[11] while the majority of abdominal wall allotransplant recipients were pretreated with alemtuzumab.[12] Induction immunosuppressive protocol in the first human face allotransplant was based on ATG.[2]

13.2.4.2 Desensitization Agents

Antibodies can also be used to neutralize the deleterious effects of antihuman leukocyte antigen (anti-HLA) antibodies which develop as a result of sensitization to HLA. Anti-HLA can prevent successful transplantation for a prolonged period of time or in the worst case scenario pose a near exclusionary barrier to transplantation.

Current desensitization treatments consist of intravenous immunoglobulin (IVIg) or combination of plasmapheresis and IVIg. Pretransplant treatment with rituximab, a monoclonal anti-CD20 antibody, has shown some promising results reducing allosensitization and increasing a chance of successful transplantation.[13,14] To our knowledge there have been no reports of desensitization regimens in CTA. However, development and introduction of desensitizing agents may prove of particular importance in CTA because a majority of severely disfigured patients have received multiple blood transfusions or have been treated with skin allografts and therefore at increased risk of sensitization.

13.2.4.3 Antirejection Agents

Antibodies can also be used to treat severe, steroid-resistant, and refractory acute rejection episodes. A number of antibodies used in induction therapy are also used for this particular indication. Muromonab-CD3 is highly effective in reversing acute rejection, but its poor tolerability has limited its use.[15] CAMPATH-1H, a specific and highly potent immunosuppressive antibody, has recently been gaining interest as both an induction agent as well as an effective antirejection drug.[16] Anti-IL-2R antibodies, although sporadically used against acute rejection,[11] are generally assumed to be inefficient in halting an ongoing acute rejection.

13.2.4.4 Antibody-Mediated Rejection Therapies

AMR is a recently described and unique form of acute rejection that is mainly mediated by antibody driven responses. This form of antibody-mediated rejection has failed to show response to immunosuppressive treatments targeting T cells, and hence has rekindled interest in the pathophysiological role of B cells and innate immunity, specifically complement activation. Current therapies against AMR have been tailored to reduce effects of anti-HLA sensitization and block complement action by administering high-dose IVIg, rituximab, and plasmapheresis plus anticytomegalovirus (CMV)-IgG therapy.[17] Furthermore, combination of rituximab with muromonab-CD3, corticosteroids, or plasmapheresis and antithymocyte globulin[18,19] has proven an effective treatment against AMR in solid organ transplantation.

Due to their important role as physical and immunological barriers to the outside world, our skin, as well as other epithelial barrier tissues, is highly immunogenic. Hence, it could be argued that composite tissue allotransplants involving a skin or mucosal component would be prone to acute rejection. Indeed, approximately 70% of human hand transplant recipients experienced one or more acute rejection episodes[11] as did the first facial transplant recipient.[2] A majority of these cases were reversed with standard immunosuppressive regimens consisting of high-dose pulse corticosteroids and increase in maintenance immunosuppressive therapy. Some of the recurring rejections were treated with addition of ATG or basiliximab. Only one case of acute rejection has been described as steroid and ATG resistant, but proved to be amenable to CAMPATH-1H therapy.[11]

It is unclear whether and to which extent AMR may play a role in CTA. On he basis of the experiences from human hand and abdominal wall allotransplants only the most severe cases of rejection were associated with CD20 (B cell) positive immunostaining.[20] Nevertheless, the magnitude and clinical consequences of AMR in CTA could be important, and the efficacy of current anti-AMR protocols in solid organ transplantation are worth consideration, especially when transplanting tissues containing skin and/or mucosa.

The use of antibodies in transplantation is an emerging concept. Specifically in CTA, there has been little use for them. However, they hold great promise as we continue to explore ways of reducing morbidity and mortality secondary to lifelong immunosuppression.

In the next section, we review antibodies currently in use in the field of transplantation and their potential application in CTA.

13.3 Antibody-Based Immunosuppressive Agents: Mechanism of Action, Clinical Efficacy, and Safety Profiles

13.3.1 Polyclonal Antibodies

Antilymphocyte, and more specifically antithymocyte globulins are purified polyclonal immunoglobulin G (IgG) antibodies originating from animal serum (e.g., rabitt, horse).that can cause complement-mediated cytolysis and cell-mediated opsonization. While they primarily target T cells, their specificity is not quite distinct and they exert effects on various other cell types including B cells, neutrophils, and platelets. Also, in addition to their antirejection properties, they may provide benefit by inhibiting the proliferation of EBV-infected lymphoblastoid cells. Their potency and safety profiles vary greatly depending on the immunogen and species of origin.[21,22] Thus, rabbit-derived antithymocyte globulin (Thymoglobulin®) is for example more potent and its effects long-lasting than that of equine-derived antithymocyte globulin (ATGAM®).[21,23]

Due to their high immunogenicity, a wide range of adverse events have been associated with polyclonal antibodies. The most frequently reported is the "cytokine release syndrome,", which presents with symptoms such as fever, chills, leukopenia, thrombocytopenia, and tachycardia.[24,25]

When studied for their effect on infection, polyclonal antibodies were not found to be associated with higher CMV infection rates,[21] but did confirm a significantly increased risk of posttransplant lymphoproliferative disorder (PTLD).[23,26]

Experience in CTA, and in particular human hand transplants, have shown a pattern of adverse effects similar to those described in solid organ transplantation. Although we lack data linking specific adverse events with administered induction or antirejection therapy, approximately 1/3 of patients developed CMV infections and one patient was diagnosed with cytokine release syndrome; no malignancies have been reported to date.[11]

13.3.2 Monoclonal Antibodies

Monoclonal antibodies derive their name from hybridoma clones that are capable of producing one single immunoglobulin population directed toward exactly predefined epitopes. Their high specificity and stability have become key resources in therapeutic treatment of various immunological disorders, malignancies, and transplantation medicine. Of special interest among the monoclonal antibodies are Muromonab-CD3 (anti-CD3), basiliximab (anti-IL-2 receptor, anti-CD25), almetuzumab (CAMPATH-1H, anti-CD52), and rituximab (anti-CD20). As discussed above, they are primarily used in induction and antirejection therapeutic protocols. In this section, antibodies are ordered according to epitope specificity.

13.3.3 Anti-CD3 Antibody (Muromonab-CD3)

Muromonab-CD3 was the first mAb used to prevent acute rejection in solid organ transplantation.[27] It is the only commercially available monoclonal T-cell depleting induction agent that was found to be significantly more effective in reversing acute rejection than corticosteroid therapy alone.[28] When used as an induction agent, Muromonab-CD3 has efficacies similar to polyclonal antibodies.[29,30] Muromonab-CD3 is a murine monoclonal antibody of the IgG2a isotype that targets CD3. CD3 is a 17–20 kDa molecule that is part of a multimolecular complex found only on mature T cells and medullary thymocytes.[31] By binding to CD3, Muromonab-CD3 blocks mitogenic T-cell activation and function. The postulated mechanism of action is thought to be based on the selective removal of CD3 by internalization. In spite of its promise, Muromonab-CD3 has been associated with significant toxicity, thereby limiting its use in transplantation medicine. Most patients developed cytokine release syndrome after the initial two or three doses with symptoms ranging from very mild to shock-like reactions and involvement of the central nervous system. Furthermore, studies investigating connections between Muromonab-CD3 and lymphoproliferative disorders have shown that the relative risk of PTLD is increased by approximately 70%.[32]

A decision to introduce Muromonab-CD3 as a treatment option in CTA should balance these side effects with its great potency.

13.3.4 Anti-CD25 Antibodies (Basiliximab, Daclizumab): IL-2 Receptor-Directed Antibodies

The interleukin-2 receptor antagonists (IL-2RAs) basiliximab and daclizumab have gained considerable clinical attention since their introduction in the mid-1990s. Initially introduced as an adjunctive to the core immunosuppressive maintenance therapies (CNIs), both basiliximab and daclizumab have recently demonstrated their potency and clinical importance as induction agents. IL-2R antagonists bind in a highly specific manner to CD25, an α subunit of the trimer (α, β, and γ subunits) cell surface receptor IL-2R. As a result, T-cell-mediated cytokine production is inhibited. Furthermore, their highly specific biological intervention is based on fact that CD25 (α subunit) is expressed only on activated T cells, hence leaving resting T cells unaffected. However, selective blockade with an IL-2R agent does not prevent other cytokines from still activating T cells.

Basiliximab is a chimeric antibody that includes the entire variable region of the original murine anti-CD25 antibody. Daclizumab is a humanized antibody in which the hypervariable region was framed out of the murine antibody and the remainder of the molecule was based on human origin. Their pharmacokinetic and pharmacodynamic characteristics are comparable and seem to be equipotent.[33,34] A number of multicenter, randomized, placebo-controlled studies with basiliximab and daclizumab in combination with a CNI (cyclosporine or tacrolimus) have demonstrated a significant, 30–40%, relative reduction in the incidence of biopsy-proven acute rejection when compared with placebo.[35,36] Head-to-head comparison in efficacy between anti-IL2R antibodies and lymphocyte-depleting antibodies in solid organ transplantation suggest that patients at normal or low immunological risk do not exhibit significant difference in acute rejection incidence.[24,25,37] However, in high-risk transplant patients, anti-IL2R induction appears to be inferior to lymphocyte depleting antibodies resulting in an increased risk of acute rejection.

In contrast to the high incidence of reported adverse effects with lymphocyte-depleting agents,[24] anti-IL2R antibodies have proven to be very safe and virtually void of any typical immunosuppresion-associated adverse events.[35,38] Posttransplantation infection rates, including CMV infection,[39] seem to be comparable to placebo.[35,36,40] Furthermore, virally driven malignancies like PTLD do not appear to be affected by either of the anti-IL2R antibodies.[26,39]

IL2 receptor antagonists have demonstrated remarkable efficacy in reducing acute rejection episodes pared with excellent tolerability and safety. These characteristics have rendered anti-IL2 antibodies into an appealing drug category in transplantation medicine. Approximately 30% of human hand transplant recipients have been treated with anti-IL2R antibodies as induction therapy.

13.3.5 Anti-CD52 Antibody (CAMPATH-1H; Alemtuzumab)

Alemtuzumab (CAMPATH-1H) was first developed for the treatment of conventional therapy (fludarabine) resistant chronic B cell lymphocytic leukemia.[41] Recently, a growing appreciation of its specificity and potential led to its introduction in the treatment of rheumatoid arthritis,[42] scleroderma,[43] multiple sclerosis,[44] as well as its use as an induction and antirejection agent in transplantation medicine.

Alemtuzumab is a humanized murine IgG1 monoclonal antibody that includes a humanized variable region. It reacts with the GPI-anchored dodecapeptide CD52, an abundantly expressed protein on the surface of many mononuclear cells, including T and B lymphocytes, NK cells, monocytes, and macrophages.[45] Its profound and sustained lymphocyte-depleting effect is conveyed through the ability of alemtuzumab to fix and activate complement, and hence permit controlled lymphocyte (especially T cell) lysis.

In transplantation, alemtuzumab was first used in the late 1990s as induction therapy in renal transplantation along with CNI (cyclosporine)[46,47] with promising results. Recently, early trial results utilizing alemtuzumab as an induction agent have demonstrated good patient and graft survival and remarkable acute rejection reduction rates in short-term follow-up studies.[48–50] The only long-term study we are aware of included a relatively small number of patients, thus preventing definitive statements regarding long-term efficacy and safety.[51] Nevertheless, the results described in this study are promising. Potent immunosuppression by alemtuzumab significantly delayed acute rejection, but did not result in a reduction of adverse events, including infection and PTLD. Patient and graft survival were similar to conventional triple therapy. Other studies show a surprising lack of serious infection despite the profound and long-lasting lymphocyte depleting effect.[52,53] Recently, there has been some concern regarding an increased rate of autoimmune disease in patients treated with alemtuzumab, in particular Graves' disease in patients with MS.[54,55]

In CTA, alemtuzumab has been successfully used as induction therapy in abdominal wall transplants, a part of complex intestinal or multivisceral transplantation. Abdominal wall transplantation was performed in eight patients, four as a part of intestinal and four as a part of multivisceral transplantation, with alemtuzumab used as an induction agent in seven out of eight patients. Two deaths and one graft failure due to infarction were reported, with five intact and viable abdominal grafts, all in patients who received alemtuzumab.[12] In human hand transplantation, alemtuzumab has been used successfully to reverse steroid- and ATG-resistant acute rejection in the case of a bilateral hand allotransplant.[11,56] We are not aware of any other studies in CTA using alemtuzumab as induction or antirejection therapy. The relatively frequent use of alemtuzumab as induction therapy in abdominal wall transplants as opposed to other CTA procedures can be explained by early positive results with this agent in visceral transplantation.[57]

13.3.6 Anti-CD20 Antibody (Rituximab)

Rituximab is a high-affinity anti-CD20 monoclonal antibody directed against the B-cell compartment. Rituximab was approved in late 1990s by the FDA for the treatment of refractory or relapsed B-cell non-Hodgkin lymphoma,[58,59] and lately it is being used experimentally for the treatment of other immuno-related diseases such as rheumatoid arthritis[60,61] and systemic lupus erythematosus.[62]

In the setting of transplantation medicine, rituximab gained considerable interest when novel mechanisms of allograft injury, e.g., refractory acute rejection based on the presence and immunological activity of CD20+ B cells, were recognized. Recently, rituximab has gained further interest, as reports indicate that rituximab can be effective at treating posttransplant lymphoproliferative disorder[63] and can be effective at desensitizing refractory HLA-sensitized patients[13] as well as recipients of ABO-incompatible transplants.[14]

Rituximab is a chimeric murine/human monoclonal antibody composed of a human kappa light and IgG1 heavy chain constant region, and a variable light and heavy chain of murine origin.[64] It reacts with CD20, a hydrophobic transmembrane protein encountered on pre-B and mature B cells,[65] and inhibits B-cell proliferation and induces B-cell apoptosis. The proposed mechanism of selective CD20+ B-cell depletion include complement-dependent cytotoxicity (CDCC), and the induction of apoptosis and antibody-dependent cellular cytotoxicity (ADCC) by natural killer (NK) cells and macrophages.[64]

While T cells have traditionally been associated with acute rejection, an analysis of a substantial proportion of steroid-resistant and refractory rejection episodes indicated that CD20+ B cells, and their immunological effects, may be an underlying cause in these nonresponsive acute rejection episodes.[66] Although the number of treated patients is small, published reports of rituximab as a treatment for humoral rejection are promising[67,68] especially considering that some of them did not respond to highly potent, traditional antirejection treatment.[18]

Rituximab has also been used in severely HLA-sensitized patients with high PRA levels,[13] historically a group of patients with increased rejection and allograft failure rates. Early results from kidney and heart/lung transplantation are encouraging.[69,70] In addition, use of rituximab has been described in successful solid organ transplantation across ABO-incompatible barriers, with and without historically required splenectomy.[14,71–73] Virally driven malignancies and aggressive involvement of CD20+ B cells, especially in PTLD, has opened another potential treatment avenue for rituximab in transplantation medicine. Initial results are promising and demonstrate great efficacy of rituximab monotherapy in PTLD patients.[63]

Side effects associated with the use of rituximab have been mainly caused by cytokine release syndrome as a reaction to first dose administration, and more so in lymphoma patients[74] than transplant patients.[60] While no clear viral, bacterial, or fungal infection rate increases have been associated with the use of rituximab,[60] there are some concerns regarding hepatitis B reactivation.[75]

To our knowledge there have been no reports of CTA implementing rituximab in their transplantation protocols. However, if initial results in solid organ transplantation prove substantial, use of rituximab in CTA may gain an important place in the treatment of severe cases of antibody-mediated acute rejection.[20] Furthermore, in the novel field of CTA, where the lack of donor organ availability is even more pronounced than in solid organ transplantation, and where potential transplant recipients are typically HLA-sensitized as a consequence of previous treatments (i.e., blood transfusions and skin allografts), effective desensitization therapies may prove invaluable.

13.3.7 Costimulation Blockade (CD40-CD154; CD28-CD80/CD86 and CTLA-4)

The costimulatory pathway is of paramount importance in triggering T-cell activation, proliferation, and effector function. Indeed, sole activation of naïve T cells via their T-cell receptor (TCR), in the absence of any costimulatory signals, induces anergy or apoptosis.[76] While many costimulatory pathways have been identified, the best characterized families of costimulatory molecules includes the immunoglobulin (Ig) superfamily (CD28-CD80/CD86 and CTLA-4), the tumor necrosis factor (TNF)/tumor necrosis factor receptor (TNFR) family (CD40-CD154), and the integrin family (CD11a).[77] Observed effects of costimulatory molecules may differ substantially, as different costimulatory pathways modulate T-cell responses toward increased induction or reduction of T-cell activation.

CD40 belongs to the TNFR superfamily and can be found on B cells, macrophages, dendritic cells, and epithelial cells in the thymus.[78] Upon activation CD40 promotes B-cell activation and DC survival, most likely through NFκB-mediated effects such as increased expression of CD80, CD86, ICAM-1 (adhesion molecule), and the production of IL12.[79] The ligand for CD40 is CD154. It can be found in two forms, namely as a type II integral membrane protein or as a soluble cytokine. Its expression on T cells is also modulated through the CD28 costimulatory pathway.

Despite impressive experimental evidence (reduction of acute rejection, long-term allograft acceptance, and even tolerance) in nonhuman primates,[80–85] clinical trials with anti-CD154 antibodies were halted due to unexpected thromboembolic events and increased rejection rates.[82,86] New anti-CD154 antibodies (IDEC-131) have been generated targeting different epitopes, thus hopefully rendering them inert to the coagulation cascade.[87] CD40 has also been explored as a target for antibody therapy. Although primarily developed to propagate an agonistic effect and to boost the immune response, recent evidence has shown that some of the anti-CD40 mAb's may prove beneficial in transplantation. Chi220, a chimeric anti-CD40 mAb, was able to establish transient B-cell depletion and increase allograft survival in certain experimental settings.[88] Further research is required to see whether this approach will live up to its initial promise.

CD28 shows a pattern of constitutive expression on almost all T-helper cells (CD4+) and a majority of cytotoxic T cells (CD8+).[89] Activation of the CD28 receptor, with concomitant TCR-mediated signals, plays a pivotal role in orchestrating

T-cell differentiation into T helper cells and proliferation of already activated T cells, while at the same time stimulating B-cell antibody production and dendritic cells (DC) survival.[90,91] In addition, recent evidence has implicated CD28 signaling as a controlling pathway in "resting" immune homeostasis through its action on thymic development and peripheral homeostasis of regulatory T cells.[92] Interference with the CD28:CD80/CD86 costimulatory pathway enhances antiapoptotic effects, clonal expansion, and altered cytokine secretion.[93]

Initial studies examining the effects of CD28:CD80/CD86 pathway blockade showed impressive results ranging from prevention of acute allograft rejection to induction of donor-specific tolerance in certain models.[94,95] Monoclonal antibodies against CD80 and CD86 successfully delayed renal allograft rejection in nonhuman primates with and without CNI and steroid-based maintenance therapy.[96,97] In addition, a Phase I study in human renal transplant recipients concluded that anti-CD80 and CD86 (h1F1 and h3D1) antibodies were safe and effective when used in conjunction with cyclosporine, mycophenolate mofetil, and steroids maintenance therapy.[99]

It is important to point out that combined blockade of CD80 and CD86 proved to be superior in delaying rejection when compared with blockades of CD80 or CD86 alone.[97] A possible explanation for this observation might be sought in allograft rejection dynamics with CD86 signaling involved in early and CD80 in late rejection. Furthermore, and of special interest for skin-containing CTA, are the results obtained from CD80/CD86 double-knockout transgenic mice which are unable to reject cardiac, but able to readily reject skin allografts,[99,100] possibly through activation of an alternative costimulatory pathway.

Alternatively, monoclonal antibodies that block CD28 have also exhibited a potent inhibition of acute and chronic rejection, regulatory T-cell induction, and tolerance in rodent animal models.[101]

Another method of interfering with the CD28:CD80/CD86 pathway is by using cytotoxic lymphocyte antigen-4 (CTLA-4). Like CD28, CTLA-4 binds to CD80 and CD86, but with a 10- to 20-fold higher affinity. Unlike CD28, CTLA-4 expression is induced upon T-cell activation in a feedback loop aimed at decreasing T-cell activation, IL2-IL2R expression, and at suppressing antigen presenting DCs.[90,102,103] Furthermore, CTLA-4 appears to play an important role in T regulatory cell homeostasis.[104]

During the initiation of a T-cell-mediated immune response, CD86 and CD80 are the primary binding ligands to CD28, whereas CTLA-4 consequently modulates the T-cell-mediated immune response.[93,105] In addition, there seems to exist a difference in affinity and avidity of CD86 toward CD28, whereas CD80 is more inclined toward binding with CTLA-4.[106]

A therapeutic approach targeting interactions of CD28 with CD80 and CD86 has led to the generation of CTLA-4Ig, a fusion protein combining the extracellular binding domain of CTLA-4 with the Fc portion of IgG1. Unfortunately, although the initial results obtained in rodent models have shown to prevent the development of T-cell-mediated humoral and cellular responses as well as chronic rejection,[107] the same effects were significantly less effective in nonhuman primate models.[83]

However, the appealing central role of CTLA-4 led to the development of more potent CTLA4-Ig variants, eventually resulting in belatacept (LEA29Y), a CTLA-4Ig fusion protein with increased binding affinity and avidity for both CD86 and CD80. When studied in nonhuman primate models, belatacept, either as monotherapy or in combination with common immunosuppressive maintenance regimens, was able to prevent acute rejection and extend renal allograft survival.[108] Furthermore, belatacept prevented antidonor antibody formation, and hence possibly diminished the chance of chronic rejection, while at the same time increasing the chance of successful retransplantation when and if required.[108] A study comparing belatacept to regular immunosuppressive maintenance in human renal allograft transplants demonstrated equivalent efficacy in preventing acute rejection.[109] More importantly, CNI-induced side effects (nephropathy) were not encountered in patients treated with belatacept, an observation that may be predictive for long-term allograft outcome.

While many additional costimulatory pathways have been described, the results of blocking a particular costimulatory pathway are not always predictable and depend on the nature of the experimental model. Therefore, it remains to be determined whether and which of those pathways will prove to be viable candidates for future antibody drug development.

13.4 Conclusion

Historically, following the discoveries and the recognition of the pivotal role played by T cells in orchestrating allograft rejection, a common goal of immunosuppressive drugs was and is to exert potent, intense, and prolonged T-cell suppression. As mentioned earlier, current immunosuppressive drugs have proved their ability of inhibiting the activation of T cells, but at the cost of penalizing the entire immune system. Consequently, the emphasis in transplantation research has been on immunomodulation, rather than the currently imposed (pan) immunosuppression.

The tactics of immunomodulation focus on the inhibition and/or stimulation of select T-cell populations. Antibodies are ideal molecules to achieve this goal. They can be generated against virtually every protein, which is especially interesting when that protein has an extracellular domain in the membrane of T cells. Thus, antibodies can bind specific populations and either block interaction with the targeted protein or destroy the target cell via cellular immune responses.

A closer look at (monoclonal) antibody-based induction, antirejection, and maintenance immunosuppressive therapy reveals its potential to reduce or even eliminate the need for calcineurin inhibitors and/or steroids in organ transplantation.[24,25,27,109] While regimen trends have historically flown naturally from solid organ transplantation to CTA, it remains unclear how to optimally advance antibody-based therapies into the field of CTA. CTA surgeons are reluctant to test new antibody-based therapies in a field that in and of itself is experimental.[2,11]

It is our opinion that (monoclonal) antibodies will gradually gain acceptance by their potency when used in extreme conditions. For example, all acute rejection episodes treated with (monoclonal) antibodies were successfully reversed, even in the case of steroid resistant rejection.[11,12,56] Furthermore, susceptibility to acute rejection may arise from the high number of HLA sensitized patients (due to blood transfusions or previous skin allografts in CTA candidates) and very low number of available donor tissue (complicating the immunologic donor–receptor match). Recent studies with some of the antibodies used as desensitization agents have shown promising results and might prove of value in CTA donation.

However, as with most modulating processes, the use of (monoclonal) antibodies does not provide an unidirectional and finite response as evidenced by recent results showing elimination of potentially tolerance-inducing regulatory T cells.[110]

The ultimate goal of immunomodulation is transplantation tolerance. Although it is out of the scope of this chapter to discuss transplantation tolerance in detail, it is important to note that there is compelling evidence showing the potential of some monoclonal antibodies to modulate the immune system toward tolerance. Molecules targeted by these monoclonal antibodies belong to the groups of coreceptor, costimulatory, external, and internal adhesion molecules.[111] In spite of their promise, it is unlikely that transplantation tolerance will become a clinical reality any time soon. Until then, we believe that the field of transplantation medicine should be shifted toward "near" tolerance using monoclonal antibodies to modulate the immune system followed by low-dose immunosuppression. We also feel that, if proven successful, "near" tolerance approach may reshape the ethical question surrounding the field of CTA, and tip the balance of the risk-benefit equation in favor of its benefits.

References

1. J. M. Dubernard, et al., Human hand allograft: report on first 6 months, *Lancet* **353**(9161), 315–20 (1999).
2. B. Devauchelle, et al., First human face allograft: early report, *Lancet* **368**(9531), 203–9 (2006).
3. E. T. Ustuner, et al., Swine composite tissue allotransplant model for preclinical hand transplant studies, *Microsurgery* **20**(8), 400–6 (2000).
4. J. L. Gowans, G. D. Mc, and D. M. Cowen, Initiation of immune responses by small lymphocytes, *Nature* **196,** 651–5 (1962).
5. D. D. McGregor and J. L. Gowans, Survival of homografts of skin in rats depleted of lymphocytes by chronic drainage from the thoracic duct, *Lancet* **15,** 629–32 (1964).
6. E. M. Lance and P. B. Medawar, Survival of skin heterografts under treatment with antilymphocytic serum, *Lancet* **1**(7553), 1174–6 (1968).
7. E. M. Lance and P. Medawar, Quantitative studies on tissue transplantation immunity. IX. Induction of tolerance with antilymphocytic serum, *Proc R Soc Lond B Biol Sci* **173**(33), 447–73 (1969).
8. E. M.Lance and P. B. Medawar, Immunosuppressive effects of heterologous antilymphocyte serum in monkeys, *Lancet* **1**(7639), 167–70 (1970).

9. G. Kohler and C. Milstein, Continuous cultures of fused cells secreting antibody of predefined specificity, *Nature* **256**(5517), 495–7 (1975).
10. S. P. Cobbold, et al., Therapy with monoclonal antibodies by elimination of T-cell subsets in vivo, *Nature* **312**(5994), 548–51 (1984).
11. M. Lanzetta, et al., The international registry on hand and composite tissue transplantation, *Transplantation* **79**(9), 1210–4 (2005).
12. D. M. Levi, et al., Transplantation of the abdominal wall, *Lancet* **361**(9376), 2173–6 (2003).
13. J. M. Gloor, et al., Overcoming a positive crossmatch in living-donor kidney transplantation, *Am J Transplant* **3**(8), 1017–23 (2003).
14. G. Tyden, et al., ABO incompatible kidney transplantations without splenectomy, using antigen-specific immunoadsorption and rituximab, *Am J Transplant* **5**(1), 145–8 (2005).
15. B. Nashan, Antibody induction therapy in renal transplant patients receiving calcineurin-inhibitor immunosuppressive regimens: a comparative review, *BioDrugs* **19**(1), 39–46 (2005).
16. H. Waldmann and G. Hale, CAMPATH: from concept to clinic, *Philos Trans R Soc Lond B Biol Sci* **360**(1461), 1707–11 (2005).
17. T. Tanaka, et al., Correlation between the Banff 97 classification of renal allograft biopsies and clinical outcome, *Transpl Int* **17**(2), 59–64 (2004).
18. Y. T. Becker, et al., Rituximab as treatment for refractory kidney transplant rejection, *Am J Transplant* **4**(6), 996–1001 (2004).
19. M. Alausa, et al., Refractory acute kidney transplant rejection with CD20 graft infiltrates and successful therapy with rituximab, *Clin Transplant* **19**(1), 137–40 (2005).
20. L. C. Cendales, et al., Composite tissue allotransplantation: classification of clinical acute skin rejection, *Transplantation* **80**(12), 1676–80 (2005).
21. D. C. Brennan, et al., A randomized, double-blinded comparison of Thymoglobulin versus Atgam for induction immunosuppressive therapy in adult renal transplant recipients, *Transplantation* **67**(7), 1011–8 (1999).
22. A. O. Gaber, et al., Results of the double-blind, randomized, multicenter, phase III clinical trial of Thymoglobulin versus Atgam in the treatment of acute graft rejection episodes after renal transplantation, *Transplantation* **66**(1), 29–37 (1998).
23. K. L. Hardinger, et al., Five-year follow up of thymoglobulin versus ATGAM induction in adult renal transplantation, *Transplantation* **78**(1), 136–41 (2004).
24. Y. Lebranchu, et al., Immunoprophylaxis with basiliximab compared with antithymocyte globulin in renal transplant patients receiving MMF-containing triple therapy, *Am J Transplant* **2**(1), 48–56 (2002).
25. H. Sollinger, et al., Basiliximab versus antithymocyte globulin for prevention of acute renal allograft rejection, *Transplantation* **72**(12), 1915–9 (2001).
26. G. Opelz and B. Dohler, Lymphomas after solid organ transplantation: a collaborative transplant study report, *Am J Transplant* **4**(2), 222–30 (2004).
27. R. L. Kirkman, et al., A randomized prospective trial of anti-Tac monoclonal antibody in human renal transplantation, *Transplantation* **51**(1), 107–13 (1991).
28. Ortho Multicenter Transplant Study Group, A randomized clinical trial of OKT3 monoclonal antibody for acute rejection of cadaveric renal transplants, *N Engl J Med* **313**(6), 337–42 (1985).
29. E. H. Cole, et al., A comparison of rabbit antithymocyte serum and OKT3 as prophylaxis against renal allograft rejection, *Transplantation* **57**(1), 60–7 (1994).
30. J. M. Grino, et al., Antilymphocyte globulin versus OKT3 induction therapy in cadaveric kidney transplantation: a prospective randomized study, *Am J Kidney Dis* **20**(6), 603–10 (1992).
31. D. J. Norman, Mechanisms of action and overview of OKT3, *Ther Drug Monit* **17**(6), 615–20 (1995).
32. R. T. Bustami, et al., Immunosuppression and the risk of post-transplant malignancy among cadaveric first kidney transplant recipients, *Am J Transplant* **4**(1), 87–93 (2004).
33. D. Adu, et al., Interleukin-2 receptor monoclonal antibodies in renal transplantation: meta-analysis of randomised trials, *BMJ* **326**(7393), 789 (2003).

34. T. M. Chapman and G. M. Keating, Basiliximab: a review of its use as induction therapy in renal transplantation, *Drugs* **63**(24), 803–35 (2003).
35. B. Nashan, et al., Randomised trial of basiliximab versus placebo for control of acute cellular rejection in renal allograft recipients. CHIB 201 International Study Group, *Lancet* **350**(9086), 1193–8 (1997).
36. C. Ponticelli, et al., A randomized, double-blind trial of basiliximab immunoprophylaxis plus riple therapy in kidney transplant recipients, *Transplantation* **72**(7), 1261–7 (2001).
37. G. Mourad, et al., Sequential protocols using basiliximab versus antithymocyte globulins in renal-transplant patients receiving mycophenolate mofetil and steroids, *Transplantation* **78**(4), 584–90 (2004).
38. F. Vincenti, et al., Interleukin-2-receptor blockade with daclizumab to prevent acute rejection in renal transplantation. Daclizumab Triple Therapy Study Group, *N Engl J Med* **338**(3), 161–5 (1998).
39. A. C. Webster, et al., Interleukin 2 receptor antagonists for renal transplant recipients: a meta-analysis of randomized trials, *Transplantation* **77**(2), 166–76 (2004).
40. J. G. Lawen, et al., Randomized double-blind study of immunoprophylaxis with basiliximab, a chimeric anti-interleukin-2 receptor monoclonal antibody, in combination with mycophenolate mofetil-containing triple therapy in renal transplantation, *Transplantation* **75**(1), 37–43 (2003).
41. M. J. Keating, et al., Therapeutic role of alemtuzumab (Campath-1H) in patients who have failed fludarabine: results of a large international study, *Blood* **99**(10), 3554–61 (2002).
42. E. L. Matteson, et al., Treatment of active refractory rheumatoid arthritis with humanized monoclonal antibody CAMPATH-1H administered by daily subcutaneous injection, *Arthritis Rheum* **38**(9), 1187–93 (1995).
43. J. D. Isaacs, et al., Monoclonal antibody therapy of diffuse cutaneous scleroderma with CAMPATH-1H, *J Rheumatol* **23**(6), 1103–6 (1996).
44. T. Moreau, et al., Preliminary evidence from magnetic resonance imaging for reduction in disease activity after lymphocyte depletion in multiple sclerosis, *Lancet* **344**(8918), 298–301 (1994).
45. M. Q. Xia, et al., Characterization of the CAMPATH-1 (CDw52) antigen: biochemical analysis and cDNA cloning reveal an unusually small peptide backbone, *Eur J Immunol* **21**(7), 1677–84 (1991).
46. R. Calne, et al., Prope tolerance, perioperative campath 1H, and low-dose cyclosporin monotherapy in renal allograft recipients, *Lancet* **351**(9117), 1701–2 (1998).
47. R. Calne, et al., Campath IH allows low-dose cyclosporine monotherapy in 31 cadaveric renal allograft recipients, *Transplantation* **68**(10), 1613–6 (1999).
48. G. Ciancio, et al., The use of Campath-1H as induction therapy in renal transplantation: preliminary results, *Transplantation* **78**(3), 426–33 (2004).
49. A. D. Kirk, et al., Results from a human renal allograft tolerance trial evaluating the humanized CD52-specific monoclonal antibody alemtuzumab (CAMPATH-1H), *Transplantation* **76**(1), 120–9 (2003).
50. A. G. Tzakis, et al., Preliminary experience with alemtuzumab (Campath-1H) and low-dose tacrolimus immunosuppression in adult liver transplantation, *Transplantation* **77**(8), 1209–14 (2004).
51. C. J. Watson, et al., Alemtuzumab (CAMPATH 1H) induction therapy in cadaveric kidney transplantation – efficacy and safety at five years, *Am J Transplant* **5**(6), 1347–53 (2005).
52. S. K. Malek, et al., Campath-1H induction and the incidence of infectious complications in adult renal transplantation, *Transplantation* **81**(1), 17–20 (2006).
53. F. P. Silveira, et al., Bloodstream infections in organ transplant recipients receiving alemtuzumab: no evidence of occurrence of organisms typically associated with profound T cell depletion, *J Infect* **53**(4), 241–7 (2006).
54. A. J. Coles, et al., Pulsed monoclonal antibody treatment and autoimmune thyroid disease in multiple sclerosis, *Lancet* **354**(9191), 1691–5 (1999).
55. A. Paolillo, et al., Quantitative MRI in patients with secondary progressive MS treated with monoclonal antibody Campath 1H, *Neurology* **53**(4), 751–7 (1999).

56. S. Schneeberger, et al., Steroid- and ATG-resistant rejection after double forearm transplantation responds to Campath-1H, *Am J Transplant* **4**(8), 1372–4 (2004).
57. A. G. Tzakis, et al., Alemtuzumab (Campath-1H) combined with tacrolimus in intestinal and multivisceral transplantation, *Transplantation* **75**(9), 1512–7 (2003).
58. B. Coiffier, et al., Rituximab (anti-CD20 monoclonal antibody) for the treatment of patients with relapsing or refractory aggressive lymphoma: a multicenter phase II study, *Blood* **92**(6), 1927–32 (1998).
59. D. G. Maloney, et al., Phase I clinical trial using escalating single-dose infusion of chimeric anti-CD20 monoclonal antibody (IDEC-C2B8) in patients with recurrent B-cell lymphoma, *Blood* **84**(8), 2457–66 (1994).
60. J. C. Edwards, M. J. Leandro, and G. Cambridge, B lymphocyte depletion therapy with rituximab in rheumatoid arthritis, *Rheum Dis Clin North Am* **30**(2), 393–403, viii (2004).
61. C. M. Ng, et al., Population pharmacokinetics of rituximab (anti-CD20 monoclonal antibody) in rheumatoid arthritis patients during a phase II clinical trial, *J Clin Pharmacol* **45**(7), 792–801 (2005).
62. J. H. Anolik, et al., The relationship of FcgammaRIIIa genotype to degree of B cell depletion by rituximab in the treatment of systemic lupus erythematosus, *Arthritis Rheum* **48**(2), 455–9 (2003).
63. S. Norin, et al., Posttransplant lymphoma – a single-center experience of 500 liver transplantations, *Med Oncol* **21**(3), 273–84 (2004).
64. M. E. Reff, et al., Depletion of B cells in vivo by a chimeric mouse human monoclonal antibody to CD20, *Blood* **83**(2), 435–45 (1994).
65. L. M. Nadler, et al., A unique cell surface antigen identifying lymphoid malignancies of B cell origin, *J Clin Invest* **67**(1), 134–40 (1981).
66. M. Sarwal, et al., Molecular heterogeneity in acute renal allograft rejection identified by DNA microarray profiling, *N Engl J Med* **349**(2), 125–38 (2003).
67. J. M. Aranda, Jr., et al., Anti-CD20 monoclonal antibody (rituximab) therapy for acute cardiac humoral rejection: a case report, *Transplantation* **73**(6), 907–10 (2002).
68. H. E. Garrett, Jr., et al., Treatment of vascular rejection with rituximab in cardiac transplantation, *J Heart Lung Transplant* **24**(9), 1337–42 (2005).
69. I. C. Balfour, et al., Use of rituximab to decrease panel-reactive antibodies, *J Heart Lung Transplant* **24**(5), 628–30 (2005).
70. C. A. Vieira, et al., Rituximab for reduction of anti-HLA antibodies in patients awaiting renal transplantation: 1. Safety, pharmacodynamics, and pharmacokinetics, *Transplantation* **77**(4), 542–8 (2004).
71. T. Sawada, et al., Preconditioning regimen consisting of anti-CD20 monoclonal antibody infusions, splenectomy and DFPP-enabled non-responders to undergo ABO-incompatible kidney transplantation, *Clin Transplant* **18**(3), 254–60 (2004).
72. C. J. Sonnenday, et al., Plasmapheresis, CMV hyperimmune globulin, and anti-CD20 allow ABO-incompatible renal transplantation without splenectomy, *Am J Transplant* **4**(8), 1315–22 (2004).
73. M. Usuda, et al., Successful use of anti-CD20 monoclonal antibody (rituximab) for ABO-incompatible living-related liver transplantation, *Transplantation* **79**(1), 12–6 (2005).
74. A. Agarwal, et al., Rituximab, anti-CD20, induces in vivo cytokine release but does not impair ex vivo T-cell responses, *Am J Transplant* **4**(8), 1357–60 (2004).
75. Y. Tsutsumi, et al., Reactivation of hepatitis B virus with rituximab, *Expert Opin Drug Saf* **4**(3), 599–608 (2005).
76. R. H. Schwartz, A cell culture model for T lymphocyte clonal anergy, *Science* **248**(4961), 1349–56.
77. L. Biancone, I. Deambrosis, and G. Camussi, Lymphocyte costimulatory receptors in renal disease and transplantation, *J Nephrol* **15**(1), 7–16 (2002).
78. C. P. Larsen and T. C. Pearson, The CD40 pathway in allograft rejection, acceptance, and tolerance, *Curr Opin Immunol* **9**(5), 641–7 (1997).

79. H. Gudmundsdottir and L. A. Turka, T cell costimulatory blockade: new therapies for transplant rejection, *J Am Soc Nephrol* **10**(6), 1356–65 (1999).
80. W. W. Hancock, et al., Costimulatory function and expression of CD40 ligand, CD80, and CD86 in vascularized murine cardiac allograft rejection, *Proc Natl Acad Sci U S A* **93**(24), 13967–72 (1996).
81. N. S. Kenyon, et al., Long-term survival and function of intrahepatic islet allografts in rhesus monkeys treated with humanized anti-CD154, *Proc Natl Acad Sci U S A* **96**(14), 8132–7 (1999).
82. A. D. Kirk, et al., Treatment with humanized monoclonal antibody against CD154 prevents acute renal allograft rejection in nonhuman primates, *Nat Med* **5**(6), 686–93 (1999).
83. A. D. Kirk, et al., CTLA4-Ig and anti-CD40 ligand prevent renal allograft rejection in primates, *Proc Natl Acad Sci U S A* **94**(16), 8789–94 (1997).
84. C. P. Larsen, et al., Long-term acceptance of skin and cardiac allografts after blocking CD40 and CD28 pathways, *Nature* **381**(6581), 434–8 (1996).
85. D. C. Parker, et al., Survival of mouse pancreatic islet allografts in recipients treated with allogeneic small lymphocytes and antibody to CD40 ligand, Proc Natl Acad Sci U S A 92(21), 9560–4 (1995).
86. T. Kanmaz, et al., Monotherapy with the novel human anti-CD154 monoclonal antibody ABI793 in rhesus monkey renal transplantation model, *Transplantation* **77**(6), 914–20 (2004).
87. E. H. Preston, et al., IDEC-131 (anti-CD154), sirolimus and donor-specific transfusion facilitate operational tolerance in non-human primates, *Am J Transplant* **5**(5), 1032–41 (2005).
88. A. B. Adams, et al., Development of a chimeric anti-CD40 monoclonal antibody that synergizes with LEA29Y to prolong islet allograft survival, *J Immunol* **174**(1), 542–50 (2005).
89. J. A. Gross, E. Callas, and J. P. Allison, Identification and distribution of the costimulatory receptor CD28 in the mouse, *J Immunol* **149**(2), 380–8 (1992).
90. M. L. Alegre, K. A. Frauwirth, and C. B. Thompson, T-cell regulation by CD28 and CTLA-4, *Nat Rev Immunol* **1**(3), 220–8 (2001).
91. C. Orabona, et al., CD28 induces immunostimulatory signals in dendritic cells via CD80 and CD86, *Nat Immunol* **5**(11), 1134–42 (2004).
92. Q. Tang, et al., Cutting edge: CD28 controls peripheral homeostasis of CD4+CD25+ regulatory T cells, *J Immunol* **171**(7), 3348–52 (2003).
93. A. J. McAdam, A. N. Schweitzer, and A. H. Sharpe, The role of B7 co-stimulation in activation and differentiation of CD4+ and CD8+ T cells, *Immunol Rev* **165**, 231–47 (1998).
94. T. C. Pearson, et al., Transplantation tolerance induced by CTLA4-Ig, *Transplantation* **57**(12), 1701–6 (1994).
95. L. A. Turka, et al., T-cell activation by the CD28 ligand B7 is required for cardiac allograft rejection in vivo, *Proc Natl Acad Sci U S A* **89**(22), 11102–5 (1992).
96. T. Birsan, et al., Treatment with humanized monoclonal antibodies against CD80 and CD86 combined with sirolimus prolongs renal allograft survival in cynomolgus monkeys, *Transplantation* **75**(12), 2106–13 (2003).
97. A. D. Kirk, et al., Induction therapy with monoclonal antibodies specific for CD80 and CD86 delays the onset of acute renal allograft rejection in non-human primates, *Transplantation* **72**(3), 377–84 (2001).
98. F. Vincenti, What's in the pipeline? New immunosuppressive drugs in transplantation, *Am J Transplant* **2**(10), 898–903 (2002).
99. D. A. Mandelbrot, et al., Expression of B7 molecules in recipient, not donor, mice determines the survival of cardiac allografts, *J Immunol* **163**(7), 3753–7 (1999).
100. G. L. Szot, et al., Absence of host B7 expression is sufficient for long-term murine vascularized heart allograft survival, *Transplantation* **69**(5), 904–9 (2000).
101. F. Haspot, et al., Anti-CD28 antibody-induced kidney allograft tolerance related to tryptophan degradation and TCR class II B7 regulatory cells, *Am J Transplant* **5**(10), 2339–48 (2005).

102. C. A. Chambers, M. S. Kuhns, and J. P. Allison, Cytotoxic T lymphocyte antigen-4 (CTLA-4) regulates primary and secondary peptide-specific CD4(+) T cell responses, *Proc Natl Acad Sci U S A* **96**(15), 8603–8 (1999).
103. M. F. Krummel and J. P. Allison, CD28 and CTLA-4 have opposing effects on the response of T cells to stimulation, *J Exp Med* **182**(2), 459–65 (1999).
104. D. H. Munn, M. D. Sharma, and A. L. Mellor, Ligation of B7-1/B7-2 by human CD4+ T cells triggers indoleamine 2,3-dioxygenase activity in dendritic cells, *J Immunol* **172**(7), 4100–10 (2004).
105. K. S. Kim, et al., CD28-B7-mediated T cell costimulation in chronic cardiac allograft rejection: differential role of B7-1 in initiation versus progression of graft arteriosclerosis, *Am J Pathol* **158**(3), 977–86 (2001).
106. T. Pentcheva-Hoang, et al., B7-1 and B7-2 selectively recruit CTLA-4 and CD28 to the immunological synapse, *Immunity* **21**(3), 401–13 (2004).
107. H. Azuma, et al., Blockade of T-cell costimulation prevents development of experimental chronic renal allograft rejection, *Proc Natl Acad Sci U S A* **93**(22), 12439–44 (1996).
108. C. P. Larsen, et al., Rational development of LEA29Y (belatacept), a high-affinity variant of CTLA4-Ig with potent immunosuppressive properties, *Am J Transplant* **5**(3), 443–53 (2005).
109. F. Vincenti, et al., Costimulation blockade with belatacept in renal transplantation, *N Engl J Med* **353**(8), 770–81 (2005).
110. L. Graca, et al., Antibody-induced transplantation tolerance: the role of dominant regulation, *Immunol Res* **28**(3), 181–91 (2003).
111. H. Waldmann, et al., Therapeutic aspects of tolerance, *Curr Opin Pharmacol* **1**(4), 392–7 (2001).

Section IV

Chapter 14
World Experience of Hand Transplantation-Independent Assessment

W. P. Andrew Lee, Justin M. Sacks, and Elaine K. Horibe

14.1 Introduction

Human hand transplantation, in the modern era of immunosuppression, began in 1998 when the first case was performed in Lyon, France.[1] Since that time multiple hand transplants have been performed around the world.[2-6] The peak incidence was in 2000 with seven hand transplants, four being unilateral and three bilateral (Fig. 14.1). Through 2003, 18 hand transplants had been confirmed. Following an approximately 3-year hiatus with no reported hand transplants, two additional transplants were performed in 2006. Two patients, whose hand allografts had been removed because of rejection, underwent the original operations in 1998 and 1999.

In 2003, the primary author received the Sterling Bunnell Traveling Fellowship from the American Society for Surgery of the Hand. A general surgeon in San Francisco, Dr. Sterling Bunnell, revolutionized hand surgery by incorporating aspects of orthopedics, plastic surgery, and general surgery into the care of the hand. His textbook *Surgery of the Hand*, published in 1944, is considered a classic in the field of surgery of the hand and upper extremity. In 1946, he helped found the oldest medical specialty society in the United States – the American Society for Surgery of the Hand – and became its first President.

The stated goals of the Sterling Bunnell Traveling Fellowship were to develop international and national relations and to foster principles of scholarship. In accordance with these goals, the primary author embarked upon a worldwide tour to study the clinical outcomes of hand transplantations in a systematic and objective manner. Six transplant centers, where 14 confirmed hand-transplant cases had been performed, were visited, including Lyon, Louisville, Guangzhou, Brussels, Milan, and Innsbruck.[7] Of the 14 patients who had received hand transplants in these centers, the author evaluated 11 in 2003. Three other centers in China (Guangxi and Harbin) and Malaysia were not visited (Table 14.1).

Despite the numerous reports from individual transplant centers, the results of these hand transplants had not been assessed in a standardized and independent manner. The author sought to evaluate the transplant recipients objectively with the common parameters in motor and sensory functions accepted in the subspecialty of hand surgery. The Michigan Hand Outcome questionnaires were administered

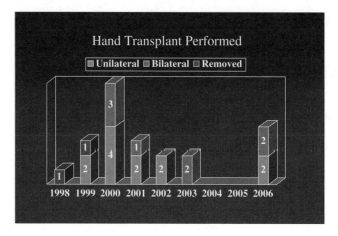

Fig. 14.1 Since 1998 there have been at least 30 confirmed hand transplants in 22 recipients. As shown in this graph of the number of cases per year, the peak incidence was in 2000. Eight of the total cases (marked in blue) have been bilateral and hand transplants, and two of the earlier transplants (marked in red) have been removed

Table 14.1 The senior author visited six centers, where 14 transplants had been performed

	Performed	Surviving	Visited
Lyon	3	2	2
Louisville	2	2	2
Guangzhou	3	2	3
Milan	3	3	1
Innsbruck	2	2	2
Brussels	1	1	1
Total	14	12	11

Among those patients, 12 still had viable allografts in 2003 and 11 were examined.

where permitted. Finally, the author asked the recipients the same questions regarding their subjective assessment of the hand-transplant experience.

14.2 Recipients

Patients selected for hand transplantation were typically young, with age at the time of hand transplant ranging from 21 to 46 years. The ages were evenly distributed among the three decades of early adulthood. They presented with severe disability secondary to the loss of one or both hands. Of the 14 hand-transplant recipients at the time in 2003, all were men. Five out of the 14 patients received bilateral hand transplants. Of the nine unilateral transplants that were visited, eight were performed to replace the dominant hand, and one to replace the nondominant hand.

The time intervals between amputation injury and hand transplantation were variable and ranged from 1 to 15 years, with a median of 4 years. There were 11 patients with amputations in the distal forearm, two in the middle forearm and one in the proximal forearm. The bilateral hand transplant performed in Innsbruck in 2003 was at a level close to the elbow. Range of allograft ischemia time was between 2 and 10 h, with a median of 7 h (Table 14.2).

Human leukocyte antigen (HLA) matching was tested in all 14 cases. Six transplants did not contain any HLA matching. Two recipients contained one HLA match and the rest of the transplants were performed with some degree of HLA matching between the donor and recipient (Fig. 14.2). The allografts were matched for bone size, gender, and skin color for recipient needs.

Systemic immunosuppression was administered to prevent the rejection of the transplanted hands. The typical core regimen consisted of an induction agent of polyclonal

Table 14.2 Hand-transplant recipients' characteristics

Age	21–46 years
Sex	Male: 14
Bilateral	5
Unilateral	Eight dominant hands, one nondominant hand
Time since injury	1–15 years (median 4 years)
Forearm amputation level	Distal 11, middle 2, proximal 1
Ischemic time	2–10 h (median 7 h)

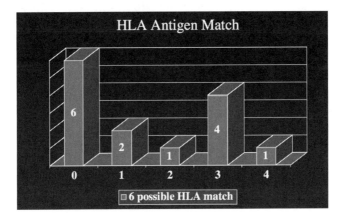

Fig. 14.2 Human leukocyte antigen (HLA) matching was obtained in all cases. The majority of the transplants[6] did not contain any HLA matching

(ATG) or monoclonal antibody (Basiliximab, Thymoglobulin), steroid, FK-506, and the antiproliferative agent mycophenolate mofetil (MMF). Side effects from immunosuppression included cytolomegalovirus (CMV) and fungal infections and reversible neutropenia. Many patients developed transient hyperglycemia requiring insulin treatment, and at least one recipient has developed sustained insulin-dependent diabetes. Cushing's syndrome and weight gain from systemic steroid, dermatitis, and mood swings were observed. One patient developed avascular necrosis of bilateral hip joints requiring hip replacement. None of these side effects to date, however, had been life threatening.

Acute rejection was common among all hand-transplant recipients (Fig. 14.3). All but one patient have had at least one episode of skin rejection characterized by rash and evidence of lymphocytic infiltrates on biopsy. To effectively treat acute rejection episodes, additional immunosuppression was used, including injection of systemic steroids or the use of topical steroids or topical tacrolimus. Newer agents such as rapamycin, the monoclonal antibody, Simulect (monoclonal antibody against CD25, the high-affinity chain of IL-2 receptor), and Campath-1H (anti-CD52 monoclonal antibody) had also been used. In the bilateral forearm transplant patient in Innsbruck, Campath-1H was used to reverse seemingly refractory rejection when it appeared that allograft removal was inevitable.

14.3 USA (Transplants 1999 and 2001)

In January 1999 and February 2001, two unilateral hand transplantations were performed at the University of Louisville in Kentucky, USA by a team led by Dr. Warren Breidenbach. The longest surviving transplanted hand, then at 4 years in 2003, belonged to a 37-year-old American. The patient, formerly a paramedic,

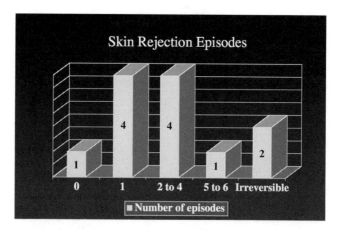

Fig. 14.3 Number of skin rejection episodes among recipients. Most of them had one to four episodes of rejection. Two had irreversible episodes that resulted in amputation of the allograft

reported using his transplanted left hand in many daily activities and was at the time a paramedic instructor. There was no donor HLA match. Ischemia time was 6h and 10min. The patient received induction therapy of Basiliximab and was maintained on an immunosuppressive regimen of prednisone, tacrolimus, and MMF. The patient converted from CMV negative to positive despite gancyclovir treatment and in addition developed a tinea (ringworm) infection. The patient's last episode of acute rejection, at the time of visit in 2003, was three and a half years earlier.

Motor function revealed a wrist range of motion (ROM) at 65° and 35° in active extension and flexion, respectively. ROM at the metacarpalphalangeal (MP) joint was found to be 30°/90°, and 0°/75° and 0°/45° at the proximal interphalangeal (PIP) joint and distal interphalangeal (DIP) joint, respectively. There was no active motion observed at the thumb interphalangeal (IP) joint. There was a palpable contraction of thenar muscles upon attempted thumb abduction; however, there was very weak active thumb palmar abduction and adduction against gravity. The patient reported being able to feel the examiners pin touch "50% of the time" in moving two-point discrimination and could accurately localize the digit upon touch. Previously, according to the patient, he was confused among the median nerve-innervated digits, and among the ulnar-innervated digits. A Tinel's sign, evidence of progressing nerve regeneration, was elicited in the distal palm.

Given the opportunity to discuss his experience following hand transplantation, the patient felt subjectively that his function had "plateaued." He stated the hand transplant had greatly improved his body image, and proudly spoke of being able to applaud with both hands for his son at a karate contest. According to the patient, the most significant disappointment was the medication side effects. He was treated for CMV diarrhea and concomitant weight loss.

The second Louisville patient was a married man aged 40 who underwent a unilateral hand transplant to his left hand in 2001. There was no donor HLA match. He received Basiliximab as an induction agent followed by prednisone and FK-506 for maintenance therapy. His MMF was converted to rapamycin due to recurrent rejection episodes.

This patient had six episodes of acute rejection, with the first not being promptly treated secondary to a lack of lymphocytic infiltration on skin biopsy. Steroids and thymoglobulin were used to reverse the rejection process. Elevated blood glucose manifested itself as diabetes, which was treated with oral hypoglycemics. Avascular necrosis of both the patients' hips developed secondary to steroid use. At the time of examination in 2003, the patient's last previous episode of rejection was one and a half years earlier.

Functional evaluation of the transplanted hand revealed 45° and 55° of active extension and flexion at the wrist, respectively. A pulp to palm distance of greater than 3cm was observed upon composite finger flexion. A brachioradialis (BR) to flexor pollicis longus (FPL) tendon transfer was performed in this patient augmenting active motion at the thumb IP joint to 75°. Thumb abduction, as well as finger abduction and adduction, were absent. Moving two-point discrimination was absent, and the patient was confused among median nerve or ulnar nerve innervated digits upon digital localization. The patient reported protective sensibility against extreme temperatures.

This patient formerly worked in construction and at time of interview was self-employed as a construction manager. He was engaged in activities such as snowmobile, motorcycle riding, and vigorous housework. He also confirmed benefits in the perception of his own body image. He had raised the mirrors at home after loss of his hand so he would not see his amputation stump. After the transplant, he reported lowering the mirrors back to normal levels. His most significant disappointments included medication side effects, which additionally had included alterations in mood, and most significantly, the time required away from his home for various medical treatment.

14.4 Belgium (Transplant 2002)

The only hand-transplant patient evaluated not to have experienced any overt acute rejection was a 23-year-old Belgian recipient of unilateral right-dominant hand allograft. His transplant team leader, Dr. Frederic Schuind, was most forthcoming in offering information and medical data. At the time of the visit, 1 year had elapsed since the hand transplant. The traumatic amputation of this patient's hand had taken place about 18 months before the transplantation. Prior to the hand transplant the patient was utilizing a myoelectric prosthesis with relatively good function.

The hand donor was a 27-year old with a 3/6 HLA match. This hand was harvested before the internal organs from the donor with total ischemia time being 6 h and 7 min. Induction therapy with ATG was initiated and the patient was continued on a maintenance regimen of FK-506, MMF, and prednisolone. Transient diabetes was observed requiring insulin for 3 days. There was a rash for 8 days following hand transplant. There had been no clinically observable episodes of acute rejection. However, perivasculitis was observed histologically at 15 months, which resolved spontaneously. The patient experienced severe depression for about 1 day after the transplant requesting removal of the hand allograft. However, the depression resolved spontaneously.

Upon questioning the patient reported that he now had two hands with a normal appearance. However, he only expected the function of his hand to be better than the prosthesis in "3 to 5 years." The most significant disappointment was the lack of a "normal life" secondary to his rigorous hand therapy schedule.

14.5 Austria (Transplants 2000 and 2003)

Two hand transplantations were performed at the University Hospital in Innsbruck, Austria in 2000 and 2003. Bilateral transplants were performed on both patients. Team members included Dr. Milomir Ninkovic, Dr. Stefan Schneeberger, and the team leader and Surgery Chairman, Dr. Raimund Margreiter.

The first hand-transplant recipient in Austria was a police officer who had lost both hands from a bomb explosion. He actively sought hand transplant following the accident in 1994, and had his wishes fulfilled 6 years later. An intelligent and extremely motivated man, he performed daily hand exercises for up to 7 h throughout the first year after transplant.

Prior to the transplants, the patient had use of prosthesis with adequate myoelectric function. The patient's amputation level was above the wrist in both of his arms. The donor hands contained a 0/6 HLA match. The patient did not receive any irradiation prior to transplant. Ischemia time was 3 h with four teams performing the operation. Bone fixation was performed first followed by arterial and then venous anastomosis.

Complications from the surgical procedure at the time of visit were limited to partial skin necrosis of one of the hand transplants requiring split thickness skin grafting 3 weeks postoperatively. In addition, an arterio-venous fistula became evident in the proximal forearm requiring surgical ligation 8 months postoperatively.

Immunosuppressive therapy consisted of both an induction and maintenance regimen. Antithymocyte globulin (ATG) was given as the induction agent for 4 days starting prior to transplantation. A maintenance regimen consisted of prednisone starting at 25 mg and being tapered over 3 years to 5 mg/day. At the time of visit in 2003, the patient had been off steroids for 2 months. Initial maintenance, in addition to steroids, consisted of FK-506 and MMF. The latter was eventually discontinued and replaced by rapamycin two and a half years postoperatively. Medication side effects at the time of visit included hyperglycemia, which did not require insulin. Skin rejection was observed at postoperative day 55 and reversed with steroids. There was a similar episode of skin rejection on postoperative day 188, which was treated with topical FK-506.

At the time of visit in September 2003, three and a half years had passed since the bilateral transplants. The patient was working as a police dispatch officer. This was his job before the transplant in 2000.

He showed convincing recovery of intrinsic muscle function, a finding seen in only one other patient visited. The pulp to palmar crease distance was 1 cm upon finger flexion. The patient had active motion in both thumb IP joints along with active motion at the MPs, PIPs and DIPs, bilaterally. Thumb abduction was evident on the right side with the left starting to reveal contraction of the muscle (Fig. 14.4). This patient's hand therapy consisted of an inpatient regimen for 2 months followed by therapy sessions for 6–7 h weekly for 1 year. At the time of visit, hand therapy was being performed for 1 h a day.

In the patient's words, his work capacity improved profoundly after the transplants as a police dispatch. He was able to write, dress, and attend to personal hygiene. He had many hobbies, and was leaving after the author's interview to go on a 20,000 km motorcycle trip. According to the patient, the most significant benefits from his hand transplantation were the ability to "feel" his environment with his hands and the enhanced ability to engage in social interactions. Asked to state the most significant disappointment, the patient responded, "none at all."

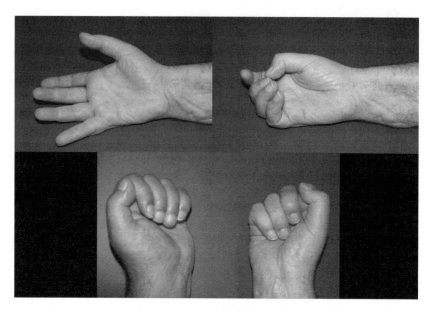

Fig. 14.4 First hand-transplant recipient in Austria, 540 days posttransplantation. The pictures demonstrate true recovery of intrinsic muscles function

The second Austrian hand-transplant patient, a 41-year-old man, received bilateral transplant at the proximal forearm level 6–8 cm below elbow. The HLA match was 2/6 between donor and recipient. Induction therapy consisting of ATG was administered starting prior to transplant for 4 days. Donor ischemia time was 2.5 h. Maintenance therapy consisted of prednisone, FK-506, and MMF. Gancyclovir was discontinued secondary to neutropenia with the patient remaining CMV positive without any evidence of clinical disease. Skin necrosis was observed at 3 weeks postoperatively requiring split-thickness skin grafts.

Rejection episodes were observed multiple times immediately following the transplant. Skin rejection was observed at 9 days postoperatively, which was treated with intravenous and topical steroids. Skin rejection was again observed on postoperative day 46, which was treated with both steroids and an IL-2 Ab (Simulect). He developed a third episode of skin rejection at 3 months postoperatively that was refractory to both high-dose steroids and ATG, but eventually was reversed with Campath-1H, a potent anti-CD52 monoclonal antibody. At the time of his evaluation, he was an inpatient receiving nearly constant therapy to prevent acute rejection.

This Austrian patient was interviewed 7 months following his hand transplant. At the visit he was unable to localize any of his digits but reported a Tinel's sign in the proximal forearm. No discrimination to fine touch was experienced but the patient reported being able to sense temperature difference. The patient had active

ROM at the MP, PIP, and DIP joints bilaterally. The pulp to palm distance was 6 cm. The patient did not have any ROM in either of his thumbs at the time of interview.

This patient felt the most significant benefit of the transplant was sensation and improved techniques in his ability to perform aspects of personal hygiene. The patient did not feel that there were any significant disappointments with the transplant procedure because he felt that, "nothing was unexpected." For him the decision to proceed with the hand transplants, regardless of the rejection episodes and immunosuppressive medications, was the right decision for himself. His recommendation for other hand potential hand-transplant recipients was neutral and felt, similarly to the first Austrian transplant, that this was the right decision for himself.

14.6 China (Transplants 1999, 1999, and 2000)

In March 2003, at the time of the first author's visit to China, three hand-transplants procedures had been performed in Guangzhou, China. The first two were unilateral in 1999 followed by a bilateral hand transplant in 2000.

The first two hand transplants were performed in September 1999. One patient was a 44-year-old farmer who had lost his dominant right hand in a fishing explosion 2 years prior to the hand transplant. The amputation level was 3 cm proximal to the wrist. The transplanted hand was from a donor who was a 4/6 HLA match. The patient received 8 Gy of irradiation for 30 min prior to the transplant procedure and received ATG for 1 week as an induction agent. Maintenance therapy was prednisone, FK-506, MMF, and topical steroids.

At the time of the interview in 2003, 1 year had passed since his transplanted hand had been removed. According to the patient his initial function had been "almost normal" at the wrist and hand. Thumb abduction began 6 months postoperatively. At 6 months, the patient was able play badminton and basketball followed by bicycle riding and the use of the parallel bars at 10 months. He was able to write and type at the computer keyboard at 1 year. The most significant benefit he felt from the transplant procedure was the increased function that he was able to obtain with the transplanted hand.

Unfortunately, two and a half years following the initial hand transplant the graft had to be removed secondary to pain and ischemic necrosis. According to his surgeons, the patient's hand developed severe rash refractory to steroid or antifungal agent. Subcutaneous cortisone injections were administered by the dermatologists at the hospital, which resulted in apparent graft vessel thrombosis and severe ischemic pain necessitating allograft removal (Fig. 14.5). Despite his initial positive functional return, the patient stated that he would not undergo another hand transplant. He felt that the pain he experienced posttransplant was worse than the initial injury.

The second transplant patient from China was a married 30-year-old farmer who lost his dominant right hand from a traumatic amputation secondary to a farming

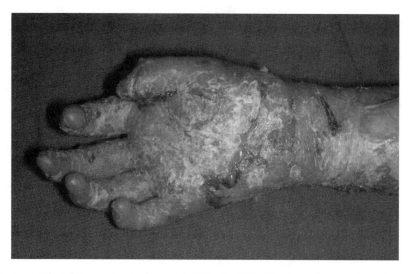

Fig. 14.5 First hand transplant performed in China in 1999. The allograft presented with severe and refractory rash due to cutaneous rejection, two and a half year after the transplantation. Subcutaneous cortisone injections were administered, which apparently resulted in vessel thrombosis and severe ischemic pain, leading to allograft removal

accident. An unsuccessful replantation attempt was performed. The final amputation level was 3 cm proximal to the wrist. The transplanted hand was from a donor who was a 3/6 HLA match. The patient did not receive irradiation prior to the transplant. Ischemia time was 7 h. The induction agent was ATG for 1 week followed by prednisone, FK-506, MMF, and topical steroids. Immunosuppressive side effects included dyspepsia and dysphoria. In addition, transient hyperglycemia requiring insulin developed.

Postoperative complications from the transplant included vasospasm and a revision of the venous anastomosis with a vein graft. A tenolysis, neurolysis and removal of hardware-plate were performed at 7 months postoperatively. Subclinical rejection was observed in the form of lymphocytic infiltrates in the dermis, muscle, vessel wall, and epineurium of the hand allograft at the time of hardware removal based on biopsies specimens obtained.

This patient had one of the best functional returns observed with recovery of intrinsic muscle function. Motion at the wrist was 75° at both active extension and flexion. Significant motion at the MP, PIP, and DIP joints was observed. The patient exhibited both thumb abduction and adduction, however, with limitation. At two and a half years following the patient's right-hand transplant, he was able to perform various common functional activities with some limited restrictions (Fig. 14.6). The patient was able to dress himself and unbutton his clothes. He was able to write with his right hand and hold chopsticks while eating. In addition, he

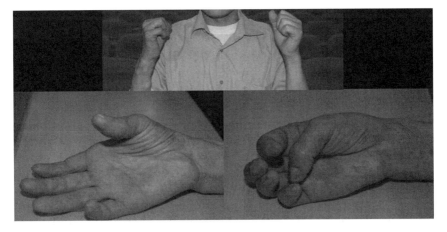

Fig. 14.6 Second hand transplant performed in China. This patient had one of the best functional returns observed with convincing recovery of intrinsic muscle function at two and a half years following the patient's right-hand transplant

was able to play Mah-jong and poker. His was working as a "security guard' at the time of the visit.

The most significant benefit he felt from his hand transplant was his self-reliance. The patient felt this had helped contribute to his current marriage with his wife. This union eventually led to a successful pregnancy. However, the patient was disappointed by the side effects incurred from the use of immunosuppressive medications.

The third Chinese transplant recipient was a former police officer who had lost both his hands and sustained eye injuries in a bomb accident less than 2 years prior to his hand transplant. The amputation level was at the mid-forearms. Preoperative irradiation was administered at 8 Gy for 30 min. Ischemia time for the right donor hand was 9 h and 8 h for the left. The patient received ATG as an induction agent followed by FK-506, MMF, and prednisone. Fluocinolone was administered as a topical ointment to prevent local skin rejection. There were no significant immunosuppressive side effects reported by the patient.

Upon examination, at two and a half years posttransplant, there was no evidence of intrinsic muscle function in either of the hands. Motion at the wrist was 15°/0° on the right and 15°/5° on the left to extension and flexion, respectively. Motion at the MP, PIP, and DIP joints in both hands showed limited movement to active flexion. Digit localization was considered 100%. The patient reported recovery of proprioception and observed "good" sensation in his right hand greater than the left.

When assessed for subjective comments he was extremely positive. He reported being able to use a fork and a computer mouse. He relied less on his wife for assistance and was independent in the bathroom in the summer time (without heavy clothing). The most significant benefit reported by the patient was concerning the intimate benefits of the hand transplant in his ability to have a daughter. He did not have any significant disappointments.

14.7 France (Transplants 2000 and 2003)

A visit to Lyon, France was made in September 2003 where both bilateral hand-transplant recipients were evaluated. The first hand transplant in the modern era of immunosuppression was performed in 1998 by the same transplant team, ultimately resulting in rejection attributed to noncompliance with immunosuppressive medications. This patient was not interviewed.

The first bilateral hand-transplant patient from Lyon was a 36-year-old right-hand-dominant man who had last both his hands in a blast injury secondary to a fireworks accident 4 years previously. The amputation was 3 cm above the wrist bilaterally. The procedure in 2000 was the first bilateral hand transplant performed in the world. The donor hands were obtained from an 18-year-old male with 0/6 HLA matches. Ischemia time for the hand transplantation was 8 h.

The recipient did not receive any irradiation prior to transplantation. Thymoglobulin was given as an induction agent followed by FK-506, MMF, and steroids for immunosuppression. Simulect was administered on POD 12 and 20. Medication side effects were limited to hyperglycemia treated with insulin for 35 days, serum sickness on POD 8, and some mild headache and confusion in the immediate postoperative period.

There were no major complications reported at the time of interview in 2003, three and a half years following transplantation. Episodes of rejection noted were maculopapular lesions found on the left hand on POD 53 and 82. Biopsies of these lesions showed dermal lymphocytic infiltrates of recipient origin, which resolved after 2 weeks with increased systemic and topical administration. Subsequently, there had been no clinically evident episodes of acute rejection.

Functional evaluation revealed significant gains in hand motion. The patient was able to extend and flex his wrist (+40°/60° right, +55°/+5° left) and move his PIP (0°/90°) and DIP (0°/60°) joints. However, MP flexion was minimum and there was no significant palmar abduction of thumbs or finger abduction or adduction. Digit localization upon touch was 100% accurate. This patient's hand therapy had consisted of inpatient work for the first month followed two to three times per day for the following year.

In the three and a half years since the transplant, this French patient felt that the transplant had made his life better than what he previously experienced with the prosthesis. He could dress more effectively on his own and his personal hygiene had improved. He could eat without assistance, use the computer and telephone, and even begin to write (Fig. 14.7). He enjoyed driving a car, riding a bicycle, and even dribbling a basketball. He lived alone, went out socially, and worked at an ecology preservation site. He stated that he did not accept the transplanted hands as his own until a few months after surgery. However, he had no significant disappointments.

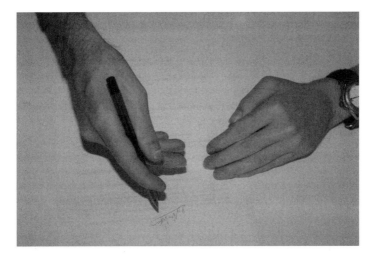

Fig. 14.7 French recipient of bilateral hand transplants demonstrating his ability to write, three and a half years posttransplantation

He was happy to lead a "normal simple life." He felt that his hand function would continue to improve.

The second bilateral transplant performed in Lyon involved a 22-year-old patient from Turkey, the youngest recipient of a hand transplant. An industrial farm machine caused the injury resulting in the loss of both hands. The interview of this patient was conducted through an Italian surgeon, who spoke French to the patient's wife, who then translated the questions in Turkish to her husband.

The donor hands were received from a 45-year-old man who was a 1/6 HLA match. The recipient amputation level was 14. cm below the right elbow and 24 cm below the left elbow. Hand-transplant ischemia time was 6 h. The patient did not receive any preoperative irradiation. An induction agent of Thymoglobulin was given followed by FK-506, mycophenolate, and Solumedrol. An IL-2 inhibitor was given twice for a rejection episode on POD 86. The only medication side effect as of the time of the interview was a transient rise in serum creatinine levels, which had resolved.

Surgical complications involved a left ulnar artery thrombosis on POD 1 that was revised. In addition, left ulnar bone osteomyelitis was diagnosed with intraoperative bone cultures revealing *Staphylococcus aureus*. This was treated with plate removal and intravenous antibiotics even with radiographic evidence of nonunion. Upon physical examination 4 months after his bilateral hand transplants, there was little objective functional motor return.

This patient had a most attentive wife, who was at his side nearly all the time. When asked about her assessment of hand transplant, she appreciated his greater autonomy in eating and using the toilet. However, she wondered if the results would be worth, in her words through translation, all the "complexity and efforts."

14.8 Italy (Transplants 2000, 2001, and 2002)

Between 2000 and 2002 there had been three hand transplants performed in Milan, Italy. The author was able to evaluate the second Italian transplant patient along with his hand surgeon, Dr. Marco Lanzetta. The patient was at that time a 32-year-old right-hand-dominant man who had lost his right hand in an explosion almost 5 years previously. The hand transplant had taken place 2 years before in 2001.

The explosion injury left the patient with an amputation level at the wrist. The donor hand was a 3/6 HLA match. The patient did not receive irradiation prior to the transplant and was treated with an induction agent followed by steroids, FK-506, and MMF for immunosuppression. There were no significant side effects secondary to immunosuppressive medications, other than vomiting from the antiviral agents.

The patient at time of interview was participating in a therapy regimen every other week. He had regained limited PIP and DIP joint mobility in his index and middle fingers, while the ring and small finger interphalangeal joint motion was minimal at the time of evaluation. The thumb did not have any observable palmar abduction or opposition. There was no observable finger abduction or adduction. However, positive findings on EMG were observed correlating to some muscle function return.

Two years after his right-hand transplant, the patient had been able to return to work to his syringe-manufacturing factory. He felt that the most significant benefit was being "balanced." His most significant disappointment was that he expected "faster movement." He wanted to advise future transplant recipients to be "patient" with functional progress.

14.9 Conclusions

Independent assessment of the hand-transplant recipients documented the motor and sensory function of the hand allografts in a standardized and objective manner. In addition, valuable psychological perspectives were attained from these transplant recipients. Taken together these results represent a composite sketch of the early hand-transplant recipients.

It was through these individual visits of hand-transplant recipients that the intensity of hand therapy performed was revealed. Patients typically stayed in the hospital for the first 1–2 months for nearly daylong therapy. This daily rehabilitation continued as an outpatient for at least another 6–12 months, followed by weekly or more frequent sessions after 1 year (Table 14.3).

The range of motion of the wrist, fingers, and thumb were assessed in all the transplanted hands. Although significant mobility was achieved, none approached "normal" range of motion in uninjured joints. The patients who were evaluated had a mean active wrist extension of about 40°, and active wrist flexion of 33°. Total

Table 14.3 Posttransplant hand therapy

First 1–2 months (inpatient)	6–7 h/day
First 6–12 months	5–6 times/week
After 12 months	1–3 times/week

finger flexion was 174°, with an extension lag averaging 35°. The distance from pulp to distal palmar crease showed a wide range between 1 and 7 cm, with a mean of 3.7 cm. The recovery of intrinsic muscle function was generally poor. A few patients had palpable contraction of their transplanted thenar muscles, but no active palmar abduction. Upon examination, only two patients, one in China and one in Austria, had significant thumb abduction or opposition against gravity. Thumb adduction, as well as finger abduction and adduction, was severely limited in all patients at the time of evaluation in 2003.

Sensory findings showed nearly uniform return of protective sensation, as all but one patient reported return of protective sensibility in the digits. Six of the patients were able to accurately localize digits upon touch, and two were confused among median or ulnar nerve innervated digits. Although two patients had inconsistent two-point discrimination between 12 and 15 mm, the great majority could not distinguish two points that were 15 mm apart (Table 14.4).

Consistently found in this hand-transplant population was the desire to return to a "normal" life. Overall, 9 of 11 hand-transplant patients had returned to modified job tasks. Of those patients who have had transplants for more than a year, all but one had returned to work. These results could have reflected a selection bias in that the most motivated patients were chosen for these initial hand transplants.

In terms of objective measurements of functional outcome, a few patients had Carroll's test performed, with results (63, 48 in Louisville, 72, 64 in Guangzhou) comparable to average and above-average scores after hand replants. The Michigan Hand Questionnaire was administered to two patients in Brussels and Innsbruck. On a scale of 100, the results were noted for complete lack of pain, activities of daily living comparable to preoperative carpal tunnel patients at 72.3, a high aesthetic score of 93.8, and an overall high score of 76.9.

At the conclusion of each interview, the question was asked what the patient regarded as the greatest benefit of their respective hand transplant was. Of the unilateral recipients, four cited improved body image and enhanced ability to engage in social interactions, three cited increased hand function, and two cited greater self-reliance. The results were different for the bilateral hand recipients. Two cited the ability to "feel" their world again, including touching their wives or children, and three cited greater self-reliance as the most significant benefits.

The patients were then asked if there were any disappointments. Four answered none, four mentioned less function than they had hoped in the transplanted hands, three mentioned side effects from medications, and two mentioned the length of recovery and rehabilitation. However, only one patient interviewed stated he would not go through the procedure again. Unfortunately, that patient had lost his hand secondary to rejection and ischemic pain.

Table 14.4 Functional and sensory assessment of hand allografts

	Mean active mobility (deg.)
Wrist extension	40.4
Wrist flexion	33.2
Total finger flexion	173.8
Finger extension lag	35.4
Pulp to palm	3.7 cm
Digital localization	6/10 patients
Two-point discrimination	>15 mm, 8/10 patients

In summary, 11 patients with 16 transplanted hands were evaluated. There were successes, and there were failures. No serious adverse effects had been encountered from immunosuppression; yet, additional medications were required in some cases with unknown long-term efficacy or side effects. Limited functional returns had been observed, but any effect of chronic rejection was too early to determine at the time in 2003. We do know, however, that each transplant represents a human story of needs and hopes. What was gleaned by the author from this independent assessment was that hand transplantation stands to benefit the lives of patients and their families, yet its future belongs in further research to achieve better function and minimize systemic immunosuppression.[8]

References

1. J. M. Deeryard, E. Owen, G, Herzberg, et al., Human hand allograft: report on first 6 months, *Lancet* **353**(9161), 1315–1320 (1999).
2. J. W. Jones Jr., E. T. Ustuner, M. Zdichavsky, et al., Long-term survival of an extremity composite tissue allograft with FK506-mycophenolate mofetil therapy, *Surgery* **126**(2), 384–388 (1999).
3. C. G. Francois, W. C. Breidenbach, C. Maldonado, Hand transplantation: comparisons and observations of the first four clinical cases, *Microsurgery* **20**(8), 360–371 (2000).
4. J. M. Dubernard, P. Petruzzo, M. Lanzetta, et al., Functional results of the first human double-hand transplantation, *Ann Surg* **238**(1), 128–136 (2003).
5. J. W. Jones, S. A. Gruber, J. H. Barker, W. C. Breidenbach, Successful hand transplantation. One-year follow-up. Louisville Hand Transplant Team, *N Engl J Med.* **343**(7), 468–473 (2000).
6. G. Pei, L. Gu, L. Yu, [A preliminary report of two cases of human hand allograft], *Zhonghua Yi Xue Za Zhi* **80**(6), 417–421 (2000).
7. M. Lanzetta, P. Petruzzo, R. Margreiter, et al., The international registry on hand and composite tissue transplantation, *Transplantation* **79**(9), 1210–1214 (2005).
8. W. P. Lee, Composite tissue transplantation: more science and patience needed, *Plast Reconstr Surg* **107**(4), 1066–1070 (2001).

Chapter 15
Hand Transplantation: Lyon Experience

Palmina Petruzzo, Emmanuel Morelon, Jean Kanitakis, Lionel Badet,
Assia Eljaafari, Marco Lanzetta, Earl Owen, and Jean-Michel Dubernard

15.1 Introduction

The first right hand and the first bilateral hand transplantation were performed in Lyon (France) on September 23, 1998[1] and on January 13, 2000,[2] respectively; then a second bilateral hand transplantation was performed on April 30, 2003.[3] These cases of hand transplantation demonstrated that it was possible to perform composite tissue allografts.

The immunosuppressive protocol used for all French patients included an induction therapy (antithymocyte globulins, prednisone, tacrolimus, and mycophenolate mofetil) and a maintenance therapy (prednisone 5 mg/d, tacrolimus with blood levels between 5 and 10 ng/ml, and mycophenolate mofetil 2 g/d).

The results achieved in the first case of hand allotransplantation showed the feasibility of the surgical technique, the efficacy of the immunosuppressive protocol, the limited adverse effects, and the importance of patient's compliance and rehabilitation to ensure graft viability and functional recovery.[4] The recipient of the first single hand transplantation, a 48-year-old-man from New Zealand, whose right arm was accidentally amputated in 1984, received the hand from a 41-year-old brain-dead man. They presented the same blood group and several HLA mismatches, negative T- and B-cell cross-match. During the first months the patient presented a well-vascularized hand graft with normal skin and fast nerve regeneration which resulted in protective and useful sensation. He was able to perform the majority of daily activities (such as gripping a glass or writing) with his grafted right hand. At this time he presented a transient hyperglycemia and a Herpes virus infection as side effects of his immunosuppressive treatment, and 8 weeks after transplantation an acute rejection episode characterized by erythematous maculopapular lesions disseminated on the transplanted hand, which regressed increasing the oral dose of steroids and using topical immunosuppressants, such as tacrolimus and clobetasol creams.

During this period the patient adhered to his immunosuppressive treatment and physiotherapy protocol. Later, he adhered to the treatment transiently before discontinuing it completely. During month 15, posttransplantation signs of rejection appeared over the skin of the grafted hand and the lesions progressively worsened.

They were remarkably similar to those seen in chronic lichenoid cutaneous graft-versus-host-disease. At the patient's request he was amputated in London on March 2, 2001 (29 months after his transplantation). After amputation various tissue specimens were studied[5] confirming that the more severe pathologic alterations (inflammatory infiltrate and necrosis) were present at skin level. The other tissues showed milder, if any, alterations. A lymphocytic infiltrate of moderate density forming loose perivascular aggregates was shown in the vicinity of muscles and tendons.

Although the results achieved in this first case showed the feasibility of hand allotransplantation, we also learned the great importance of patient compliance to immunosuppressive treatment and physiotherapy as well as his motivation. Remarkably and somehow unexpectedly, the progression of this rejection process appeared slow although the long treatment-free period and the signs were mainly in the skin and few in deeper tissue. Consequently, it can be speculated that if the patient had started his treatment, the rejection process could have been reversed. Indeed, although hand allograft contains the most antigenic tissue (skin), its immunogenicity might be reduced or modified at long term.

For all these reasons in January 2000 we performed the first bilateral hand allograft. The recipient was a 33-year-old man who suffered a bilateral amputation of hands after a blast injury in 1996. The donor was an 18-year-old man, 5 HLA A, B, DR mismatches, negative T and B cell cross-match.

The recipient of the second bilateral hand transplantation performed in April 2003 was a 21-year-old man who underwent amputation of the right forearm and left hand after a crash injury in 2000. The donor was a 48-year-old man, 4 HLA A, B, DR mismatches, negative T and B cell cross-match.

Both patients received the above-cited immunosuppressive treatment and the same rehabilitation program which started 12 h after surgery. It was intensive (twice a day) and included physiotherapy, electro-stimulation, and occupational therapy for the first 12–18 months and continued even after the first bilateral hand transplanted patient returned to work.

During the first month posttransplantation the first recipient of bilateral hand transplantation presented hyperglycemia and serum sickness while the second bilateral hand transplanted patient suffered thrombosis of the right ulnar artery the very first postoperative day and 6 months later an osteomyelitis of left ulna, which disappeared after immediate osteosynthesis removal and an antibiotic treatment for 6 months.

These complications were successfully solved and the bilateral hand transplanted patients did not present any other complication correlated to the immunosuppressive treatment.

The first recipient presented two episodes of acute rejection on days 53 and 82[6] and the second patient on days 57 and 86.[3] Macroscopically the patients developed asymptomatic skin lesions varying from faint pink macules to erythematous, slightly infiltrated scaly papules. In both cases skin biopsies revealed a perivascular dermal inflammatory infiltrate made of lymphocytes of recipient's origin, expressing mainly the CD3+/CD4+ or the CD3+/CD8+ phenotype, mixed with a low percentage of FoxP3+ Treg cells. These changes corresponded to rejection grades

I and II, according to a score recently defined.[7] Therefore oral prednisone dose was increased while clobetasol and tacrolimus cream were applied topically. Both episodes resolved clinically and histologically within 10–15 days. Thereafter they did not show other macroscopic or histological signs of acute rejection. Besides these episodes of rejection, the skin presented a normal structure.

In the cases of bilateral hand transplantation the same immunosuppressive protocol used in the first case of hand transplantation showed its efficacy and safety. Indeed, some side effects, such as transient hyperglycemia, were evidenced only in the first period after transplantation and they could be avoided by decreasing the doses of immunosuppressive drugs as it has been done in the second recipient. The second patient presented an infectious complication, which regressed with the appropriate antibiotic therapy. In the majority of cases the toxicity of these drugs is related to the dose and no overimmunosuppression is necessary in hand transplantation. Indeed, in both patients two episodes of acute rejection were reported only in the first 3 months after transplantation and were easily reversed.[3]

Functional recovery is the final goal in upper extremity transplantation. It is a long and complex process, which not only involves preservation of the viability of neural, muscular, and sensory end-organ components, but also appropriate and timely reinnervation of neural targets and several degrees of cortical reorganization. The functional outcome expected in limb transplantation is believed to be related to the level of amputation; indeed, our experience shows earlier results in the case of amputation at wrist level. However, late functional outcome appears very encouraging also at forearm level as demonstrated by the results achieved in the second recipient of bilateral hand transplantation, who presented a forearm amputation on the right side.

Both recipients of bilateral hand transplantation showed a relevant sensorimotor recovery during the entire period of the follow-up, particularly of sensibility and activity of intrinsic muscles. Sensitivity recovery was shown in both bilateral hand grafted patients with normal pain and cold sensations, without dysesthesia or cold intolerance. In our experience, recovery of intrinsic muscles started later and evolved slowly compared to extrinsic muscles. Although both patients presented a relatively limited range of motion of their joints, particularly of the wrist, because of fibrosis and adherences with a certain degree of impaired function and a diminished muscular power, they are able to perform the majority of daily activities and live a normal social life.

In the first case motor recovery started with extrinsic muscle function (at present M4+, except for finger extensor which is M3+ on both sides) allowing the patient to grasp large objects as well as to pinch. Intrinsic muscular function began only at a later stage and at 6 years after transplantation a variable degree of muscle activity was present, particularly at level of thumb opposition, hand lumbrical, and interossei. Motor recovery began with extrinsic muscle function also in the second case (3 years after transplantation it was M3+ on the right hand and M4+ on the left hand). Function of intrinsic muscles was observed by 6 months and it was between 3 and 4 on the left and 2 on the right at 2 years after transplantation. Electromyography confirmed these results in both patients.

In both cases, recognition of small objects was possible using shape, contour, and temperature criteria; manual dexterity was tested by specific tests such as the Minnesota and Caroll tests, which showed a normal capacity of reaching, grasping, moving, positioning, and turning the objects although there was an impairment to lateral pinch and bimanual grasp in the first recipient. It is remarkable that both patients were able to perform the majority of daily activities by the first year after transplantation. The first recipient started to work in March 2003. The second patient did not resume work merely because of language difficulties.

Both recipients presented a pretransplant right-dominant hand; however in the posttransplant period the first patient still has a right-dominant hand while in the second patient the left hand became dominant.

fMRI was performed before and after transplantation at different time points of the follow-up in both bilateral hand grafted patients and the results showed that hand transplantation resulted in global remodelling of the limb cortical map, reversing the functional reorganization induced by the amputation.[8] The spatial trajectory of these activations in time further indicates that the cortical rearrangement takes place in an orderly manner: the hand and arm representations tend to return to their original cortical locus. Hence, brain plasticity seems to be accomplished with reference to a preamputation body representation. Thus, peripheral input can modify cortical hand organization in sensorimotor regions. It is important to note that subsequent fMRI exams performed at 12 and 18 months after the graft showed no changes in the cortical map. This suggests that once hand neurons have reached their targets brain plasticity processes in the motor areas become stable.

The studies with the Cyber glove[9] in the first grafted patient showed his ability to perform complex movements involving intersegmental coordination 2 years after transplantation, while he presented normal anticipatory adjustments of hand shape before contact after 3 years. These results show a degree of motor coordination in bilateral hand grafted patients.

The first patient was exhaustively evaluated 5 years after transplantation: using the parameters proposed by Chen[10] the score was II (good); the evaluation performed during the follow-up[2] was based on the score proposed by Tamai and modified by Ipsen,[11] which was the same at 5 years after transplantation (good for the right hand and fair for the left hand), and the Dash score[12] was 18. Moreover, the score of the International Registry on Hand and Composite Tissue Transplantation[13] – IRHCTT – was excellent on both sides. All these scores were the same at 6 years after transplantation.

The second case was evaluated on the basis of the score proposed by the IRHCTT and it was good on both sides at 2 years after transplantation while Dash score was 18.66.

It is interesting to note that recovery of sensibility and the aesthetic aspect of the grafted hands are very important issues for hand transplantation recipients. For this reason the IRHCTT adopted an own comprehensive functional evaluation system and score as the favorable social, aesthetic, and psychological impact on the patients' well-being must be taken into consideration. These motivations explain the better evaluation of the first case of bilateral hand transplantation obtained with the IRHCTT score compared to that of Chen or Tamai, modified by Ipsen. Although at 7 years after transplantation this patient showed a better self-confidence and a major ability to perform a lot of daily activities, the functional evaluation is the same except for a slight improvement of electromyography results and sensitivity tests, at 5 and 6 years after transplantation.

The rehabilitation program as well as patient compliance seems to condition the functional recovery and for this reason our rehabilitation program started early and was complex. On the basis of our experience, muscular power and range of motion should be improved with steady and targeted exercises. The patients need strong motivation, not usually required in solid organ transplant recipients, as the results follow a rigorous protocol of physiotherapy.

In conclusion, on the basis of our experience and that of other teams[14], we believe that 8 years after the first hand transplantation the achieved results are very encouraging as major adverse effects due to surgery and immunosuppressive regimen did not occur and the patients' quality of life improved considerably, although patient compliance and motivation are indispensable.

References

1. J. M. Dubernard, E. Owen, G. Herzberg, M. Lanzetta, X. Martin, H. Kapila, M. Dawahra, N. S. Hakim, Human hand allograft: report on first 6 months, *Lancet* **353**, 1315–1320 (1999).
2. J. M. Dubernard, P. Petruzzo, M. Lanzetta, H. Parmentier, X. Martin, M. Dawahra, et al., Functional results of the first human double-hand transplantation, *Ann Surg* **238**(1), 128–136 (2003).
3. P. Petruzzo, L. Badet, A. Gazarian, M. Lanzetta, H. Parmentier, J. Kanitakis, A. Sirigu, X. Martin, J. M. Dubernard, Bilateral hand transplantation: six years after the first case, *Am J Transpl* **6**, 1–7 (2006).
4. J. M. Dubernard, E. Owen, N. Lefrancois, P. Petruzzo, X. Martin, M. Dawahra, D. Jullien, J. Kanitakis, C. Frances, X. Preville, L. Gebuhrer, N. Hakim, M. Lanzetta, H. Kapila, G. Herzberg, J. P. Revillard, First human hand transplantation: case report, *Transpl Int* **13**(Suppl 1), S521–524 (2000).
5. J. Kanitakis, D. Jullien, P. Petruzzo, N. Hakim, A. Claudy, J. P. Revillard, E. Owen, J. M. Dubernard, Clinicopathologic features of graft rejection of the first human hand allograft, *Transplantation* **27**(4), 688–693 (2003).
6. J. Kanitakis, P. Petruzzo, D. Jullien, L. Badet, M. C. Dezza, A. Claudy, M. Lanzetta, N. Hakim, E. Owen, J. M. Dubernard, Pathological score for the evaluation of allograft rejection in human hand (composite tissue) allotransplantation, *Eur J Dermatol* **15**(4), 235–238 (2005).
7. P. Petruzzo, J. P. Revillard, J. Kanitakis, M. Lanzetta, N. Hakim, N. Lefrançois, et al., First human double hand transplantation: efficacy of a conventional immunosuppressive protocol, *Clin Transplant* **17**(5), 455–460 (2003).
8. P. Giraux, A. Sirigu, F. Schneider, J. M. Dubernard, Functional cortical reorganization after transplantation of both hands as revealed by fMRI. *Nat Neurosci* **4**, 691–692 (2001).
9. P. Giraux, A. Cheylus, J. R. Duhamel, P. Petruzzo, J. M. Dubernard, A. Sirigu, Motor recovery after bilateral hand transplantation: a two year follow-up study [abstract]. *Transplantation* **74**(4), 63 (2002).

10. Z.-W. Chen, V. E. Meyer, H. E. Kleinert, R. W. Beasley, Present indications and contraindications for replantation as reflected by l ong-term functional results, *Orthop Clin North Am* **12**, 849–870 (1981).
11. T. Ipsen, L. Lundkvist, T. Barfred, J. Pless, Principles of evaluation and results in microsurgical treatment of major limb amputations: a follow-up study of 26 consecutive cases 1978–1987, *Scand J Plast Reconstr Hand Surg* **24**, 775–780 (1990).
12. D. C. Beaton, J. N. Katz, A. H. Fossel, J. G. Wright, V. Tarasuk, C. Bombardier, Measuring the whole or the parts? Validity, reliability, and responsiveness of the disabilities of the arm, shoulder and hand outcome measure in different regions of the extremity, *J Hand Ther* **14**, 128–146 (2001).
13. M. Lanzetta, P. Petruzzo, R. Margreiter, J. M. Dubernard, F. Schuind, W. Breidenbach, et al. The International Registry on Hand and Composite Tissue *Transplantation* 15;79(9):1210–1214 (2005).
14. M. Lanzetta, P. Petruzzo, J. M. Dubernard, R. Margreiter, W. Breidenbach, et al. Second report (1998–2006) of the International Registry of Hand and Composite Tissue Transplantation. *Transpl Immunol* Jul; 18(1):1–6 (2007).

Chapter 16
Hand Transplantation: The Louisville Experience

Vijay S. Gorantla and Warren C. Breidenbach III

16.1 Evolution of the Louisville Hand Transplant Program

In February 1964, Dr. Roberto Gilbert Elizalde performed a right forearm transplant on a 28-year-old sailor with a blast injury, laying the foundation to the field of hand transplantation.[1,2] However, it was not until September 1991, that the first conference on composite tissue allotransplantation (CTA) was held in Washington, DC to "determine the clinical feasibility of transplanting limbs in patients with limb loss" and the "direction in which clinically oriented limb transplantation research should head."[3] In June 1996, we organized a team of surgeons comprising hand, plastic, and transplant specialties along with members representing transplant psychiatry, pathology, tissue typing, hand therapy, and organ procurement. This constituted the Louisville Hand Transplant team. In November 1997, the First International Symposium on Composite Tissue Allotransplantation was convened in Louisville, Kentucky. The goal of this meeting was to discuss the "scientific, clinical and ethical barriers standing in the way of performing the first human hand transplant." International experts at the meeting predicted that limb allotransplantation was not far from "becoming a clinical reality."[4] In September 1998, 34 years after the first hand transplant, surgeons in Lyon, France, performed the world's second hand transplant.[5,6]

The first hand transplant performed in Ecuador rejected acutely at 2 weeks due to primitive immunosuppression (azathioprine and prednisone)[7] and the second hand transplant performed in France rejected after 2 years due to medication noncompliance and withdrawal.[8] In January 1999, we performed the first unilateral hand transplant in the United States in Louisville, Kentucky.[9] At 8 years after surgery, our first patient is the recipient of the first successful and longest surviving hand transplant in the world. In February 2001 and November 2006, we performed two more transplants at our center. We discuss here in our experience with hand transplantation in the three American patients.

16.2 Patient profiles

16.2.1 Patient 1

He was a 37-year-old Caucasian male, paramedic by occupation, who lost his left-dominant hand in 1985 due to a blast injury. Since the amputation, he used an Otto-Bock myoelectric prosthesis (Otto Bock, Inc., Minneapolis, USA). His medical history was significant for Type II insulin-dependent diabetes diagnosed in 1988, but had no complications secondary to this disease. He had been a smoker for 20 years and quit in 1996. He had no other medical or psychiatric problems. He was married with two children. He was transplanted in January 1999, 13 years following his amputation.

16.2.2 Patient 2

He was a 36-year-old Caucasian male, seamless gutter installer by occupation, who lost his left nondominant hand in 1996 in a blast injury. Since the amputation, he used a cable-hook prosthesis. His medical history was noncontributory and he had no psychiatric problems. He was a nonsmoker, married with three children. He was transplanted in February 2001, 5 years following his amputation.

16.2.3 Patient 3

He was a 54-year-old Caucasian male, product supervisor by occupation, who lost his right-dominant hand in 1972 in a machine press injury. Since the amputation, he used a cable-hook prosthesis. His medical history was significant for mitral valve prolapse and a spontaneous pneoumothorax without any psychiatric issues. He was a nonsmoker, married with four children and nine grandchildren. He was transplanted in November 2006, 34 years following his amputation.

16.3 Scientific Rationale for the Louisville Experiment

Experimental trials in the early 1990s aiming at prolongation of limb transplant survival in rodent and primate models using cyclosporine monotherapy were uniformly unsuccessful.[10–17] In 1996, it was Benhaim and colleagues who showed that a combination of cyclosporine with mycophenolate mofetil (MMF) could successfully prolong rat hindlimb allograft survival.[18] In 1998, using two different combination regimens comprising of cyclosporine, MMF, prednisone,[19] and tacrolimus, MMF, prednisone,[20] we demonstrated long-term survival of fully mismatched limb allografts in a large animal porcine model. In addition to data from small and large animal studies, we based our rationale to proceed with clinical trials of hand transplantation using modern triple immunosuppression on the following existing evidence: (1) all individual component tissues of the hand, including skin, muscle, tendons, vessels, nerve, bone, and joint, were successfully transplanted in humans[21]; (2) the availability of novel immunosuppressive drugs that have improved efficacy and lower risk profiles;[22] (3) better expertise with drug dosing and fine-tuning of immunosuppressive drug combinations based on years of experience with solid organ transplantation, and, most importantly; (4) improved prophylaxis and treatment of opportunistic fungal or viral infections (such as *Pneumocystis carinii* and cytomegalovirus [CMV]); and (4) improved therapies for posttransplant malignancies (such as rituximab for posttransplant lymphoproliferative disorder [PTLD]).

16.4 Ethical Considerations

We consulted leading ethicists for advice on formulating our ethical guidelines for an innovative procedure like hand transplant.[23] We adapted Moore's criteria to our program and addressed the following questions:

1. What is the scientific basis of the innovation? The existing literature revealed that limb CTAs were successfully prolonged on modern combination immunosuppression in small animal models. We could achieve prolongation of CTA survival in our preclinical large animal model using a similar immunosuppressive regimen as used in solid organs like kidney. Also, most components of a clinical CTA were successfully transplanted on modern immunosuppression with extended survival.
2. What is the skill and experience of the team ("field strength")? Our institutional strengths lay in our very productive plastic surgery research laboratories, a strong multiorgan transplant division, a well-equipped tissue typing/pathology facility, an experienced transplant psychiatry team, and importantly, a hand surgery program renowned for its high volume of upper extremity replants and a track record of innovations in the field.
3. What is the ethical climate of the institution? As part of an external and internal review process, we invited prominent ethicists like Dr. Mark Siegler (University of Chicago) and Dr. Paul Simmons (University of Louisville) along with others in the field to examine the ethical climate and determine its suitability to perform the procedure.
4. Is the program "transparent" in terms of open display, public evaluation, and public and professional discussions? We declared our intention to proceed with the procedure through open announcements in the lay and professional

media, and via debates/presentations at scientific meetings and specialty symposia prior to clinical application. Our ethical practices have been reviewed and critiqued by the scientific community and have established the credibility of our program.

16.5 Recipient and Donor Selection

As there were no available standards for selection of hand-transplant donors and recipients, we based our criteria on solid organ transplant experience. Though most criteria were similar to that established in solid organs, significant differences existed in certain areas of selection of hand-transplant recipients and donors.

Prospective hand recipient criteria differed in four areas from solid-organ recipient criteria:

1. *Prosthetic use.* We required our potential recipients to at least have attempted prosthetic use prior to transplant. This criterion allows us a successful exit strategy in event of posttransplant complications.
2. *Age or recipient.* Recipients less than 18 years of age were excluded due to issues of informed consent and the potentially increased risk of PTLD. Recipients older than 65 years of age were excluded due to vascular concerns, increased incidence of comorbidities, limited years of potential gain from the transplant, and decreased nerve regeneration.
3. *Health state/comorbid diseases.* Recipients with severe comorbid states, like major organ failure, were excluded. We also considered blindness to be an absolute contraindication, since sensory return in a transplanted hand is delayed and/or absent in the early phase and sight provides the only means of protecting the hand during that time.
4. *Amputation level.* We selected our patients based on the level of amputation which was appropriate to allow motor function from the recipient musculature. This included patients with a level distal to mid-forearm but proximal to wrist (Figs. 16.1–16.3).

Prospective hand donor criteria differed from solid-organ donor criteria in four areas:

1. *Donor selection.* Skin color, tone, hairiness, gender, and race were matched between the donor and recipient. Bone size was also matched for successful osteosynthesis.
2. *Medical history.* We excluded donors with history of congenital or connective tissue disorders, peripheral neuropathy, and traumatic deformities. Unlike solid organ transplants, we believe that any history of malignancy in the donor, even remote, is an absolute contraindication for hand transplants. The risk of transmitting a malignancy, no matter how minute, is unacceptable in this nonlife-saving transplant.

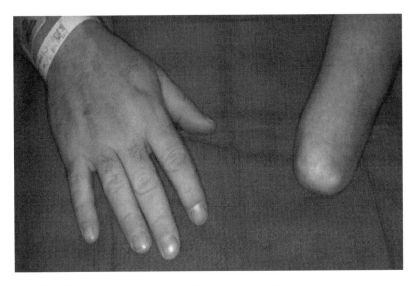

Fig. 16.1 The First American Transplant Patient - Amputation Level

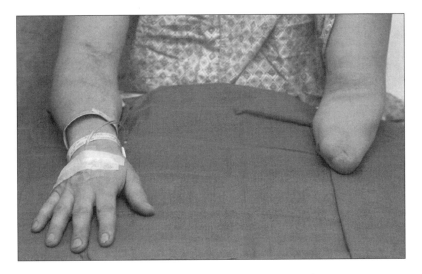

Fig. 16.2 The Second American Transplant Patient - Amputation Level

3. *Organ recovery.* The timing of donor-hand procurement was integrated in the sequence of solid-organ procurement. Our protocol was to dissect the hand last (following organs) and retrieve the donor graft first.
4. *Consent.* As part of the consenting process, we offered families the option of forearm prosthesis to enable open casket funerals.

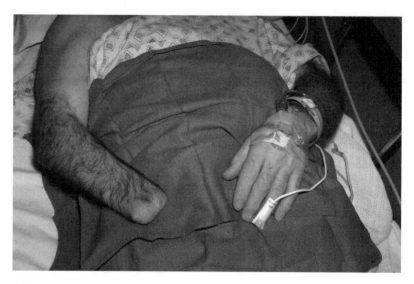

Fig. 16.3 The Third American Transplant Patient - Amputation Level

16.6 Recipient Recruitment

We enrolled patients based on referrals, a website (http://www.handtransplant.com), and word of mouth. Following a preliminary phone interview by the transplant coordinator, interested subjects were sent a screening consent form. Upon completion of the consent, subjects were medically screened for eligibility criteria. The screening procedures involved physical and laboratory examinations, comprehensive psychiatric evaluations, and assessment of medical insurance status. All subject data was reviewed by the Louisville Hand Transplant patient selection committee. Those subjects considered to be eligible were then invited to review the informed consent for the procedure. Following extensive education regarding the transplantation procedure, immunosuppression protocol, complications and risks involved, and completion of the consent process, the potential recipient was waitlisted for a suitable donor.

16.6.1 Medical Screening of Potential Recipients

This included a complete medical history and physical examination; routine laboratory studies; blood typing and cross-matching; human leukocyte antigen (HLA) typing; testing for panel-reactive antibodies; and serology for Epstein–Barr virus, cytomegalovirus, HIV, and viral hepatitis. Other tests included radiography (to plan for osteosynthesis), angiography (to exclude abnormal vascular patterns), electromyography, and nerve conduction velocity.

16.6.2 Psychiatric Evaluation

Our patients underwent a thorough psychiatric consultation prior to their transplantation.[24–26] This consisted of a general clinical interview along with comprehensive evaluation of emotional and cognitive preparedness for transplant, decision-making capacity, and history of medical compliance. Issues specific to hand transplantation were separately addressed. These included degree of motivation and level of realistic expectations regarding posttransplant outcomes, potential for psychological regression, perceived body-image adaptation, and anticipated comfort with the cadaver hand. In addition to the consultation and interview, our patients were also subjected to the Rorschach and the Thematic Apperception tests. Factors like family support, social, and financial issues were also carefully examined. The patients and their spouses met with a transplant social worker for assessment of the social system available to support the patient during transplantation and the posttransplant rehabilitation period.

16.6.3 Assessment of Insurance Coverage

All costs related to obtaining the donor limb, the surgery and hospital fees, post-transplant medications, postoperative visits, and physical therapy visits for the first 3 months were covered by Jewish Hospital and Kleinert, Kutz and Associates. As recipients would be responsible for posttransplant medications, follow-up evaluations, and lab work after their discharge, we sought assurance from the subject's insurance company that standard of care coverage will not be affected. This was done before the patient was enrolled. Patients without insurance and/or financial security were excluded from the selection process.

16.6.4 Informed Consent

The final stage of patient recruitment involved completion of a clear and extensive informed consent by the potential recipient. In addition to obtaining a written consent, we also filmed the consenting for our records to ensure that due diligence was followed during the process. The consent addressed all the components of the procedure including pre-, intra- and postoperative risks (including graft failure and death), immunosuppressive protocol and complications (including rejection of graft, serious infections, cancer, metabolic side effects, and life-threatening adverse events), psychosocial risks of the procedure, available alternatives to hand transplantation, and exit strategies like amputation in the event of complications.

16.7 Donor Procurement

We worked with our local organ procurement organization (OPO) to identify potential hand donors and inform families of the opportunity to donate. Our local OPO, upon receiving information from a hospital of a case of probable brain death, sent representatives to approach the patient's family to attempt consent for donation. The donor family was assured of confidentiality during the donation process and the OPO paid for all donation-related expenses incurred following declaration of brain death. In cases of approved family consent, the OPO then initiated the process of donor evaluation and organized hand procurement. Irrespective of geographic location, once we had a suitable donor identified by the local OPO, we dispatched our donor retrieval team via charter flight to procure the limb. We simultaneously notified the recipient and arranged for his transportation to our hand transplant center. Our OPO ensured that selection of potential hand donors was in accordance to the criteria established by the Louisville Hand Transplant team. If the donor was unstable, the hand dissection was performed following organ dissection. However, before cross-clamping of aorta, the hand team commenced dissection and retrieved the limb prior to organ retrieval. Upon completion of hand retrieval, the OPO fitted the donor body with a cosmetic prosthesis, allowing the family the option of an open-casket funeral. Following retrieval, the limb (wrapped in moist sterile gauze) was transported in a sterile container (provided by the OPO) with iced water at 4–6 °C. During transport, the limb was continuously perfused by cold University of Wisconsin (UW) solution through a brachial artery cannula.

16.8 Operative Procedure

We had two teams working in tandem to minimize the cold ischemia time. The recipient team worked on preparing the distal stump and tagging vessels, nerves, and tendons. The donor team worked on the back table to prepare the donor limb for transplant. The limb was trimmed of excess skin, flaps were planned, and bone, tendon, and nerves lengths cut per estimates determined by the extent of tissue loss in the recipient. The UW fluid was replaced with chilled lactated ringers so that it was flushed out of the donor graft.

The technical aspects of hand transplantation were the same as replantation except for a few differences. As prolonged warm ischemia could potentiate inflammatory responses and acute rejection in hand transplants,[27] we followed the order of bone–artery–few veins–tendon–nerve–remaining veins (BAVTNV) in our procedure. In doing so we gave priority to bone fixation and early vascular anastomosis. The ulna was plated dorsally and the radius ventrally using an 8-hole, 3.5-mm dynamic compression plate for osteosynthesis. We anastomosed at least two main arteries and at least one or two veins (remaining veins completed later). At this point, the decision for the need for tendon transfers or grafts was made as necessary.

If sufficient tendon length was available on the recipient and donor, a Pulvertaft weave was chosen as it is superior to an end-to-end repair. Strong tendon repair was ensured to enable early, active postoperative range of motion (ROM). Donor and recipient incisions were offset by 90 ° to achieve optimal skin closure without tension. The limb was immobilized in a long arm splint following the surgery.

16.9 Immunosuppressive Regimen

16.9.1 Induction Immunosuppression

Basiliximab (Simulect, Novartis Pharmaceutical Corp, East Hanover, NJ), an interleukin-2 receptor blocking antibody was given perioperatively in Patients 1 and 2 while alemtuzumab (Campath 1H, Millennium Pharmaceutical Corp, Cambridge, MA), a monoclonal antibody that blocks the CD52 receptor was used in Patient 3.

16.9.2 Maintenance Immunosuppression

Maintenance therapy in Patient 1 was with tacrolimus (FK506; Prograf, Astellas, Deerfield, IL), MMF (CellCept, Roche, Nutley, NJ) and prednisone. In Patient 2, MMF was replaced with sirolimus (Rapamycin, Rapamune, Wyeth-Ayerst Labs, Philadelphia, PA) and tacrolimus dose reduced at 4 weeks after surgery. Tacrolimus was started at the same time as basiliximab induction. Target levels for tacrolimus were 10–15 ng/ml during months 1–6, then 5–10 ng/ml thereafter. Dosing adjustments were made if the 12-h trough is >20% above or below the target range. Twelve-hour whole-blood trough concentrations were measured with the Incstar ProTrac II enzyme-linked immunosorbent assay (Diasorin, Stillwater, MN). MMF was also begun before surgery, with the dose subsequently adjusted to maintain trough plasma concentrations of mycophenolic acid between 3 and 5 ng/ml (as measured with the EMIT 2000 assay [Dade Behring, Deerfield, IL]), with a maximal daily dose of 3 g. MMF doses were adjusted based on white cell count (at counts <4.0, MMF dose was reduced 50%, and at counts <2.5, MMF was discontinued). Five hundred milligrams of intravenous (IV) methylprednisolone (Solumedrol) was administered intraoperatively; tapering doses were given orally, beginning on the first postoperative day (at 2 mg/kg/d, which was decreased to 10 mg/d by month 3). Patient 2 received 500 mg methylprednisolone given IV 1 h before alemtuzumab induction. He did not receive oral steroid maintenance.

For prophylaxis against CMV, 5 mg of ganciclovir/kg (Cytovene, Hoffmann-La Roche, Nutley, NJ) was given intravenously every 12 h while the patient was hospitalized, followed by oral therapy (1,000 mg t.i.d) until 3 months after transplantation.

Currently, the maintenance doses of the patients have been modified to the following levels. Patient 1 is on 3 mg b.i.d. tacrolimus oral, 500 mg q.i.d. of MMF oral, and 5 mg/d of prednisone oral. Patient 2 is on 2–4 mg b.i.d. tacrolimus oral, 3 mg/d of sirolimus oral and 10 mg/d of prednisone oral. Patient 3 is on 2.5–3.5 mg b.i.d tacrolimus oral and 500 mg b.i.d. of MMF oral. He is not on systemic steroids.

16.10 Posttransplant Rehabilitation

On the basis of our experience with replantation, we developed a treatment protocol for postoperative management of the transplanted hand.[28,29] Once the viability of the transplanted limb is guaranteed, the focus of rehabilitation becomes the restoration of normal form and function which includes the ability to perform physical, psychosocial, vocational, and recreational activities. We advocate early mobilization of the transplanted limb, if possible within 24–48 h. This reduces edema and stiffness, as well as prevention of an intrinsic-minus hand and claw deformities. During surgery it is of paramount importance to perform three procedures that will enhance success of the early mobilization/bracing program. These include proper hemostasis and ligation of vessels not used for transplantation to prevent hematoma, scrupulous removal of devascularized/functionless tissue to reduce the risk of infection or postoperative fibrosis, and keeping bone fixation hardware to a minimum to avoid interference with early extensor tendon gliding over the dorsum of the hand.

We developed a dynamic crane extension outrigger splint that mimics intrinsic function of the hand (Fig. 16.4).[30] It positions the hand appropriately and allows for

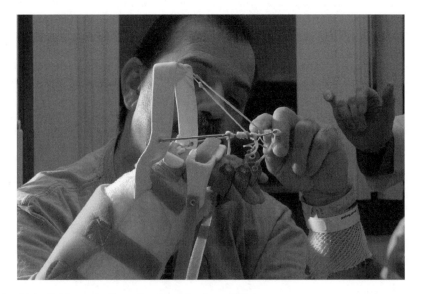

Fig. 16.4 The Dynamic Crane Extension Outrigger Splint

initiation of exercise. The wrist is positioned in slight extension; the metacarpophalangeal joints in 50–70° of flexion; the interphalangeal joints held at 0°, and the thumb is held in a balance between radial and palmar abduction (by light dynamic extension). This splint differs from others as it reduces the force on the repaired fingers, as much of the force of the elastic rubber-bands is dissipated into the crane outrigger and the tower base, minimizing risk of tendon rupture. To date we have not had any ruptures with this device. At approximately 4–5 weeks postsurgery, and depending upon bony healing, wrist and forearm ROM is initiated within a hand-based anticlaw splint. From 8 to 12 weeks postsurgery, other therapeutic modalities are added depending upon the level of healing and usage gained at that time. At 12 weeks postsurgery a dynamic wrist extension splint is applied by connecting it to the anticlaw splint. This aids in strengthening of the wrist flexors and extensors by allowing wrist flexion against resistance and assistive active extension. This splint is used three to four times a day for 15–30 min. It helps strengthen the repaired tendons and muscles by increasing flexor strength and balancing the antagonistic muscle groups. Light weights are used to isolate and strengthen specific muscle groups such as the wrist flexor and extensors. Its use is alternated with the crane-extension outrigger splint. The anticlaw splint is worn alone when exercises are not being performed. Function at the metacarpal level may be improved by early use of the dynamic crane outrigger splint with a metacarpophalangeal joint extension block. Promoting early protective active motion and blocking metacarpophalangeal joint extension help achieve a hand with an intrinsic-plus posture and coordinated grasping. Tenolysis may be needed in some patients, but it should not be performed until 6 months after surgery.

16.11 Assessment of Outcomes

16.11.1 *Functional Evaluation*

We used the Carroll test as a means of evaluating integrated upper extremity and global hand function. It utilizes a series of 33 tasks scored by two independent observers. A maximum of 99 points are available for scoring.[31] On the Carroll test, outcomes are considered excellent if the score is ≥85, good for scores between 75 and 84, fair for scores of 51–74, and poor for scores lower than 51. Grip strength was measured using a Jamar dynamometer and pinch strength (tip, three-jaw chuck and key pinch) was measured using a pinchometer. ROM including total active and passive ROM was measured according to guidelines of the ASSH. Tinel's sign was assessed until it advanced to the fingertips. Thereafter, Semmes Weinstein monofilament testing (for pressure threshold of slowly adapting receptors), vibration (30 and 250 cps), and static and moving 2-point discrimination (for number of innervated receptors) were performed as previously reported.[32] For data reporting to the international registry, we used the International Registry

Score (IRS) to assess the patients.[33] The IRS measures six parameters that each test several areas. Each area is assigned a point value that varies by outcome. The total possible score on the IRS system is 100. Final outcomes are graded as Poor (0–30 points), Fair (31–60 points), Good (61–80 points), and Excellent (81–100 points).

16.11.2 Assessment for Rejection, Graft Versus Host Disease and Immunomonitoring

Skin and muscle biopsies were obtained when clinically indicated by visible signs of rejection (maculopapular rash, edema, scaling, or blistering) and according to the institutional review board protocol on days 0, 5, 7, 10, 14, 21, and 30 and monthly thereafter. Scoring for acute rejection (AR) was accomplished using grading criteria developed in our preclinical model.[34] Important clinical endpoints of AR included edema, erythema, escharification, and necrosis. Biopsies were also examined for evidence of chronic rejection (CR).[35] Endpoints for CR included evidence of intimal hyperplasia and subintimal foamy histiocytes in the vessels of the skin or muscle. Clinical diagnosis of graft versus host disease (GVHD) was based on previously described criteria.[36] Donor chimerism and cell phenotype were assessed by monoclonal antibodies specific for host or donor class I antigens.[37] The antibody panel consisted of control antibodies plus antibodies specific for T cells (CD3, CD4, CD8), B cells (CD19), NK cells (CD56), and myeloid markers (CD33, CD45) [CD stands for Cluster of Differentiation].

16.11.3 Psychosocial Evaluation

As in the pretransplant evaluation, recipients were subjected to psychiatric assessment at yearly follow-up.

16.12 Summary of Outcomes in the American Patients

16.12.1 Allograft Survival

At the time of writing this chapter, Patients 1 and 2 underwent evaluation at 7 and 5 years. Patient 3 was evaluated at 3 months following transplantation. The present allograft survival is 8 years for Patient 1, 6 years for Patient 2, and 4 months for Patient 3.

16.12.2 Function

16.12.2.1 Patient 1

Carroll score is 72/99 (Fair), and the IRS score is 90/100 (Excellent). He can perform tasks requiring fine skills and coordination. He can pick up tiny ball bearings, checkers, poker chips, tie shoe laces, write, and even sign his name. He can also throw and catch a ball. Though he can dress himself, buttoning his clothes is still difficult. Total active ROM has shown variable improvement over the years and he has full passive finger extension and flexion (most increases in index finger ROM). Motor function in transplanted intrinsics has improved with notable increases in index finger abduction. Arthritis at the carpometacarpal joint was limiting thumb abduction. However, joint motion improved with use of an abduction splint. Grip strength (at second setting on Jamar dynamometer) is 15 lb, lateral pinch is 5 lb, and power of lift with the transplanted hand is 60 lb. He now demonstrates 3-point pinch of 7 lb.

Semmes–Weinstein monofilament testing indicates sensation in the normal has returned to normal range (2.83) in all finger tips. Static two-point discrimination showed significant improvement in index and ring fingers. Moving two-point discrimination has shown most improvement in thumb, index, and long fingers. Touch localization (to tips of thumb, long, ring, and small finger), stereognosis, temperature, and vibration sensation (256 cps) have returned. Tinel's is strongest at the tips of index and small fingers. Sweating is still absent.

16.12.2.2 Patient 2

Carroll score is 42/99 (Poor), and the IRS score is 50/100 (Fair). He can perform tasks like turning pages, throwing and catching a ball, picking up poker chips, turning door knobs, and pouring water out of a jug with ease. Finer tasks are more difficult. Total active motion has also shown similar variability at testing but has been less than that observed in Patient 1. Wrist and forearm ROMs have remained the same as that at previous follow-up. There is persistence of extrinsic flexor and extensor tightness. There is still no 3-point pinch.

Semmes–Weinstein monofilament testing reveals loss of protective sensation at finger tips (4.56). Localization patterns have changed and he can perceive a stimulus but still cannot discriminate. Dorsal web space testing reveals diminished light touch (3.61). Sweating, temperature, and vibration sensation (256 cps) have returned. Tinel's has advanced to the tip of the small finger. He can detect smooth and rough surfaces and edges but still does not have stereognosis.

16.12.2.3 Patient 3

Functional information is not yet available in this patient.

16.12.3 Acute Rejection, Chronic Rejection, GVHD, and Immunomonitoring

16.12.3.1 Patient 1

Three episodes of clinical rejection were observed at 51, 143, and 204 days after surgery with biopsy confirmation of Grade 2–3 AR. Though he has been Grade 1 on occasional biopsies, he had not had a histologically confirmed clinical rejection episode (Grade 3) since the 7-month time point. At most recent follow-up, transplant biopsy from distal ulnar aspect showed no evidence of cellular AR. Transplant biopsy from distal radial aspect revealed no cellular AR (Grade 0). Mild solar elastosis and actinic changes present. Overlying epidermis and dermal adnexae were histologically unremarkable. No epithelial necrosis, granulomatous inflammation, or viral cytopathic effect was noted. There was no clinical or histopathological evidence of CR or GVHD. Immunomonitoring did not reveal evidence of either macro- or microchimerism.

16.12.3.2 Patient 2

He had biopsy confirmed AR on day 10 (Grade 1) and day 21 (Grade 2) both of which responded to 500 mg of intravenous methylprednisolone (Solumedrol). On day 50, AR recurred (Grade 3) and was treated with rabbit antithymocyte globulin (Thymoglobulin, Genzyme, Cambridge, MA). On day 77, he had a relapse of AR (Grade 2) that responded to topical treatment with tacrolimus (Protopic, Astellas, Nutley, NJ) and clobetasol creams. On day 90, skin biopsy confirmed Grade 2 AR (Fig. 16.5). It responded poorly to intravenous methylprednisolone or topical drug treatment but cleared on repeat Thymoglobulin infusion. Histologically, he continues to have episodes of steroid-resistant AR despite ongoing immunosuppression. His most recent Grade 2–3 AR episode was as 4 years. At most recent follow-up, transplant biopsy from medial distal radial aspect of dorsum revealed focal mild cellular AR (Grade 1). Chronic perivascular inflammation with chronic perifolliculitis was noted in mid and superficial dermis. Dermal adnexae and superficial epidermis were histologically normal. There was no clinical or histopathological evidence of CR or GVHD. Immunomonitoring did not reveal evidence of either macro- or microchimerism.

16.12.3.3 Patient 3

He had a Grade 3 AR episode on day 56 postoperative that resolved with topical clobetasol and tacrolimus cream. There was no evidence of clinical AR at the time of his discharge from the hospital at 3 months. No signs of GVHD were noted. Results of immunomonitoring were not available.

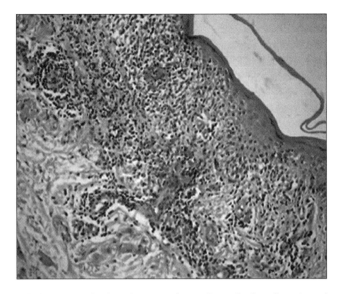

Fig. 16.5 Grade 2 Acute Rejection demonstrating perivascular lymphocytic and eosinophilic infiltration and periadnexal interphase reaction

16.12.4 Psychosocial Status

All patients were found to have a high level of personality organization and motivation with significant psychological strengths, and adjusted very well to their transplants. They felt that having a transplant helped them to become "whole," to overcome work limitations and be able to physically express emotions to their families. In general, the patients felt that the transplant facilitated mastery of physical and psychological trauma of amputation and restored the human touch in communication and close relationships.

16.13 Complications

16.13.1 Patient 1

This patient was seronegative for CMV prior to transplant (donor was seropositive). He was culture positive for CMV infection at 150 days after transplant and completely recovered upon extended treatment for 90 days with ganciclovir [Cytovene, Hoffmann-La Roche, Nutley, NJ]. He had an episode of Tinea in the first year that was treated with terbinafine (Lamisil, Sandoz, East Hanover, NJ) cream.

16.13.2 Patient 2

At 21 days after transplant, he developed hyperglycemia that responded well to metformin (Glucophage, Bristol-Myers-Squibb, Park Ave, New York, NY). To reduce the risk of tacrolimus-induced hyperglycemia, his tacrolimus dose was reduced to 4 mg b.i.d. orally, and sirolimus was added to his regimen at a dose of 3 mg/d orally. The latest results of glycosylated hemoglobin (HbA1c) showed his levels to be 5.6. He, however, developed hypercholesterolemia shortly after starting sirolimus. This was treated with atorvastatin (Lipitor, Pfizer, Cambridge, MA). At 210 days after surgery, he developed community-acquired pneumonia that was successfully treated. The most severe complication in Patient 2 was avascular necrosis of the hips. Stage III avascular necrosis involving the right femoral head and neck and Stage II avascular necrosis limited to left femoral head as confirmed by MRI was diagnosed at 28 months after transplant. He is pain free and mobile following total hip arthroplasty on the right hip and is currently being considered for an arthroplasty on the left side.

16.14 Conclusion

Outcomes in Patients 1 and 2 have confirmed that intermediate to long-term survival of hand transplants is possible using a standard immunosuppressive drug regimen as used in solid-organ transplants. Function is superior to that obtained by prostheses and both patients have returned to professional activities. Both patients had more than one episode of AR in the first year. AR was mostly responsive to bolus steroids (Patient 1) or depletional agents (Patient 2). Complications in these two patients ranged from minor fungal infections to CMV[38] and osteonecrosis. None of the complications have been fatal. No life-threatening opportunistic infections, GVHD or lymphomas were observed.[39] Patient 2 represents the longest-standing amputee to be transplanted in the world. He is one of the three patients in the world whose induction regimen consisted of alemtuzumab. His maintenance regimen is tacrolimus and MMF, making him the first hand recipient in the world on a protocol that completely eliminates systemic steroids.

None of our patients demonstrated evidence of macro- or microchimerism (the presence of donor-derived cells in recipient tissues).[40] We did not observe any histopathologic evidence of CR in our patients.

At the time of this publication, 35 hands have been transplanted in 27 patients between 1998 and 2007 (http://www.handregistry.com). Of these, 23 transplants were performed in 16 recipients in the USA and Europe. Additionally, 14 hands were transplanted onto 11 patients in China. All patients were male except for one patient, and a total of nine unilateral and six bilateral transplants were performed. With the exception of this single loss of the French transplant, the combined US and European experience has shown an allograft survival of greater than 95%.

No patient has yet lost his hand while on immunosuppression. Lack of immunosuppression (due to inability to pay for medication) led to the poor outcomes in the Chinese patients. At the Sixth International Symposium on Hand and Composite Tissue Allotransplantation, Tucson, AZ, January 2006, it was announced that out of 14 hands transplanted, the majority were lost to CR.

In addition to the Chinese reports of CR, there were early reports of the same by the French team in their first patient.[41-45] However, in later reports, the French have carefully distanced themselves from their prior statements regarding CR.[8] Notably, neither the French nor the Chinese have provided histologic evidence that confirms the classic pathologic features of this condition. This has only worsened the confusion regarding this phenomenon and increased the debate within the misinformed hand and transplant community. However, it is important to remember that, as confirmed in kidney transplants, younger recipient age, older donor age, male sex, higher panel reactive antibody status, greater HLA mismatch, and cadaver donor could potentially increase the risk of CR.[46] As most patients around the world fulfill these criteria to varying extent, it is possible that some of them could eventually develop CR. The long-term results in our patients and the remaining world hand transplants will definitively answer this issue.

In spite of highly encouraging preliminary outcomes of hand transplantation, there will always be critics as long as there are severe complications such as diabetes and avascular necrosis. These debates are guaranteed to continue until we can satisfactorily and reliably reduce risk and improve outcomes. Though tolerance to composite tissue is the ideal goal that we must all strive for, development of novel protocols that minimize maintenance immunosuppression and allow steroid avoidance is the immediate priority in hand transplants.[47,48]

On the horizon, are new drugs which bring the possibility of markedly reducing maintenance immunosuppression.[49] Right now, there are monoclonal antibodies like alemtuzumab, which when used at induction for kidney transplants result in a steroid-free maintenance therapy.[50] The acute rejection rate is higher with these protocols but the long-term complications (based on solid-organ data) will presumably be less. The next ethical debate that faces hand transplantation is whether these and other new induction techniques should be used. Although they hold the promise of reducing the long-term complications, they may be associated with higher rate of acute rejection. How much longer do we continue to use standard immunosuppression in hand transplant with its already established complication rate as opposed to embracing new drugs/protocols with only short-term clinical testing but with excellent results?

References

1. Anonymous, Historic cadaver-to-man hand transplant, *Med. World News* **5**(6), 60 (1964).
2. Anonymous, Helping hand, *Time* **83**(10), 42 (1964).
3. K. S. Black, C. W. Hewitt, *Report: Composite Tissue Transplantation Workshop*. Washington, DC: Department of Veterans Affairs, Rehabilitation Research and Development Service (1991).

4. J. H. Barker, J. W. Jones, W. C. Breidenbach, Closing remarks. Proceedings of the International Symposium on Composite Tissue Allotransplantation, Louisville, Kentucky, *Transplant. Proc. (Special Issue)* **30**, 2787 (1998).
5. J. M. Dubernard, E. Owen, G. Herzberg, et al., Human hand allograft: report on first 6 months, *Lancet* **1**, 1315 (1999).
6. J. M. Dubernard, E. Owen, N. Lefrancois, et al., First human hand transplantation. Case report, *Transpl. Int.* **13**, 521 (2000).
7. Anon, Hand transplanted from cadaver is reamputated, *Med. Trib. Med. News* **5**, 20 (1964).
8. J. Kanitakis, D. Jullien, P. Petruzzo, et al., Clinicopathologic features of graft rejection of the first human hand allograft, Transplantation **76**(4), 688–693 (2003).
9. J. W. Jones, S. A. Gruber, J. H. Barker, et al., Successful hand transplantation. One-year follow-up. Louisville Hand Transplant Team, *N. Engl. J. Med.* **343**, 468 (2000).
10. K. S. Black, C. W. Hewitt, J. S. Hwang, et al., Dose response of cyclosporine-treated composite tissue allografts in a strong histocompatible rat model, *Transplant. Proc.* **20**, 266 (1988).
11. S. K. Kim, S. Aziz, P. Oyer, et al., Use of cyclosporine A in allotransplantation of rat limbs, *Ann. Plast. Surg.* **12**, 249 (1984).
12. W. D. Fritz, W. M. Swartz, S. Rose, et al., Limb allografts in rats immunosuppressed with cyclosporine A, *Ann. Surg.* **199**, 211 (1984).
13. Z. Min, N. F. Jones, Limb transplantation in rats: immunosuppression with FK-506, *J. Hand Surg.* **20A**(1), 77 (1995).
14. R. K. Daniel, E. P. Egerszegi, D. D. Samulack, et al., Tissue transplants in primates for upper extremity reconstruction: a preliminary report, *J. Hand Surg.* **11A**(1), 1 (1986).
15. G. B. Stark, W. M. Swartz, K. Narayanan, et al., Hand transplantation in baboons. *Transplant. Proc.* **19**, 3968 (1987).
16. S. E. R. Hovius, H. P. J. D. Stevens, P. W. M. van Nierop, et al., Allogeneic transplantation of the radial side of the hand in the rhesus monkey: I. Technical aspects, *Plast. Reconstr. Surg.* **89**, 700 (1992).
17. E. P. Egerszegi, D. D. Samulack, R. K. Daniel, Experimental models in primates for reconstructive surgery utilizing tissue transplants, *Ann. Plast. Surg.* **13**, 423 (1984).
18. P. Benhaim, J. P. Anthony, L. Ferreira, et al., Use of combination of low-dose cyclosporine and RS-61443 in a rat hindlimb model of composite tissue allotransplantation, *Transplantation* **61**, 527 (1996).
19. E T. Üstüner, M. Zdichavsky, X. Ren, et al., Long-term composite tissue allograft survival in a porcine model with cyclosporine/mycophenolate mofetil therapy, *Transplantation* **66**, 1581 (1998).
20. J. W. Jones Jr., E. T. Üstüner, M. Zdichavsky, et al., Long-term survival of an extremity composite tissue allograft with FK506-mycophenolate mofetil therapy, *Surgery* **126**, 384 (1999).
21. V. S. Gorantla, C. Maldonado, J. Frank, et al., Composite tissue allotransplantation (CTA): current status and future insights, *Eur. J. Trauma* **27**, 267 (2001).
22. V. S. Gorantla, J. H. Barker, J. W. Jones Jr., et al., Immunosuppressive agents in transplantation: mechanisms of action and current anti-rejection strategies, *Microsurgery* **20**(8), 420 (2000).
23. G. R. Tobin, W. C. Breidenbach, M. M. Klapheke, F. R. Bentley, D. J. Pidwell, P. D. Simmons, Ethical considerations in the early composite tissue allograft experience: a review of the Louisville Ethics Program, *Transplant. Proc.* **37**(2), 1392–1395 (2005).
24. M. M. Klapheke, The role of the psychiatrist in organ transplantation, *Bull. Menninger Clin.* **63**(1), 13–39 (1999).
25. M. M. Klapheke, C. Marcell, G. Taliaferro, B. Creamer, Psychiatric assessment of candidates for hand transplantation, *Microsurgery* **20**(8), 453–457 (2000).
26. M. Klapheke, Transplantation of the human hand: psychiatric considerations, *Bull. Menninger Clin.* **63**, 159–173 (1999).
27. A. K. Qayumi, M. N. Nikbakht-Sangari, D. V. Godin, et al., The relationship of ischemia-reperfusion injury of transplanted lung and the up-regulation of major histocompatibility complex II on host peripheral lymphocytes, *J. Thorac. Cardiovasc. Surg.* **115**(5), 978 (1998).

28. L. R. Scheker, A. Hodges, Brace and rehabilitation after replantation and revascularization, *Hand Clin.* **17**(3), 473–480 (2001).
29. L. R. Scheker, S. P. Chesher, D. T. Netscher, et al., Functional results of dynamic splinting after transmetacarpal, wrist, and distal forearm replantation, *J. Hand Surg. [Br]* **20**(5), 584–590 (1995).
30. A. Hodges, S. Chesher, S. Feranda, Hand transplantation: rehabilitation. Case report, *Microsurgery* **20**, 389 (2000).
31. D. Carroll, A quantitative test of upper extremity function, *J. Chron. Dis.* **18**, 479 (1965).
32. J. Bell-Krotoski, S. Weinstein, C. Weinstein, Testing sensibility, including touch-pressure, two-point discrimination, point localization, and vibration, *J. Hand Ther.* **6**(2), 114–123 (1993).
33. M. Lanzetta, P. Petruzzo, R. Margreiter, et al., The international registry on hand and composite tissue transplantation, *Transplantation* **79**(9), 1210–1214 (2005).
34. M. Zdichavsky, J. W. Jones, E. T. Ustuner, et al., Scoring of skin rejection in a swine composite tissue allograft model, *J. Surg. Res.* **85**(1), 1–8 (1999).
35. H. Shirwan, Chronic allograft rejection. Do the Th2 cells preferentially induced by indirect alloantigen recognition play a dominant role? *Transplantation* **68**(6), 715–726 (1999).
36. J. L. Ferrara, H. J. Deeg, Graft-versus-host disease, *N. Engl. J. Med.* **324**(10), 667–674 (1991).
37. K. A. Prabhune, V. S. Gorantla, C. Maldonado, et al., Mixed allogeneic chimerism and tolerance to composite tissue allografts, *Microsurgery* **20**, 441 (2000).
38. S. Schneeberger, S. Lucchina, M. Lanzetta, et al., Cytomegalovirus-related complications in human hand transplantation, *Transplantation* **80**(4), 441–447 (2005).
39. S. Baumeister, C. Kleist, B. Dohler, et al., Risks of allogeneic hand transplantation, *Microsurgery* **24**(2), 98–103 (2004).
40. D. K. Granger, W. C. Breidenbach, D. J. Pidwell, et al., Lack of donor hyporesponsiveness and donor chimerism after clinical transplantation of the hand, *Transplantation* **74**(11), 1624–1630 (2002).
41. P. Petruzzo, J. M. Dubernard, 2001, Hand transplantation: Lyon experience. In: Dubernard J. M., ed. *Composite Tissue Allografts*. Paris: John Libbey Eurotext, p. 63.
42. Lefrancois N, 2001, Immunosuppression in hand allograft. In: Dubernard J. M., ed. *Composite Tissue Allografts*. Paris: John Libbey Eurotext, p. 71.
43. Hakim N, 2001, Immunosuppression in composite tissue allograft. In: Dubernard J. M., ed. *Composite Tissue Allografts*. Paris: John Libbey Eurotext, p. 17.
44. Kanitakis J, Jullien D, 2001, Pathology of the skin after hand allografting. In: Dubernard J. M., ed. *Composite Tissue Allografts*. Paris: John Libbey Eurotext, p. 71.
45. P. Petruzzo, L. Badet, M. Lanzetta, J. M. Dubernard, Concerns on clinical application of composite tissue allotransplantation, *Acta Chir. Belg.* **104**, 266–271 (2004).
46. A. Matas, Chronic rejection in renal transplant recipients – risk factors and correlates, *Clin. Transpl.* **8**(3), 332 (1994).
47. W. C. Breidenbach, G. R. Tobin II, V. S. Gorantla, et al., A position statement in support of hand transplantation, *J. Hand Surg. [Am]* **27**(5), 760 (2002).
48. H. D. Kvernmo, V. S. Gorantla, R. N. Gonzalez, W. C. Breidenbach, Hand transplantation. A future clinical option? *Acta Orthop. Scand.* **76**(1), 14 (2005).
49. T. E. Starzl, N. Murase, K. Abu-Elmagd, et al., Tolerogenic immunosuppression for organ transplantation, *Lancet* **361**(9368), 1502–1510 (2003).
50. R. Shapiro, A. Basu, H. Tan, E. Gray, et al., Kidney transplantation under minimal immunosuppression after pretransplant lymphoid depletion with thymoglobulin or Campath, *J. Am. Coll. Surg.* **200**, 505 (2005).

Chapter 17
Hand Transplantation: The Innsbruck Experience

Stefan Schneeberger, Marina Ninkovic, and Raimund Margreiter

17.1 Introduction

Hand transplantation is currently the most controversially discussed issue in the field of clinical transplantation. After the first hand of the "new era" was transplanted in Lyon in 1998, the debate on whether hand transplantation is justified or not resulted in numerous debates in the scientific press and the public media. Subjective conclusions and recommendations rather than a scientific evaluation of the current results have resulted in polarization between those pro and those contra hand transplantation.[1-6] Initial fears that the transplanted limbs might be irreversibly rejected early after transplantation and that function would be poor were disproved. Instead, 100% graft survival at 1 year after hand transplantation is superior to the outcome achieved in any type of solid organ transplantation.[7] However, the side effects related to the immunosuppressive treatment, the uncertain long-term outcome, the limited number of recipients meeting the required criteria together with the high cost of surgery, rehabilitation, and immunosuppression may be responsible for the decreased activity seen in this field in recent years.

For some authors, the induction of graft-specific tolerance represents a prerequisite for commencing such a transplant program.[5] Even if it is unlikely that induction of full tolerance toward an allograft will be achieved in the near future, long-term acceptance has been realized in solid organ transplantation. Therefore, we felt that clinical hand transplantation represents a therapeutic option for select patients who have lost both hands/forearms. The surgical procedure as well as the long-term immunosuppression needs to be carefully weighed against the expected benefits of such a nonlife-saving procedure. In this chapter we report on the experience made in Innsbruck with hand and forearm transplantation and outline aspects of particular importance in this field.

17.2 Inclusion/Exclusion Criteria

Hand transplantation in its current stage is not a therapy for all patients suffering from loss of a hand or forearm but represents an option for a very select group. Specific criteria were therefore defined for selection of limb-transplant recipient candidates, and a large number of patients were denied a hand transplant because one or more criteria were not met.[8-10] At our institution, candidates were classified as nontransplantable because of, e.g., a neurinoma proximal to the amputation level, amputation proximal to the elbow, or loss of hands in a suicide attempt.[11]

The first clear inclusion criterion for patient selection is a strong desire by the candidate. Additional criteria are defined based on anatomic requirements and experience with solid organ transplantation (Table 17.1). In summary, a patient having lost a hand or forearm is considered a good candidate when he is between 18 and 55 years old, physically and mentally healthy and able to understand the complexity of such a procedure. In addition, extraordinary compliance and the motivation to undergo an operation followed by 2 years of painstaking and intensive rehabilitation are required. For the time being, we consider only loss of both hands/forearms to be a good indication for transplantation. We fear the outcome after single hand transplantation might be regarded unsatisfactory as the patient would certainly compare the function of the graft with that of his own hand.

Most limb transplants were performed at the level of the distal forearm or wrist.[7,12-15] In these cases, forearm muscles are of recipient origin and the intact motor function allows early active motion and cortical (re)integration. Intrinsic muscle function and sensitivity recommence later, when nerve regeneration reaches the respective muscles. In two patients, the level of amputation was the proximal forearm, and in one of our patients donor forearm muscles were transplanted and fixed to the recipient humerus.

17.3 Pretransplant Evaluations

Careful selection of donor and recipient as well as detailed preparation of surgery, immunosuppressive protocol, postoperative monitoring, and rehabilitation program were performed ahead of transplantation. Preparations aimed to maximize functional outcome, achieve long-term graft survival, and minimize side effects and tumor risk. The utmost attention was paid to the patient's informed consent. Every potential problem that might arise in the postoperative period and, in particular, side effects of systemic immunosuppression were extensively discussed with all candidates.

Table 17.1 Criteria for patient selection for hand transplantation in Innsbruck

Inclusion criteria	Exclusion criteria
Patient desire and compliance	Malignancy in the past 10 years
>18 years, <55 years	Infection (temporarily)
Bilateral loss of hand or forearm	Neurinoma far proximal of amputation level
Normal function of all vital organs	Blindness
Psychologically healthy and stable	IDDM
Intact social background	
Ability to understand the complexity of the procedure including potential consequences	

For stumps investigation patients underwent CT scan, angio CT, angiography, magnetic resonance imaging, ultrasound for clarification of bone length, muscle, blood vessel, and nerve status. Using these findings a protocol was designed for the surgical intervention and the planned type of reconstruction was carried out in a corpse. To exclude malignancies and infections, patients underwent gastrointestinal, dental, and oropharyngeal examination.

17.4 Recipients

Two patients were selected to undergo hand/forearm transplantation. The first patient was a 47-year-old male police officer who had lost both hands at the wrist when he attempted to deactivate a bomb in 1994. Both eyes were injured in the bomb blast, resulting in a significant decrease in visual acuity of the left eye. Myoelectrical prostheses enabled the patient to perform desk work, but he was unhappy with the loss of sensitivity, loss of body integrity, limited motor capacity, and the cosmetic appearance of his prosthesis and already requested a hand transplantation shortly after the accident.[15]

In the second case, a 41-year-old athletic male had lost both forearms at a level just below the elbow in a high-voltage electric current accident. The use of myoelectrical prostheses allowed him to reach a fair level of satisfaction, but, for similar reasons as for the first patient, he requested a bilateral transplant. In March 2000, he became the first patient to receive a bilateral forearm transplant.[16]

As we considered reversibility of the surgical intervention a prerequisite, precautions were made to facilitate the use of myoelectrical prostheses in the case of graft loss. This could become necessary, e.g., in the case of an irreversible acute rejection, chronic rejection, a malignant tumor, or a life-threatening infection as well as at the patient's request in case of an unsatisfactory functional outcome.

Our first patient was negative for CMV and EBV and had 5% panel-reactive HLA antibodies. The second patient was positive for CMV but negative for EBV and had no panel-reactive HLA antibodies.

17.5 Donors and Surgery

Donors were matched with recipients for blood group, gender, age, bone size, and cosmetic appearance. Serological testing for hepatitis B and C, HIV, lues, and toxoplasmosis was negative. There was a six HLA antigen mismatch in the first and a four antigen mismatch with the donor in the second recipient. The lymphocytotoxic cross-match was negative in both cases. Both donors were negative for EBV but positive for CMV. Despite presumed-consent legislation in Austria, consent for hand donation was requested from the donor families. Donor brain death had occurred in both cases after intracerebral/subarachnoidal bleeding.

The first hand transplantation in Innsbruck was performed in March 2000, 5 years and 6 months after amputation. Simultaneous preparation of donor limbs and recipient stumps in adjacent theatres kept ischemia time short (150 and 170 min for right and left hand, respectively). All anatomic structures were dissected under tourniquet control in donor and recipient. The forearms were then perfused with cold University of Wisconsin solution. Next, all structures were dissected and forearm bones osteotomized at the mid-forearm. After wound closure the recipient's cosmetic prostheses were fitted to the donor.

Reconstruction of bones, radial and ulnar artery, cephalic and basilic vein, hand and finger flexors and extensors, ulnar, median, and radial nerves was performed simultaneously on both sides. After skin closure, an autologous split-thickness skin graft was placed on the left forearm to cover a small defect. Some tendons had to be repaired en masse or by transpositioning.

The far more complex surgical procedure in the second patient was performed in February 2003. In contrast to the first case, this operation included transposition and fixation of forearm muscles to the recipient's humerus in addition to reconstruction of bones, nerves, vessels, and skin. Skin closure was performed at the elbow level. Cold ischemia time was again kept particularly short (155 and 153 min).

Donor and recipient operations were performed by members of the Department of Plastic and Reconstructive Surgery (H. Piza, M. Ninkovic, and H. Hussl) and hand surgeons of the Department of Traumatology (S. Pechlaner, M. Gabl. M. Lutz, and M. Blauth).

17.6 Rehabilitation

The primary goals of early rehabilitation after hand transplantation are to control swelling and pain, prevent joint stiffness and adhesions, and achieve good motility without jeopardizing the healing process. "Early Protective Motion – EPM" has shown favorable results in hand replantation. A similar program was therefore introduced after hand transplantation.[17] Exercises permitted maintenance of optimal ligament lengths and balance in tension between flexors and extensors. Long-term treatment aims for motor reeducation and sensitivity training. Sensory reeducation was given high priority, and therefore the specific cognitive exercise program described by Perfetti was introduced as a cornerstone of rehabilitation.[18] Occupational therapy focused on sensory stimulation of the hands and forearms as well as on activities related to work and daily living.

Rehabilitation was started on postoperative day 3. Exercises for intrinsic muscle as well as maintenance of joint positions were started after 3 weeks. Electrical stimulation of thenar and hypothenar muscles together with electromyographic biofeedback training were introduced at weeks 3 and 9, respectively. Occupational therapy and active finger movements were started 1 week later.

Different types of positioning and functional thermoplastic splints, such as night and daytime splints and passive and active splints, were employed to protect the transplanted hands, avoid retraction, and facilitate rehabilitation.

As the first patient was transplanted at the wrist level and the second patient was given two forearms including forearm muscles, a major difference in recovery of hand function was expected. Corresponding treatment protocol as well as the applied therapeutic methods were chosen according to specific personal requirements and adjusted for functional progress and clinical situation.

17.7 Immunosuppression and Infection Prophylaxis

The immunosuppressive protocols were designed on the basis of regimens applied in solid organ transplantation. They were adapted to reflect the clinical situation and the patient's particular immunosuppression requirements at different stages posttransplantation.

Immunosuppression in each patient included induction therapy with antithymocyte globulin at a dosage of 2.5 or 5 mg/kg for 4 days. Prior to revascularization, patients received 500/750 mg methylprednisolone. Mycophenolate mofetil (MMF) was started at 2 g/day. On subsequent days, 250 and 125 mg methylprednisolone were given. Prednisolone was then rapidly tapered to 25 mg on day 8, and further gradually tapered to 5 mg at 2 years. Tacrolimus was administered to achieve trough levels of 15 ng/ml during the first 2 months, 12 ng/ml by month 6, 10 ng by one-and-a-half years after transplantation and 8 ng/ml thereafter. In addition, patients maintained on 2 g MMF.[15,16]

At 30 and 24 months after transplantation, when recovery of graft function had reached a high level, sirolimus/everolimus was started at 2/1.75 mg/day and adjusted to achieve trough levels of 6–8 ng/ml. Simultaneously, tacrolimus was reduced. In the first patient, steroids and tacrolimus were then tapered and finally withdrawn.[19]

Patients received broad-spectrum antibiotics during the early postoperative period. Trimethoprim/sulfamethoxazol was given for 18 months as prophylaxis for *Pneumocystis carinii* pneumonia. For CMV prophylaxis, GCV (10 mg/kg) i.v. was administered for 1 week and 3 × 1,000 mg gancyclovir (GCV) or 900 mg valgancyclovir (ValGCV) orally thereafter.

17.8 Results

17.8.1 Surgery

In both patients a small area of the transplanted skin became necrotic at the proximal site of the graft and required an autologous skin graft. In the hand-transplant recipient multiple arteriovenous fistulas caused swelling and required ligation. The time course of bone healing after transplantation was equivalent to that for replantation, but bone healing in the first patient was delayed after fracture of the radial bone of the graft in an accident. The forearm transplant recipient underwent a cosmetic surgical intervention for correction of scars. Otherwise, no surgical complications were observed, skin healing did not differ much from that of replants and nerve regeneration was faster than usually seen in replantation.

17.8.2 Infection

The postoperative course was complicated by CMV infection in both patients.[20]

The first patient was transplanted in a high-risk CMV-mismatch situation. Despite GCV prophylaxis, CMV infection was detected on day 34. The virus was effectively eradicated with foscarnet, but when oral GCV was restarted, a second breakthrough infection was observed. Virus replication was associated with fever and malaise. The patient finally became negative for CMV after two courses of cidofovir. CMV markers have remained negative since then.

For the forearm-transplant recipient, donor/recipient CMV status was pos/pos. On day 137 the patient developed CMV infection. Cidofovir therapy was commenced together with anti-CMV hyperimmunoglobulin. This treatment resulted in a lasting response, but was accompanied by edema in both transplanted forearms, possibly attributable to the hydration protocol accompanying the drug. The edema disappeared spontaneously a few weeks later.

Papilloma virus-associated skin lesions on the back of both hands occurred at 9 months after forearm transplantation (Fig. 17.1). Topical application of cidofovir ointment caused regression of these lesions and only a few warts persisted without further progression in size or number. A cutaneous mycosis infection at the lower limb was observed at 2 years, but responded to local excision and a short course of amphotericin followed by itraconazole. No additional infectious complications and notably no bacterial infection occurred throughout the observation period.

17.8.3 Immunosuppression and Rejection

In the first patient a disseminated erythema and papulous lesions occurred on day 55 after transplantation. Histology demonstrated perivascular and interstitial mononuclear cell infiltrates (Fig. 17.2). The episode was consistent with acute rejection grade II according to the established classification for rejection of the skin in CTAs (Table 17.2).[16] Lesions disappeared after treatment with methylprednisolone given on three consecutive days and topical treatment with tacrolimus and steroids. On day 188 a spotted erythema recurred (histology: rejection grade I), but promptly

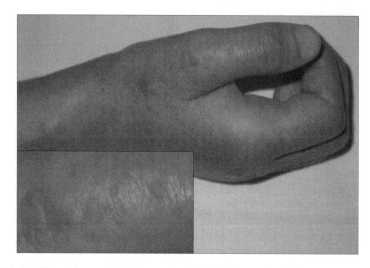

Fig. 17.1 Papilloma virus-associated warts at the back of both hands at 9 months after double forearm transplantation

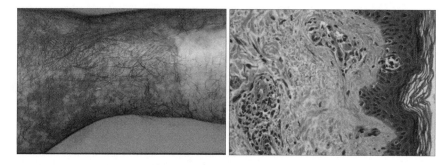

Fig. 17.2 Disseminated erythema and papulous lesions as signs of rejection at 55 days after hand transplantation. Histology demonstrated perivascular and interstitial mononuclear cell infiltrates

Table 17.2 Grading for skin rejection in hand transplantation

Rejection severity	Grade	Histology
Minimal rejection	Grade I	Perivascular lymphocytic and eosinophilic infiltrates
Mild rejection	Grade II	Additional interphase reaction in epidermis and/or adnexal structures
Moderate rejection	Grade III	Diffuse lymphocytic infiltration of epidermis and dermis
Severe rejection	Grade IVa	Necrosis of single keratinocyte and focal dermal–epidermal separation
	Grade IVb	Necrosis and loss of the epidermis

responded to local tacrolimus therapy. A third rejection episode (grade II) was observed upon reduction of immunosuppression at 4 years after transplantation. Transient administration of tacrolimus resulted in restitution of normal skin. Subsequently, tacrolimus was again withdrawn and rapamycin (trough levels 4–8 ng/ml) and MMF (2 g) were sufficient to prevent additional rejections.[19]

In our second case, maculopapular cutaneous lesions occurred as early as day 10 after transplantation. Punch biopsies revealed a lymphocytic perivascular infiltrate indicative for mild rejection (grade I). The rejection promptly responded to 3 × 500 mg methylprednisolone and topical steroids. Lesions recurring on both forearms on day 46, with biopsy again showing low-grade rejection (grade I), were treated with 2 ×20 mg basiliximab. On day 95, a third rejection episode occurred and steroid treatment failed to reverse rejection.[16] Blisters occurring in superficial epidermal layers and in particular in the basal membrane resulted in epidermal desquamation (grade IVa, Fig. 17.4). Skin biopsies showed extensive lymphocytic infiltrates in dermis and epidermis together with apoptotic and necrotic keratinocytes. Immunohistochemistry identified the majority of infiltrating cells as CD3-positive T lymphocytes together with 5% B lymphocytes. ATG administered for 4 days neither prevented progression of rejection nor changed characteristics of the infiltrate. Subsequently, Campath-1H was administered at 20 mg i.v. on day 109 and again on day 110. Simultaneously, MMF was discontinued and FK506 reduced to achieve trough levels of 10–15 ng/ml. In response, skin normalized completely within 2 weeks.[16] Differential blood cell count confirmed almost complete elimination of lymphocytes (0–0.5%). When repopulation of lymphocytes was observed 5 months later, rapamycin was started. A fourth rejection again required treatment with Campath-1H. Thereafter, two additional rejection episodes were encountered when the relatively high IS was lowered, but both episodes responded to systemic methylprednisolone treatment and transient tacrolimus increase. After 30 months, everolimus (trough level 4–6 ng/ml) together with tacrolimus (trough level 10 ng/ml) and steroids were able to prevent further rejections.

Nephrotoxicity as reflected by an increase in urea and creatinine was observed in the first patient at 24 months after transplantation, but complete recovery was achieved after conversion from tacrolimus to rapamycin. HBA1c levels were transiently elevated in both patients and required oral antidiabetic therapy with pioglitazon-hydrochloride in one patient. In our forearm recipient, repetitive headache required treatment with amitryptilin. MMF was well tolerated without any gastrointestinal side effects. An increase in weight in one patient might have been caused at least in part by steroids.

17.8.4 Chimerism

As a certain amount of bone marrow is transplanted together with a hand or forearm, the recipients' blood was tested weekly for donor cells using the gene print STR Systems-vWA during the first year. When alleles of the von Willebrand gene were compared with alleles in donor and recipient blood taken before transplantation, it became apparent that no donor cells were present in the recipients' blood at any time.[15]

Regular hair regrowth on the hands and forearms occurred at 1 year after transplantation in the first patient (Fig. 17.3). The very uniform pattern of hair growth on donor and recipient skin caused us to ask whether regrowth might be of recipient origin. Analysis of donor and recipient hair extracted at close proximity to the skin suture level, however, clearly demonstrated that no chimerism was present in the samples analyzed.[19]

17.8.5 Function

Various scoring systems such as Tinel's sign, the Semmes–Weinstein monofilaments test, hot and cold temperature test, Weber static two-point discrimination test, Dellon moving two-point discrimination test, pinch gauge test, shape/texture identification test, volumetric analysis, manual muscle strength testing using MRC muscle power grading, range of motion (ROM) measurement, grip strength using Jamar dynamometer, Kapandji opposition testing, visual analog scale, tactile and kinesthetic test after Perfetti, ADL, Nine Hole Peg Test, Disability of Arm, Shoulder and Hand Questionnaire (DASH), and Hand Transplantation Comprehensive Outcome Questionnaire (IRSS) were applied for functional assessment and documentation of hand function. Compound motor action potentials were recorded for the abductor pollicis brevis and abductor digiti minimi muscles. Compound sensory action potentials were recorded for the index and fifth fingers using band electrodes.

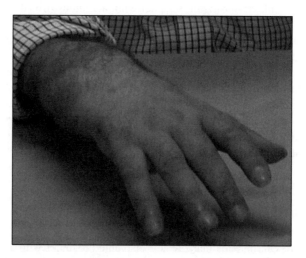

Fig. 17.3 Uniform hair regrowth after double hand transplantation. Despite uniformity between donor and recipient hair, regrowth on the graft was of donor origin

In the hand-transplant recipient regenerating nerves reached the center of the palm at 3 months and the finger tips at 6 months. Active range of motion (AROM) of the wrist joint developed progressively for the first 12 months. By day 270 the patient was able to perform supination and pronation, 50° in wrist extension and 20° in palmar flexion. Active finger ROM continued to improve for both hands after the first postoperative year.[15] After the third year, overall finger ROM remained stable with some minor improvements. As compared with normal ROM, AROM is 61.1% for the right wrist joint and 49.3% for the left wrist joint, 69.9% for the finger joints of the right hand and 59.2% for those of the left hand. Overall, average AROM in both hands is 60.1%.

Intrinsic muscle activity was first observed at 4 months and improved during the subsequent 3 years. Reinnervation was confirmed by electromyography. Thumb opposition improved during the first 3 years after transplantation and remained stable thereafter.[19]

At 1 year, the patient had a grip strength of 14.0 kg in his right and 8.5 kg in his left hand. Thereafter, overall strength remained stable with some minor improvements. In contrast, tip, key, and three-fingered pinch constantly improved during a 5-year observation period. At 5 years, tip pinch is 1 kg for the right and 0.8 kg for the left side. Key pinch is 1.8 kg and 2.7 kg for the right and the left hand, respectively; chuck pinch is 1.3 kg for the right and 1 kg for the left side.[19]

Sensitivity to pain and thermal discrimination were present in both hands at 1 year. Two-point discrimination showed sensory function to improve in most fingers during the first 3 years.[19] Nerve conduction studies demonstrated motor and sensory reinnervation to various degrees in both hands. Six months after transplantation electromyographic signs of reinnervation were identified in the left hand. One year after transplantation, reinnervation was also seen in the right abductor digiti minimi muscle and the abductor pollicis brevis in both hands. Reinnervation progressed and long-duration polyphasic potentials were recorded after 3 years. A certain loss of motor units was seen in all muscles studied.[19]

Cortical responses were recorded after stimulation of the left and right index and fifth fingers; no potentials were recorded over Erb's point or C5. Latencies of the cortical responses were prolonged, but amplitudes were within normal range.[21]

The results 30 months after forearm transplantation in our second case show an ongoing increase in AROM of wrist, MCP, and IP joints on both sides. The improvement shows some significant differences related to side and joint. AROM of the right wrist is 85° and on the left side 80°. Total AROM for the index finger is 170° on the right side and 225° on the left side, respectively. Hand function is now slightly superior to the function the patient had with myoelectrical prostheses. Muscle strength of the right and left M. interosseus dors. is 1 and 2–3 kg, respectively. The muscle power of the M. interosseus palm. is 4 kg on the both sides. Extrinsic muscle power is still increasing in all muscles. Discrimination for cold was detected at 6 months and discrimination for hot 2 months later, although overall sensitivity remains rather poor with a moving two-point discrimination of > 15 mm on both sides. The functional outcome at 3 years after transplantation has been published recently.

17.8.6 Imagery

At 1 year after transplantation, ultrasound, CT angiography, and angiography demonstrated normal blood flow through the radial and ulnar arteries in the left hand and forearm in our first patient. In the right forearm the radial artery was occluded at the level of the retinaculum flexorum, and the distal part of the radial artery beyond the occlusion was perfused retrograde via the arcus palmaris profundus (Fig. 17.4, 19). The left superficial palmar arch was occluded. Surprisingly, at 4 years posttransplantation the left radial artery was seen to be recanalized and the deep palmaric arch was perfused in an orthograde manner (Fig. 17.4, 19). On both sides, kinking of radial and ulnar arteries was caused by excess length of the grafted vessels. As mentioned earlier, multiple arteriovenous fistulas occurred at 6 months and were ligated. No additional radiomorphologic changes were observed during the first 3 years.

17.8.7 Patient Satisfaction

For both patients transplanted in Innsbruck, a sense of body integrity was achieved as the transplanted hands/forearms were fully integrated in the patients' appearance

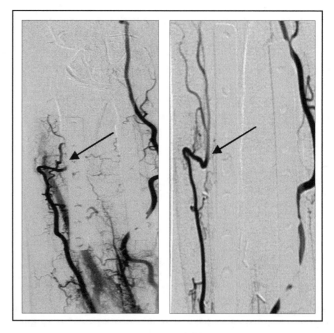

Fig. 17.4 *Left*: Radial artery of the right forearm occluded at the level of the retinaculum flexorum at 1 year after hand transplantation. *Right*: At 4 years the left radial artery is recanalized

and regarded as their own. They are satisfied with the functional and the cosmetic outcome. Both patients' capacity for social contact as well as for intimacy with a partner has improved.

The function regained by the hand transplant recipient is much better than what that he had with myoelectrical prostheses, while functional recovery in the forearm transplant recipient is still making slow progress and presently slightly superior to prosthetic function. In the hand-transplant recipient, overall achieved motor function is >60% of normal. Together with the high degree of sensitivity without cold intolerance, hand function enables the patient to perform activities he could not perform with his myoelectrical prostheses. Not only he can manage advanced activities of daily life such as buttoning his shirt or picking up small coins from a flat surface, but also his self-confidence and interaction with his surroundings have improved profoundly. No signs of chronic rejection or loss of function have been observed so far.[19] The patient considers his daily life "completely normal" and remains highly active in his job as a police officer. His new hands enabled him to undertake transcontinental motorcycle trips. The envisaged goal has thus been achieved and, from the patient's view, the decision to undergo transplantation was absolutely justified. In numerous presentations organized by him he has demonstrated to the public the highly satisfactory outcome after hand transplantation.

The forearm recipient is satisfied with the current result but experienced multiple rejections and side effects before a stable situation was finally achieved. At 30 months after transplantation, he is now rejection-free and has no side effects whatsoever. The major shortcomings are the lack of discriminative sensation and muscle fatigue after prolonged forearm motor activity.

However, defining the benefit of such a procedure is difficult and several aspects need to be taken into consideration. Of particular relevance for patient satisfaction are social integrity, self-esteem, body integrity, and the ability to interact by touching, hugging, caressing, or any form of intimacy with a partner. The ability to objectively assess these activities, feelings, and impressions as well as personal satisfaction, however, is limited, because interindividual differences do not permit sufficient comparability. It is therefore the patient's albeit subjective view of whether and how hand transplantation has improved his quality of life which is the decisive factor in answering the question whether such a procedure was successful and justified. Further, such a judgment is strongly dependent on the particular time frame, and evaluations made at different times give rise to different conclusions.

17.9 What's Important and What's Not

The principal goals of hand transplantation are to achieve motor function superior to that of myoelectrical prostheses together with a discriminative sensation sufficient for tactile sensation in advanced motor activities and social interaction. Moreover, patient satisfaction and improved social integration are factors justifying such a cost- and labor-intensive procedure.

The individual outcome after hand transplantation ranges from failure (loss of the transplanted hand) to hand function reaching approximately 65–70% of that of a normal hand, namely better than the function achieved after many hand replantations. Within that range, different outcomes with different patient satisfactions have been observed at different centers, for which a multitude of variables might be responsible. After evaluating numerous candidates for hand transplantation and acquiring clinical experience in two cases, we believe the following aspects are of utmost importance for satisfactory outcome and should therefore be considered when planning human hand transplantation.

1. Profound psychological stability together with the ability to understand the complexity of the therapeutic modality is a prerequisite. The patient must understand that daily intensive training is necessary for nerve and muscle regeneration and reintegration of the hand in the cerebral cortex. In addition, a sound social background is essential. Furthermore, the patient must be informed in detail about every potential risk associated with the procedure including the short- and long-term side effects of immunosuppression and he needs time to consider his decision after detailed information.
2. Each individual case requires a precise protocol and in some cases specific surgical training of novel reconstruction techniques. With regard to anatomic prerequisites, amputation at the wrist or not far above is better than at a higher level where forearm muscles have to be transplanted as functional components. Whether good results can be achieved with forearm transplantation or transplantation of a limb above the elbow cannot be answered at this stage. In the first forearm-transplant recipient muscle degeneration due to initial lack of reinnervation seems to be one of the key limiting factors.
3. After loss of both hands at a distal level, hand transplantation can produce results that are far superior to those obtained with myoelectrical prostheses. Satisfactory results have also been achieved with single hand transplantation, but comparison of graft function with that of the patient's own hand might prompt dissatisfaction. With regard to the dominant or nondominant hand, the plasticity of the brain, which has been shown after hand transplantation, might be relevant: a certain time after loss of the dominant hand, the nondominant hand might well be considered "dominant" as the motor cortex can reorganize itself in response to changed peripheral inputs.[22] A difference between dominant and nondominant hand transplantation might therefore be of little relevance.
4. Standard immunosuppressive treatment can prevent the loss of a hand transplant due to rejection in most but probably not all recipients. Induction therapy with ATG or Campath-1H may help prevent early rejection and keep maintenance immunosuppression low. Tacrolimus should be part of the immunosuppressive regime during the first 2 years since it has been shown to accelerate nerve regeneration. A triple therapy including steroids and MMF seems to be effective in preventing acute rejection in that time frame. Steroids should then be tapered and finally withdrawn. Later, calcineurin inhibitors should be replaced with a TOR-inhibitor. As the skin is constantly available for visual inspection and is the

major compartment affected by acute rejection, we believe that immunosuppression should be reduced to determine the minimum required to prevent rejection and thus minimize the risk for tumors and infection.

5. Muscles are sensitive to ischemia, and damage such as interstitial edema, microvascular constriction, or damage of myocyte membranes already results in muscle dysfunction after 2.5 h of (warm) ischemia.[23] Although cold flush and preservation with UW (or similar) solutions might limit myocyte damage, short ischemia time is desirable. We therefore aimed to minimize ischemia and performed donor and recipient operations simultaneously. This approach permitted ischemia to be kept at 150–170 min.

6. An interdisciplinary approach by surgeons and the rehabilitation team is of utmost importance. This allows for an individualized rehabilitation program flexible enough to be adapted for surgical complications, infection, episodes of acute rejection as well as slow or fast progress in recovery of function. For best results we recommend that rehabilitation be commenced on day 1 posttransplantation and continue with intensive and long-lasting therapy. Patient compliance and steady teamwork are prerequisites for successful hand/forearm transplantation.

7. Although the number of patients who have received a limb transplant is still small, complications related to CMV have been observed at many centers.[20] A hand from a CMV-positive donor may contain a larger viral load than, e.g., the kidney, liver, or heart, as the significant mass of endothelium and hematopoietic precursor cells from the bone marrow may host latent CMV. In addition, high-level immunosuppression and a poor HLA match limit T-cell response and complicate interaction between donor antigen-presenting cells and recipient CD8-positive cells required for virus control. On the basis of these findings avoidance of CMV mismatch transplantation was proposed. In addition, anti-CMV prophylaxis with ValGCV for 6 months in combination with anti-CMV hyperimmunoglobulin should be mandatory after transplantation of a hand from a CMV-positive donor.[20] For treatment of CMV infection, immunosuppression should be transiently reduced in addition to GCV/ValGCV treatment. The two more toxic drugs foscarnet and cidofovir should be used as a third-line intervention. Despite the limited number of patients transplanted to date, CMV and its correlation with acute rejection seems to be an important issue in hand transplantation.

8. Central or peripheral chimerism has been repeatedly demonstrated to contribute to tolerance induction in experimental models and even in humans. However, stable chimerism has not been conclusively demonstrated in any hand-transplant recipient. We therefore consider the bone marrow content of a hand or forearm transplant not to be of major clinical relevance.

9. Graft survival and function early after hand transplantation is good. It remains unknown, however, whether long-term survival is limited by chronic rejection. The longest surviving hand was transplanted 6 years and 9 months ago in Louisville, USA.[13] To date, no signs of chronic rejection whatsoever have been reported for this or any other hand transplant.[7,19] However, this issue remains a

major concern and is one of the reasons why the initial number of hand transplants performed per year decreased after 2000 (see http://www.handregistry.com).

(10) The number of patients living with a transplanted hand is still low, and it is unlikely that the number of transplants will increase exponentially in the next few years. It is therefore of utmost importance that patient data be collected and evaluated by an international registry (IRHCTT) to improve the definition of factors influencing outcome. These data can be used to design recommendations, guidelines, and future clinical protocols.

17.10 Conclusion

In Innsbruck, two hands and two forearms have been transplanted. Three and six rejection episodes were observed, one of which was resistant to steroids and ATG. An acceptable level of immunosuppression was able to prevent irreversible and early chronic rejection. No chimerism but accelerated nerve regeneration and reinnervation of intrinsic muscles were observed. A high degree of motility in addition to good sensitivity was achieved with extensive physiotherapy in our first patient, whereas in the second patient the outcome after double forearm transplantation is less favorable.

In conclusion, hand transplantation can be performed successfully with an acceptable risk in select patients. However, careful weighing of the potential benefits against the enormous effort and the risk of infection and malignancy on an individual basis remains important. For the outcome after forearm transplantation, no definite conclusions can be drawn to date. Observations made in our forearm transplant recipient suggest that reinnervation and reactivation of muscle function are far more complex than in hand transplantation.

References

1. S. E. Edgell, S. J. McCabe, W. C. Breidenbach, W. P. Neace, A. S. LaJoie, T. D. Abell, Different reference frames can lead to different hand transplantation decisions by patients and physicians, *J Hand Surg [Am]* **26**(2), 196–200 (2001).
2. S. McCabe, G. Rodocker, K. Julliard, W. Breidenbach, C. Marcel, M. V. Shirbacheh, J. Barker, Using decision analysis to aid in the introduction of upper extremity transplantation, *Transplant Proc* **30**, 2783–2786 (1998).
3. N. F. Jones, Concerns about human hand transplantation in the 21st century, *J Hand Surg [Am]* **27**(5), 771–787 (2002).
4. S. Hettiaratchy, M. A. Randolph, F. Petit, W. P. Lee, P. E. Butler, Composite tissue allotransplantation – a new era in plastic surgery? *Br J Plast Surg* **57**(5), 381–391 (2004).
5. W. P. Lee, Composite tissue transplantation: more science and patience needed, *Plast Reconstr Surg* **107**(4), 1066–1070 (2001).
6. S. Hettiaratchy, P. E. Butler, W. P. Lee, Lessons from hand transplantations, *Lancet* **357**(9255), 494–495 (2001).

7. M. Lanzetta, P. Petruzzo, R. Margreiter, J. M. Dubernard, F. Schuind, W. Breidenbach, S. Lucchina, S. Schneeberger, C. van Holder, D. Granger, G. Pei, J. Zhao, X. Zhang, The international registry on hand and composite tissue transplantation, *Transplantation* **79**(9), 1210–1214 (2005).
8. P. Petruzzo, L. Badet, M. Lanzetta, J. M. Dubernard, Concerns on clinical application of composite tissue allotransplantation, *Acta Chir Belg* **104**, 266–271 (2004).
9. M. Lanzetta, P. Petruzzo, G. Vitale, S. Lucchina, E. R. Owen, J. M. Dubernard, N. Hakim, H. Kapila, Human hand transplantation: what have we learned? *Transplant Proc* **36**, 664–668 (2004).
10. G. Germann, Bilateral hand transplantation – indication and rationale, *J Hand Surg [Br]* **26**, 521 (2001).
11. S. Schneeberger, B. Zelger, M. Ninkovic, R. Margreiter, Transplantation of the hand, *Transplant Rev* 100–107 (2005).
12. J. M. Dubernard, E. Owen, G. Herzberg, M. Lanzetta, X. Martin, H. Kapila, M. Dawahra, N. S. Hakim, Human hand allograft: report on first 6 months, *Lancet* **353**(9161), 1315–1320 (1999).
13. J. W. Jones, S. A. Gruber, J. H. Barker, W. C. Breidenbach, Successful hand transplantation. One-year follow-up. Louisville Hand Transplant Team, *N Engl J Med* **343**, 468–473 (2000).
14. J. M. Dubernard, P. Petruzzo, M. Lanzetta, H. Parmentier, X. Martin, M. Dawahra, N. S. Hakim, E. Owen, Functional results of the first human double-hand transplantation, *Ann Surg* **238**, 128–136 (2003).
15. R. Margreiter, G. Brandacher, M. Ninkovic, W. Steurer, A. Kreczy, S. Schneeberger, A double-hand transplant can be worth the effort! *Transplantation* **74**, 85–90 (2002).
16. S. Schneeberger, A. Kreczy, G. Brandacher, W. Steurer, R. Margreiter, Steroid- and ATG-resistant rejection after double forearm transplantation responds to campath-1H, *Am J Transplant* **4**, 1372–1374 (2004).
17. L. R. Scheker, A. Hodges, Brace and rehabilitation after replantation and revascularization, *Hand Clin* **17**, 473 (2001).
18. G. F. Salvini, C. C. Perfetti, A new method of rehabilitation of the hand in hemiplegic patients. (preliminary results) *Riv Neurobiol.* **17**(1), 11–20 (1971).
19. S. Schneeberger, M. Ninkovic, M. Gabl, M. Ninkovic, H. Hussl, M. Rieger, W. Loescher, B. Zelger, G. Brandacher, H. Bonatti, T. Hautz, C. Boesmueller, H. Piza-Katzer, R. Margreiter, First forearm transplantation outcome at 3 years. *Amer J Transplant* **7**(7), 1753–62 (2007 July).
20. S. Schneeberger, M. Ninkovic, H. Piza-Katzer, M. Gabl, H. Hussl, M. Rieger, W. Loescher, B. Zelger, G. Brandacher, M. Ninkovic, H. Bonatti, C. Boesmueller, W. Mark, R. Margreiter, Status 5 years after bilateral hand transplantation, *Am J Transplant.* **6**(4): 834–41 (2006).
21. S. Schneeberger, S. Lucchina, M. Lanzetta, G. Brandacher, C. Bosmuller, W. Steurer, F. Baldanti, C. Dezza, R. Margreiter, H. Bonatti, Cytomegalovirus-related complications in human hand transplantation, *Transplantation* **80**(4), 441–447 (2005).
22. C. Brenneis, W. N. Loscher, K. E. Egger, T. Benke, M. Schocke, M. F. Gabl, G. Wechselberger, S. Felber, S. Pechlaner, R. Margreiter, H. Piza-Katzer, W. Poewe, Cortical motor activa-tion patterns following hand transplantation and replantation, *J Hand Surg [Br]* **30**(5), 530–533 (2005).
23. P. Giraux, A. Sirigu, F. Schneider, J. M. Dubernard, Cortical reorganization in motor cortex after graft of both hands, *Nat Neurosci* **4**, 691–692 (2001).
24. J. Nanobashvili, C. Neumayer, A. Fugl, A. Punz, R. Blumer, M. Prager, M. Mittlbock, H. Gruber, P. Polterauer, E. Roth, T. Malinski, I. Huk, Ischemia/reperfusion injury of skeletal muscle: plasma taurine as a measure of tissue damage, *Surgery* **133**, 91–100 (2003).
25. M. R. Costanzo, D. C. Naftel, M. R. Pritzker, J. K. Heilman 3rd, J. P. Boehmer, S. C. Brozena, G. W. Dec, H. O. Ventura, J. K. Kirklin, R. C. Bourge, L. W. Miller, Heart transplant coronary artery disease detected by coronary angiography: a multiinstitutional study of preoperative donor and recipient risk factors. Cardiac Transplant Research Database, *J Heart Lung Transplant* **17**, 744–753 (1998).
26. H. J. Eisen, E. M. Tuzcu, R. Dorent, J. Kobashigawa, D. Mancini, H. A. Valantine-von Kaeppler, R. C. Starling, K. Sorensen, M. Hummel, J. M. Lind, K. H. Abeywickrama,

P. Bernhardt; RAD B253 Study Group, Everolimus for the prevention of allograft rejection and vasculopathy in cardiac-transplant recipients, *N Engl J Med* **349**(9), 847–858 (2003).
27. D. Mancini, S. Pinney, D. Burkhoff, J. LaManca, S. Itescu, E. Burke, N. Edwards, M. Oz, A. R. Marks, Use of rapamycin slows progression of cardiac transplantation vasculopathy, *Circulation* **108**(1), 48–53 (2003).
28. J. C. Ruiz, J. M. Campistol, J. M. Grinyo, A. Mota, D. Prats, J. A. Gutierrez, A. C. Henriques, J. R. Pinto, J. Garcia, J. M. Morales, J. M. Gomez, M. Arias, Early cyclosporine a withdrawal in kidney-transplant recipients receiving sirolimus prevents progression of chronic pathologic allograft lesions, *Transplantation* **78**(9), 1312–1318 (2004).
29. T. S. Ikonen, J. F. Gummert, M. Hayase, Y. Honda, B. Hausen, U. Christians, G. J. Berry, P. G. Yock, R. E. Morris, Sirolimus (rapamycin) halts and reverses progression of allograft vascular disease in non-human primates, *Transplantation* **70**(6), 969–975 (2000).
30. J. M. Campistol, A. Gutierrez-Dalmau, J. V. Torregrosa, Conversion to sirolimus: a successful treatment for posttransplantation Kaposi's sarcoma, *Transplantation* **77**(5), 760–762 (2004).
31. G. E. Koehl, J. Andrassy, M. Guba, S. Richter, A. Kroemer, M. N. Scherer, M. Steinbauer, C. Graeb, H. J. Schlitt, K. W. Jauch, E. K. Geissler, Rapamycin protects allografts from rejection while simultaneously attacking tumors in immunosuppressed mice, *Transplantation* **77**(9), 1319–1326 (2004).
32. M. Guba, P. von Breitenbuch, M. Steinbauer, G. Koehl, S. Flegel, M. Hornung, C. J. Bruns, C. Zuelke, S. Farkas, M. Anthuber, K. W. Jauch, E. K. Geissler, Rapamycin inhibits primary and metastatic tumor growth by antiangiogenesis: involvement of vascular endothelial growth factor, *Nat Med* **8**(2), 128–135 (2002).

Section V

Chapter 18
Vascularized Bone Marrow Transplantation

Chau Y. Tai, Louise F. Strande, Hidetoshi Suzuki, Martha S. Matthews, Chad R. Gordon, and Charles W. Hewitt

18.1 Introduction

18.1.1 The Chimera

The classic description of the Chimera since the days of ancient Greece dating to Homer was a beast with the head of a lion, the body of a goat, and the tail of a serpent. The concept of this mythical creature – one animal made from parts of others – remained the epitome of modern transplantation, symbolizing the American Society of Transplant Surgeons.

Among patients with solid organ transplants (SOTs), long-term acceptances of allografts without immunosuppression were the exceptions rather than the rule. Even with good control of acute rejection episodes, chronic rejection of allografts remains dauntingly frequent. On the other side of the spectrum, chronic graft-versus-host disease (GVHD) still plague patients who survived the initial morbidities of bone marrow transplantation (BMT). These clinical "chimeras" lack full tolerance to the graft, and graft or host failure rates remained high.

The concept of chimerism generally divides into two categories. Macrochimerism refers to a state where levels of donor cells are easily detectable by flow cytometry, and microchimerism refers to presence of donor cells detectable by molecular techniques such as polymerase chain reaction (PCR). These categories are somewhat arbitrary, a spectrum describing the same state – coexistence of donor and recipient cells. The more important point relates to tolerance – Does chimerism lead to tolerance? One of the key potential utilities of the vascularized bone marrow transplant (VBMT) is to maintain T-cell chimerism as a mechanism for tolerance, and research is going on to unlock the puzzle of a true chimera.

18.1.2 Tolerance

"Tolerance" refers to the failure to mount an immune response to an antigen. Natural or "self" tolerance prevents the body from attacking its own antigens, as seen in autoimmune diseases. Both T and B cells have immunologic tolerance, though it is the T cell that has the more dominant role in regulation. Central tolerance refers to the maturation of T cells in the thymus with negative selection of cells that recognizes self-epitopes. After emigration from the thymus, peripheral tolerance occurs by ignorance, suppression, anergy, or split tolerance. In the context of VBMT, both central and peripheral tolerance mechanisms may be present since donor cells from the marrow migrated to the thymus as well as peripheral lymphoid tissues.

18.1.3 Composite Tissue Transplant

Upper extremity reconstruction using composite tissue allotransplantation (CTA) is now a clinical reality. The primary controversy is the lifelong immunosuppression and its potential side effects for an elective transplantation. This provides even further impetus for researchers toward donor specific tolerance that permits CTA survival without long-term immunosuppression. Early limb-transplant experiments quickly noted the viability of the bone marrow compartment and its possible contribution to maintaining chimerism and tolerance in recipients.[1] In clinical hand transplantations, however, no evidence of chimerism or donor hyporesponsiveness has been noted.[2] Currently, there is no consensus on the role of the VBMT within a CTA.

18.1.4 Vascularized Bone Marrow Transplant

The VBMT is a unique component within the CTA that contains both bone marrow and stromal cells within a skeletal support. It differs from cellular BMT by its vascular dependence, and the presence of its supportive stromal environment renders it independent of an engraftment period. It differs from an SOT by the abundance of immature immune regulatory cells within the graft, where other SOTs are composed primarily of matured somatic cells.

Multiple studies in animal models suggested an immunomodulatory role for transplanted bone marrow cells in tolerance induction, with prolongation of pancreatic islet grafts, lung allografts, small bowel grafts, hindlimb grafts, and indefinite survival of cardiac grafts.[3] The underlying theme in these experiments was that chimerism induced by donor bone marrow cells modulated the host's response to the transplant and facilitated the development of donor-specific tolerance. More specifically, the marrow's stromal cells also appear to have a significant suppressive effect of alloreactivity.[4] Rather than contributing to GVHD, the VBMT may be beneficial to overall allograft survival.

Other than its potential role in a CTA, the rapid repopulation kinetics of the VBMT in an irradiated host makes it an attractive adjunct to cellular BMT.[5] This topic is further discussed in Dr. Olszewski's chapter.

18.2 Chimerism and Tolerance

18.2.1 Is the Establishment of Chimerism a Prerequisite to Tolerance?

For many years, host adaptation to cellular bone marrow transplantation and solid organ transplantation has been thought to occur via different mechanisms. In an eloquent review by Dr. Starzl, he unified the immunological concepts between cellular marrow transplant and SOT.[6] Rather than operating on different mechanisms, the immunological interplay between donor and recipient, GVHD and rejection, are expressions on a continuum depending on the origin of the majority cellular population – strong host response produces rejection, strong donor response results in GVHD (Fig. 18.1). All transplanted recipients are chimeras.

18.2.1.1 Experimental Evidence

In the laboratory, chimeric animals can be created with immune manipulation by means of radiation and/or immunosuppression. Multiple protocols have been devised. The simplest protocol uses lethal total body irradiation, and reconstitution with a mix of T-cell-depleted (TCD) syngeneic and allogeneic bone marrow. Chimeric mice produced in this manner showed hyporesponsiveness to subsequent donor skin allografts but not full tolerance.[7] In rats, mixed hematopoietic chimerism similarly created induced donor-specific tolerance sufficient for lung allografts.[8]

To avoid toxicities from lethal and sublethal irradiation preconditioning, researchers sought after clinically applicable nonmyeloablative approaches. The introduction of costimulation blockade allowed production of a mixed chimera with donor-specific tolerance in mice.[9,10] Improving on this regimen, addition of rapamycin increased the establishment of stable chimerism and skin allograft tolerance to 93%.[11] Concerned with the potential thromboembolic complications associated with anti-CD40L, Luo et al. were able to induce stable chimerism in mice using

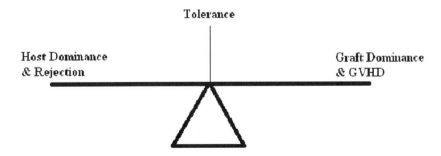

Fig. 18.1 Immune balance between graft and host

sirolimus and lymphocyte-depleting antibodies with BMT that accepted donor islet transplants.[12] Skin allograft tolerance was not tested in this experiment.

Chimerism alone does not guarantee donor-specific tolerance in mice. Umemura et al. found that high levels of chimerism can be attained in sublethally irradiated B10.A mice given either CD4 knockout (KO) or CD8 KO BMT.[13] These chimeras rejected donor skin allograft, and adoptive transfer of donor T cells restored donor-specific allograft tolerance. Supporting the importance of donor T cell in tolerance induction, Xu et al. used a nonmyeloablative conditioning regimen in mice and demonstrated that donor skin allograft tolerance strictly correlated with early production of donor T cells in the chimeric recipients.[14] Additionally, long-lasting and stable mixed chimerism of around 85% was maintained only in the early donor T-cell producing group.

In the rat, a nonmyeloablative protocol using CTLA4-Ig, tacrolimus, low-dose irradiation (300 cGy), and antilymphocyte-serum produced chimeras via TCD BMT that were fully tolerant of a subsequent hindlimb CTA without additional immunosuppression.[15] Despite TCD, T-cell, B-cell, and macrophage donor chimerism were demonstrated by flow cytometry post BMT.

In larger animals, mixed chimerism has been established in the miniature swine after using a nonmyeloablative TCD conditioning.[16] Subsequent donor-specific cardiac allografts achieved long-term survival without chronic rejection, though indefinite donor skin grafts survival was achieved only in one of four animals.[17]

The relationship of chimerism and tolerance in composite tissue transplantation is a little more complex. In a hindlimb model using chimeric rats (ACI → WF), Prabhune et al. found full acceptance of an irradiated ACI limb.[18] However, without irradiation, the ACI limb caused GVHD in the chimeric recipients. Lymphadenectomy of the graft limb eliminated GVHD and allowed indefinite graft survival, and the authors concluded that it was the mature lymphocytic load, not the bone marrow, that contributed to GVHD in CTA in the chimeric rat.[19]

Larger animal studies in the miniature swine by Mathes et al. found that tolerance to a musculoskeletal allograft was not associated with chimerism within the bone marrow compartments.[20] Pig allelic antigen was used as the allograft marker in MHC-matched, minor-antigen-mismatched pairs treated with a 12-day course of cyclosporine. In this study, the graft's bone marrow compartment was sequentially repopulated by host cells over time to a level undetectable by flow cytometry ($<0.1\%$), while the muscle and bone graft as a whole survived without signs of rejection. However, the level of "tolerance" achieved in the swine model did not tolerate a free skin or vascularized skin allograft component, and all animals rejected the skin components in a delayed fashion.[21]

Studies on "chimerism" need to be interpreted cautiously, since presence of chimerism is subjected to detection sensitivity. A newer technique, the PCR-flow assay, utilizes the amplification power of PCR combined with flow cytometry technology to identify discrete cellular subsets in renal transplant patients.[22] Investigators found low levels of donor cells in the iliac bone marrow of renal transplant recipient but not in the peripheral circulation, confirming the interplay of cells between donor and host even in SOT patients.

Thus, in the laboratory, animals with peripheral chimerism detectable by flow cytometry are reproducible by multiple methods. Donor-specific tolerance in these chimeras required the presence of donor T-cell production in the recipient. However, mature lymphocytes from a naive donor can still cause GVHD in the chimeric host, indicating an immune transition period between both host and donor is needed. Meanwhile, the bone marrow component appeared to be well tolerated.

18.2.1.2 Chimerism and Solid Organ Graft Prolongation

Spurred on by the laboratory results, clinical trials of augmenting chimerism using donor bone marrow to achieve better tolerance of SOTs have been attempted. Simultaneous infusion of bone marrow cells in unconditioned kidney transplant recipients transplantations did not demonstrate conclusive improvement in survival of the patient or graft compared with historic controls (85 versus 76%), but the authors noted a trend toward decreased chronic allograft neuropathy.[23] However, multiple variables compounded these findings, including but not limited to the type of immunosuppressant used, lack of recipient preconditioning, and combination with islet or pancreas grafts.

When attempted in liver recipient, more acute rejection episodes occurred in the BM-infused group, but patient and graft survival was higher at 6 year follow-up in the study group, suggesting potential better long-term outcome.[24] In cardiac-transplant patients, patient survival was similar (86 and 87% at 3 years) but the proportion of patients free from grade 3A rejection was higher in the study group (64 versus 40%, $p = 0.03$).[25] In lung transplant recipients, infusion of donor bone marrow did not affect survival, but is associated with a lower rate of obliterative bronchiolitis.[26] Simple infusion of BMT with SOT did not appear to significantly improve outcome in the above studies.

However, tolerance for SOT in conjunction with same donor allogeneic BMT have been achieved in case reports. Sellers et al. reported a patient with chronic myelogenous leukemia who was successfully treated with BMT from an HLA-identical sibling.[27] Seven years later she developed end-stage renal disease and a renal transplant was performed from the same donor without any postoperative immunosuppression. Interestingly, glucocorticoids were not used in this patient because of her diabetes. Buhler et al. reported two patients with end-stage renal disease secondary to multiple myelomas that were treated with combined bone marrow and kidney transplantation. Transient lymphohematopoietic chimerism was demonstrated, and no rejection episodes have occurred 2 and 4 years after withdrawal of immunosuppression.[28] These reports proved the possibility of true clinical chimeras and research continues to investigate the donor and recipient conditions that will lead to reproducible results. Current NIH phase I study at Massachusetts General Hospital combines bone marrow and renal transplantations to treat patients with multiple myeloma with associated renal failure. It appears that proper recipient conditioning can lead to SOT tolerance without immunosuppression.

Stepping back to look at current research findings for transplant tolerance, a clear theme emerges: Appropriate conditions (not yet completely defined) can allow the key players from donor and host (likely T-cell population) to "talk" to one another, to arrive at a state of mutual immune acceptance. Ablative conditioning to establish chimerism is not justifiable for patient who only needs an SOT, and alternate nonmyeloablative approaches with newer immunosuppressants are undergoing investigation.

18.2.1.3 Chimerism in Bone Marrow Transplantation

The emphasis on the T-cell population for chimerism and tolerance in SOT recipients cannot be readily applied to BMT patients. As mentioned earlier, there are reports of individuals who underwent BMT successfully were able to accept subsequent donor-specific organs without immunosuppression.[27,28] However, these are exceptions rather than the rule. The morbidity and mortalities associated with a myeloablative protocol are high, since the treatment was targeted to eliminate the host's dysfunctional lymphohemopoietic system. Chronic GVHD and long-term immunodeficiency still threatens patients who survive the initial transplant and high incidences of early and late infection occur even in patients with successful engraftment and minimal GVHD.[29] In vitro analysis of T cells obtained in patients after BMT showed that transplanted T cells expressed little or no PHA-induced GM-CSF message, even up to 18 months posttransplant.[30]

The chimerism achieved in successful BMT tend to be donor dominant as desired, since recovery of defective host cells also indicates relapse of disease. By evaluating the time to achieve full donor chimerism using sensitive PCR technology, Balon et al. found that early complete donor chimerism was an indicator for severe chronic GVHD.[32] In the case of BMT, chimerism is clearly not an indicator for tolerance.

To reduce incidence and severity of GVHD, TCD was commonly employed. However, T-cell depletion was also associated with relapse of leukemia.[32] A recent multicenter clinical trial confirmed the earlier reports. This study evaluated TCD versus methotrexate and cyclosporine immunosuppression for BMT patients with lymphohemopoietic malignancy.[33] Investigators found no difference in disease-free survival at 3 years. In the TCD group, initial hospitalization was reduced with more rapid neutrophil recovery and less grade III–IV acute GVHD. However, the risk of chronic myelogenous leukemia relapse was significantly higher in the TCD group (20 versus 7%, $p = 0.009$), and more cytomegalovirus infections were noted (28 versus 17%, $p = 0.023$).

T-cell chimerism in BMT patients is a difficult balancing act. The treatment for BMT patients aimed at eliminating defective host bone marrow cells and these protocols also permanently alter the host stromal environment with significant morbidity.

18.2.1.4 Summary

In summary, chimerism of the peripheral cells alone does not reflect the level of tolerance achieved. Just as chimerism exists on a spectrum, tolerance appears to do so as well, though the two conditions are not parallel to each other. As stated earlier, all transplanted recipients by definition are chimeras. Full tolerance is not necessary for chimerism to exist, just sufficient tolerance to allow graft viability is required. An animal can be tolerant of an SOT but not tolerant of the skin component. Conversely, a high level of chimerism does not guarantee tolerance. Research is still going on to identify the key players, the regulatory cells from both donor and recipient that orchestrate tolerance. Cellular communication must occur for immune transition and reeducation. Perhaps then more specifically, the chimerism of the regulatory cells is the state desired for allograft tolerance.

Chimerism exists without tolerance, such as in our immunosuppressed SOT and BMT patients. However, tolerance cannot exist without at least a period of chimerism. In the case of CTA of the extremity with a significant skin component, full tolerance is the desired goal.

18.2.2 The Stromal Cell

It is now established the plasticity of the stromal (aka mesenchymal) cells enable differentiation to a variety of tissues, inclusive of the skeletal components (chondrocytes, osteoblasts, reticular cells, adipocytes) as well as nonskeletal tissues (neural, vascular, myogenic, hepatic).[34,35] However, in context of BMT, whether the stromal element is replaced by donor cells was debated.[36–38] The stromal component was glaringly absent in conventional BMT, and although transfused bone marrow cells eventually engrafted, the altered stromal environment from ablative conditioning did not function normally.

Preclinical research by Ikehara's group brought to attention the contribution of stromal cells in enhancing engraftment of BMT in mice.[39,40] In comparing mice transplanted with and without bone grafts, Li et al. demonstrated evidence of donor marrow stromal cell migration to the recipient's thymus as well participation in positive selection.[41] Other researchers have shown cotransplantation of marrow stromal cells in mice-prevented lethal GVHD.[4]

In addition to its possible role in central tolerance, stromal cells may also provide an environment for peripheral tolerance. In vitro study of human marrow stromal cells showed no proliferative response when cocultured with allogeneic peripheral blood monocytes.[42] They express MHC I and II antigens but not CD80, 86, or 40 costimulatory molecules. Cocultures with stimulated T cells also suppressed their activity. This has important implications for VBMT which brings a vascularized stromal environment to the recipient.

On the basis of the encouraging laboratory results, multiple clinical applications were subsequently reported. Koc et al. infused cultured-expanded mesenchymal stem cells along with BMT in breast cancer patients requiring bone marrow transplant and found more rapid neutrophil recovery.[43] Cahill et al. used both culture-expanded stromal cells with intraperitoneal and intramedullary bone grafts in conjunction with BMT to treat patients with infantile hypophosphatasia, Hunter syndrome, and autoimmune disease.[44] All patients demonstrated clinical improvement, and donor chimerism in bone-biopsy specimens despite negative peripheral-blood chimerism.

The role of the stromal cell within a CTA is not fully established. Rat studies found that VBMT (in form of a limb allograft) prolonged survival of a free skin allograft compared with bone marrow cells and other vascularized components of the limb.[45] The authors concluded that the VBMT facilitated induction of immunologic tolerance, though the mechanism was not specified. Lukomska's group demonstrated chimerism of specifically the bone marrow stromal cells in syngeneic sex-mismatched rats when transplanted with a VBMT (in form of hindlimb) that was not seen in BMT-infused group.[46] This correlated with earlier reports by Hewitt et al. of bone marrow chimerism in VBMT hindlimb recipients, though the stromal component was not specifically assayed.[1]

Combining the known laboratory and clinical results regarding the stromal environment, the question still remains – Does the stromal environment provide the stage for tolerant induction? Current findings strongly suggest a role for the stromal cell, in addition to the T cell, in orchestrating the immune adaptations in allogeneic transplantation. We await results of current and future research efforts in elucidating the interactions and mechanisms within the bone marrow stroma.

18.3 Vascularized Bone Marrow Transplant Models

A popular legend of the patron Saints Cosmas and Damian described their healing of a Christian verger diseased with an ulcerated leg by transplantation with the leg of a moor. It was certainly an attractive concept, and orthotopic transplantation of the limb became a widely used model for study of CTA, providing researcher with results on form and function of the graft. Within the CTA model was the VBMT. Researchers quickly noted that it was not only a structural support for the limb, but the bone marrow component was viable and has immune modulatory potential for the entire graft. Thus, CTA research laid the groundwork for VBMT.

18.3.1 Hindlimb

In the 1960s, investigators were already studying the allotransplantation of extremities. One of the first models was performed in dogs, consisting of an orthotopic transplantation at the midthigh level.[47] Without the current immunosuppressants available, these experiments showed the technical feasibility of limb replantation but with inevitable rejection in allografts.

18.3.1.1 Rat

One of the first reports of limb allotransplantation in the rat was by Doi in 1979 (Fig. 18.2).[48] He demonstrated the technical feasibility and superiority of using the rat model for CTA research, and defined common features of composite tissue rejection. However, the immunosuppressive agents used were either ineffective in delaying rejection (6-mercaptopurine, prednisolone) or delayed rejection but caused toxicity (azathioprine and prednisolone).

The discovery of cyclosporine (CsA) in the 1970s was a huge catapult to transplantation research.[49] By this time microsurgical equipment and techniques were refined and available, and in the early 1980s, Black and Hewitt et al. demonstrated significant prolongation of hindlimb allotransplantation in the rat using CsA across

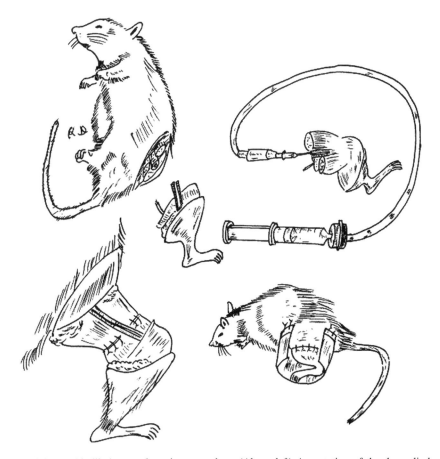

Fig. 18.2 Rat hindlimb transplantation procedure. (*Above left*) Amputation of the donor limb. (*Above right*) Irrigation of the donor limb through a micropore filter. (*Below left*) The microneurovascular anastomoses. (*Below right*) Application of the aluminum splint. (From Doi[48] with permission)

a semiallogeneic barrier LBN → LEW.[50,51] Allogeneic orthotopic and heterotopic hindlimb transplant both demonstrated survival as long as CsA was administered.[52,53] Hewitt et al. then showed peripheral blood chimerism and indefinite survival of the CTA in a fraction of the semiallogeneic transplant recipients after CsA withdrawal, and noted normal appearing bone marrow compartment in the donor limb.[1] The authors suggested a role for the donor bone marrow in achievement of tolerance.

The multiple antigenic components in a limb transplant made it difficult to clearly evaluate the vascularized bone marrow portion. Lee et al. separated the vascularized tissue components into skin, subcutaneous tissues, muscle, bone (represented by the knee joint), and blood vessel portions.[54] All vascularized tissues tested elicited a more rapid rejection response compared to the whole limb transplant. This delayed rejection was thought to be possible due to a "consumption" phenomenon as the immune system was overloaded with a large antigenic load. Alternatively, the bone marrow component with the femur was not evaluated.

Buttemeyer et al. developed a grading system for rejection of the component tissues in CTA.[55] Recapitulating findings of previous researchers, they found that the skin component elicited strongest rejection response, followed by muscle, bone, and cartilage.

To try to understand the immunologic effect of the VBMT portion within a CTA, Tsuchida, Usui, and Uede compared vascularized skin, muscle, and joint components to a whole limb transplant.[45] The animals were administered low-dose FK-506 and simultaneous free skin graft was transplanted. The authors found that the skin allograft survival was prolonged only in the whole limb allograft group and concluded that the VBMT affected skin allografts survival. With the presence of other tissues in the whole limb transplant, an isolated VBMT model would perhaps yield cleaner data to their study.

18.3.1.2 Mouse

The multiple advantages of a mouse model in transplantation research are well recognized. The availability of well-defined inbred strains, genetically engineered animals (transgenic and knock-out), and monoclonal antibodies specific to mice provide researchers the ability to dissect out complex immune mechanisms. Lower capital and housing costs are also considerations. However, their small vessel sizes and fragile physiology prohibited limb transplantation research in the mouse until recently.

In 1999, Zhang et al. published an orthotopic hindlimb transplantation model in the mouse using end-to-end anastomoses of the femoral vessels.[56] A couple of years later, Tung et al. developed a heterotopic limb and composite-tissue transplant models.[57] Single agent immunosuppression using CD40 costimulation blockade up to 60 days significantly prolonged allograft survival the musculoskeletal portion of the limb allograft, whereas the skin component was rejected in a delayed fashion.[58] Although tolerance was not achieved secondary to chronic rejection in this mouse model, the prolonged survival of the VBMT component echoed previous research results in rats, and opened exciting new potentials in CTA research using targeted monoclonal antibody immunosuppression.

Most recently, Foster and Liu provided technical simplifications to the orthotopic hindlimb model using the "cuff" technique.[59] Simplifying the technical demands hopefully will further expedite the research efforts in CTA.

18.3.2 Sternum

Noting the need for a purer VBMT model than the hindlimb allograft, Santiago et al. published their sternum transplant model in 1999.[60] Syngeneic and allogeneic models were established, and a 30-day course of FK-506 prevented rejection with demonstration of chimerism by flow cytometry, and histology demonstrated a viable marrow compartment. The donor procedural descriptions and illustrations were kindly provided by Dr. Sergio Santiago (Fig. 18.3a–d). The graft vessels were then anastomosed to the respective intra-abdominal vessels in an end-to-side fashion.

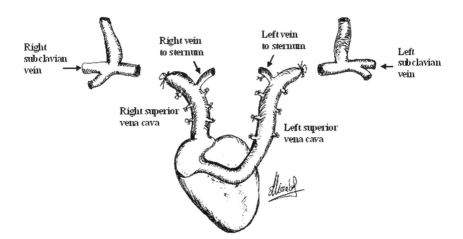

Fig. 18.3 Donor operation of the sternal model of vascularized bone marrow transplantation. (Courtesy of Dr. Sergio Santiago, University of Miami School of Medicine.) (**a**) The superior vena cava (SVC) is dissected on both sides up to the formation of the brachiocephalic veins and all draining veins are individually tied with 8/0 silk and divided except for the vein draining the sternum. (**b**) The SVC is divided distal to the preserved vein and a veno-venous end-to-side anastomosis is carried out between the left and right SVC using 11-0 nylon continuous sutures. This results in a single venous orifice for anastomosis to the recipient vena cava. (**c**) Posterior view of sternal graft with vessels. The ribs were divided on both sides of the sternum 0.5 cm away from the lateral sternal border. An end-to-side anastomosis (ESA) was performed between the left and right superior vena cava (SVC). Both carotid and subclavian arteries and brachiocephalic veins were ligated and divided. (**d**) The arteries supplying the sternum are taken with the aortic arch, leaving the proximal end of the arch open for the arterial anastomosis

(continued)

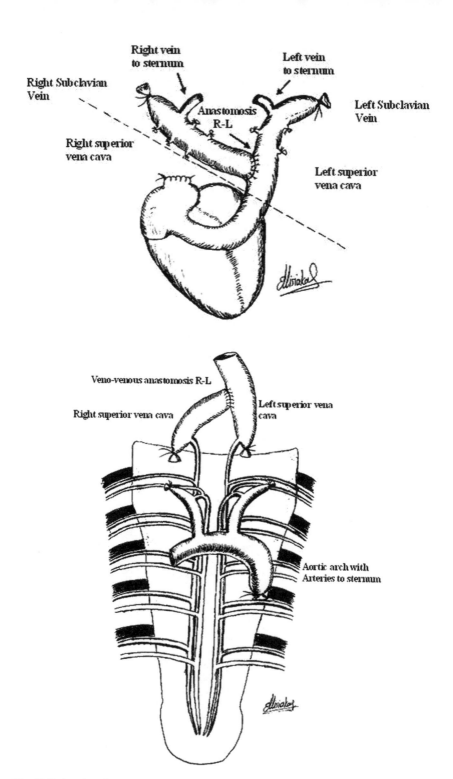

Fig. 18.3 (continued)

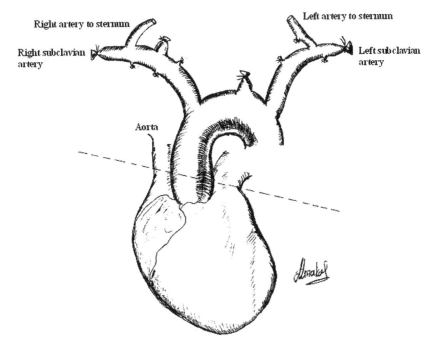

Fig. 18.3 (continued)

18.3.3 Femur

Shortly following the sternum model, Suzuki et al. published an isolated VBMT (iVBMT) model using the femur based on nutrient vessels from the femoral artery and vein anastomosed to the aorta and vena cava.[61] Since usage of the abdominal vessels for the iVBMT made simultaneous and/or subsequent SOTs more difficult, an extraperitoneal model was also developed in the same laboratory.[62]

18.3.4 Procedure for Graft Harvest

The limb is approached from the medial aspect. A generous incision is made from the groin to below the knee. The superficial vessels (epigastric to the fat pad and saphenous to the lower extremity) are divided. Reflection of the gracilis and semi-membranous muscles off the tibial attachment with division of the supplying vessels reveals the length of the femoral vessel. Detachment of the gastrocnemius at its origin allows better visualization of the popliteal area.

The three nutrient vessels are then isolated by detachment of muscular origins and preservation of nutrient vessels that arborize in the periosteum (Fig. 18.4a). Proximally, the lateral circumflex femoral sends a relatively constant nutrient

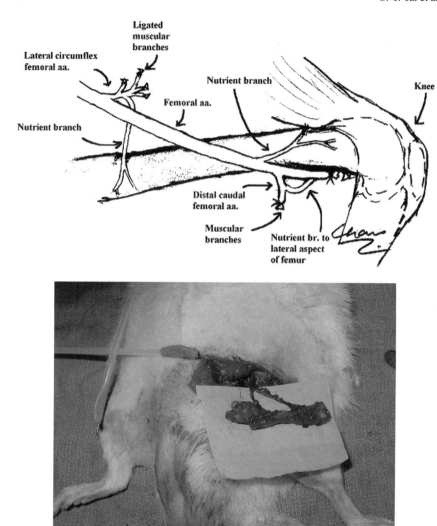

Fig. 18.4 Graft harvest procedure for the femoral isolated vascularized bone marrow transplant model. (**a**) The three nutrient vessels identified and isolated in situ prior to disarticulation. (**b**) The isolated vascularized bone marrow graft after disarticulation, still attached to the donor and perfusing in situ

branch straight down to the femur. This branch was not seen in only 1 of the 50 animals dissected. All other branches from the lateral circumflex to the lateral muscles are carefully identified and divided, taking care not to injure the nutrient vessel by traction or thermal injury. Distally, the next two branches are near popliteal artery. The distal caudal femoral artery sends branches to the flexors, and constant nutrient branch winds around the posterior aspect of femur to vascularize the femur on the lateral aspect. Muscular branches are divided, and the popliteal artery is ligated and divided distal to the distal caudal femoral take-off. At the anterior side of the femur, around the same level of the distal caudal femoral artery take off, a small branch runs along and into the periosteum while also giving off a branch to the sartorius lying just anteriorly. This branch is kept whenever possible.

After identification and isolation of the nutrient vessels, the femur is disarticulated at the knee. Residual muscular attachments are released, and finally disarticulated at the acetabulum. The graft is left perfusing in situ until the recipient site is ready for anastomosis (Fig. 18.4b). In the extraperitoneal model, anastomosis to the recipient femoral vessels was straight forward in an end-to-end fashion, and the graft was placed in a subcutaneous pocket in the abdomen.

Syngeneic and allogeneic transplant results echoed Santiago's results. Syngeneic grafts demonstrated normal architecture of the marrow compartment at explant, while allogeneic grafts showed progressive fibrosis in the bone marrow with loss of cellular constituents.

Experiments across a semiallogeneic LEW → LBN barrier was performed to study GVHD without the rejection component and immunosuppression.[63] Surprisingly, the experimental animals did not demonstrate any clinical or histopathologic signs of GVHD. When lethally irradiated, the isolated VBMT was able to reconstitute the semiallogeneic host lymphohematopoetic system, also without GVHD. These recipients also demonstrated chimerism and accepted donor free skin grafts, while maintaining third party skin graft rejection.[64] Additional studies across a fully allogeneic barrier and simultaneous studies with solid organ grafts are underway to better characterize the mechanisms of the isolated VBMT.

18.4 Future Studies

The VBMT is a marriage of paradigms, a solid organ graft that can function as cellular bone marrow graft, and carries with it stromal cells with untapped pluripotent and immunomodulatory potentials. Although current data on the VBMT are still preliminary, applications in the fields of BMT, SOT, and CTA warrant further investigations.

In BMT, preparative protocols obligatorily target the bone marrow components, and in addition to the lymphohematopoetic elements, the stromal cells also suffer irreparable damage. Utilization of a VBMT has the advantage of (1) immediate start of reconstitution without an engraftment period, (2) its own stromal milieu to provide and support cell renewal, and (3) providing an immunomodulatory environment for tolerance induction. The main disadvantages are the possible morbidities associated with surgical procedures in donor and recipient, though in well-controlled situations the risks are minimized.

SOT without long-term immunosuppression is the goal of allotransplantation. The immunomodulatory potentials of the VBMT have been suggested based on studies evaluating separate components of a CTA. Cotransplantation of SOT with an isolated VBMT is a clear next step in this investigation.

Just as VBMT stemmed from CTA research, its ultimate application back in CTA would change the utilization of composite tissue grafts. A main opposition to CTA currently is the morbidities required in lifelong immunosuppression since full tolerance to all tissue components including skin is not yet feasible in humans today. Many researchers believe in preconditioning of the recipient, conceptually rendering the host "immune neutral" for the initial period that allows introduction of donor antigens, sets the stage for donor and recipient communication, and then allows development of a new order of immune integrity. In the coming years of research, we strive to answer the question – Can the VBMT component within the CTA induce tolerance under appropriate conditions?

References

1. C. W. Hewitt, R. Ramsamooj, M. P. Patel, B. Yazdi, B. M. Achauer, K. S. Black, Development of stable mixed T cell chimerism and transplantation tolerance without immune modulation in recipients of vascularized bone marrow allografts, *Transplantation* **50**, 766 (1990).
2. D. K. Granger, W. C. Briedenbach, D. J. Pidwell, J. W. Jones, L. A. Baxter-Lowe, C. L. Kaufman, Lack of donor hyporesponsiveness and donor chimerism after clinical transplantation of the hand, *Transplantation* **74**, 1624 (2002).
3. P. Girman, J. Kriz, E. Dovolilova, E. Cihalova, F. Saudek, The effect of bone marrow transplantation on survival of allogeneic pancreatic islets with short-term tacrolimus conditioning in rats, *Ann Transplant* **6**, 43 (2002).
4. N. G. Chung, D. C. Jeong, S. J. Park, et al., Cotransplantation of marrow stromal cells may prevent lethal graft-versus-host disease in major histocompatibility complex mismatched murine hematopoietic stem cell transplantation, *Int J Hematol* **30**, 370 (2004).
5. S. Janczewska, A. Ziolkowska, M. Durlik, W. L. Olszewski, B. Lukomska, Fast lymphoid reconstitution after vascularized bone marrow transplantation in lethally irradiated rats, *Transplantation* **68**, 201 (1999).
6. T. E. Starzl, Chimerism and tolerance in transplantation, *Proc Natl Acad Sci U S A* **101** Suppl 2, 14607 (2004).
7. S. T. Ildstad, D. H. Sachs, Reconstitution with syngeneic plus allogeneic or xenogeneic bone marrow leads to specific acceptance of allografts or xenografts, *Nature* **307**, 168 (1984).
8. S. M. Pham, S. N. Mitruka, W. Youm, et al., Mixed hematopoietic chimerism induces donor-specific tolerance for lung allografts in rodents, *Am J Respir Crit Care Med* **1**, 199 (1999).
9. T. Werkele, J. Kurtz, H. Ito, et al., Allogeneic bone marrow transplantation with co-stimulatory blockade induces macrochimerism and tolerance without cytoreductive host treatment, *Nat Med* **6**, 464 (2000).
10. M. M. Durham, A. W. Bingaman, A. B. Adams, et al., Cutting edge: administration of anti-CD40 ligand and donor bone marrow leads to hemopoietic chimerism and donor-specific tolerance without cytoreductive conditioning, *J Immunol* **165**, 1 (2000).
11. C. Domenig, A. Sanchez-Fueyo, J. Kurtz, et al., Roles of deletion and regulation in creating mixed chimerism and allograft tolerance using a nonlymphoablative irradiation-free protocol, *J Immunol* **175**, 51 (2005).
12. B. Luo, S. A. Nanji, C. D. Schur, R. L. Pawlick, C. C. Anderson, A. M. J. Shapiro, Robust tolerance to fully allogeneic islet transplants achieved by chimerism with minimal conditioning, *Transplantation* **80**, 370 (2005).
13. A. Umemura, H. Morita, X. C. Li, et al., Dissociation of hemopoietic chimerism and allograft tolerance after allogeneic bone marrow transplantation. *J Immunol* **167**, 3043 (2001).

14. H. Xu, P. M. Chilton, Y. Huang, C. L. Schanie, S. T. Ildstad, Production of donor T cells is critical for induction of donor-specific tolerance and maintenance of chimerism, *J Immunol* **172**, 1463 (2004).
15. R. D. Foster, S. Pham, S. Li, A. Aitouche, Long-term acceptance of composite tissue allografts through mixed chimerism and CD28 blockade, *Transplantation* **76**, 988 (2003).
16. C. A. Huang, Y. Fuchimoto, R. Scheier-Dolberg, M. C. Murphy, D. M. Neville Jr., D. H. Sachs, Stable mixed chimerism and tolerance using a nonmyeloablative preparative regimen in a large-animal model, *J Clin Invest* **105**, 173 (2003).
17. M. L. Schwarze, M. T. Menard, Y. Fuchimoto, et al., Mixed hematopoietic chimerism induces long-term tolerance to cardiac allografts in miniature swine, *Ann Thorac Surg* **70**, 131 (2000).
18. K. A. Prabhune, V. S. Gorantla, G. Perez-Abadia, et al., Composite tissue allotransplantation in chimeric hosts part II. A clinically relevant protocol to induce tolerance in a rat model, *Transplantation* **76**, 1548 (2003).
19. P. C. R. Brouha, G. Perez-Abadia, C. Francois, et al., Lymphadenectomy prior to rat hind limb allotransplantation prevents graft-versus-host disease in chimeric hosts. *Transplant Int* **17**, 341 (2004).
20. D. W. Mathes, M. A. Randolph, J. L. Bourget, et al., Recipient bone marrow engraftment in donor tissue after long-term tolerance to a composite tissue allograft, *Transplantation* **73**, 1880 (2002).
21. D. W. Mathes, M. A. Randolph, M. G. Solari, et al., Split tolerance to a composite tissue allograft in a swine model, *Transplantation* **75**, 25 (2003).
22. R. Garcia-Morales, V. Esquenazi, K. Zucker, et al., An assessment of the effects of cadaver donor bone marrow on kidney allograft recipient blood cell chimerism by a novel technique combining PCR and flow cytometry, *Transplantation* **62**, 1149 (1996).
23. R. Shapiro, A. S. Rao, R. J. Corry, et al., Kidney transplantation with bone marrow augmentation: five-year outcomes, *Transpant Proc* **33**, 1134 (2001).
24. A. S. Rao, I. Dvorchik, F. Dodson, et al., Donor bone marrow infusion in liver recipients: effect on the occurrence of acute cellular rejection, *Transplant Proc* **33**, 1352 (2001).
25. S. M. Pham, A. S. Rao, A. Zeevi, et al., A clinical trial combining donor bone marrow infusion and heart transplantation: intermediate-term results, *J Thorac Cardiovasc Surg* **119**, 673 (2001).
26. S. M. Pham, A. S. Rao, A. Zeevi, et al., Effects of donor bone marrow infusion in clinical lung transplantation, *Ann Thorac Surg* **69**, 345 (2000).
27. M. T. Sellers, M. H. Deierhoi, J. J. Curtis, et al., Tolerance in renal transplantation after allogeneic bone marrow transplantation – 6-year follow-up, *Transplantation* **71**, 1681 (2001).
28. L. H. Buhler, T. R. Spitzer, M. Sykes, et al., Induction of kidney allograft tolerance after transient lymphohematopoietic chimerism in patients with multiple myeloma and end-stage renal disease, *Transplantation* **74**, 1405 (2002).
29. E. C. Williamson, M. R. Millar, C. G. Steward, et al., Infections in adults undergoing unrelated donor bone marrow transplantation, *Br J Haematol* **104**, 560 (1999).
30. S. Thomas, S. C. Clark, J. M. Rappeport, D. G. Nathan, S. G. Emerson, Deficient T cell granulocyte-macrophage colony stimulating factor production in allogeneic bone marrow transplant recipients, *Transplantation* **49**, 703 (1990).
31. A. Devergie, J. Reiffers, J. P. Vernant, et al., Long-term follow-up after bone marrow transplantation of chronic myelogenous leukemia: factors associated with relapse, *Bone Marrow Transplant* **5**, 379 (1990).
32. J. Balon, K. Halaburda, M. Bieniaszewska, et al., Early complete donor hematopoietic chimerism in peripheral blood indicates the risk of extensive graft-versus-host disease, *Bone Marrow Transplant* **35**, 1083 (2005).
33. J. E. Wagner, J. S. Thompson, S. L. Carter, N. A. Kernan, Effect of graft-versus-host disease prophylaxis on 3-year disease-free survival in recipients of unrelated donor bone marrow (T-cell Depletion Trial): a multi-centre, randomised phase II-III trial, *Lancet* **366**, 733 (2005).

34. P. Bianco, M. Riminucci, S. Gronthos, P. G. Robey, Bone marrow stromal stem cells: nature, biology, and potential applications, *Stem Cells* **19**, 180 (2001).
35. S. N. Shu, L. Wei, J. H. Wang, Y. T. Zhan, H. S. Chen, Y. Wang, Hepatic differentiation capability of rat bone marrow-derived mesenchymal stem cells and hematopoietic stem cells, *World J Gastroenterol* **10**, 2818 (2004).
36. P. J. Simmons, D. Przepiorka, E. D. Thomas, B. Torok-Storb, Host origin of marrow stromal cells following allogeneic bone marrow transplantation, *Nature* **328**, 429 (1987).
37. A. Keating, J. W. Singer, P. D. Killen, et al., Donor origin of the in vitro haematopoietic microenvironment after marrow transplantation in man, *Nature* **298**, 280 (1982).
38. O. N. Koc, C. Peters, P. Aubourg, et al., Bone marrow-derived mesenchymal stem cells remain host-derived despite successful hematopoietic engraftment after allogeneic transplantation in patients with lysosomal and peroxisomal storage diseases, *Exp Hematol* **27**, 1675 (1999).
39. T. Ishida, M. Inaba, H. Hisha, et al., Requirement of donor-derived stromal cells in the bone marrow for successful allogeneic bone marrow transplantation. Complete prevention of recurrence of autoimmune diseases in MRL/MP-Ipr/Ipr mice by transplantation of bone marrow plus bones (stromal cells) from the same donor, *J Immunol* **152**, 3119 (1994).
40. H. Hisha, T. Nishino, M. Kawamura, S. Adachi, S. Ikehara, Successful bone marrow transplantation by bone grafts in chimeric-resistant combination, *Exp Hematol* **23**, 347 (1995).
41. Y. Li, H. Hisha, M. Inaba, et al., Evidence for migration of donor bone marrow stromal cells into recipient thymus after bone marrow transplantation plus bone grafts: a role of stromal cells in positive selection, *Exp Hematol* **28**, 950 (2000).
42. W. T. Tse, J. D. Pendleton, W. M. Beyer, M. C. Egalka, E. C. Guinan, Suppression of allogeneic T-cell proliferation by human marrow stromal cells: implications in transplantation, *Transplantation* **75**, 389 (2003).
43. O. N. Koc, S. L. Gerson, B. W. Cooper, et al., Rapid hematopoietic recovery after coinfusion of autologous-blood stem cells and culture-expanded marrow mesenchymal stem cells in advanced breast cancer patients receiving high-dose chemotherapy, *J Clin Oncol* **18**, 307 (2000).
44. R. A. Cahill, O. Y. Jones, M. Klemperer, et al., Replacement of recipient stromal/mesenchymal cells after bone marrow transplantation using bone fragments and cultured osteoblast-like cells, *Biol Blood Marrow Transplant* **10**, 709 (2004).
45. Y. Tsuchida, M. Usui, T. Uede, Vascularized bone-marrow allotransplantation in rats prolongs the survival of simultaneously grafted alloskin, *J Reconstr Microsurg* **18**, 289 (2002).
46. B. Lukomska, S. Janczewska, B. Interewicz, M. Wisniewski, Engraftment of donor-derived stromal cells stimulates fast hematopoietic repopulation of vascularized bone marrow transplant recipients, *Transplant Proc* **33**, 1757 (2001).
47. R. M. Goldwyn, P. M. Beach, D. Feldman, R. E. Wilam, Canine limb homotransplantations, *Plast Reconstr Surg* **37**, 184 (1966).
48. K. Doi, Homotransplantation of limbs in rats. A preliminary report on an experimental study with no specific immunosuppressive drugs, *Plast Reconstr Surg* **64**, 613 (1979).
49. J. F. Borel, C. Feurer, H. U. Gubler, H. Stahelin, Biological effects of cyclosporin A: a new antilymphocytic agent, *Agents Actions* **6**, 468 (1976).
50. K. S. Black, C. W. Hewitt, L. A. Fraser, et al., Cosmas and Damian in the laboratory, *N Engl J Med* **306**, 368 (1982).
51. K. S. Black, C. W. Hewitt, L. A. Fraser, et al., Composite tissue (limb) allografts in rats. II. Indefinite survival using low-dose cyclosporine, *Transplantation* **39**, 365 (1985).
52. S. K. Kim, S. Aziz, P. Oyer, V. R. Hentz, Use of cyclosporine A in allotransplantation of rat limbs, *Ann Plast Surg* **12**, 249 (1984).
53. W. D. Fritz, W. M. Swartz, S. Rose, J. W. Futrell, E. Klein, Limb allografts in rats immunosuppressed with cyclosporine A, *Ann Surg* **199**, 211 (1984).
54. W. P. Lee, M. J. Yaremchuk, Y. C. Pan, M. A. Randolph, C. M. Tan, A. J. Weiland, Relative antigenicity of components of a vascularized limb allograft, *Plast Reconstr Surg* **87**, 401 (1991).
55. R. Buttemeyer, N. J. Jones, Z. Min, U. Rao, Rejection of the component tissues of limb allografts in rats immunosuppressed with FK-506 and cyclosporine, *Plast Reconstr Surg* **97**, 139 (1994).

56. F. Zhang, D. Y. Shi, Z. Kryger, et al., Development of a mouse limb transplantation model, *Microsurgery* **19**, 209 (1999).
57. T. H. Tung, T. Mohanakumar, S. E. Mackinnon, Development of a mouse model for heterotopic limb and composite-tissue transplantation, *J Reconstr Microsurg* **17**, 267 (2001).
58. T. H. Tung, S. E. Mackinnon, T. Mohanakumar, Long-term limb allograft survival using anti-CD40L antibody in a murine model, *Transplantation* **75**, 644 (2003).
59. R. D. Foster, T. Liu, Orthotopic hindlimb transplantation in the mouse, *J Reconstr Microsurg* **19**, 49 (2003).
60. S. F. Santiago, W. de Faria, T. F. Khan, et al., Heterotopic sternum transplant in rats: a new model of a vascularized bone marrow transplantation, *Microsurgery* **19**, 330 (1999).
61. H. Suzuki, N. Patel, M. S. Matthews, A. J. DelRossi, E. J. Doolin, C. W. Hewitt, Vascularized bone marrow transplantation: a new surgical approach using isolated femoral bone/bone marrow, *J Surg Res* **89**, 176 (2000).
62. C. Y. Tai, M. A. France, L. F. Strande, et al., Extraperitoneal isolated vascularized bone marrow transplant model in the rat, *Transplantation* **75**, 1591 (2003).
63. C. Y. Tai, L. F. Strande, R. Eydelman, et al., Absence of graft-versus-host disease in the isolated vascularized bone marrow transplant, *Transplantation* **77**, 316 (2004).
64. C. Y. Tai, L. F. Strande, V. Lounev, et al., Vascularzied bone marrow transplantation: a new surgical approach to bone marrow transplantation induces immunological tolerance, *Am J Transplant* **5** Suppl, 366 (2005).

Chapter 19
Vascularized Bone Marrow Transplantation: Pathology of Composite Tissue Transplantation-Induced Graft-Versus-Host-Disease

Rajen Ramsamooj and Charles W. Hewitt

19.1 Background

Composite tissue allografts (CTAs) represent the transplantation of several tissue types including integumentary, musculoskeletal, cutaneous, and hematopoietic elements. The rat hindlimb CTA using a parental limb to an F_1 hybrid host actually represents a vascularized bone marrow transplant model.[1] The hindlimb CTA provides transplantation of precursor hematolymphoid (bone marrow) and mature (blood and lymph nodes) elements by a surgical approach along with transfer of their syngeneic/supportive microenvironments. Immediate engraftment with and without immune modulation has been previously shown.[2-7]

By comparison, other bone marrow transplant models have a finite rate of engraftment failures of which none have been reported with the hindlimb CTA/vascularized bone marrow transplant. There are significant advantages to the transplantation of composite tissues when considering bone marrow transplantation. Compared with other methods of bone marrow transplantation,[8-10] CTAs allow immediate engraftment of donor lymphoid cells with development of donor-specific lymphoid chimerism.[4,5,7]

Chimerism produces two profound effects in the hybrid recipient of a parental limb. These are the development of donor-specific immune tolerance and graft-versus-host-disease (GVHD). The tolerant animals showed significantly lower levels of donor-specific T-cell chimerism.[1] Mechanisms of host-specific tolerance are associated with the fate of the chimeric T-cell populations. A curious phenomenon occurs during the first 30 days postvascularized bone marrow transplantation (VBMT). These animals become polyclonal, self-, and host-specifically responsive in *in vitro* studies.[11] These results are similar to the immune reactivity associated with GVHD in other models.[12-14] This initial dysregulated immune response is later replaced by polyclonal unresponsiveness at 100 days and host-specific unresponsiveness at 200 days.[11] Thus, this initial immune dysregulation in the tolerant animals is associated with a stable low-level mixed chimerism. It appears as though the chimeric environment supports the development of suppressor circuits and thus host-specific tolerance.

Unfortunately, the converse of tolerance, when considering VBMT, is GVHD. This undesired outcome is associated with unstable higher levels of donor chimerism. In the recipient animal, these chimeric T cells become effector cells that lead to the development of GVHD. In murine studies, evidence of GVHD correlates with the presence of increased levels of donor CD8+ lymphocytes.[15] Thus it follows that the depletion of the CD8+ cells would decrease the chance of developing GVHD,[15] but there is an increased risk of graft failure.[15–17]

19.2 Gross Clinical Aspects of VBMT

The majority of recipients (60–70%) of parental to F_1 hybrid rat hindlimbs are tolerant. They thrive after allograft transplantation. Weight gain is at the usual rate and they remain in excellent health.[18] The minority develops GVHD. GVHD is best described as a cachectic wasting syndrome of dermatitis, enteritis, and hepatitis. The dermatitis takes on the form of a macular erythematous rash that can involve any part of the body. In the rat hindlimb model, though, the most affected areas include the ears, nose, and genitalia (Fig. 19.1). In the initial stages of the disease, there is an erythematous appearance to the skin. There is concomitant alopecia. In the later stages, the rash changes to a lichen planus-like rash that eventually becomes sclerotic.

The enteritis is manifested clinically as profound diarrhea and weight loss with loss of appetite. In the rat hindlimb CTA/VBMT, average weight loss ranges from 25 to 40% of original weight at the time of transplantation.[18]

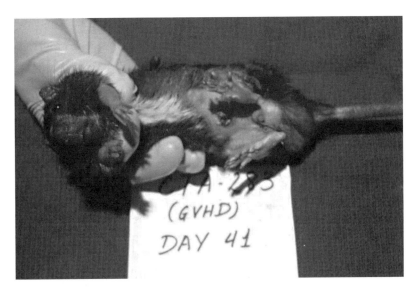

Fig. 19.1 Graft-versus-host-disease in a LEW to LBN CTA/VBMT recipient. LEW to LBN composite tissue allograft/vascularized bone marrow transplant undergoing one-way donor antihost graft-versus-host disease day 41 posttransplant (*See Color Plates*)

The hepatitis component is usually detected by abnormal bilirubin levels and/or the presence of jaundice which is not readily apparent in the rat hindlimb CTA. In human bone marrow transplantation, these parameters are easily determined and/or observed with serum liver enzyme tests such as bilirubin, etc. Yet, in animal models this component is typically not clinically relevant.

19.3 Acute and Chronic GVHD

All animals that develop GVHD in the hindlimb CTA/VBMT model eventually die of the disease within an average of 163 days posttransplantation.[18] A curious phenomenon occurs in the development of the disease. Two distinct groups designated as acute and chronic develop. In general, the acute group shows a significantly greater weight loss over a shorter period of time compared to the chronic group.[18] In addition, the onset of the precipitous weight loss occurs earlier in the course of the disease.

Acute and chronic GVHD is not unique to the rat hindlimb CTA/VBMT model. In fact, these two groups have been described in other models as well as human GVHD associated with bone marrow transplantation. It is generally accepted that acute and chronic GVHD represents two distinct disease/immunologic processes. The mechanisms of this dichotomy are beyond the scope of this chapter. Nevertheless, numerous studies in mouse models have shown that there are two separate pathways, at least from an immune response aspect, and that acute GVHD does not beget chronic GVHD. In humans, acute and chronic GVHD is arbitrarily defined as a GVHD crisis occurring before 100 days for the former and after 100 days for the latter.[19]

In general, acute GVHD is regarded as an abrupt onset of dermatitis, enteritis, and/or hepatitis that is immediately life threatening. Conversely, chronic GVHD is typically thought to be a more sclerosing process.

19.4 Histopathology

19.4.1 Skin

GVHD in the skin and mucosal surfaces is characterized by a lichenoid inflammation at the dermal–epidermal junction. The inflammatory infiltrate is composed almost exclusively of mature lymphocytes. This inflammatory infiltrate is most pronounced in the early stages of the disease. There is concomitant dyskeratosis and individually necrotic keratinocytes are associated with this inflammation.[18] There is usually inflammation and destruction of the adnexal structures. As the disease progresses there is replacement of the inflammation by dense sclerosis at dermal–epidermal junction.

19.4.2 Liver

When considering GVHD, there is typically a prominent infiltrate that appears almost identical to a viral hepatitis. That is, there is a prominent portal inflammatory infiltrate of mature lymphocytes. The inflammation can extend beyond the limiting plate (active hepatitis). The inflammation usually surrounds the vessels within the portal tracts and may show endothelialitis. But, the more diagnostic histopathologic feature is bile duct damage.[18] The changes can range from mild ductulitis, which is composed of intraepithelial lymphocytes, to complete bile duct damage. There is epithelial damage consisting of irregularly shaped bile ducts with vacuolization of the nuclei.

19.4.3 Gastro-Intestinal Tract

Unlike the liver and skin, lymphocytic inflammation is usually not a prominent feature. The sine qua non of GVHD in the GI tract is apoptosis. Histologically, apoptosis is best characterized as a ballooned crypt cell containing a pyknotic, karyorrhectic nucleus.[18] The apoptosis can range from single cells involving individual crypts to complete necrosis of the bowel wall with ulceration and granulation tissue. Fibrosis of the bowel wall may or may not be present.

19.4.4 Other Tissues

The bone marrow of recipients of rat hindlimb CTA/VBMT shows several interesting findings. Typically, there is increased cellularity in those animals developing GVHD compared to the tolerant animals in both the transplanted and contralateral limbs.[20] By immunohistochemistry, *in situ* TGF-beta expression is significantly increased in the CTA/VBMT chimeras who develop GVHD. This increased expression is present in both the transplanted and contralateral limbs. When considering the transplanted versus contralateral limb, there is an increased level of TGF-beta in the contralateral versus transplanted limb marrow in the animals that are tolerant. Although *in situ* TGF-beta expression was present in the tolerant animals, the level of immunostaining is less than that in the GVHD animals.[20,21]

These findings suggest an important mechanism involving the immuno-modulator, TGF-beta. The differences in the GVHD and tolerant CTA chimeras, with regard to TGF-beta expression, suggest an auto-/allo-immune dysregulation that occurs in GVHD CTA/VBMT chimeras. The lower level of TGF-beta expression in the tolerant versus GVHD animals may also support the maintenance of tolerance in these chimeras.

19.5 Conclusion

F_1 hybrid recipients of parental rat hindlimb CTA and therefore vascularized bone marrow transplants develop one of several outcomes. All of these CTA/VBMT develop donor-specific lymphoid chimerism. The level of this chimerism, to some extent, determines whether or not these animals develop tolerance or GVHD. Studies of this model have shown that stable low levels of mixed donor chimerism are associated with tolerance. Conversely, GVHD is linked to higher unstable levels of donor chimerism.

The pathology associated with CTA/VBMT induced is best described as a syndrome of dermatitis, hepatitis, and enteritis. The CTA/VBMT recipients developed characteristic clinical and histopathological findings of GVHD. With respect to the immunomodulator TGF-beta, GVHD was associated with high levels of in situ expression in the bone marrow compared with the tolerant animals. Thus, TGF-beta may represent a mechanism of tolerance and immune dysregulation associated with CTA/VBMT and GVHD.

References

1. C. W. Hewitt, R. Ramsamooj, M. Patel, et al. Development of stable mixed T cell chimerism and transplantation tolerance without immune modulation in recipients of vascularized bone marrow allografts, *Transplantation* **50**, 766–772 (1990).
2. K. S. Black, C. W. Hewitt, L. A. Fraser, et al. Composite tissue (limb) allografts in rats: II. Indefinite survival using low dose cyclosporine. *Transplantation* **39**, 365–386 (1985).
3. C. W. Hewitt, K.S. Black, L. A. Fraser, et al. Composite tissue (limb) allografts in rats: I. Dose dependent increase in survival with cyclosporine. *Transplantation* **39**, 360–364, (1985).
4. C. W. Hewitt, K. S. Black, D. F. Dowdy, et al. Composite tissue (limb) allografts in rats: III. Development of donor-host lymphoid chimeras in long-term survivors. *Transplantation* **41**, 39–43 (1986).
5. C. W. Hewitt, K. S. Black, L. E. Henson, et al. Lymphocyte chimerism in a full allogeneic composite tissue (rat limb) allograft model prolonged with cyclosporine. *Transplant Proc* **20**, 272–278 (1988).
6. L. E. Henson, C. W. Hewitt, K. S. Black. Use of regression analysis and the complement-dependent cytotoxicity typing assay for predicting lymphoid chimerism. *J Immunol Methods* **114**, 139–144 (1988).
7. C. W. Hewitt, K. S. Black, R. Ramsamooj, et al. Lymphoid chimerism and graft-versus-host disease (GVHD) in rat-limb composite tissue allograft recipients. *FASEB J* **3**, 5233 (1989).
8. E. D. Thomas, C. D. Buckner, R. A. Cliff, et al. Marrow transplantation for acute non-lymphoblastic leukemia in first remission period. *N Engl J Med* **301**, 597–599 (1979).
9. G. W. Santos. Bone marrow transplantation. *Adv Intern Med* **24**, 157–182 (1979).
10. W. E. Beschorner, P. J. Tutschka, G. W. Santos. Chronic graft-versus-host-disease in the rat radiation chimera. I. Clinical features, hematology, histology, and immunopathology in long-term chimeras. *Transplantation* **33**, 393–399 (1982).
11. R. Ramsamooj, R. Lull, M. P. Patel, et al. Mechanisms of alloimmune tolerance associated with mixed chimerism induced by vascularized bone marrow transplants. *Cell Transpl* **11**, 683–693 (2002).

12. A. G. Rolink, T. Radaszkiewicz, F. Melchers. The autoantigen-binding B cell repertoire of normal and of chronically graft versus host disease mice. *J Exp Med* **165**, 1675–1687 (1987).
13. S. Luzuy, J. Merino, H. Engers, et al. Autoimmunity after induction of neonatal to alloantigens: Role of B cell chimerism and F1 donor B cell activation. *J Immunol* **146**, 4420–4426 (1986).
14. D. B. Wilson. Idiotypic regulation of T cells in graft-versus-host-disease and autoimmunity. *Immunol Rev* **107**, 159–177 (1989).
15. R. Korngold, J. Sprent. Variable capacity of L3T4+ T cells to cause lethal graft-versus-host disease across minor histocompatibility barriers in mice. *J Exp Med* **165**, 1552–1564 (1987).
16. B. L. Hamilton. L3T4-positive T cells participate in the induction of graft-versus-host-disease in response to minor histocompatibility antigens. *J Immunol* **139**, 2511–2515 (1987).
17. R. L. Truitt, A. A. Atasoylu. Contribution of CD4+ and CD8+ T cells to graft-versus-host disease and graft-versus leukemia reactivity after transplantation of MHC-compatible bone marrow. *Bone Marrow Transplant* **8**, 51–58 (1991).
18. R. Ramsamooj, R. Llull, K. S. Black, et al. Composite tissue allografts in rats: IV. Pathological manifestations of graft-versus-host-disease (GVHD) in recipients of vascularized bone marrow allografts. *Plast Reconstr Surg* **104(5)**, 1365–1371 (1999).
19. M. R. Wick, S. B. Moore, D. A. Gastineau, et al. Immunologic, clinical and pathologic aspects of human graft-versus-host disease. *Mayo Clin Proc* **58**, 603–612 (1983).
20. C. W. Hewitt, M. J. Englese, L. D. Tatem, et al. Graft-versus-host-disease in extremity transplantation: Digital image analysis of bone marrow *in situ*. *Ann Plastic Surg* **35**, 108–112 (1995).
21. R. Ramsamooj, R. Llull, L. D. Tatem, et al. Graft versus host disease in extremity transplantation: Digital image analysis of bone marrow and TGF-β expression in situ using a novel 3-D microscope. *Transplant Proc* **28**, 2029–2031 (1996).

Chapter 20
Immune Cell Redistribution After Vascularized Bone Marrow Transplantation

Waldemar L. Olszewski and Marek Durlik

20.1 Introduction

The specificity of a limb transplant lies in its anatomy. It is a graft of an organ, in analogy to the kidney or heart transplant, but in addition, it is a graft of bone marrow (BM) whose cells (BMC) do not only proliferate and mature in the graft but also migrate to the recipient bone marrow cavities and lymphoid organs (LO). Thus, the immune contact between the donor and recipient takes place not only in the graft itself but also in the recipient's immune organs, where the released BMC home. The BMC released from the graft may also home in other tissues, especially those with direct contact with environment as skin, gut, and lungs. Interestingly, there have been reports that the donor bone marrow cells may survive in the allogeneic recipient and create a state of cellular microchimerism.[1] Microchimerisms are, according to some researchers, linked with the development of partial tolerance to donor alloantigens.[2-6] This is a controversial issue with a number of observations supporting and negating the concept of microchimerism as a causative factor in prolongation of survival of organ allograft transplanted concomitantly with bone marrow. Another problem is the graft-versus-host reaction developing after bone marrow transplantation. There are reports providing evidence for lack of the graft-versus-host reaction after limb transplantation.[7-12]

The transplanted limb is a source of BMC. The in-bone BM is a tissue where the hemopoietic cells remain in a spatial functional relationship with the stromal cells, in contrast to the intravenously transplanted BMC suspension deprived of stromal cells. This means that the hemopoietic cells contained in the bone graft can physiologically mature after transplantation and can be released to the recipient circulation together with the hemopoietic cytokines produced by BM stromal cells. The main unknowns are the rate of release of BMC from the transplanted bone, homing sites of the released BMC, the speed of population of recipient BM cavities and LO by donor cells, the functional capacity of the homing donor hemopoietic cells in producing mature blood cells in the recipient, the rejection rate of donor BMC rejected by the allogeneic recipient, the probability of donor in BMC to evoke the graft-versus-host reaction, and finally survival of the BMC homing in the recipient tissues and creating a state of microchimerism.

20.2 Distribution of Donor BMC in Recipient Tissues

20.2.1 Distribution of BMC Released from il-BMTx in Syngeneic Recipient

To study the topographical distribution of BMC released from the in limb-bone marrow transplantation (il-BMTx), the in-bone BMC were labelled with ^{51}Cr and transplanted with the hindlimb to a syngeneic recipient (Fig. 20.1). There was a high accumulation rate of BM cell radioactivity in recipient BM (Fig. 20.2). High levels of radioactivity were also found in the gut, spleen, mesenteric lymph node (MLN), and liver. The pattern of distribution was specific for migrating BMC but different from that of the thoracic duct lymphocytes (TDL). The TDL migrate preponderantly to the liver and spleen. As a normal BM contains only about 10% of lymphocytes, the high rate of BMC accumulating in the lymphoid organs indicates that not only the lymphoid but also the nonlymphoid lineage BMC home to the lymphoid tissues.[13] There were no differences in the BM accumulation rate of ^{51}Cr-labeled BMC 4 and 24h after transplantation. This observation suggests that the BM homing cells do not recirculate and remain at their site of destination to fulfil their tasks.[13]

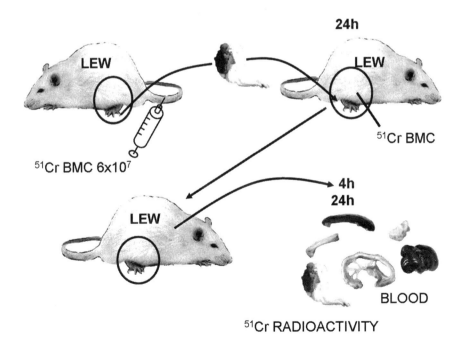

Fig. 20.1 Schematic presentation of in vivo labeling of BMC in hindlimb for studies of BMC distribution. LEW rat received iv ^{51}Cr-labeled BMC, 24h later his limb containing radioactive BMC was transplanted to a syngeneic recipient. Four or 24h after transplantation radioactivity was measured in recipient BM and lymphoid organs

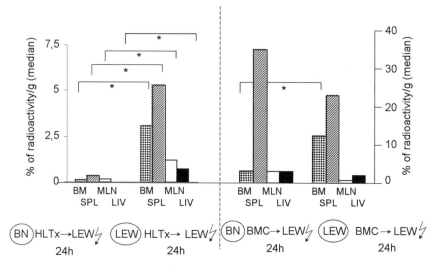

Fig. 20.2 Distribution of BMC from the transplanted hindlimb. *Left panel* – HLTx, *right panel* – iv-BMC (intravenous isolated bone marrow cell) infusion. Only a few allogeneic BMC populated recipient BM cavities and lymphoid organs after HLTx compared with syngeneic combination. Low number of allogeneic cells was caused by "allogeneic elimination." Note high number of BMC in recipient tissues after iv-BMC bolus injection. Interestingly, repopulation of recipient BM was faster after HLTx than iv-BMC infusion

20.2.2 The Effect of In Limb-Bone Marrow Transplantation on the Syngeneic Nonirradiated Recipient BM and (LO) Cellularity

Ten days after il-BMTx to a syngeneic nonirradiated recipient, the BMC yield from recipient tibia was three times higher than in the control rats (Fig. 20.3).[14] The frequency of erythroid BMC subsets reached normal values. There was a slightly higher percentage of segmented neutrophiles and lower percentage of juvenile forms and metamyelocytes than in an intact animal. However, an evident decrease in BM lymphocyte percentage was observed. Subsequently, a decrease in the BMC yield was observed within 30 days, however, its level still remained statistically higher than in the control rats. On day 30, the percentages of myeloid line cells and lymphocytes returned to control values. The spleen and MLN weight and cell yield did not differ on day 10 and 30 from the control values. Also, there were no changes in the frequency of peripheral blood cells.

The overshoot of BMC volume observed after il-BMTx should be accounted for by signals promoting BMC proliferation, presumably originating not only from BM cavities but also from the infiltrating cells accumulating in the healing anastomotic wound of the transplanted limb. Another factor responsible for the crowding effect may be the lack of space for the donor BMC due to the presence of recipient own BMC. The crowding effect seems to be responsible for the temporary suppression of neutrophil and lymphocyte maturation.

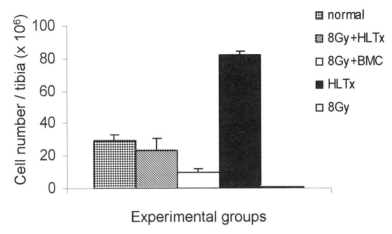

Fig 20.3 Repopulation of tibial BM cavity 10 days after syngeneic hindlimb transplantation (HLTx). Data show the number of retrieved BMC. HLTx to irradiated rats led to total repopulation of recipient tibia and was more effective than iv infusion of BMC suspension. Transplantation to a nonirradiated recipient brought about "crowding effect"

20.2.3 *The Effect of il-BMCTx on the Syngeneic Irradiated Recipient BM and LO Cellularity*

The effect of il-BMtx was studied in the 8-Gy irradiated rats with a follow-up period of 10 and 30 days.[14–18] Total repopulation of recipient BM cavities was observed already on day 10. The recipient tibia cell yield did not differ from that of control animals (Fig. 20.3). The percentage of juvenile neutrophils and myeloblasts was higher and of lymphocytes lower than in controls. There were no differences in the differential picture of the BM erythroid, myeloid, and lymphoid lines compared with control animals. After 30 days, the tibia BMC yield rose above that of 10 days and remained higher than in the control rats. There were no differences in the frequencies of the BM subsets compared with controls.[19]

The il-BMTx is a transplantation of BMC together with stromal cells in their natural spatial relationship. This allows immediate resumption of the hemopoietic activity of the transplant. Moreover, cells released from the graft retain full migratory capacity from the bone cavity and homing in recipient BM and LO. The production of cytokines by graft stromal cells seems to remain unimpaired. The hemopoietic cytokines may upregulate the process of proliferation and maturation of graft BMC in a situation of high demand for blood cells by the recipient. Released into circulation, the cytokines may also have a remote regulatory effect on LO, facilitating their colonization and replenishment by lineage precursors from the transplanted BM.

20.3 In Vitro Responsiveness of BM Lymphocytes in il-BMTx Recipients

The BM contains around 10% of lymphocytes. The in vitro responsiveness to phytohemagglutinin (PHA) of the whole population of BMC harvested on day 10 after il-BMTx from recipient tibia was slightly above control values. Recipient's sera had a slight, but statistically nonsignificant, additive stimulatory effect at higher concentrations. The supernatants from 24-h cultures of BMC from recipients of il-BMTx had only a slight enhancing effect on PHA stimulation of normal BMC.[20]

The responding population belonged to the BM lymphocytes. Their responsiveness was close to normal. This observation points to the functional reconstitution of the BM lymphocyte subset already on day 10 after il-BMTx. The level of responsiveness of BMC in the presence of recipients' sera was low. This indicates that at that time point recipient sera did not contain cytokines that would activate BMC proliferation. Similarly, the supernatant from recipient BMC culture did not contain stimulatory factors for normal BMC. These observations may suggest that the recipient reconstituted BM was on day 10 already in a "quiescent" state. The cell yield gradually decreased.

20.4 In Vitro Responsiveness of MLN Lymphocyte in il-BMTx Recipients

The MLN cell yield in the il-BMTx recipients was on day 10 significantly lower than in control rats.[19,20] The phenotypical evaluation of MLN population showed slightly less of CD43 and CD4 cells. The responsiveness of MLN lymphocytes to PHA, concavalin A (ConA), and pokeweed mitogen (PWM) did not differ from the controls. Sera from the reconstituting rats did not possess stimulatory effect on the MLN lymphocytes in culture, neither had the supernatants from the cultured recipient BMC.[20] These results suggest that 10 days after il-BMTx, the lymph node phenotypical and functional population returned to a normal level.

20.5 Histology of Recipient LO Repopulated by il-BMTx

Histological evaluation of thymus, spleen, and MLN (Fig. 20.4) revealed on day 10 total restoration of the cellular architecture of these organs. Repopulation of T cells was first seen in the paracortical areas of MLN and perarteriolar sheets of spleen. The B-cell repopulation was less evident in MLN germinal centers and around spleen T areas.[17] On day 30, repopulation was completed.[17,18]

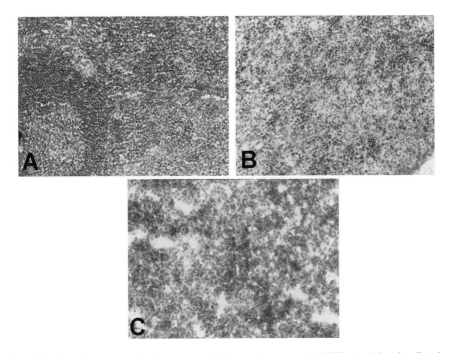

Fig 20.4 Recipient mesenteric lymph node 10 days after syngeneic HLTx (recipient irradiated 8 Gy). (**a**) HLTx, (**b**) iv-BMC in suspension, (**c**) Control, no transplant. HE stain, ×200

Full repopulation of lymphoid organs 10 days after il-BMTx indicates that maturation of BM lymphocyte precursors and their migration to the periphery was completed. The speed of restoration of normal architecture of nodes, spleen, and thymus again suggests that BM transplanted as tissue can resume its function immediately after transplantation. Replacement of recipient by donor dendritic cells was seen in nonlymphoid organs (Fig. 20.5).

20.6 Peripheral Blood Cell Subsets

The concentration of blood nucleated cells was on day 10 lower than in control rats. The subset analysis of peripheral blood cells labelled with anti-CD90 (stem cells), CD43 (leukocytes and lymphocytes), CD4 (helper cells), CD8 (cytotoxic cells), and SIg (mostly B cells) antibody showed lower concentration of CD90, CD4, and SIg cells.[18]

In contrast to the lymph node cell population, the blood lymphocyte subsets did not reach normal counts 10 days after il-BMTx. This was most evident in the B-cell population. This suggests defects in release of freshly maturing lymphocytes in BM and LO.

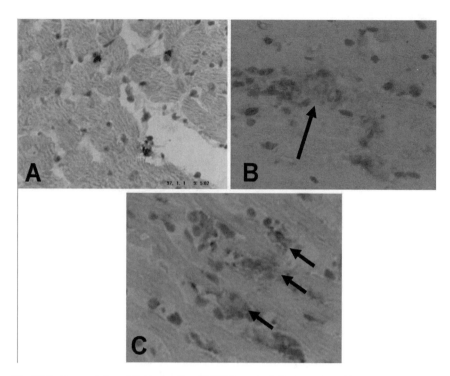

Fig. 20.5 Repopulation of 8-Gy-irradiated LEW heart by BN donor dendritic cells 14 days after transplantation of BN hindlimb. (**a**) Control, no transplant, (**b**) BN-specific OX27 cells (*arrow*), (**c**) OX6 (class II) cells mostly of donor origin (*arrows*). HE stain, ×200

20.7 Distribution of BMC Released from il-BMTx in Allogeneic Recipient

Migration of the il-BMtx cells was studied from BN to LEW rats. Twenty-four hours after il-BMTx, homing to the recipient BM, spleen (SPL), and MLN was found significantly lower than in a respective syngeneic model (Fig. 20.2).[21] It was seven times lower in the BM, two times lower in the SPL, and three times lower in the MLN. Interestingly, the level of the "allogeneic elimination" effect after il-BMTx was low and less pronounced than usually seen after iv-BMCTx. This phenomenon, mediated by NK cells, can be explained by a limited access of these cells to the graft cells contained in the BM cavities.

Irradiation did not abrogate the "allogeneic effect" of early BMC elimination. The values of homing to BM, SPL, and MLN remained at the same level after il-BMTx in the irradiated and nonirradiated rats. These data suggest that the recipient cells responsible for allogeneic BM cell elimination are highly radioresistant.

Pretreatment of allogeneic recipients with anti-asialo-GM1 antiserum (AAGM1) abrogated the allogeneic elimination effect.[21] This observation proves that the NK cells, sensitive to AAGM1, mediated the process of allogeneic but not syngeneic BMC elimination.

20.7.1 Phenotypes of BMC Populating Allogeneic Recipient BM After il-BMTx

The BMC from BN il-HLTx transplanted to 8-Gy-irradiated LEW populated recipient BM cavities. On day 3 after transplantation, the total BN population (OX27) in LEW BM reached 8% to increase by day 7 to 19% (Fig. 20.6). The concentration of donor T and B lymphocytes (W3/13, OX12), stem cells (OX7), granulocytes (HIS48), leukocyte common antigen-positive cells (LCA) (OX33), NK (CD56), and macrophages (ED1) ranged between 4 and 6%. A decrease of donor cell concentration in recipient BM was observed on day 30 and thereafter.

Distribution of recirculating and nonrecirculating BM populations was evaluated. The percentage of donor T lymphocytes, stem and NK cells, and migrating OX62 cells equalled that of recipient already on day 3 (Fig. 20.7). In contrast, the nonrecirculating leukocytes (W3/13), granulocytes and erythroid cells (HIS48), LCA (OX33), and OX43 cells populated recipient BM at a low rate (Fig. 20.8).

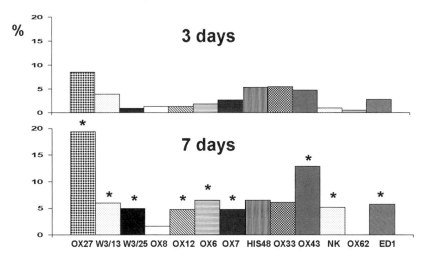

Fig. 20.6 The percentage of donor phenotypes populating irradiated allogeneic recipient hindlimb BM cavities 3 and 7 days after (HLTx). *OX 27* antigen specific for donor; *W3/13* leukocytes including T cells; *W3/25* helper cells; *OX8* cytotoxic cells; *OX12* B cells; *OX7* thymocytes, stem cells; *HIS48* granulocytes, erythoid cells; *OX33* LCA, leukocyte common antigen; *OX43* leukocytes, NK cells; *NK* natural killers; *OX62* migrating dendritic cells; *ED1, ED5* macrophages

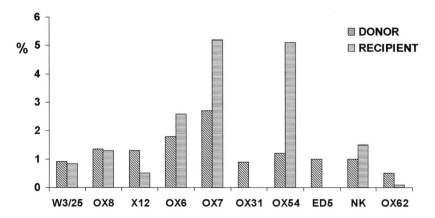

Fig. 20.7 Comparison of frequency of donor and irradiated allogeneic recipient cell phenotypes in recipient BM cavities 3 days after donor HLTx. Recirculating population. Note fast population of recipient and donor cell subsets reaching recipient levels

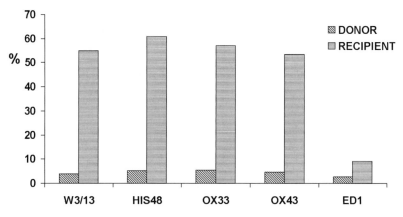

Fig. 20.8 Comparison of frequency of donor and irradiated allogeneic recipient cell phenotypes in recipient BM cavities 3 days after donor HLTx. Nonrecirculating population. Note low level of donor cells compared with recipient population

20.8 Microchimerism in Allogeneic il-BMTx in Immunosuppressed Recipient

To detect the BMC of BN donor origin in the CsA-treated LEW recipient organs after il-BMTx, recipient BM, blood, spleen, and MLN cells were harvested on day 30 or 100 after transplantation and stained with OX27 monoclonal antibody specific for BN but not LEW class I antigens. A few BN cells were found in BM, MLN, SPL, and blood.[22,23]

The consequence of il-BMTx is the presence of donor immune cells in the recipient lymphoid tissues. The donor cells persisting in recipient tissues were detectable both after 30 and 100 days. The question as to whether the presence of donor cells was a proof of tolerance to donor antigens or the transplanted BM cells survived together with the limb graft under the effect of cyclosporin A, remains so far unanswered.

20.9 Donor DNA Distribution (Noncellular Microchimerism) in Allogeneic il-BMTx Nonimmunosuppressed and Immunosuppressed Recipients

The male BN il-BMTx to female LEW were performed without or with CsA administration. The observation period lasted for 30 days, followed by a 70-day period without CsA. Recipient blood cells, BMC, MLN lymphocytes, spleen, liver, and skin were tested for the presence of donor SRY nucleotide before and after rejection. Donor DNA was hardly detected in recipient tissues as long as the graft was not undergoing rejection.[24] Following rejection, donor DNA was found at high levels in all recipient tissues (Fig. 20.9).

These findings indicate that the detected donor DNA originated from the destructed graft tissues and to a lesser extent from the donor cells homing to recipient organs. Cellular microchimerism was present from the day of grafting with a tendency to decrease in course of time, whereas increasing levels of donor DNA appeared at the time of rejection and were maintained for many weeks. This study has evidently shown that il-BMTx is connected with dissemination of the donor genetic material in recipient tissues. The biological importance of this finding requires elucidation.

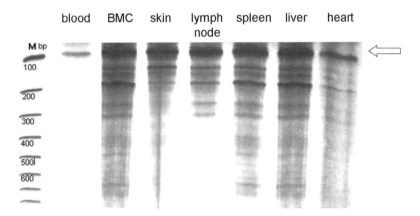

Fig. 20.9 Donor hindlimb transplant DNA was detected in all recipient tissues 7 days after HLTx including the nonlymphoid tissues (skin, heart). Much less donor DNA in blood cells compared with tissues

20.10 Conclusions

The BMC contained in the vascularized limb transplant are released from the graft and home to the recipient BM and LO. The number of released cells is low but sufficient to repopulate an irradiated (cytoablated) recipient within 10 days.

Transplantation of limb to a syngeneic nonirradiated recipient brings about "crowding" of BM and suppression of granulocyte and lymphocyte maturation.

Transplantation of limb to a syngeneic irradiated recipient results in total repopulation of BM and LO within 10 days. The restoration of BM and LO cellularity to normal levels ensues, whereas blood lymphocyte population reveals chronic deficiency in some subsets.

Transplantation of allogeneic limb to an immunosuppressed recipient brings about repopulation of BM and LO and a state of microchimerism. Partial elimination of transplanted allogeneic BM cells is mediated by recipient NK cells. Recirculating population replenishes recipient BM within 3 days whereas the nonrecirculating cells enter BM at a lower rate. Donor DNA can be detected in recipient lymphoid and nonlymphoid tissues at the time of rejection.

References

1. T.E. Starzl, A.J. Demetris, N. Murase, S. Ildstad, C. Ricordi, and M. Trucco, Cell migration, chimerism, and graft acceptance, *Lancet* **339**, 1579–1582 (1992).
2. J. Kanitakis, D. Jullien, A. Claudy, J.P. Revillard, and J.M. Dubernard, Microchimerism in a human hand allograft, *Lancet* **354**, 1820–1821 (1999).
3. C.W. Hewitt, R. Ramsamooj, M.P. Patel, B. Yazdi, B.M. Achauer, and K.S. Black, Development of stable mixed T cell chimerism and transplantation tolerance without immune modulation in recipients of vascularized bone marrow allografts, *Transplantation* **50**, 766–772 (1990).
4. R.D. Foster, L. Fan, M. Niepp, et al., Mixed allogeneic chimeras as a model for tolerance induction in composite tissue allografts: chimeric stability and functional recovery, *Surg. Forum* **52**, 605 (2001).
5. M. Vossen, V. Gorantla, G. Perez-Abadia, et al., Vascularized bone marrow transplantation: fact or fiction? *Surg. Forum* **525**, (2001).
6. A. Umemura, H. Morita, X.C. Li, S. Tahan, A.P. Monaco, and T. Maki, Dissociation of hemopoietic chimerism and allograft tolerance after allogeneic bone marrow transplantation, *J. Immunol.* **167**, 3043–3048 (2001).
7. R. Llull, N. Murase, Q. Ye, R. Manez, A.J. Demetris, V. Fournier, and T.E. Starzl, Vascularized bone marrow transplantation in rats: evidence for amplification of hematolymphoid chimerism and freedom from graft-versus-host reaction, *Transpl. Proc.* **27**(1), 164–165 (1995).
8. R. Llull, N. Murase, A.J. Demetris, Q. Ye, R. Manez, and T.E. Starzl, Multilineage ampliafication of graft-vs-host disease-resistant chimerism following rat vascularized bone marrow allotransplantation, *Transpl. Proc.* **27**(4), 2363–2364 (1995).
9. R. Ramsamooj, R. Llull, L.D. Tatem, K.S. Black, V. Lotano, R.M. Dalsey, C.T. Born, W.G. DeLong, and C.W. Hewitt, Graft-versus-host disease in limb transplantation: digital image analysis of bone marrow and TGF-β expression in situ using a novel 3-D microscope, *Transpl. Proc.* **28**, 2029–2031 (1996).
10. V. Gorantla, G. Perez-Abadia, K. Prabhune, H. Orhun, R. Majzoub, T. Kakoulidis, C. Maldonado, G. Anderson, L. Ogden, W. Breidenbach, S. Ildstad, and J. Barker, Composite tissue allografts: tolerance induction without graft-versus-host disease, *Plast. Surg.* **51**, 578–579 (2000).

11. S.P. Hiotis, K.L. Wnuk, W.A. Blumenthals, S.A. Halaris, and R.A. Good, Successful limb transplantation across a multi-minor barrier facilitated by preceding engraftment of T-cell-purged donor and recipient bone marrow, *Transpl. Proc.* **31**, 692–693 (1999).
12. P.C. Brouha, G. Perez-Abadia, C.G. Francois, V. Gorantla, M. Vossen, L.A. Laurentin-Perez, C. Maldonado, G. Anderson, M. Kon, and J.H. Barker, Prevention of graft-versus-host disease in chimeric hosts by lymph node removal prior to limb allotransplantation, *Surg. Forum* **52**, 527 (2001).
13. M. Durlik, B. Lukomska, A. Namyslowski, E. Cybulska, S. Janczewska, and W.L. Olszewski, The kinetics of seeding of syngeneic cells from vascularized bone marrow grafts, *Transpl. Proc.* **29**, 2008–2009 (1997).
14. W.L. Olszewski, B. Lukomska, M. Durlik, and A. Ziembinski, Bone marrow in bone versus bone marrow cell suspension transplant, *Transpl. Proc.* **24**(6), 3002–3003 (1992).
15. M. Durlik, B. Lukomska, M. Morzycka-Michalik, and W.L. Olszewski, Bone marrow reconstitution in irradiated rats receiving syngeneic hind limb graft, *Eur. Sur. Res.* **23**(Suppl 1), 30 (1991).
16. B. Lukomska, M. Durlik, M. Morzycka-Michalik, and W.L. Olszewski, Transplantation of vascularized bone marrow, *Transpl. Proc.* **23**(1), 887–888 (1991).
17. W.L. Olszewski, B. Lukomska, M. Durlik, A. Namyslowski, and E. Cybulska, Bone marrow cells transplanted in suspension or in vascularized bone graft repopulate not only bone marrow but also lymphoid organs, *Transpl. Proc.* **26**(6), 3319–3320 (1994).
18. S. Janczewska, A. Ziolkowska, M. Durlik, W.L. Olszewski, and B. Lukomska, Fast lymphoid reconstitution after vascularized bone marrow transplantation in lethally irradiated rats, *Transplantation* **68**(2), 201–209 (1999).
19. B. Lukomska, S. Janczewska, M. Durlik, and W.L. Olszewski, Kinetics of bone marrow repopulation in lethally irradiated rats after transplantation of vascularized bone marrow in syngeneic hind limb, *Ann. Transpl.* **5**(1), 14–20 (2000).
20. B. Lukomska, M. Durlik, E. Cybulska, and W.L. Olszewski, Comparative analysis of immunological reconstitution induced by vascularized bone marrow versus bone marrow cell transplantation, *Transpl. Int.* **9**, S492–S496 (1996).
21. W.L. Olszewski, B. Lukomska, M. Durlik, A. Namyslowski, D. Laszuk, and E. Cybulska, Nonspecific rapid elimination of transplanted allogeneic bone marrow cells, *Transpl. Proc.* **29**, 2073–2074 (1997).
22. M. Durlik, B. Lukomska, A. Namyslowski, S. Janczewska, E. Cybulska, and W.L. Olszewski, Long-term survival of limb allografts after weaning of cyclosporine: possible role of microchimerism, *Transpl. Proc.* **29**, 1226–1227 (1997).
23. M. Durlik, B. Lukomska, P. Religa, H. Ziolkowska, A. Namyslowski, S. Janczewska, E. Cybulska, J. Soin, Z. Gaciong, and W.L. Olszewski, Tolerance induction following allogeneic vascularized bone marrow transplantation – the possible role of microchimerism, *Transpl. Int.* **11**, S229–S302 (1998).
24. W.L. Olszewski, M. Durlik, B. Lukomska, P. Religa, H. Ziolkowska, S. Janczewska, E. Cybulska, J. Soin, Z. Gaciong, and B. Interewicz, Donor DNA can be detected in recipient tissues during rejection of allograft, *Transpl. Int.* **13**, S461–S464 (2000).

Section VI

Chapter 21
Vascularized Knee Transplantation

Michael Diefenbeck and Gunther O. Hofmann

21.1 Introduction and History

The allogeneic grafting of total joints has been a matter of discussion for almost a century. In 1908, Erich Lexer[1,2] reported the first transplantation of a human knee joint. The grafting of human joint and tissue were performed without organ preservation techniques, without vascular pedicles and graft reperfusion. Transplantation immunology and the phenomenon of acute and chronic rejection were unknown, as well as immunosuppressive drugs and antibiotics. Hence, Lexer's attempts were doomed to fail.

Meanwhile, various groups have performed experimental vascularized knee joint transplantations in different animal models using various immunosuppressive protocols.[3–8]

The encouraging results of our first vascularized transplantations of human femoral diaphyses[9,10] in combination with growing experience in composite tissue allotransplantation (CTA) has led to the start of our clinical transplantation program of vascularized knee joints in 1996.[11,12] Six transplantations have been performed since.

21.2 Indication

The indication has not changed over the last years. Grafting might be considered in massive destruction of bone and soft tissue of the knee joint by severe trauma and/or infection. In addition, the complete loss of the extensor apparatus (patella, patella ligament, quadriceps tendon) has to be present, which makes the implantation of a total knee arthroplasty (TKA) impossible.[13] The only alternatives to transplantation remain above knee amputation or arthrodesis with shortening of the leg. Arthrodesis might result in a stable, weight-supporting leg, but mobility at the level of the former knee joint is definitely lost. Transplantations have been limited to patients younger than 35 years. Due to the strict inclusion criteria, the last knee transplantation was done in April 2002.

21.3 Trauma Management

Massive traumatic or infectious destruction of the knee joint had led to large segmental defects in all our cases. A standardized protocol was used for the treatment of infection and preparation for transplantation.

21.3.1 Eradication of Infection and Soft Tissue Coverage

This is a prerequisite for grafting. It is achieved by radical debridement including the removal of all necrotic bone and soft tissue. Stabilization of bony defects is performed by external fixators or intramedullary arthrodesis nails. Soft tissue management employs techniques like vacuum assisted closure (VAC)[14] or temporal wound closure.

After successful treatment of infection, skin and soft tissue defects are closed by local (e.g. gastrocnemius) or free pedicle flaps (e.g. latissimus dorsi). This procedure may be combined with a switch in the fixation technique.

21.3.2 Preparation for Transplantation

At this stage, the osseous defect including the joint defect is microbiological aseptic and temporarily stabilized with an articulating knee spacer made of polyethylene (Fig. 21.1). A soft tissue expander is additionally placed inside the former knee joint cavity. Assisted passive motion and isometric exercises are possible and necessary to avoid contractions and muscular atrophy. If the defect is too large for a hinge arthroplasty, an intramedullary arthrodesis nail can be used for fixation (Fig. 21.2). After informed consent, the patient is placed on the waiting list.

21.4 Transplantation

21.4.1 Bone Allograft Procurent

The knee joints were harvested in accordance with standard organ procurement guidelines used in multiorgan donation (MOD). All MODs were allocated by the Transplantation Centre of the University of Munich respecting their established standard criteria for organ acceptance. MODs older than 45 years or those who had an accident involving the same leg were excluded. For additional safety reasons, MODs that had received blood substitutes or fresh-frozen plasma had been excluded as well.

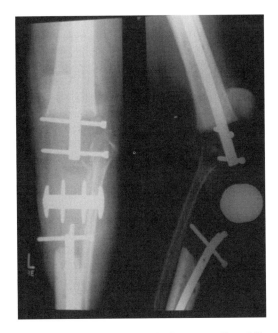

Fig. 21.1 The osseous defect including the knee joint is temporarily stabilized with an articulating knee spacer

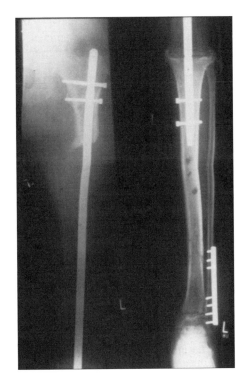

Fig. 21.2 Osseous defect (length 44 cm) stabilized with an intramedullary arthrodesis nail

Harvesting of the knee joint included perfusion of the external iliac artery with 4-1 University of Wisconsin (UW) solution at 4 °C, dissection of the femoral artery and vein distally to the proximal level of the adductor canal, transection of the muscles, and osteotomy of femur, tibia and fibula. The graft was stored in sterile conditions in three layers of plastic bags at 4 °C. Cold ischemia time ranged from 18 to 25 h.

21.4.2 Back-Table Allograft Preparation

In back-table preparation the allograft was dissected from surrounding soft tissue. The quadriceps tendon and the articular capsula remained intact. All vessels perfusing the muscles were ligated, while the vessels to the bone were carefully preserved.

Finally, the graft's arterial pedicle was perfused with methylene blue to verify the adequate perfusion of the graft (Fig. 21.3).

21.4.3 Transplantation Procedure

For transplantation, a frontal S-shaped incision from the medial thigh crossing over the former knee joint to the lateral calf was used to expose the recipient site. The hinge arthroplasty device or the intramedullary arthrodesis nail was removed. The

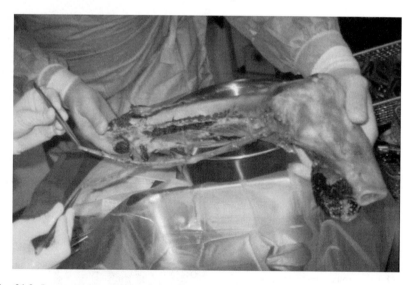

Fig. 21.3 Intraoperative picture of the allograft consisting of knee joint with intact capsula, femur, tibia, quadriceps tendon, vascular pedicle and sentinel skin graft

internal fixation of the graft was performed using an antegrad femoral and a retrograde tibial interlocking compression nail.

The graft's vessels were anastomosed to the recipient's superficial femoral artery and vein using end-to-side technique. Reperfusion was started immediately and the graft's quadriceps tendon was inserted into the quadriceps muscle of the recipient.

21.4.4 *Histocompatibility and Immunosuppression*

All transplantations were performed with AB0-compatible grafts. HLA profiles were determined but not matched due to logistic restrictions in donor acquisition. Cross-matching excluded preformed cytotoxic antibodies and avoided hyperacute rejection in all cases.

Immunosuppression was started immediately after reperfusion of the graft and consisted of a quadruple induction therapy in the first five cases for the first 3 days (Cyclosporine A, 1, 5 mg/kg bw i.v.; azathioprine, 1.5 mg/kg bw i.v.; antithymocyte globulin, 4 mg/kg bw i.v.; and methylprednisolone, 250 mg).

During the first week, methylprednisolone was reduced stepwise. Immunosuppression was continued with an oral double-drug maintenance therapy with cyclosporine A (CsA, 6 mg/kg bw) and azathioprine (1.0 mg/kg bw). After 6 months, the regime consisted of a CsA monotherapy.

In the sixth case FK 506 (tacrolimus; 10 mg p.o.) and mycophenolate mofetil (MMF; 2 g p. o.) were used in the quadruple induction therapy instead of CsA and azathioprine, following the immunosuppressive regime used in hand-transplantation.[15,16] Oral double-drug maintenance therapy was continued with MMF (2 g p.o.) and FK 506 (tacrolimus) with a serum level between 8 and 10 µg/l.

21.5 Follow-Up

Different technical methods are employed for the follow-up of the transplanted patients:

- *Clinical chemistry*: White blood cell count, C-reactive protein and procalcitonine level to monitor inflammation; cyclosporine or FK 506 level to control immunosuppression
- Angiography by DSA-technique in the first week after transplantation to demonstrate macroperfusion of the graft's arterial pedicle
- Duplex sonography in the follow-up of the graft's perfusion
- Scintigraphy by SPECT technique to evaluate the microcirculation of the graft[17]
- Conventional radiographs to monitor bone healing and osseous integration of the grafted bone

- Arthroscopy 6 months after transplantation or in case of suspected rejection to take biopsies of the synovial membrane, the cartilage and the grafted bone
- Clinical examination every 2 months in our outpatient clinic

21.6 Results

To date, six allogeneic transplantations of vascularized human knee joints have been performed. Preliminary outcomes and follow-ups have been published in detail elsewhere.[11–13,18–21] In the following, each patient is described separately. After the first five cases, immunosuppression and some technical details have been changed.

21.6.1 Patient 1

The first grafting was done on the April 27, 1996. There where no early intra- or postoperative complications. Excellent macrocirculation of the graft was shown by duplex sonography and angiography. Undisturbed microcirculation and intact cellular metabolism were demonstrated by scintigraphy and SPECT technique. Wounds healed on first intention. The patient was discharged after 2 weeks, completely mobilized using two crutches, partly weight bearing. Radiographs showed complete integration of the transplanted knee after 6 months. Full range of motion was found in clinical examination after 12 month.

At 15-month postgrafting, the patient complained about pain and reduced range of motion of the grafted joint. The knee showed clinical signs of inflammation. We interpreted the signs as a rejection crisis. SPECT showed an increased accumulation of tracer in the subcartilaginous zone of the graft. Biopsy of synovial membrane revealed vital and perfused tissue; however, there were signs of perivascular infiltration of lymphocytes. Subsequently, the patient developed an occlusion of the allograft's vascular pedicle (duplex sonography) and transplant failure. Immunosuppression was discontinued and the patient received a TKA using the graft as bone stock, which resulted in good stability as well as mobility.

In 2002, a periprosthetic infection occurred. Despite surgical and antibiotic treatment, a chronic infection of the TKA developed. Confronted with a severe sepsis with the beginning of a multiorgan failure (MOF), above knee amputation could not be avoided in 2004.

21.6.2 Patient 2

Transplantation (Nov 1996) and postoperative treatment were without any major complications. The patient had a stable joint, was able to walk, to do sports and had returned to work. During a personal crisis in 1999, the patient stopped to take his immunosuppressive medication. Acute rejection occurred and most parts of the graft were lost. A TKA was performed using the remaining graft as bone stock. Later an implant-related infection was diagnosed. On request of the patient, above knee amputation was done in July 2001.

21.6.3 Patient 3

One week after grafting in December 1996, a surgical site infect of the allograft was noticed. In spite of antibiotic therapy, reduction of the immunosuppressive regime and aggressive surgical debridement, infection persisted. Immunosuppression had to be discontinued and the allograft removed 5 weeks after transplantation. When infection was controlled, again a temporary, articulating spacer was implanted and the patient scheduled for the next transplantation. Due to difficulties in the geometric match (small size of the recipient's knee), a donor could not be found within a year. After discussing the options with the patient and his relatives, the patient agreed upon an arthrodesis of the knee, bridging the bone defect with a callus distraction in Ilizarov's technique. The procedure took 3 years in total, resulting in a stable and full-weight bearing leg.

21.6.4 Patient 4

The fourth grafting took place in July 1997. Two years following transplantation, the patient developed a stress fracture of the tibial plateau of the grafted knee joint whilst running downstairs. On admission, SPECT revealed no tracer uptake of the whole graft. We decided to perform a TKA using parts of the remaining allogeneic bone as bone stock. Postoperatively, the patient had a stable joint, good mobility, was able to walk and returned to work. In March 2000, 3 years after transplantation, a periprosthetic infection occurred. The patient did not want further surgical treatment for control of the infection and, on his request, the leg was amputated.

21.6.5 Patient 5

The first year postgrafting in February 1998 was uneventful. At 14 months a stress fracture of the lateral tibia plateau was detected. A TKA was performed, using the remaining graft as bone stock. The patient was discharged with full range of motion and no signs of infection. Eighteen months later a periprosthetic fracture following a fall onto the knee was diagnosed. The femoral part of the TKA was removed and a custom-made femoral part implanted. At 5 years the patient reinjured his grafted knee sustaining a patella fracture. Open reduction and internal fixation with screws failed, so that the patella ligament had to be replaced by a fascia lata plastic. Late rejection led to a necrotic bone stock, which became infected. The graft had to be removed and an intramedullary arthrodesis had to be performed, resulting in a shortening of the leg by 8 cm.

21.6.6 Patient 6

In the sixth patient, a block of donor skin and subcutaneous tissue was harvested in combination with the graft and inserted into the skin of the recipient to monitor early signs of graft rejection (sentinel skin graft).

One and a half years after transplantation the patient was mobilized with full-weight bearing and had returned to his previous job. Radiography showed the complete osseous integration of the graft (Figs. 21.4 and 21.5) The range of motion (ROM) of the left knee was 0–0–90 (Fig. 21.6). The allogeneic block of skin completely integrated in the recipient's skin (Fig. 21.7). Arthroscopy showed vital cartilage without degeneration, intact menisci and ligaments.

Two years and 4 months after transplantation, the patient noticed redness and itching pain of the sentinel skin graft at his lateral tight (Fig. 21.8).
Recognizing the inflammation of the grafted skin and soft tissue, we suspected a rejection crisis and took skin biopsies.
Histological examination showed acute cellular rejection. We started treatment with steroids.

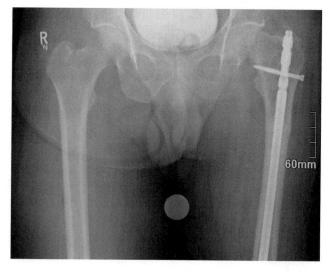

Fig. 21.4 Radiography of pelvis 1.5 years after transplantation: stable bony union between graft and host left femur

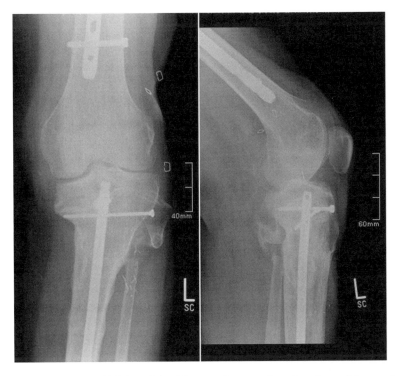

Fig. 21.5 Radiography of left knee joint 1.5 years after transplantation: the graft is completely osseous integrated

Two days later an arthroscopy of the grafted knee was performed and biopsies taken.
Histology showed the same signs of acute rejection than in the skin biopsy.
With steroid therapy the inflammation of the grafted skin vanished (Fig. 21.9).
Angiography of the left leg showed a well-perfused knee graft with reticular vessel (Fig. 21.10).

Despite continuous immunosuppression, the graft was rejected and above knee amputation had to be performed in 2006. In the first histopathologic examinations of the graft we found signs of a chronic vasculopathy.

21.7 Discussion and Overview

Analysing the first five cases retrospectively, two main complications can be found: reoccurrence of infection and late rejection.

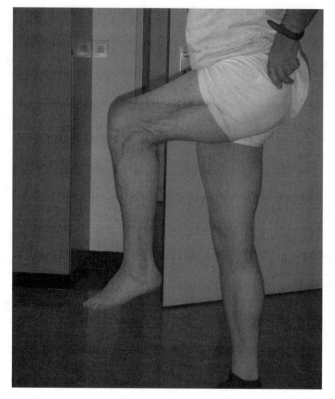

Fig. 21.6 Clinical examination after 1.5 years showing good range of motion

21.7.1 Recurrence of Infection

Despite the fact that microbiological examination of biopsies taken before grafting showed no growth of bacteria, in one case infection recurred immediately postoperative. Persisting bacteria might have not been detected and, supported by immunosuppression, osteomyelitis was reactivated.

Control of infection during immunosuppresion was not possible, so it had to be reduced and the transplants were rejected. After discussing this topic, we decided to change our immunosuppressive regime in the sixth case.

21.7.2 Late Rejection

In three patients, necrosis of the grafted bones and stress fractures were found after 15, 16 and 24 month, respectively.

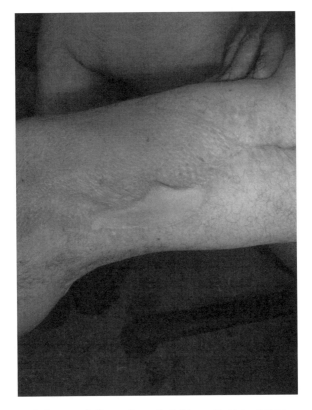

Fig. 21.7 Completely integrated allogeneic sentinel skin graft at lateral tight

Contrary to transplantation of parenchymal organs, where graft failure is noticed by reduced organ function and laboratory examinations, rejection in grafted joints seems to be occult for a period of time. From intraoperative and histological examinations, it seems that vascular rejection leads to ischemic necrosis of soft tissue and vital bone cells. After rejection, only the avital bone matrix remains, which stays integrated in the recipient's bone. This matrix is predisposed for fractures, explaining why stress fractures were the first signs of rejection found in our cases.

In hand transplantation, rejection can be monitored by a change of the colour of the skin.[22] So far, we were only able to monitor rejection by indirect methods like scintigraphy, SPECT or biopsies. To improve the monitoring of rejection, we decided to harvest a block of skin and subcutaneous tissue with a vascular pedicel together with the graft and integrate the allogeneic skin in the recipient's skin. The same technique was used by Lanzetta and colleagues in their hand transplantation project, where an additional full-thickness skin was transplanted onto the left hip area. The skin served as a source of biopsies and as an additional area to monitor rejection, hence called "distant sentinel skin graft."[23]

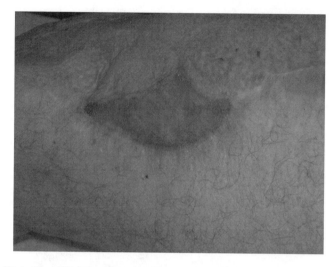

Fig. 21.8 Clinical examination: redness of the sentinel skin graft 3 years posttransplantation

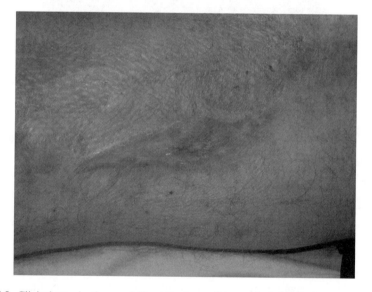

Fig. 21.9 Clinical examination: vanishing of redness of the sentinel skin graft

In patient 6, the immunosuppressive regime was changed and "sentinel skin" grafted. The first sign of acute rejection in this patient was redness of the "sentinel skin." Biopsies of synovia and "sentinel skin" showed the same signs of cellular rejection, proving that the grafted skin can be used as a monitor of rejection. In this patient, acute rejection was overcome by treatment with corticoids.

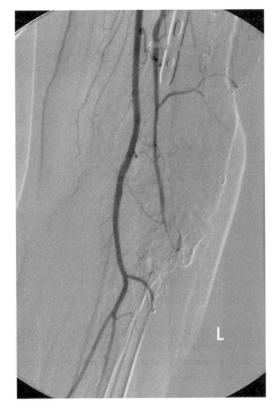

Fig. 21.10 Angiography (DSA) of left lower extremity showing good perfusion of the graft 3 years after transplantation

21.8 Summary

In summary, vascularized transplantation of knee joint allografts is technically feasible. In our cases, the indication was a complete destruction of the knee joint and the extensor mechanism, where the only alternatives above knee amputation or arthrodesis remain. Intramedullary nailing resulted in complete integration of the graft. Acute rejection can be monitored by grafted allogeneic skin (sentinel skin graft). Infection and late rejection lead to graft failure. Thus, the question remains, which immunosuppressive regime is able to prevent late rejection. For the future, the procedure should remain limited to clinical study design.

References

1. E. Lexer, Substitution of whole or half joints from freshly amputated extremities by free plastic operation, *Surg Gynecol Obstet* **6**, 601–607 (1908).
2. E. Lexer, Joint transplantation and arthroplasty, *Surg Gynecol Obstet* **40**, 782–809 (1925).

3. K. Doi, G. De Santis, D. J. Singer, et al., The effects of immunosuppression on vascularised allografts, *J Bone Joint Surg* **71B**, 576–582 (1989).
4. P. C. Innis, M. A. Randolph, J. P. Paskert, et al., Vascularized bone allografts: In vitro assessment of cell-mediated and humeral responses, *Plast Reconstr Surg* **87**, 315–325 (1991).
5. D. Schäfer, R. Rosso, R. Fricker, et al., Functional and morphological results of vascularized total knee transplantation under cyclosporine A as compared to autologous vascularized knee replantation, *Surg Forum* **44**, 597–607 (1983).
6. W. P. A. Lee, Y. C. Pan, S. Kesmarky, et al., Experimental orthotopic transplantation of vascularized skeletal allografts: Functional assessment and long-term survival, *Plast Reconst Surg* **95**, 336–353 (1995).
7. M. I. Boyer, J. S. Danska, L. Nolan, et al., Microvascular transplantation of physeal allografts, *J Bone Joint Surg* **77B**, 806–814 (1995).
8. R. Rosso, D. Schäfer, R. Fricker, et al., Functional and morphological outcome of knee joint transplantation in dogs depends on control of rejection, *Transplantation* **63**, 1723–1733 (1997).
9. G. O. Hofmann, M. H. Kirschner, V. Bühren, et al., Allogeneic vascularized transplantation of a human femoral diaphisis under cyclosporine A immunosuppression, *Transpl Int* **8**, 418–419 (1995).
10. M. H. Kirschner, G. O. Hofmann, Vorläufige Ergebnisse der Transplantation allogener gefäßgestieleter Femurdiaphysen unter Immunosuppression. *Transplantations medizin* **8**, 48–53 (1996).
11. G. O. Hofmann, M. H. Kirschner, F. D. Wagner, et al., First vascularized knee joint transplantation in man. *Tex Med* **8**, 46–47 (1996).
12. G. O. Hofmann, M. H. Kirschner, F. D. Wagner, et al., Allogeneic vascularized grafting of a human knee joint with postoperative immunosuppression, *Arch Orthop Trauma Surg* **116**, 125–128 (1997).
13. G. O. Hofmann, M. H. Kirschner, F. D. Wagner, et al., Allogeneic vascularized transplantation of human femoral diaphysis and total knee joints – first clinical experiences, *Transplant Proc* **30**, 2754–2761 (1998).
14. L. X. Web, New techniques in wound management: Vacuum-assisted wound closure, *J Am Acad Orthop Surg* **10**, 303–311 (2002).
15. J. W. Jones, S. A. Gruber, J. H. Barker, W. C. Breidenbach, Successful hand transplantation. One-year follow up. Louisville Hand Transplant Team, *N Engl J Med* **343**, 468–473 (2000).
16. J. M. Dubernard, P. Henry, H. Parmentier, B. Vallet, D. Vial, L. Badet, P. Petruzzo, N. Lefrancois, M. Lanzetta, E. Oen, N. Hakim, First transplantation of two hands: Results after 18 months, *Ann Chir* **127**, 19–25 (2002).
17. M. H. Kirschner, N. Manthey, K. Tasch, A. Nehrlich, K. Hahn, G. O. Hofmann, Use of three phase bone scans and SPECT in the follow up of patients with allogeneic vascularized femur transplants, *Nuclear Med Commun* **20**, 517–524 (1999).
18. G. O. Hofmann, M. H. Kirschner,, L. Brauns, F. D. Wagner, W. Land, V. Bühren, Vascularized knee joint transplantation in men: A report on the first cases, *Transplant Int* **11**, 487–490 (1998)
19. G. O. Hofmann, M. H. Kirschner, F. D. Wagner, L. Brauns, O. Gonschorek, V. Bühren, Allogeneic vascularized grafting of human knee joints under postoperative immunosuppression of the recipients, *World J Surg* **22**, 818–823 (1998).
20. M. H. Kirschner, L. Brauns, O. Gonschorek, V. Bühren, G. O. Hofmann, Vascularized knee joint transplantation in man: The first two year experience, *Eu J Surg* **166**, 320–327 (2000).
21. G. O. Hofmann, M. H. Kirschner, Clinical experience in allogeneic vascularized bone and joint allografting, *Microsurg* **20**, 375–383 (2000).
22. J. M. Dubernard, E. Owen, N. Lefrancois, P. Petruzzo, X. Martin, M. Dawahra, D. Jullien, J. Kanitakis, C. Frances, X. Preville, L. Gebuhrer, N. Hakim, N. Lanzetta, H. Kapila, G. Herzberg, J. P. Revillard, First human hand transplantation. Case report, *Transpl Int* **13**, Suppl 1, S521–S524 (2000).
23. M. Lanzetta, P. Petruzzo, G. Vitale, S. Lucchina, E. R. Owen, J. M. Dubernard, N. Hakim, H. Kapila. Human hand transplantation: What have we learned? *Transplant Proc* **36**, 664–668 (2004).

Chapter 22
Tracheal Transplantation

Gabriel M. Marta and Walter Klepetko

22.1 Introduction

The human trachea has a length of approximately 10–13 cm (average 11.8 cm) of which only a maximum of 6.5 cm or 50% of its total length can safely be resected and reanastomosed. However, the thoracic surgeon is often confronted with localized tracheal tumors or long segment stenosis exceeding this resection limits. To reconstruct these long tracheal segment defects, an adequate substitute material is needed.

In 2002, Grillo imagined the ideal conduit. According to him, this tracheal substitute must fulfill the following requirements: (1) should be a laterally rigid but longitudinally flexible tube; (2) must be initially airtight and should not dislocate or erode over the time; (3) should be biocompatible, nontoxic, nonimmunogenic, and noncarcinogenic so that infection, erosion, chronic inflammation, or granulation tissue formation should be avoided; (4) it should provide or facilitate epithelial resurfacing; (5) should present a surface of ciliated respiratory epithelium, which is a desirable but not an essential requirement; (6) the reconstruction technique should be surgically straightforward and the results predictably successful; (7) the need of immunosuppressive therapy is undesirable since most patients requiring tracheal reconstruction have malignant tumors; and (8) should be a permanent solution.[1]

On the basis of the used replacement material, the same author organized the numerous proposed techniques into five groups of trials: (1) foreign materials with different technical modifications to avoid implantation complications; (2) use of nonviable tissues, including fixed trachea; (3) adaptation and transfer of autogenous tissues with or without scaffolding of foreign materials as patches or tubes; (4) tissue engineering; (5) transplantation of allografts with and without immunosuppressive therapy, preservation, and vascularization procedures (see Table 22.1).[1]

So far none of the current available artificial materials can provide these biological qualities so that the use of human tracheal allografts currently remains the most promising technical option for reconstruction of long segmental tracheal defects.

Unfortunately, the human trachea lacks a well-defined blood supply that would allow a simple surgical transfer with direct revascularization. Therefore, the problem of tracheal transplantation is not only an immunological one but also a technical one.

Table 22.1 Tracheal reconstruction and replacement techniques

(1) Foreign materials
    (a) Solid prostheses
    (b) Porous prostheses
(2) Nonviable tissues (bioprostheses)
(3) Autogenous tissues
    (a) Free grafts with and without foreign material support
    (b) Vascularized autogenous tissue flaps
    (c) Autogenous tube construction
(4) Tissue engineering
(5) Tracheal transplantation
    (a) Nonrevascularized grafts
        Fresh, devascularized autografts
        Fresh, devascularized allografts
        Preserved, devascularized allografts
    (a) Vascularized grafts
        Fresh, indirectly vascularized autografts
        Fresh or preserved and indirectly vascularized allografts
        Direct revascularized allografts

22.2 History

The late nineteenth century can be considered as the beginning of experimental and clinical tracheal resection and repair. During the first half of the twentieth century few examples of limited tracheal resections and primary anastomosis, mostly cervical, as well as staged cervical repairs were reported. In 1909, Nowakowski used local skin flaps to close small defects of the cervical trachea in human patients.

Burket reported, in 1918, successful transplantation of fresh autografts consisting of three- to nine-ring segments in dogs.

At mid-century, the generally held belief was that a safe tracheal resection and primary anastomosis can be achieved only if the resected segment does not exceed 2 cm.[2,3] The experimental studies from the 1950s and 1960s widely extended these limits. It became generally accepted that approximately 50% of the adult and 33% of child trachea can be surgical removed and safely primary reanastomosed without the use of any prosthesis or graft.[4-7] Belsey reconstructed, in 1943, a tracheal wall defect with fascia lata reinforced with a coil of steel wire.[3]

Skin and cartilage were used, in 1945, by Crafoord and Lindgren to repair a cervical tracheal defect. In 1949, Rob and Bateman reported a partial resection of the tracheal wall with reconstruction by means of autologous material supported by a synthetic material.[2] However, these procedures were frequently complicated by fistula, mediastinal infections, and stenosis.

In the 1950s, the use of wire-supported dermal grafts to widen bronchi and trachea was often reported.[8] Unfortunately, the use of larger dermal grafts for tracheal defects repair was frequently unsuccessful. In the same year, Jackson and colleagues failed in repair of extensive defects using partly de-epithelized,

Merthiolate-treated and cold-preserved canine allografts. In 1952, Davies and coworkers reported also negative results with the use of fresh, devascularized canine allografts preserved in Tyrode's solution or 4% formaldehyde.

In 1979, Rose and colleagues published the first allogenic tracheal transplantation in a human.[9] The donor trachea was first heterotopically implanted into the recipient sternocleidomastoid muscle and transferred into the orthotopic position after 3 weeks.

Herberhold and colleagues introduced, in 1979, the use of a cryopreserved tracheal homograft for treatment of long segment tracheal defects in adults.[10]

The "slide tracheoplasty" technique described by Tsang and Goldstraw in 1989[11] and successfully used by Grillo,[12] beginning with 1994, constitutes a landmark in the treatment of congenital tracheal long segment stenosis.

Messineo in 1991, Levashov in 1993, and Nakanishi in 1995 demonstrated that omental wrapping allowed fresh tracheal autografts to recover from the early ischemic changes as new vessels connected to the graft.[13–15]

Khalil-Marzouk and Cooper in 1993[16] and Macchiarini and colleagues in 1994[17] reported two experimental techniques of direct revascularization using a composite thyrotracheal allograft in dogs. However, despite the positive reported experimental results, these methods where never used in humans.

Backer and colleagues described and developed, in 1998, a technique for repairing congenital tracheal stenosis using a free tracheal autograft with or without pericardial augmentation.[18]

In 2004, a successful human case of heterotopic tracheal allotransplantation and omentum wrapping in the abdomen was described and published by Klepetko and coworkers.[19]

22.3 Anatomy of the Trachea

The human trachea is a posterior flattened tube consisting of a fibro-muscular membrane and 18–22 cartilaginous rings (corresponding approximately to two rings per centimeter). The cartilages represent two-thirds of the tracheal circumference and give the human trachea its lateral rigidity. In the surface anatomy, the trachea extends almost vertically in the midline from the cricoid cartilage to the sternal angle, inclining slightly to the right. In 1968, Mulliken et al. pointed out that, when the neck is flexed, the cricoid cartilage drops to the level of the thoracic inlet and the trachea becomes almost entirely mediastinal.

Anatomo-surgically the trachea is divided into a cervical and a thoracic part:
The *cervical part* is crossed *anteriorly* by the jugular arch, overlapped by the *sternohyoid* and *sternothyroid muscles* and covered by *skin, superficial* and *deep fasciae*. The *isthmus of the thyroid gland* crosses the second to fourth tracheal cartilages. Above the isthmus an *anastomotic artery* connects with the *superior thyroid arteries* and inferior to the thyroid isthmus the front of the trachea has relations with the *pretracheal fascia, inferior thyroid veins, thymic remnants,* and, if existent, with the *arteria thyroidea ima*. As an anatomical variant, the left

brachiocephalic vein may rise a little above the manubrium. In children, the cervical trachea is crossed obliquely by the brachiocephalic artery at or a little above the upper manubrial level. *Laterally*, to the cervical trachea are the lobes of the thyroid glands, the common carotid, and the inferior thyroid arteries.

The *thoracic part* descends through the superior mediastinum and is *anteriorly* related from cranial to caudal to the manubrium sterni, the attachments of the sternohyoid and sternothyroid muscles, the thymic remnants, the inferior thyroid and left brachiocephalic veins, the aortic arch, the brachiocephalic and left common carotid arteries (which diverging as they ascend in the neck become, respectively, right and left of the trachea), the deep cardiac plexus, and mediastinal lymph nodes. *Laterally,* the thoracic part is closely related on its right side to the right brachiocephalic vein, the superior vena cava, and the azygos vein; on the left side we find the aortic arch, the left common carotid, and left subclavian arteries.

Most part of the trachea is supplied by multiple branches from the inferior thyroid arteries, while its thoracic end receives its arterial branches from the bronchial arteries, which ascend to anastomose with the former. Sometimes the trachea receives arterial branches from the internal mammary artery. All the vessels supply also the esophagus. Excessive circumferential dissection with the division of the lateral pedicles during a surgical procedure can therefore easily devascularize the trachea. The *tracheal veins* end in the inferior thyroid venous plexus. The lymph vessels drain into the pretracheal and paratracheal lymph nodes.[20]

22.4 Histology of the Trachea

Histologically, the tracheal wall has a four-layer structure: an inner *mucosa*, a *submucosa*, a poorly differentiated *muscularis*, and an outer *adventitial layer*.

The *tracheal mucosa* consists of a lamina propria and a pseudostratified columnar ciliated epithelium containing six main cell types: goblet cells, ciliated cells, undifferentiated short cells or basal cells (considered as a stem cell population), type 1 and type 2 brush cells, and basal small granule cells.

Solitary lymphocytes, small nodular lymphocyte aggregates, plasma cell, macrophages, and granular leukocyte are scattered throughout the lamina propria. The *C-shaped hyaline cartilages* are bridged at the level of the open portion by connective tissue and bundles of smooth muscular fibers. The perichondrium merges with the fat-laden connective tissue of the adventitia.

The *adventitia* contains numerous blood vessels, nerves, and lymphatic vessels.[21]

22.5 Immunological Aspects of Tracheal Transplantation

Most of the tracheal transplantation experimental studies have demonstrated that, despite a minimal donor antigen expression, the tracheal cartilage remains vital and free of infiltrates, whereas in the acute posttransplant period the ciliated mucosa consistently gets sloughed and nonfunctional. The consequence is the absence of mucociliary function, followed by progressive increase in CD8+ and CD4+ infiltrates within the lamina propria.[22] Consecutively, a severe damage of the tracheal epithelium, loss of the cilia and edema of the graft occurs. Thus, it is obvious that tracheal mucosa and the lamina propria are closely associated with the rejection reaction in tracheal transplantation and serve as the target for acute rejection, compared to the tracheal cartilage which shows a very low antigenicity and can be successfully transplanted without the need of any immunosuppressant therapy.[23,24] Furthermore, the absence of B-cell infiltration suggests that there is no B-cells-mediated rejection within the graft tissue.[25]

Desquamation of the donor tracheal epithelium followed by consecutive replacement with recipient-derived epithelium, could therefore prevent rejection and omit the need for temporary or permanent immunosuppressive therapy.[26–28]

22.5.1 Tracheal Graft Reepithelialization

The majority of the experimental works in the field of tracheal transplantation have been performed with heterotopic tracheal transplant models, in which the acute rejection response is characterized by fibrosis and tracheal lumen obliteration. The recent introduction of an orthotopic tracheal transplant model provided a clinically more relevant experimental material, where rejection reaction is manifested by inflammation and consecutive fibrosis, but with absence of complete luminal obliteration.[29] This discrepancy might be based on the fact that recipient-derived reepithelization of the tracheal allograft prevents luminal obliteration in the orthotopic model compared to the heterotopic one, in which allograft fails to reepithelialize and therefore undergoes luminal obliteration.

Reepithelialization usually starts at the membranous part of the trachea proven by the rich blood supply and the diffusion of growth factors in this area. The epithelial repair is the result of tracheal basal cells migration from the remaining part of the receiver trachea to the graft, followed by proliferation and differentiation into a pseudostratified ciliated epithelium.[29] During the first 14–21 days, the allograft exists as a chimera composed of both donor- and recipient-derived epithelium and over the course of 48 days the epithelium converts to a recipient-derived phenotype.[30] The migration of basal cells into the allograft segment is dependent on the formation of lamellilopedia or cell protrusions, which serve to create focal contacts that anchor the basal cell and enable migration.[31] Such adhesions can be broken by proteolytic enzymes and inflammatory cell mediators that are abundant during allograft rejection. Thus, the administration of anti-inflammatory immunosuppressive agents prevents the secretion of inflammatory factors or modulates the expression of negative mediators. The result is a more efficient reepithelialization process as demonstrated by a higher density of morphologically normal ciliated columnar cells in the immunosuppressed recipients.

Previous published studies suggest that different factors such as the vascular endothelial growth factor (VEGF), basic fibroblast growth factor (bFGF), calcitonin gene-related peptide, and tachykinin substance P are both mitogenic and chemotactic for tracheal epithelium.[32–34] Through stimulation of nitric oxide release from the endothelial cells, these factors induce endothelium-dependent vasodilatatory responses and are implicated in the healing process through their angiogenic activities. VEGF secretion is upregulated by hypoxic stress, ischemia, and anemia. Pokharel and colleagues have demonstrated augmented expression of VEGF protein and mRNA in tracheal granulation tissue specimens after prolonged intubation in children. On the basis of the increased VEGF levels measured in the epithelial cells and magrophages that migrate to infiltrate the granulation tissue, they speculated that enhanced VEGF expression might play a pivotal role in granulation tissue development.[35] Albes and colleagues concluded, in 1994, that application of bFGF increases revascularization and results in an improved epithelial preservation.[34] Corral and associates, using a rabbit model, demonstrated the superiority of topical VEGF compared to bFGF during ischemic wound healing.[36] However, to use these factors clinically, the optimal dosage[34,37] and the drug delivery method (for example, the use of carrier-bound growth factors)[38] must be still determined.

22.5.2 Desquamation Methods

In preliminary experiments, the desquamation of the respiratory mucosa has been obtained by abrasion of the tracheal inner surface with a *plastic blade*. However, this method was soon abandoned due to insufficient removal of the mucosa and the resulting severe cartilage damage.[39] Numerous recent studies have reported excellent results in reducing the tracheal antigenicity by removing the tracheal epithelium and mixed glands by means of radiotherapy, chemical detergents treatment, preservation method (cryopreservation), or combination of the three.

Radiation of the epithelium has been used with favorable results on graft survival but with severe local tissue damages due to the high doses of irradiation needed to suppress the antigenicity of the allograft. The Kyoto University group investigated this possibility of immunosuppressant-free transplantation using high doses of Co γ irradiation (100,000 cGy) of the canine tracheal graft before transplantation. The positive results, showing no graft rejection and no adverse effects, suggested that this method could be used clinically to transplant the trachea without the use of immunosuppressive therapy.[40] In 2000, a research group from Bangkok, Thailand published successful transplantation of cryopreserved, irradiated trachea (a dose of 25 kGy) in four patients without the use of immunosuppressant medication.[41] In both studies, the high-dose irradiation did not influence the viability of the tracheal cartilage.

The use of *detergents* is another often reported technique that has proven its efficiency in eliminating cell antigens, lipids, and glycosaminoglycans and consecutively producing an epithelium-free graft without affecting the integrity of the cartilage. The detergents (i.e., the nonionic surfactant t-octylphenoxypoly-ethoxyethanol or Triton X-100) can dissolve the lipid bilayer of the epithelial cells by transforming the lipids into micelles and, thus, destroy the cell membrane and reduce the tracheal antigenicity.[39]

Favorable results of *cryopreserved allograft transplantation* have been reported in the skin, the aortic valve, the aorta, the saphenous vein, the cartilage, and the trachea. Cryopreserved tracheal allotransplantation without immunosuppression has been extensively studied in various mature animal models (dogs, piglets, rats). The majority of authors reported that the subepithelial tissue and chondrocytes kept their integrity and showed no significant inflammatory cell infiltration for a long period after transplantation with promising results for clinical applications in human patients. The tracheal graft retained its viability and continued functioning without any signs of stenosis or rejection responses as observed in fresh allografts.[42–50]

A controversial result was only reported by the Stoelben group[51] who found *no clear advantage of the cryopreservation technique in reducing tracheal allograft immunogenicity*. Despite epithelium disappearance, the tracheal lumen was occluded posttransplant by noncompact fibrous tissue, different from the inflammatory aggressive granulation tissue found in fresh allografts. Additional, the vitality of the tracheal cartilage, essential for long-term patency of the graft, was significantly reduced after short-term cryopreservation and completely destroyed after long-term cryopreservation. In fact, the cryopreserved allograft transplantation is the only method with clinical applicability.

22.5.3 Immunosuppressive Therapy

The available data regarding the necessity of an immunosuppressive therapy after tracheal transplantation, as well as the regimes to be used, not to interfere with the reepithelization process and to reduce the side effects of the immunosuppressive drugs, are still controversial.

Nakanishi concluded, in 1995, in an article published in the *Annals of Thoracic Surgery* that despite the fact that epithelial regeneration in tracheal allografts is dependent on the absence of acute rejection, high doses of cyclosporine A may simultaneously predispose to graft infections and even suppression of the epithelial regeneration process. He suggested that the use of 15 mg/kg/day of cyclosporine A for a period of 3 weeks after tracheal transplantation allows allograft epithelial regeneration and is sufficient to maintain the viability of tracheal allografts over a long-term period.[52]

In 1996, Delaere was one of the first who confirmed that cyclosporine A was effective to prevent rejection of a tracheal allograft in a rabbit model.[53]

Genden et al. reported, in 2003, that, although reepithelization occurs irrespective of the state of immunosuppression, the administration of 7 mg/kg/day of cyclosporine A (CsA) likely prevents the secretion of inflammatory factors and modulates the expression of negative mediators. These effects result in a more efficient reepithelization process, as demonstrated by a higher density of morphologically normal ciliated columnar cells in the immunosuppressed recipients.[29]

The Hashimoto group published their data in 2001 in the *Journal of Thoracic and Cardiovascular Surgery* postulating the superiority of FK506 monotherapy and of doses higher than 2.5 mg/kg/day compared to the lower dosage.[54] They also demonstrated the combined synergistic effect of cryopreservation and adequate intermittent immunosuppressive therapy in maintaining tracheal allograft viability for long periods.

However, despite positive experience with the use of different immunosuppression agents, the desirable ideal condition would be an immunosuppressant-free tracheal transplantation, especially since most of the potential candidates for a tracheal transplantation suffer from malignant tumors, where immunosuppressive therapy is contraindicated.

22.5.4 T-Cell Tolerance

The indirect allorecognition pathway, mediated by limited set of T-cells responding to a single or a few dominant donors MHC determinants, can be controlled by means of selective immune therapy which uses peptides and peptide analogues to achieve *T-cell tolerance to alloantigens*. In the last years, different independent groups published positive results in inducing tolerance to MHC-derived peptides (life-long, donor-specific unresponsiveness without the need for chronic immunosuppression) using different routes and forms of administration of these peptides in recipient rodents.

Benichou et al. reported, in 1999, a successful induction of long-term alloantigen-specific allograft survival by intrathymic injection and oral administration of rat recipients with a mixture of peptides corresponding to different polymorphic regions of donor MHC molecules.[55] In 2001, Genden et al. administrated intraportal ultraviolet B-irradiated donor alloantigen (donor splenocytes) 7 days prior to transplantation. Consecutively, the published results showed no rejection and complete normal mucociliary function in rat tracheal allograft segments.[56] Fernandez et al. reported, in 2004, positive results with intraperitoneal administration of hamster anti-CD40 ligand monoclonal antibody (MR-1) alone or in conjunction with donor-derived bone marrow cells.[57]

Negative results of a pretransplant-induced chimerism by means of intravenously administered splenocytes of donor mice were published in 2003 by Suemitsu group. They also concluded that the incomplete expected effect of their protocol may be caused by the involvement of other autoreactive-like, nonallogenic factors (infection, surgical stressor, etc.) which cannot be blocked by the designed pretreatment.[58]

22.6 Graft Revascularization Techniques

Due to the special blood supply of the trachea, revascularization of a tracheal graft remains a main problem. It can either be achieved by more complex direct revascularization techniques or by indirect revascularization methods, which rely on the ingrowth of microvessels into the graft (see Table 22.2).

22.6.1 Direct Revascularization Techniques

Until now, due to the absence of an anatomical vascular pedicle big enough to allow revascularization of a tracheal homograft by direct microvascular suture, only four different experimental techniques of successful direct revascularization have been described in the medical literature (see Table 22.2). All three techniques were developed based on the anatomical fact that the upper part of the trachea, similar to the thyroid gland, receives its arterial blood supply through branches

Table 22.2 Techniques of tracheal graft revascularization

Technique	Advantages	Disadvantages
Direct revascularization		
Composite tyro-tracheal transplant without venous drainage[16]	Preservation of arterial blood supply	No venous drainage
Heterotopic tyro-tracheal allograft with venous drainage[17]	Preservation of arterial and venous blood supply	Difficult and invasive procedure
Orthotopic tyro-tracheal allograft with venous drainage[65]	Preservation of arterial and venous blood supply; less invasive	Technically more demanding
Orthotopic thyro-tracheal allograft with "dual artery blood supply"[66]	Complete tracheo-bronchial revascularization (longer graft)	Difficult and invasive procedure
Indirect revascularization		
Omental wrapping		
Orthotopic 1-stage technique[13,69,70]	Technically more simple	Limitations in length of the graft
Split transplantation of the trachea[71]	No limitations in graft length	Possible intraluminal flap prolapse
With removal of cartilage rings[72,73]	No limitations in graft length	Technically more demanding
Heterotopic (2-stage technique)[19,74–78]	Excellent morphologic results	Temporary double location
Fascial wrapping[79,80]	Less bulky vascular carrier	No clinical relevance
Sternohyoid muscle wrapping[81]	–	No clinical relevance
Sternocleidomastoid wrapping[82]	–	No revascularization

originating from the inferior thyroid artery.[20,59,60] It was therefore postulated that the conservation of this common blood supply by preserving the tissue lateral to the trachea, containing the thyroid gland, the thyroid vessels, and all the fine branches therein, provides a vascular pedicle suited for direct revascularization of the tracheal transplant.

In 1994, Khalil-Marzouk and Cooper[16] described an experimental technique of direct revascularization of a composite tyro-tracheal allograft in adult beagle dogs (see Fig. 22.1). Revascularization was achieved by direct anastomoses of the inferior thyroid artery branches to the ipsilateral common carotid arteries, but without the creation of a venous drainage. The authors reported preservation of the tracheal cartilages and the surrounding soft tissues in five of six vascularized and immunosuppressed grafts. However, at least in theory, the lack of a venous drainage should ultimately result in infarction of the graft by means of thromboses at the arterial anastomosis and therefore the method never gained further acceptance.[61,62]

To overcome this limitation, the Macchiarini group developed, in 1994, an extensive technique of tyro-tracheal allotransplantation with venous drainage in pigs (see Fig. 22.2). The method consists of an "en bloc" cervico-thoracic exenteration of the aortic arch and its supra-aortic branches, superior vena cava, jugular

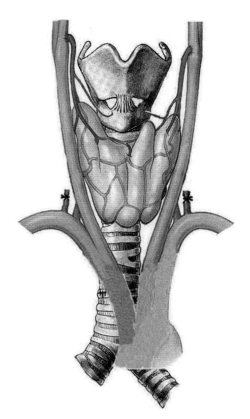

Fig. 22.1 Composite tyro-tracheal graft without venous drainage. Direct anastomosis of the inferior thyroid artery branches to the ipsilateral common carotid arteries, without a venous drainage

Fig. 22.2 Heterotopic composite tyro-tracheal allograft with venous drainage. Arterial supply of the tracheal graft is provided by the right or left subclavian artery via inferior thyroid artery and the venous drainage by the superior vena cava via the descending cervical vein

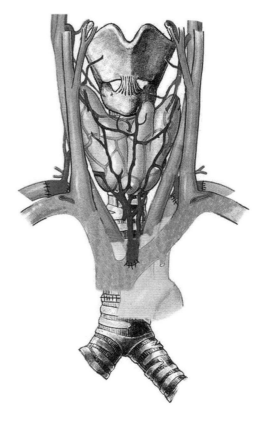

veins, subclavian vessels, thyroid gland, cervico-thoracic trachea and esophagus. The revascularization was obtained by direct anastomosis of the large arterial and venous vessels (recipient and donor subclavian artery stumps "end-to-end" anastomosis; donor superior vena cava with the recipient's brachiocephalic venous trunk end-to-side anastomosis). Thus, the arterial blood supply of the tracheal graft is provided by the right or left subclavian artery, via the inferior thyroid artery, and the venous drainage by the superior vena cava, via the descending cervical vein.[17] All tracheal grafts remained viable and had preserved or regenerated the airway epithelium.

On the basis of more recent anatomical data about the vascular perfusion territory of the inferior thyroid artery, which also include the vast majority of the cervical and upper thoracic trachea in humans,[63,64] Genden and colleagues imagined an orthotopic less invasive but technically more demanding direct revascularization technique in dogs, using the inferior thyroid artery and the internal jugular vein as the vascular supply.[65]

As a further development of these initial techniques, Macedo and colleagues suggested the "dual arterial blood supply" revascularization technique[66] which aims to ensure the viability not only of the proximal part of the trachea but also of the carinal region (see Fig. 22.3). The arterial supply of the upper 2/3 of the tracheal graft is provided by branches from the inferior thyroid artery by interposition of donor right subclavian artery into recipient cervical arterial system. In addition, an aortic patch, containing the origins of the bronchial arteries, is end-to-side anastomosed to the brachiocephalic artery of the recipient, providing the vascular supply of the inferior tracheal part, carina, and stem bronchi. The key feature of this technique is an intact bronchial vascular system able to provide a sufficient arterial blood supply of the inferior part of the tracheaobronchial graft. To protect the tiny network of paratracheal and peribronchial vessels from being injured it is important not to dissect the paratracheal and subcarinal lymph nodes and keep them attached to the graft.

Unfortunately, as claimed by Macedo himself, the "dual blood supply" technique, despite excellent positive and encouraging results, represents only "an experimental model of tracheobronchial revascularization and not a clinically relevant tracheal transplantation technique." This is also valid for the other described direct revascularization techniques, mostly due to the complexity and invasiveness of these procedures.

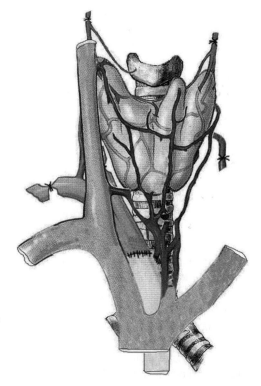

Fig. 22.3 Orthotopic tyro-tracheal allograft with dual artery blood supply. The arterial supply of the superior 2/3 of the tracheal graft is provided by branches from the inferior thyroid artery by interposition of donor right subclavian artery into recipient cervical arterial system. A preprepared aortic tube, containing the origins of the bronchial arteries, was end-to-side anastomosed to the brachiocephalic artery of the recipient providing the vascular supply of the inferior tracheal part, carina, and stem bronchi

22.6.2 Indirect Revascularization Techniques

Consequently, investigators abandoned the direct revascularization and attempted indirect methods to revascularize a tracheal graft by wrapping it in viable tissues (pedicled omentum, fascial vascular carriers, and different muscular flaps).

22.6.2.1 Greater Omentum Wrapping

From the various tissues available for wrapping tracheal allografts, the most frequently used was the greater omentum. The reason for this is anchored in the long-established experience with the use of greater omentum in general thoracic surgery, together with the omentum's unique features of easy surgical handling and excellent potential for induction of neo-angiogenesis.[67]

However, also a negative experience with omental-induced neo-angiogenesis and tracheal autografts was reported by Olech and Patterson in 1991.[68]

Two different transplantation strategies have been applied: (1) the orthothopic 1-stage procedure and (2) the heterotopic 2-stage technique.

22.6.2.1.1 The Orthotopic 1-Stage Procedure

This technique is using an immediately orthotopic reanastomosed tracheal graft, wrapped in a transposed pedicled omentum.

Baldermann and Weinblatt were the first to describe, in 1987, an orthotopic 1-stage transplantation technique of a ten-ring tracheal homograft wrapped in a transposed omental pedicle flap.[69] They reported that, due to omental circulation insufficiency, the omental graft cannot sustain chondrocyte viability and consecutively that of a tracheal autograft.

Nakanishi and colleagues extended, in 1993, the Balderman and Weinblatt experiments by investigating the maximal length of tracheal autografts wrapped in a pedicled greater omentum flap and transplanted by means of an orthotopic 1-stage technique.[70] To avoid immune reactions the authors used autografts. They were able to demonstrate that grafts exceeding a length of 4 cm frequently showed ischemia in the mid-portion but no ischemic changes at the anastomotic sites. Thus, the double blood supply of the graft, derived from the ends of the recipients' trachea and the wrapped omentum, was insufficient to maintain the viability of the tracheal cartilage.

Yokomise and colleagues,[71] as well as Murai and colleagues,[72] suggested that the ischemia of the tracheal mid-part is the result of an insufficient blood flow toward the mid-part of the graft due to the presence of the tracheal cartilage rings, which interfere with the blood supply from the omental pedicle to the submucosal tissue of the transplant.

To overcome this problem they proposed two different surgical solutions: (1) the split tracheal transplantation,[71] and (2) the partial removal of the graft cartilage rings.[72]

In case of "split tracheal transplantation" technique the long tracheal graft is longitudinally incised at its anterior cartilaginous part prior to the orthotopic transplantation. Thereafter, an omental pedicle flap is introduced into the resulted tracheal defect to facilitate blood vessel ingrowth. The reported results were positive with all animals surviving for at least 2 months. All grafts were incorporated, and none showed ischemia, stenosis, or malacia. The microscopic examination as well as the microangiography revealed neovascularization at the mid-part of the graft, promoted probably by the omental flap.[71]

The other solution proposed by Murai and colleagues in 1999[72] and republished by the Masaoka group in 2002[73] represents a more complex development of the "split tracheal transplantation" technique. This method tries to prevent a possible prolapse of the omental flap into the lumen of the transplanted trachea, though no such complication was ever mentioned by Yokomise. It consists of the complete removal of all cartilage rings with exception of the two cartilages at both ends and the one in the mid-portion of the graft. The resulting autograft is enforced with two horseshoe-shaped artificial rings placed between the remaining cartilage rings and wrapped in an omental pedicled flap primary to reimplantation. Supplementary, a silicone stent is placed inside the autograft. The reported results were similar to those published by Yokomise et al.

22.6.2.1.2 The Heterotopic 2-Stage Procedure

This procedure consists of a primary heterotopic transplantation of the tracheal graft into the greater omentum followed by transfer into the neck at a second stage together with the pedicled omentum.

Borro and colleagues in 1992[74] and Nakanishi and colleagues in 1994[75] were the first to publish positive experimental results with the heterotopic implantation of a tracheal autograft into the greater omentum primary to transplantation. Enthusiastic results with this technique were also reported by Weder et al in 1992.[76]

Li and colleagues[77,78] extensively investigated this method by harvesting a 6-ring tracheal segment as an autograft and wrapping it intraabdominal in the lower portion of the greater omentum. Two weeks later, the omental pedicled flap, together with the tracheal graft, was easily brought to the cervical area and sewed into the former defect. All dogs survived, and the tracheal grafts preserved the epithelium and cartilages. The authors concluded that the prior implantation of tracheal grafts into the greater omentum results in better preservation of its structure.

22.6.2.2 Other Wrapping Methods

Theoretically, the nature of the tissue used for wrapping is less important. Of more importance is the existence of a vascular carrier with an axial perfusion and a reliable and easily transferable vascular pedicle.

On the basis of these affirmations and searching for a vascular carrier less bulky than the greater omentum, Delaere and colleagues proposed, in 1995, the use of a vascularized sheet of thoracic fascia.[79] The Delaere technique, however, never found its way into clinical application, but remained an excellent and simple experimental model to investigate problems related to host immune tolerance and allograft rejection.

A similar technique was proposed by Hardillo et al. who used a vascularized radial forearm flap for wrapping the graft.[80]

Extremely controversial is the use of a cranially pediculated muscular wrapping. Positive results were reported by Cibantos Filho's group using a sternohyoid compound flap as vascular carrier.[81] In contrast to the above published results, Behrend and Klempnauer reported the absence of neovascularization of tracheal autografts in sheeps, despite wrapping in the right sternocleidomastoid muscle.[82]

22.7 Human Experience

In contrast to the wide experimental experience, only a limited number of tracheal transplantations in humans have been published. These clinical experiences with human tracheal transplantation include two different categories of surgical procedures: (1) transplantation of a cadaveric human homograft, and (2) tracheal reconstruction using autologous tracheal tissue (free tracheal autograft).

22.7.1 Transplantation of a Cadaveric Human Homograft

22.7.1.1 Fresh Cadaveric Human Tracheal Homograft Wrapped in Viable Tissue

Rose and colleagues were the first to publish in 1979, in *Lancet*, a case report on the heterotopic implantation of a human donor trachea that was wrapped in the sternocleidomastoid muscle and transferred into orthotopic position 3 weeks later. No immunosuppressive therapy was added. Satisfying initial results were published with no evidence of rejection, ischemia, or infection 9 weeks after transplantation. However, there is no further information regarding the long-term results.[9]

The second case of human tracheal transplantation using a cadaveric homograft was reported by Levashov and colleagues from the year 1993 and consists of a 1-stage allotransplantation of a cadaveric thoracic tracheal segment wrapped in the greater omentum in a 24-year-old female patient with idiopathic fibrosing mediastinitis. Despite the cyclosporine A and azathioprine-based immunosuppression, early rejection signs were present on the tenth postoperative day and were treated with antithymocyte globulin and loading doses of corticosteroids. However, beginning from the fourth postoperative month, progressive stenosis occurred, and the patient ultimately needed permanent stenting of the trachea. It still remains unclear whether this outcome was the result of late shrinking of the allograft because of ischemia or of underlying disease progression.[14]

In 2004, Klepetko and colleagues were the ones to confirm these experimental data and publish positive results of the indirect tracheal revascularization technique of a fresh tracheal allograft by means of omental wrapping, in human beings. In a 57-year-old patient with chronic obstructive pulmonary disease and low segment tracheal stenosis, standard bilateral sequential lung transplantation was performed with the transfer of the donor trachea into the recipient's abdomen, which was wrapped in the greater omentum and sutured into the abdominal wall, similar to a stoma. Sixty days later, the tracheal allograft presented a normal macroscopical appearance, with maintained elasticity and rigidity. The patient received a standard immunosuppressive therapy with cyclosporine A, mycophenolate mofetil, and cortisone (see Fig. 22.4).[19]

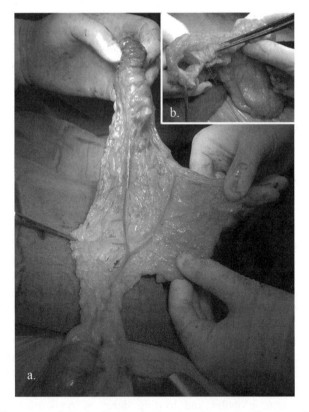

Fig. 22.4 Indirect revascularization by heterotopic omental wrapping (2-stage technique)

22.7.1.2 Cryopreserved Human Tracheal Homograft

Herberhold and colleagues introduced, in 1979, the use of *cryopreserved tracheal homografts* in treatment of long segment tracheal defects in adults, as a second option to the more popular "slide tracheoplasty."[10,83–85] The chemically treated and preserved allograft acts as a biocompatible implant with no intrinsic cellular viability. By this technique the anterior part of the receiver trachea is removed over the entire length of the stenosis leaving only the posterior tracheal wall. The cryopreserved homograft is cut to shape the defect and sutured into place using separate sutures of absorbable monofilament (see Fig. 22.5). A silastic stent is placed intraluminal for 10–12 weeks following transplantation to support the homograft until reepithelization has occurred.

The tracheal homograft has an easy availability and by incorporating the carinal part it represents an excellent replacement material for extensive repair. In addition, this procedure can be repeated if required. The major disadvantage includes the need for postoperative stenting, development of granulation tissue, and restenosis.

On the basis of the positive results regarding the immunological behavior of the tracheal grafts after cryopreservation (no further immunosuppressive therapy is needed) the tracheal cryopreserved allograft transplantation established itself as a therapeutic modality with encouraging results. After initial success with this technique in Europe, several centers in North America have also adopted the tracheal allograft transplantation.

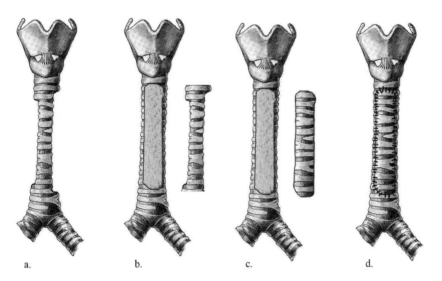

Fig. 22.5 Cryopreserved allograft transplantation. (**a, b**) The anterior part of the receiver trachea is removed over the entire length of the stenosis leaving only the posterior tracheal wall. (**c, d**)The cryopreserved homograft is cut to shape the defect and sutured into place using separate sutures of absorbable monofilament. A silastic stent is placed intra-luminal for 10–12 weeks following transplantation to support the homograft until reepithelization has occurred

The success with tracheal allograft reconstruction in adults led to extensions of this procedure to pediatric patients. Almost simultaneously, Elliot and colleagues[86] as well as Jacobs and colleagues[87] published, in 1994, their experience with *tracheal replacement in children using cadaveric cryopreserved human tracheal homograft*. In 1999, the total worldwide pediatric experience included 31 children. Tracheal allografts banks now exist in Miami, Florida, London, and Bonn.

22.7.2 Free Tracheal Autograft Transplantation

This technique includes median sternotomy and cardiopulmonary bypass support. The trachea is incised anteriorly through the area of stenosis. The mid-portion of the stenotic trachea is excised and will later be used as a free autograft. The remaining two separated ends of the trachea are end-to-end anastomosed posteriorly by means of interrupted PDS (polydiaxanone) sutures and the free autograft is trimmed and sutured in place anteriorly (see Fig. 22.6). If the autograft is not long enough to fill the anterior defect, the cranial tracheal opening can be patched with pericardium.[18,88,89]

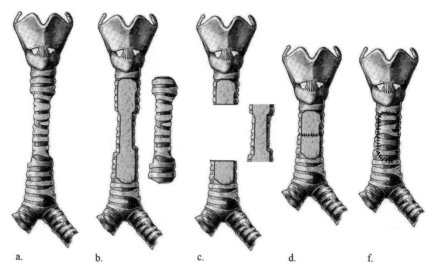

Fig. 22.6 Free autograft transplantation. (**a**) The trachea is incised anteriorly through the area of stenosis. (**b**) The mid-portion of the stenotic trachea is excised and will later be used as a free autograft. (**c–e**) The two separated ends of the trachea are end-to-end anastomosed posteriorly by means of interrupted PDS (polydiaxanone) sutures. (**f**) The free autograft is trimmed and sutured in place anteriorly. If the autograft is not long enough to fill the anterior defect, the cranial tracheal opening can be patched with pericardium

The main advantages of the tracheal autograft transplantation which made it the current procedure of choice for infants with long segment congenital tracheal stenosis in the Children's Memorial Hospital are (1) the use of readily available autologous material, (2) the procedure is reproducible and technically easy, (3) minimal tension on the suture lines, (4) architectural perfect, (5) the autograft is already lined with respiratory epithelium, (6) the cartilages maintain their intrinsic structure, and (7) there is a proven potential for growth.[88,89]

The reported survival rates are over 90% and only few patients presented recurrent granulation tissue and stenosis from exuberant scar formation as result of autograft ischemia.

22.8 Conclusion

Tracheal surgery has largely developed and matured in the last 30 years and nowadays also includes the methods of tracheal transplantation.

On the basis of the latest experimental results regarding the tracheal immunological behavior and the development of new conservation, implantation, and revascularization techniques of tracheal grafts, the reconstruction or replacement of the trachea by means of transplantation seems to be the most logic step for treatment of long segment tracheal defects, especially since none of the other reconstruction techniques (i.e., solid or porous prostheses, autogenous tissues, tissue engineering, etc.) have resulted in clinical application at large scale.

References

1. H. C. Grillo, Tracheal replacement: A critical review. *Ann Thorac Surg* **73**, 1995–2004 (2002).
2. C. G. Rob, G. H. Bateman, Reconstruction of the trachea and cervical oesophagus. *Br J Surg* **37**, 202–205 (1949).
3. R. Belsey, Resection and reconstruction of the intrathoracic trachea. *Br J Surg* **38**, 200–205 (1950).
4. D. J. Ferguson, J. J. Wild, O. H. Wangensteen, Experimental resection of the trachea. *Surgery* **28**, 597–619 (1950).
5. J. R. Cantrell, J. R. Folse, The repair of circumferential defects of the trachea by direct anastomosis: experimental evaluation. *J Thorac Cardiovasc Surg* **42**, 589–598 (1961).
6. J. Mulliken, H. C. Grillo, The limits of tracheal resection with primary anastomosis. Further anatomical studies in man. *J Thorac Cardiovasc Surg* **55**, 418–421 (1968).
7. H. C. Grillo, E. F. Dignan, T. Mirua, Extensive resection and reconstruction of mediastinal trachea without prosthesis or graft: an anatomical study in man. *J Thorac Cardiovasc Surg* **48**, 471 (1964).
8. P. W. Gebauer, Further experiences with dermal grafts for healed tuberculous stenosis of the bronchi and trachea. *J Thorac Surg* **20**, 628–651 (1950).
9. K. G. Rose, K. Sesterhenn, F. Wustrow, Tracheal allotransplantation in man. *Lancet* **1**, 433 (1979).
10. C. Herberhold, B. Franz, W. Breipohl, Chemisch-konservierte menschliche Trachea als Prothesenmaterial zur Deckung trachealer Defekte. *Laryng Rhinol* **59**, 453–457 (1980).

11. V. Tsang, A. Murday, C. Gillbe, P. Goldstraw, Slide tracheoplasty for congenital funnel-shaped tracheal stenosis. *Ann Thorac Surg* **48**, 632–635(1989).
12. H. C. Grillo, Slide tracheoplasty for long-segmentcongenital tracheal stenosis. *Ann Thorac Surg* **58**, 613–619 (1994). (Article in German).
13. A. Messineo, R. M. Filler, B. Bahoric, Successful tracheal autotransplantation with a vascularised omental flap. *J Pediatr Surg* **26**, 1296–1300 (1991).
14. Y. N. Levashov, P. K. Yablonsky, S. M. Cherny, S. V. Orlov, B. B. Shafirovsky, I. M. Kuznetzov, One stage allotransplantation of thoracic segment of the trachea in a patient with idiophatic fibrosing mediastinitis and marked tracheal stenosis. *Eur J Cardiothorac Surg* **7**, 383–386 (1993).
15. T. Takachi, T. Shirakusa, T. Shiraishi, K. Okabayashi, K. Inutsuka, K. Kawahara, R. Nakanishi, Experimental carinal autotransplantation and allotransplantation. *J Thorac Cardiovasc Surg* **110**(3), 762–767 (1995).
16. J. F. Khalil-Marzouk, J. D. Cooper, Allograft replacement of the trachea. Experimental synchronous revascularization of composite thyrotracheal transplant. *J Thorac Cardiovasc Surg* **105**, 242–246 (1993).
17. P. Macchiarini, B. Lenot, V. de Montpreville, E. Dulment, G. M. Mazmanian, M. Fattal, Heterotopic pig model for direct revascularization and venous drainage of tracheal allografts. *J Thorac Cardiovasc Surg* **108**, 1066–1075 (1994).
18. C. L. Backer, C. Mavroudis, M. E. Dunham, L. D. Holinger, Repair of congenital tracheal stenosis with a free tracheal autograft. *J Thorac Cardiovasc Surg* **115**, 869–874 (1998).
19. W. Klepetko, G. M. Marta, W. Wisser, E. Melis, A. Kocher, G. Seebacher, C. Aigner, S. Mazhar, Heterotopic tracheal transplantation with omentum wrapping in the abdominal position preserves functional and structural integrity of a human tracheal allograft. *J Thorac Cardiovasc Surg* **127**, 862–867(2004).
20. Susan Standring et al., Gray's Anatomy: *The Anatomical Basis of Clinical Practice – 39th Edition* (Elsevier Churchill Livingstone, 2005).
21. D. W. Fawcett, R. P. Jensh, *Concise Histology* (Chapman & Hall; International Thomson Publishing, 1997).
22. H. A. Cleven, E. M. Genden, T. M. Moran, Reepithelialized orthotopic tracheal allografts expand memory cytotoxic T lymphocytes but show no evidence of chronic rejection. *Transplantation* **79**, 861–868 (2005).
23. J. Bujia, E. Wilmes, C. Hammer, Class II antigenicity of human cartilage: Revelance to the use of homologous cartilage graft for reconstructive surgery. *Ann Plast Surg* **26**, 541–543 (1991).
24. Y. Liu, T. Nakamura, Y. Shimizu, H. Ueda, M. Yoshitani, T. Toba, S. Fukuda, Experimental study of blood typing in immunosuppressant-free tracheal transplantation in dogs. *Thorac Cardiov Surg* **51**, 216–220 (2003).
25. K. E. Kelly, M. I. Hertz, D. L. Mueller, T-cell and major histocompatibility complex requirements for obliterative airway disease in heterotopically transplanted murine tracheas. *Transplantation* **66**(6), 764–771 (1998).
26. T. S. Ikonen, T. R. Brazelton, G. J. Berry, R. S. Shorthouse, R. E. Morris, Epithelial re-growth is associated with inhibition of obliterative airway disease in orthotopic tracheal allografts in non-immunosuppressed rats. *Transplantation* **70**, 857–863 (2000).
27. E. M. Genden, S. Govindaraj, H. Chaboki, H. Cleven, E. Fedorova, J. S. Bromberg, L. Mayer, Reepithelization of orthotopic allografts prevents rejection after withdrawal of immunosuppression. *Ann Otol Rhinol Laryngol* **114**, 279–288 (2005).
28. E. M. Genden, P. Boros, L. Jianhua, J. S. Bromberg, L. Mayer. Orthotopic tracheal transplantation in the murine model. *Transplantation* **73**(9), 1420–1425 (2002).
29. E. M. Genden, A. Iskander, J. S. Bromberg, L. Mayer, The kinetics and pattern of tracheal allograft re-epithelization. *Am J Respir Cell Mol Biol* **28**(6), 673–681 (2003).
30. Y. Ito, H. Suzuki, Y. Hattori, B. A. H. Muhammad, T. Takahashi, K. Suzuki, T. Kazui, Complete replacement of tracheal epithelia by the host promotes spontaneous acceptance of orthotopic tracheal allografts in rats. *Transplant Proc* **36**, 2406–2412 (2004).

31. J. V. Small, K. Anderson, K. Rottner, Actin and the coordination of protrusion, attachment and retraction in cell crawling. *Biosci Rep* **16**(5), 351–368 (1996).
32. R. E. Barrow, C. Z. Wang, M. J. Evans, D. N. Herndon. Growth factors accelerate epithelial repair in sheep trachea. *Lung* **171**(6), 335–344 (1993).
33. A. Dodge-Khatami, H. W. M. Niessen, A. Baidoshvili, T. M. van Gulik, M. G. Klein, L. Eijsman, B. A. J. M. de Mol, Topical vascular endothelial growth factor in rabbit tracheal surgery: comparative effect on healing using reconstruction materials and intraluminal stents. *Eur J Cardiothorac Surg* **23**, 6–14 (2003).
34. J. M. Albes, T. Klenzer, J. Kotzerke, K. U. Thiedemann, H. J. Schafers, H. G. Borst, Improvement of tracheal autograft revascularization by means of fibroblast growth factor. *Ann Thorac Surg* **57**, 444–449 (1994).
35. R. P. Pokharel, K. Maeda, T. Yamamoto, Expression of vascular endothelial growth factor in exuberant tracheal granulation tissue in children. *J Pathol* **188**, 82–86 (1999).
36. C. J. Corral, A. Siddiqui, L. Wu, C. L. Farrell, D. Lyons, T. A. Mustoe, Vascular endothelial growth factor is more important than basic fibroblastic growth factor during ischemic wound healing. *Arch Surg* **134**, 200–205 (1999).
37. S. W. Sung, T. Won. Effects of basic fibroblast growth factor on early revascularization and epithelial regeneration in rabbit tracheal orthotopic transplantation. *Eur J Cardiothorac Surg* **19**, 14–18 (2001).
38. S. Govindaraj, R. Gordon, E. M. Genden. Effect of fibrin matrix and vascular endothelial growth factor on reepithalialization of orthotopic murine tracheal transplants. *Ann Otol Rhinol Laryngol* **113**(10), 797–804 (2004).
39. Y. Liu, T. Nakamura, Y. Yamamoto, K. Matsumoto, T. Sekine, H. Ueda, Y. Shimizu. A new tracheal bioartificial organ: evaluation of a tracheal allograft with minimal antigenicity after treatment by detergent. *ASAIO J* **46**, 536–539 (2000).
40. H. Yokomise, K. Inui, H. Wada, T. Goh, K. Yagi, S. Hitomi, M. Takahashi, High-dose irradiation prevents rejection of canine tracheal allografts. *J Thorac Cardiovasc Surg* **107**(6), 1391–1397 (1994).
41. S. Kunachak, B. Kulapaditharom, Y. Vajaradul, M. Rochanawutanon. Cryopreserved, irradiated tracheal homograft transplantation for laryngotracheal reconstruction in human beings. *Otolaryngol Head Neck Surg* **122**(6), 911–916 (2000).
42. C. Deschamps, V. F. Trastek, J. L. Ferguson, W. J. Martin, T. V. Colby, P. C. Pairolero, Cryopreservation of canine trachea: functional and histological changes. *Ann Thorac Surg* **47**, 208–212 (1989).
43. T. Tojo, K. Niwaya, N. Sawabata, K. Kushibe, K. Nezu, S. Taniguchi, Tracheal replacement with cryopreserved tracheal allograft: experiment in dogs. *Ann Thorac Surg* **66**, 209–213 (1998).
44. T. Mukaida, N. Shimizu, M. Aoe, A. Andou, H. Date, M. Okabe, M. Yamashita, S. Ichiba, Experimental study of tracheal allotransplantation with cryopreserved grafts. *J Thorac Cardiovasc Surg* **116**(2), 262–266 (1998).
45. T. Aoki, Y. Yamato, M. Tsuchida, T. Souma, K. Yoshiya, T. Watanabe, J. Hayashi, Successful tracheal transplantation using cryopreserved allografts in a rat model. *Eur J Cardiothorac Surg* **16**, 169–173 (1999).
46. K. Kushibe, K. Nezu, K. Nishizaki, M. Takahama, S. Taniguchi, Tracheal allotransplantation maintaining cartilage viability with long-term cryopreserved allografts. *Ann Thorac Surg* **71**, 1666–1669 (2001).
47. T. Muraka, J. Nakajima, N. Motomura, A. Murakami, S. Takamoto, Successful allotransplantation of cryopreserved tracheal grafts with preservation of the pars membranacea in nonhuman primates. *J Thorac Cardiovasc Surg* **123**(1), 153–160 (2002).
48. R. Nakanishi, T. Onitsuka, Y. Shigematsu, M. Hashimoto, H. Muranaka, K. Yasumoto, The immunomodulatory effect of cryopreservation in rat tracheal allotransplantation. *J Heart Lung Transplantation* **21**(8), 890–898 (2002).
49. H. Tanaka, K. Maeda, Y. Okita. Transplantation of the cryopreserved tracheal allograft in growing rabbits. *J Pediatr Surg* **38**, 1707–1711 (2003).

50. H. Yokomise, K. Inui, H. Wada, S. Hasegawa, N. Ohno, S. Hitomi, Reliable cryopreservation of trachea for one month in a new trehalose solution. *J Thorac Cardiovasc Surg* **110**, 382–385 (1995).
51. E. Stoelben, H. Harpering, J. Haberstroh, A. di Filippo, E. Wellens,. Heterotopic transplantation of cryopreserved tracheae in a rat model. *Eur J Cardiothorac Surg* **23**, 15–20 (2003).
52. R. Nakanishi, K. Yasumoto, Minimal dose of cyclosporine A for tracheal allografts. *Ann Thorac Surg* **60**, 635–639 (1995).
53. P. R. Delaere, Z. Liu, R. Sciot, W. Welvaart, The role of immunosuppression in the long-term survival of tracheal allografts. *Arch Otolaryngol Head Neck Surg* **122**, 1201–1208 (1996).
54. M. Hashimoto, R. Nakanishi, M. Umesue, H. Muranaka, M. Hachida, K. Yasumoto, Feasibility of cryppreserved tracheal xenotransplants with the use of short-course immunosuppression. *J Thorac Cardiovasc Surg* **121**(2), 241–248 (2001).
55. G. Benichou, Direct and indirect antigen recognition: the pathways to allograft immune rejection. *Front Biosci* **4**, 476–480 (1999).
56. E. M. Genden, S. E. Mackinnon, S. Yu, D. A. Hunter, M. W. Flye, Portal venous ultraviolet B-irradiated donor alloantigen prevents rejection in circumferential rat tracheal allografts. *Otolaryngol Head Neck Surg* **124**, 481–488 (2001).
57. F. G. Fernandez, B. McKane, S. H. Marshbank, A. Patterson, T. H. Mohanakumar. Inhibition of obliterative airway disease development following heterotopic murine tracheal transplantation by costimulatory molecule blockade using anti-CD40 ligand alone or in combination with donor bone marrow. *J Heart Lung Transplant* **24**(7S), 232–238 (2005).
58. R. Suemitsu, I. Yoshino, F. Shoji, M. Yamaguchi, Y. Tomita, Y. Maehara. The effects of pretreatment with donor antigen and immunosuppressive agents on fully allogenic tracheal graft. *J Surg Res* **122**(1), 8–13 (2004).
59. T. Miura, H. C. Grillo, The contribution of the inferior thyroid artery to the blood supply of the human trachea. *Surg Gynecol Obstet* **123**, 99–107 (1966).
60. J. R. Salassa, W. B. Pearson, W. Spencer-Payne, Gross and microscopical blood supply of the trachea. *Ann Thorac Surg* **24**, 100–107 (1977).
61. S. Strome, E. Sloman-Moll, J. Wu, R. B. Samonte, M. Strome, Rat model for a vascularised laryngeal allograft. *Ann Otol Rhinol Laryngol* **101**, 950–953 (1992).
62. T. Miura, H. C. Grillo, The contribution of the inferior thyroid artery to the blood supply of the human trachea. *Surg Gynecol Obstet* **99**, (1966).
63. J. Salmeron, P. J. Gannon, K. E. Blackwell, C. M. Shaari, M. L. Urken, Tracheal transplantation: superior and inferior thyroid artery perfusion territory. *Laryngoscope* **108**, 849–853 (1998).
64. C. M. Shaari, P. J. Gannon, J. Salmeron, I. Sanders, M. L. Urken, Tracheal transplantation: defining the vascular territory of the canine cranial thyroid artery. *Otolaryngol Head Neck Surg* **120**, 180–183 (1999).
65. E. M. Genden, P. J. Gannon, S. H. Smith, N. Keck, M. Deftereos, M. L. Urken, Microvascular transfer of long tracheal autograft segments in the canine model. *Laryngoscope* **112**, 439–444 (2002).
66. A. Macedo, E. Fadel, G. M. Mazmanian, V. de Montpreville, M. German-Fattal, S. Mussot, A. Chapelier, P. G. Dartevelle, Heterotopic en bloc tracheobronchial transplantation with direct revascularization in pigs. *J Thorac Cardiovasc Surg* **127**, 1593–1601 (2004).
67. E. Morgan, O. Lima, M. Goldberg, A. Ferdman, S. K. Luk, J. D. Cooper, Successful revascularization of totally ischemic bronchial autografts with omental pedicle flaps in dogs. *J Thorac Cardiovasc Surg* **84**, 204–210 (1982).
68. V. M. Olech, S. H. Keshavjee, D. W. Chamberlain, A. S. Slutsky, G. A. Patterson, Role of basic fibroblast growth factor in revascularization of rabbit tracheal autografts. *Ann Thorac Surg* **52**(2), 258–264 (1991).
69. S. C. Baldermann, G. Weinblatt, Tracheal autograft revascularization. *J Thorac Cardiovasc Surg* **94**, 434–441 (1987).
70. R. Nakanishi, T. Shirakusa, T. Mitsudomi, Maximum length of tracheal autografts in dogs. *J Thorac Cardiovasc Surg* **106**, 1081–1087 (1993).

71. H. Yokomise, K. Inui, H. Wada, M. Ueda, S. Hitomi, H. Itoh, Split transplantation of the trachea: a new operative procedure for extended tracheal resection. *J Thorac Cardiovasc Surg* **112**, 314–318 (1996).
72. K. Murai, H. Oizumi, T. Masaoka, T. Fujishima, M. Abiko, S. Shiono, Y. Shimazaki, Removal of cartilage rings of the graft and omentopexy for extended tracheal autotransplantation. *Ann Thorac Surg* **67**, 776–780 (1999).
73. T. Masaoka, H. Oizumi, T. Fujishima, Y. Naruke, S. Shiono, Y. Shimazaki, Removal of cartilage rings prevents graft stenosis in extended tracheal allotransplantation with omentopexy and immunosuppression: an experimental study. *J Heart Lung Transplant* **21**(4), 485–492 (2002).
74. J. M. Borro, M. Chirivella, C. Vila, G. Galan, M. Prieto, F. Paris, Successful revascularization of large isolated tracheal segments. *Eur J Cardiothorac Surg* **6**(11), 621–623 (1992).
75. R. Nakanishi, T. Shirakusa, T. Takachi, Omentopexy for tracheal autografts. *Ann Thorac Surg* **57**, 841–845 (1994).
76. W. Weder, D. Candinas, C. Scherer, H. Date, J. D. Cooper, Revascularization of tracheal transplants with omentum. *Helv Chir Acta* **58**(4), 533–537 (1992). (Article in German)
77. J. Li, P. Xu, H. Chen, Z. Yang, Q. Zhang, Improvement of tracheal autograft survival with transplantation into the greater omentum. *Ann Thorac Surg* **60**, 1592–1596 (1995).
78. J. Li, P. Xu, H. Chen, Successful tracheal autotransplantation with two-staged approach using the greater omentum. *Ann Thorac Surg* **64**, 199–202 (1997).
79. P. R. Delaere, Z. Y. Liu, R. Hermans, R. Sciot, L. Feenstra, Experimental tracheal allograft revascularization and transplantation. *J Thorac Cardiovasc Surg* **110**, 728–737 (1995).
80. J. A. Hardillo, V. Vander Poorten, P. R. Delaere. Transplantation of tracheal autografts: is a two-stage procedure necessary? *Acta Otorhinolaryngol Belg* **54**(1), 13–21(2000).
81. J. S. Cibantos Filho, F. V. de Mello Filho, A. D. Campos, F. Ellinguer, Viability of a 12-ring complete tracheal segment transferred in the form of a compound flap: an experimental study in dogs. *Laryngoscope* **114**(11), 1949–1952 (2004).
82. M. Behrend, R. von Wasielewski, J. Klempnauer, Failure of airway healing in an ovine autotransplantation model that includes basic fibroblast growth factor. *J Thorac Cardiovasc Surg* **124**, 231–240 (2001).
83. C. Herberhold, Transplantation of larynx and trachea in man. *Eur Arch Otorhinolaryngol* **1**(Suppl.), 247–255 (1992).
84. J. P. Jacobs, M. J. Elliott, M. P. Haw, M. Bailey, C. Herberhold, Pediatric tracheal homograft reconstruction: a novel approach to complex tracheal stenoses in children. *J Thorac Cardiovasc Surg* **112**, 1549–1560 (1996).
85. C. Herberhold, M. Stein, M. Falkenhausen, Long-term results of homograft reconstruction of the trachea in childhood. *Laryngorhinootologie* **78**, 692–696 (1999).
86. M. J. Elliott, M. P. Haw, J. P. Jacobs, C. M. Bailey, J. N. G. Evans, C. Herberhold, Successful tracheal replacement in children using cadaveric human tracheal homograft. *Eur J Cardiothorac Surg* **10**, 702–712 (1996).
87. J. P. Jacobs, J. A. Quintessenza, T. Andrews, R. P. Burke, Z. Spektor, R. E. Delius, R. J. H. Smith, M. J. Elliott, C. Herberhold, Tracheal allograft reconstruction: the total North America and worldwide pediatric experiences. *Ann Thorac Surg* **68**, 1043–1052 (1999).
88. C. L. Backer, C. Mavroudis, M. E. Dunham, L. Holinger, Intermediate-term results of the free tracheal autograft for long segment congenital tracheal stenosis. *J Pediatr Surg* **35**(6), 813–818 (2000).
89. C. L. Backer, C. Mavroudis, M. E. Gerber, L. D. Holinger, Tracheal surgery in children: an 18-year of four techniques. *Eur J Cardiothorac Surg* **19**, 777–784 (2001).

Chapter 23
Laryngeal Transplantation

Robert R. Lorenz and Marshall Strome

23.1 History

The concept of human laryngeal transplantation was first introduced into the literature in the 1960s, with experiments using the dog model by Boles,[1] Ogura,[2] and Silver.[3] In 1969, Kluyskens attempted to treat a laryngeal cancer by transplantation.[4] This transplant was subtotal, preserving recipient perichondrium to revascularize the donor organ without the use of vascular or neural anastomoses. The rapid recurrence of the tumor quashed interest in the procedure for nearly two decades.

In 1987, the senior author initiated a program to explore the potential of a total larynx transplant. The program focused on four issues crucial to successful transplantation: revascularization, reinnervation, rejection, and the ethical issues of transplanting an organ that some consider "nonvital." Utilizing the rat as a model for laryngeal transplantation, the maximum tolerated ischemia time was determined,[5] preservative solutions were investigated, stages of histological rejection were defined,[6] and immunosuppressive regimens were evaluated.[7] On January 4, 1998, a team lead by the senior author performed a total laryngeal transplantation in a man who had sustained severe laryngeal trauma in a motor vehicle accident.[8]

23.2 The Human Laryngeal Transplant

The recipient was a 40-year-old man who had suffered a crush injury to his larynx and pharynx during a motorcycle accident 20 years earlier. Despite multiple attempts at another institution to reconstruct his larynx, he remained aphonic and tracheostomal dependent. The patient underwent extensive pretransplant counseling including psychiatric evaluation, speech pathology testing, and four interviews with members of the surgical team. All of those involved agreed that the patient understood the risks and his motivation was appropriate. The procedure was approved by the Institutional Review Board of the Cleveland Clinic Foundation. After a 6-month search, a 40-year-old man, who was brain dead from a ruptured cerebral aneurysm, was identified as a suitable donor. He met all of

Laryngeal Transplantation

the predetermined criteria for acceptance in regard to HLA matching (4 of 5) and serum virology.

During the donor organ harvest, the entire pharyngolaryngeal complex, including six tracheal rings and the thyroid and parathyroid glands, was removed (Fig. 23.1). The organ complex was stored in the University of Wisconsin solution during transport until revascularization 10 h later. Prior to surgery, the recipient patient received cyclosporine, azathioprine, and methylprednisolone. After surgical exposure of the patient's severely deformed laryngeal structures but prior to their removal, perfusion to the donor organ was reestablished. The donor's right superior thyroid artery was anastomosed to that of the patient, while the proximal end of the donor's right internal jugular vein was anastomosed to the patient's right common facial vein. Blood flow through the transplanted thyroid gland, six tracheal rings, larynx, and pharynx was observed within 30 min of clamp release.

A narrow field laryngectomy was performed leaving the thyroid lobes lateralized and the hyoid bone in place. Seventy-five percent of the donor's pharynx was used to widen the patient's stenotic pharyngo-upper esophageal complex. The donor laryngeal cartilage was sutured to the hyoid bone for laryngeal elevation. Five tracheal rings were needed to reach the patient's tracheostoma. The left-sided anastomoses, which included the donor superior thyroid artery to the recipient superior thyroid artery and the donor middle thyroid donor vein to the recipient internal jugular vein, were then completed. Both superior laryngeal nerves were located and reanastomosed, but only the recipient's right recurrent laryngeal nerve could be located for reinnervation.

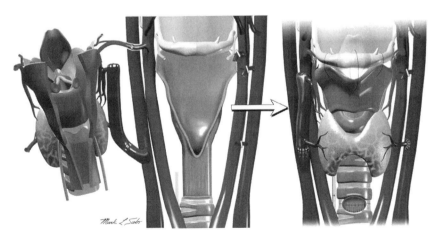

Fig. 23.1 The 1998 surgical technique of laryngeal transplantation. Anastomoses included the donor right internal jugular vein to recipient right facial vein, donor superior thyroid arteries to recipient superior thyroid arteries, and donor left middle thyroid vein to recipient left internal jugular vein. Note that both superior laryngeal nerves were anastomosed, while only the patient's right recurrent laryngeal nerve could be located for anastomosis (*See Color Plates*)

In the immediate postoperative period, the patient was maintained on muromonab-CD3, cyclosporine, methylprednisolone, and mycophenolate mofetil. Initial aspiration was controlled with glycopyrrolate and atropine, which were later discontinued. At the end of a 1-month period of observation in the hospital, the patient's transplanted trachea was normal on both endoscopy and biopsy. Fifteen months posttransplant, the patient experienced an episode of rejection that presented as a decrease in voice quality. After three daily doses of methylprednisolone 1 g/day, his larynx returned to normal. The patient is now over 8 years posttransplant and is maintained on 7.5 mg of prednisone per day, 1 g of mycophenolate mofetil daily, and 3 mg of tacrolimus per day with stable blood pressure and renal function. A second episode of rejection occurred 6 years after transplant due to laboratory error in tacrolimus values measuring levels falsely high, which resulted in decreasing the patient's medication below therapeutic levels. Laryngeal edema quickly resolved once medication levels returned to the therapeutic range.

Three months posttransplant, the supraglottis and vocal folds were sensitive to touch and purposeful swallowing returned. Subsequent barium swallows revealed no aspiration and the patient's sense of taste and smell has returned. The patient did experience three early episodes of tracheobronchitis that were successfully treated with oral amoxicillin clavulanate. At 16 weeks posttransplant, the patient inadvertently stopped his trimethoprim-sulfamethoxazole and developed *Pneumocystis carinii* pneumonia, which cleared rapidly with intravenous antibiotics. To evaluate thyroid function, a 4-h uptake of iodine-123 demonstrated 83% activity in the transplanted thyroid lobes and 17% in the patient's native thyroid. Thyroid function tests, serum calcium, and phosphate all remain within normal ranges.

The patient's first posttransplant voicing was on POD #3. (Fig. 23.2) At one month, both true vocal folds were lateral, creating a breathy voice. By 4 months, the right fold (the side of the recurrent nerve anastomosis) was midline and at 6 months the left was paramedian. Recent electromyographic (EMG) measurements have confirmed reinnervation of both folds; we believe that the left is supplied by surrounding motor nerves[9] or "field-reinnervation." Volitional cricothyroid function has been confirmed by EMG as well (Fig. 23.3a, b). Subjective and objective measures of phonation including pitch, jitter, intensity, and maximal phonation time were within the normal range at 36 months posttransplant. The patient has become a motivational speaker and reports that his quality of life has improved "immeasurably" now over 8 years posttransplantation. Laser cordotomy or sling tracheoplasty remain options for stomal management.

23.3 Animal Models of Laryngeal Transplantation

Early experiments into laryngeal transplantation in the 1960s by Boles,[1] Ogura,[2] and Silver[3] used the dog model. Berke's group applied modern microvascular techniques to extend this orthotopic model in the mid-1990s.[10] Genden's mouse model of tracheal transplantation has more recently examined the role of reepithelialization

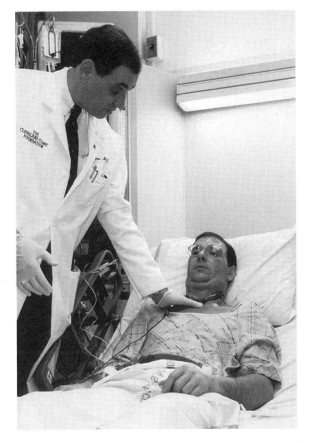

Fig. 23.2 The senior author with the first successful laryngeal transplant patient. The patient uttered his first words on postoperative day 3 after 20 years of aphonia

of the transplanted tracheal that may be extrapolatable to laryngeal work.[11] Birchall's group has developed an orthotopic pig model that is robust and allows detailed assessment of immunology in an open airway, coupled with functional reinnervation.[12] However, as with the dog, this model is expensive in time and labor and requires tracheostomy and gastrostomy, at least in the short term. These models all offer complimentary information forming the basis on which to build further understanding into laryngeal transplantation.

In our own laboratory, the rat model utilizes an arteriovenous shunt with venous outflow through the superior thyroid artery with the transplanted organ in tandem with the native airway (Fig. 23.4a–c). In 2002, the model's revisions were published, as well as a revised grading scale of rejection[13] (Fig. 23.5a–5c). With the low cost, a near 100% survivability, and a greater than 90% graft evaluability, over 2,000 rat transplants have been successfully performed to date. Furthermore, recent experiments have shown how performing a total parathyroidectomy on the recipient

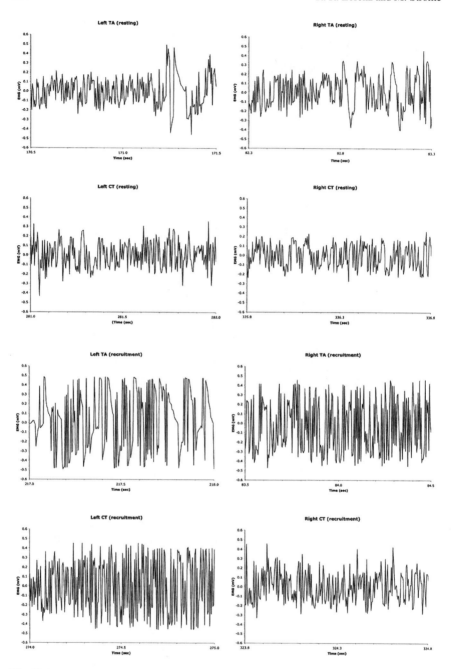

Fig. 23.3 (**a**) Resting laryngeal EMG tracings of four phonatory muscles 4 years after transplantation. (**b**) Laryngeal EMG tracings on phonation with "ee" and raising and lowering of pitch (*TA* thryoarytenoid muscle; *CT* cricothyroid muscle) (*See Color Plates*)

Laryngeal Transplantation

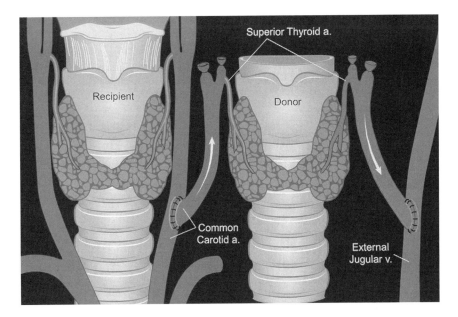

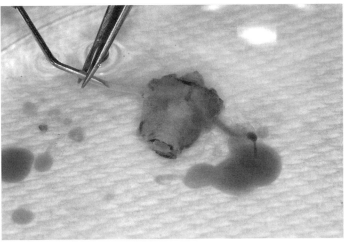

Fig. 23.4 (**a**) The rat model for laryngeal transplantation. The donor organ is placed in tandem to the recipient's airway and an arteriovenous shunt is used for venous outflow through the left superior thyroid artery. (**b**) The donor organ being flushed with Wisconsin's solution prior to revascularization (*See Color Plates*)

during transplantation can utilize the production of parathormone from the transplanted larynx as a marker of graft viability rather than having to sacrifice the animal for histologic evaluation.[14] This has allowed for a new generation of studies examining the ability to "pulse" immunosuppressives and "salvage" the organ if parathormone levels drop.

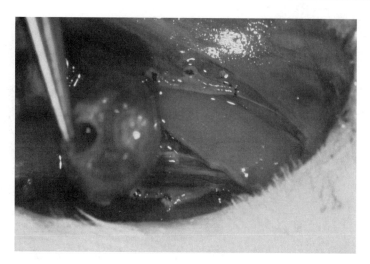

Fig. 23.4 (continued) (**c**) The donor organ being rotated superiorly in tandem in the left neck of the recipient rat. Arterial and venous anastomoses are shown as blood flow reestablished (*See Color Plates*)

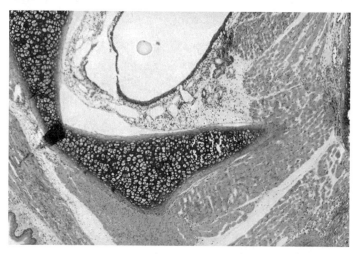

Fig. 23.5 (**a**) Histologic specimen of rat laryngeal transplant in Lewis to Lewis rat negative control after 15 days following transplantation (×5). Laryngeal architecture including epithelium, minor salivary glands, muscle, and cartilage preserved (*See Color Plates*)

Past findings using the rat laryngeal transplant model include those of Barthel et al.,[15] who studied the effect of in vitro irradiation upon the transplanted laryngotracheal complex. By administering 7.34 Gy to the organ immediately prior to transplantation, doses of cyclosporine could be reduced from 5.0 to 2.5 mg/kg with 10 out of 10 rats displaying no significant rejection at 30 days posttransplantation. These results were compared with those without radiation that demonstrated that

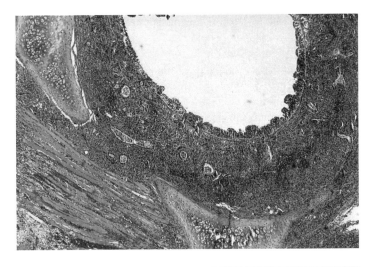

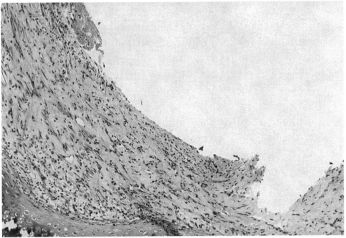

Fig. 23.5 (continued) (**b**) Histologic specimen of rat laryngeal transplant in LBN-f to Lewis rat after 7 days following transplantation without immunosuppression (×10). Tremendous infiltration of lymphocytes occurs in the subepithelial layer. (**c**) Histologic specimen of rat laryngeal transplant in LBN-f to Lewis rat after 15 days following transplantation without immunosuppression (×10). Laryngeal architecture is lost, with destruction of the epithelium and subepithelial minor salivary glands (*See Color Plates*)

with cyclosporine doses of 5.0 mg/kg, at 30 days, 33% of subjects displayed moderate rejection while an additional 33% displayed severe rejection. The authors concluded that in vitro radiation has some lasting immunosuppressive effects, perhaps reducing the number of viable "passenger" lymphocytes that accompany the transplanted organ.

Using the same model, Lorenz et al. demonstrated that by adding prednisone to cyclosporine, doses of cyclosporine could be further reduced.[16] In a multiarm study containing 220 transplantations, multiple doses of both cyclosporine and prednisone were administered and the transplanted organs were evaluated at both 15 days and 30 days posttransplantation. With the addition of 1.0 mg/kg/day of prednisone, cyclosporine doses could be reduced to 2.0 mg/kg and still demonstrate no significant rejection at 30 days posttransplantation. While this combination of low-dose cyclosporine and prednisone significantly improved graft survival when compared with cyclosporine alone at the equivalent dose, prednisone monotherapy demonstrated rates of rejection similar to no immunosuppression at all.

Haug et al. have correlated the laryngeal rejection grade, cyclosporine (CSA) concentration, and CSA intramuscular dosing.[17] Despite high variability in their CSA blood levels within groups of rats receiving cyclosporine dosed at either 1.0, 2.5, 5.0, 7.5, or 10 mg/kg/day, significantly different mean CSA concentrations were achieved among each group of five transplanted rats. While the rejection grading within the top three doses of CSA was not significantly different (5.0, 7.5, and 10 mg/kg/day), doses 2.5 or less were shown to have higher rejection grading in this blinded study. Significant pathological allograft rejection correlated with CSA concentrations below 250 ng/cm^3. This careful evaluation of drug dosing within the model established the correlation between CSA dosing, CSA levels, and graft rejection, as well as established the minimum level of CSA required to obtain optimum graft survival when used as the sole agent of immunosuppression.

When combining newer immunosuppressives within this transplantation model, Nelson et al. demonstrated that decreased levels may be used while maintaining optimum graft viability.[18] Ten experimental arms were conducted between tacrolimus alone at varying levels, and tacrolimus combined with mycophenolate mofetil at varying levels. Groups of eight to ten animals were examined at either 15 or 30 days posttransplantation. While increasing levels of tacrolimus demonstrated increasing efficacy of immunosuppression, low-dose tacrolimus, in combination with mycophenolate mofetil, achieved comparable results. Immunosuppressive investigation took an exciting step forward in 2003 with the demonstration of the ability to produce tolerance in the rat laryngeal model.[19] Akst et al. treated transplanted animals with tacrolimus and mouse anti-rat alpha beta T-cell-receptor monoclonal antibodies for only 7 days following transplant. At 100 days, all grafts demonstrated viability. Skin grafting, mixed lymphocyte reaction, and flow cytometry revealed that tolerance was neither donor specific nor related to systemic immunocompromise. Subsequent studies have utilized the parathormone production and pulsing of immunosuppressives around this 100-day time period to continue the graft survival while avoiding continuous immunosuppression. More recent studies have focused on inducing long-term tolerance, donor-derived bone marrow transplantation, dendritic cell transplantation, as well as pulsing of immunosuppressive therapy.

In other laryngeal transplantation laboratories, Genden demonstrated that a single injection of UV-B irradiated donor splenocytes was sufficient to prevent rejection in a rat tracheal graft model.[20] Birchall's group, using multiple color immunofluorescence, has described a dense, organized network of immunologically active cells in the laryngeal mucosa in both pig and man, the morphology of which suggest dendritic cells.[21,22] Human epithelial cells express MHC molecules, possibly the initiating signal for rejection. Genden has studied the role of tracheal epithelium in the rejection process. His studies of mouse tracheal grafts have shown that replacement of the epithelium by host epithelial cells prevents rejection after withdrawal of immunosuppression. The reepithelialization process was significantly quickened with the application of vascular endothelial growth factor (VEGF) carried by a fibrin matrix to the mucosa.[23]

23.4 Reinnervation Research in Laryngeal Transplantation

While the voice quality of our human laryngeal transplant recipient has remained exceptional, volitional abduction of the vocal fold is not possible given the mass reinnervation of both the abductor and adductor muscle groups by the recurrent laryngeal nerve. Therefore, he remains dependent upon a tracheostoma for his airway, and has been reticent to sacrifice voice quality with a laser cordotomy that would allow for trans-oral breathing and closure of his stoma. Clearly, reinnervation and volitional movement of the vocal folds is critical to the success and wide acceptance of laryngeal transplantation. Stavroulaki and Birchall[24] reviewed the anatomy of the laryngeal nerves in humans and in the four animal models used to study transplantation: dog, cat, rat, and pig. In reviewing the innervation of the human larynx, the authors remind us that nerve specification is more complicated than the dogma which states that the anterior recurrent laryngeal nerve is responsible for adductor function and the posterior recurrent laryngeal nerve controls abductor function. In reviewing the different correlates between the human and animal nerve anatomy, the authors even suggest that xenografting a porcine organ may become possible for restoring human phonation.

Sensory reinnervation of the transplanted dog larynx was studied by Blumin et al.[25] In a randomized, controlled study, ten dogs had their superior laryngeal nerves transected. Half of the animals had the nerves reanastomosed and all dogs were tested for laryngospasm in response to hydrochloric acid stimulation both preoperatively and 6 months postoperatively. Although none of the dogs regained normal laryngospastic responses, the reanastomosed animals exhibited protective EMG activity and coughing, while the control group exhibited no response. In our own human laryngeal transplant patient, at 3 months postoperatively, the supraglottis and vocal folds were sensitive to touch, initiating a severe cough. Stimulation through the stoma of the right side of the upper trachea elicited a sensation of touch without cough, while stimulation of the left side was not sensed.

The question arises: What happens to nerve function if transplantation is performed several years after laryngectomy? Is there a way to "bank" the recurrent nerve in the neck during tumor resection to better preserve its function later? Again using the dog model, Peterson et al.[26] attempted to answer this question. While one dog had its transected anterior and posterior branches of one recurrent nerve anastomosed to the distal ends of the ansa cervicalis, a second dog had the transected anterior branch inserted into the strap muscles while the posterior branch was transferred as a nerve-muscle pedicle to the sternothyroid muscle. Six months later, reanastomosis to the original nerve or placing the cut end into the original muscle was performed. Two weeks postoperatively, tensionometry, video and EMG testing demonstrated that both methods of "banking" successfully restored vocal fold function and electrical activity specific to abduction and adduction. The authors recommend that current patients who undergo total laryngectomy should, when it is oncologically feasible, undergo banking of the anterior and posterior recurrent laryngeal nerve branches on at least one side.

Even hemilaryngeal transplantation has been achieved in the canine model. Andrews et al.[27] resected one dog's hemilarynx including the thyroarytenoid muscle, arytenoid cartilage, and half of the thyroid cartilage. Identical structures from a littermate were then transplanted with reanastomosis of the recipient anterior RLN branch to the donor thyroarytenoid branch, along with an arytenoid adduction. Posterior cricoarytenoid and interarytenoid muscles were reapproximated with their counterparts. Postoperative immunosuppression included cyclosporine, azathioprine, and prednisone. Two months postoperatively, spontaneous EMG recordings were made detecting reinnervation potentials in the thyroarytenoid muscle corresponding to the respiratory cycle. Endoscopic exam revealed that the transplanted hemilarynx was similar in appearance to the native side, although the transplanted vocal fold remained fixed in the midline. Histologic sectioning revealed no evidence of graft rejection. The authors conclude that once immunosuppression has become more refined, hemilaryngeal transplantation may become a "theoretically ideal method of hemilaryngeal reconstruction."

23.5 Future Investigations

While the risks to transplant recipients are considered acceptable when transplantation is necessary to avoid death, in the case of nonvital organ transplantation, the institution of long-term immunosuppression and its inherent perils is more controversial. One of the largest risks is the potentiation of recurrent malignancy or a cancer de novo. While our transplantation in 1998 was performed on an ideal recipient, being a relatively fit, young trauma victim, there are only a few hundred such candidates in most countries. Other suitable though rare potential recipients would be those with large benign or low-grade malignant tumors of the larynx, or those developing laryngeal malignancy who are already on a posttransplant immunosuppression regimen. Patients who have already undergone laryngectomy for cancer might be candidates if their superior laryngeal nerves could be located, and there is no sign of recurrent cancer at 5 years or more. However, ultimately, the largest pool of patients who stand to benefit are those presenting with locally advanced laryngeal cancer, approximately 7,000 patients annually in the US.[28]

When the nonrevascularized partial laryngeal transplant was performed in 1969,[4] and again when a tongue transplant was performed in 2003, both in patients with advanced squamous cancer, both patients rapidly succumbed to recurrent disease. Therefore, an important step toward the goal of routine nonvital organ transplantation is the development of immune suppression that does not increase the risk of malignancy. Patients on chronic immunosuppression are known to have a threefold to fourfold increase in risk for development of de novo malignancies.[29]

Everolimus, a derivative of rapamycin, has been shown to have potent immunosuppressive effects as well as antiproliferative effects.[30] Belonging to the mTOR (mammalian target of rapamycin) class of immunosuppressants, everolimus blocks the translation of mRNA of critical cell cycle regulatory proteins. In addition, everolimus has been shown to inhibit the development of posttransplant lymphoproliferative disorders as well as a variety of other tumors in vitro and in vivo.[31] Recent data in our rat laryngeal transplant model have provided support for the use of everolimus as an effective immunosuppressive in laryngeal transplantation.[32,33] Everolimus' effect upon the growth of a mouse SCCa cell-line in both intradermal tumors and pulmonary metastases was more recently studied.[34] Mice received either everolimus 1 mg/kg/bid, everolimus 0.5 mg/kg/bid, cyclosporine 7.5 mg/kg/day, or no treatment. Tumors cells were injected either intradermally or pulmonary metastases were established through tail-vein injections. Everolimus showed statistically significant tumor inhibition at 1.0 mg/kg/bid and 0.5 mg/kg/day when compared with animals treated with cyclosporine and to untreated animals ($P < 0.0001$). Tumor inhibition was evident in both models studied (intradermal tumors and pulmonary metastasis generation). The authors concluded that everolimus provides potent tumor inhibition in animals inoculated with SCC VII cells by decreasing local spread of disease as well as distant metastases.

23.6 Conclusions

Now over 10 years after its attempt, successful total laryngeal transplantation has become a reality. The patient reports a vastly improved quality of life, including smell, taste, daily communication, and emotional expression through a voice that is uniquely his own. As healthy individuals, we take for granted the simple ability to clear our own nose or to express a cry with which others can empathize. But in his review of the recent larynx transplant, the reviewer, a transplant physician himself who underwent a laryngectomy 7 years earlier, stated that given the despair associated with losing his own larynx, "if I were 40 years old I would probably consider undergoing the operation myself."[35] Clearly, advances in the areas of immunosuppression and reinnervation must continue. But given the present day research in all transplanted organ systems, the day is not far off when immunosuppression without comorbidities will be a reality, and the lessons we learn today will benefit the many potential candidates for laryngeal transplantation in the future.

Acknowledgments The authors thank Mark Sabo for his artistic excellence and Mary Kalan for her assistance in preparing the manuscript.

References

1. R. Boles, Surgical replantation of the larynx in dogs: a progress report, *Laryngoscope* **76**, 1057–1067 (1966).
2. J. H. Ogura, M. Kawasaki, S. Takenouchi, e al., Replantation and transplantation of the canine larynx, *Ann Otol Rhino Laryng* **75**, 295–312 (1966).
3. G. E. Silver, P. S. Lieber, M. L. Som, Autologous transplantation of the canine larynx, *Arch Otolaryngol* **86**, 95–102 (1967).
4. P. Kluyskens, S. Ringoir, Follow-up of a human larynx transplantation, *Laryngoscope* **80**, 1244–1250 (1970).
5. M. Strome, J. Wu, S. Stome, et al., A comparison of preservation techniques in a vascularized rat laryngeal transplant model, *Laryngoscope* **104**, 666–668 (1994).
6. S. Strome, G. Brodsky, J. Darrell, et al., Histopathologic correlates of acute laryngeal allograft rejection in a rat model, *Ann Otol Rhinol Laryngol* **101**, 156–160 (1992).
7. M. Strome, S. Strome, J. Darrell, et al., The effects of cyclosporin A on transplanted rat allografts, *Laryngoscope* **103**, 394–398 (1993).
8. M. Strome, J. Stein, R. Esclamado, D. Hicks, R. R. Lorenz, W. Braun, R. Yetman, I. Eliachar, J. Mayes, Laryngeal transplantation: a case report with three-year follow-up, *N Engl J Med* **344**, 1676–1679 (2001).
9. R. R. Lorenz, D. M. Hicks, R. W. Sheilds, M. A. Fritz, M. Strome, Laryngeal nerve function after total laryngeal transplantation, *Otolaryngol – Head Neck Surg* **131**(6), 1016–1018 (2004).
10. K. F. Kevorkian, J. A. Sercarz, M. Ye, Y. M. Kim, K. H. Hong, G. S. Berke, Extended canine laryngeal preservation for transplantation, *Laryngoscope* **107**(12 Pt 1), 1623–1626 (1997).
11. E. M. Genden, A. Iskander, J. S. Bromberg, L. Mayer, The kinetics and pattern of tracheal allograft re-epithelialization, *Am J Respir Cell Mol Biol* **28**(6), 673–681 (2003).
12. M. A. Birchall, M. Bailey, E. V. Barker, H. J. Rothkotter, K. Otto, P. Macchiarini, Model for experimental revascularized laryngeal allotransplantation, *Br J Surg* **89**(11), 1470–1475 (2002).
13. R. R. Lorenz, O. Dan, M. A. Fritz, M. Strome, The rat laryngeal transplant model: technical advancements and a re-defined rejection grading system, *Ann Otol, Rhinol Laryngol* **111**(12), 1120–1127 (2002).
14. M. Nelson, O. Dan, M. Strome, Evaluation of parathyroid hormone as a functional biological marker of rat laryngeal transplant rejection, *Laryngoscope* **113**(9) (2003).
15. S. W. Barthel, O. Dan, J. Myles, et al., Effect of in vitro irradiation of donor larynges on cyclosporine requirements and rejection rates in rat laryngeal transplantation, *Ann Otol Rhinol Laryngol* **110**, 20–24 (2001).
16. R. R. Lorenz, O. Dan, M. Haug, et al., Immunosuppressive effect of irradiation in the murine laryngeal transplantation model: a controlled trial, *Ann Otol Rhinol Laryngol* **112**(8), 712–715 (2003).
17. M. Haug, O. Dan, S. Wimberley, M. Fritz, R. R. Lorenz, M. Strome, Cyclosporine dose, serum trough levels, and allograft preservation in a rat model of laryngeal transplantation, *Ann Otol Rhinol Laryngol* **112**(6), 506–510 (2003).
18. M. Nelson, M. Fritz, O. Dan, S. Worley, M. Strome, Tacrolimus and mycophenolate mofetil provide effective immunosuppression in rat laryngeal transplantation, *Laryngoscope* **113**(8), 1308–1313 (2003).
19. L. M. Akst, M. Siemionow, O. Dan, D. Izycki, M. Strome, Induction of tolerance in a rat model of laryngeal transplantation, *Transplantation* **76**(12), 1763–1770 (2003).

20. E. M. Genden, S. E. Mackinnon, S. Yu, D. A. Hunter, M. W. Flye, Portal venous ultraviolet B-irradiated donor alloantigen prevents rejection in circumferential rat tracheal allografts, *Otolaryngol Head Neck Surg* **124**(5), 481–488 (2001).
21. G. K. Gorti, M. A. Birchall, K. Haverson, P. Macchiarini, M. Bailey, A preclinical model for laryngeal transplantation: anatomy and mucosal immunology of the porcine larynx, *Transplantation* **68**(11), 1638–1642 (1999).
22. L. E. Rees, O. Ayoub, K. Haverson, M. A. Birchall, M. Bailey, Differential major histocompatibility complex class II locus expression on human laryngeal epithelium, *Clin Exp Immunol* **134**(3), 497–502 (2003).
23. S. Govindaraj, R. Gordon, E. M. Genden, Effect of fibrin matrix and vascular endothelial growth factor on re-epithelialization of orthotopic murine tracheal transplants, *Ann Otol Rhinol Laryngol* **113**(10), 797–804 (2004).
24. P. Stavroulaki, M. Birchall, Comparative study of the laryngeal innervation in humans and animal employed in laryngeal transplantation research, *J Laryngol Otol* **115**, 257–266 (2001).
25. J. H. Blumin, M. Ye, G. S. Berke, et al., Recovery of laryngeal sensation after superior laryngeal nerve anastomosis, *Laryngoscope* **109**, 1637–1641 (1999).
26. K. L. Peterson, R. J. Andrews, J. A. Sercarz, et al., Comparison of nerve banking techniques in delayed laryngeal reinnervation, *Ann Otol Rhinol Laryngol* **108**, 689–694 (1999).
27. R. J. Andrews, G. S. Berke, K. E. Blackwell, et al., Hemilaryngeal transplantation in the canine model: technique and implications, *Am J Otolaryngol* **21**, 85–91 (2000).
28. M. A. Birchall, R. R. Lorenz, E. M. Genden, B. H. Haughey, M. Siemionow, M. Strome, Laryngeal transplantation in 2005: a review, *American Journal of Transplantation* **6**(1), 20–26 (2006).
29. I. Penn, Occurrence of cancers in immunosuppressed organ transplant recipients, *Clin Transplant* 47–158 (1998).
30. R. Sedrani, S. Cottens, J. Kallen, W. L. Schuler, Chemical modification of rapamycin: the discovery of SDZ RAD, *Transpl Proc* **30**, 2192–2194 (1998).
31. A. Boulay, S. Zumstein-Mecker, C. Stephan, Antitumor efficacy of intermittent treatment schedules with the rapamycin derivative RAD001 correlates with prolonged inactivation of ribosomal protein S6 kinase 1 in peripheral blood mononuclear cells, *Cancer Res* **64**, 252–261 (2004).
32. P. D. Knott, M. Nelson, O. Dan, F. Van Lente, M. Strome, Immunosuppressive efficacy of everolimus and tacrolimus combination therapy in a rat laryngeal transplant model (submitted for publication).
33. S. S. Khariwala, P. D. Knott, O. Dan, et al., Pulsed immunosuppression with everolimus and anti-alphabeta T-cell receptor: laryngeal allograft preservation at six months. Annals of Otology, Rhinology & Laryngology. **115**(1): 74–80, 2006 Jan.
34. S. S. Khariwala, J. Kjaergaard, R. R. Lorenz, F. Van Lente, S. Shu, M. Strome, Everolimus (RAD) inhibits in vivo growth of murine squamous cell carcinoma (sec VII). Laryngoscope **116**(5): 814–820 (2006).
35. A. P. Monaco, Transplantation of the larynx: a case report that speaks for itself, *N Engl J Med* **344**, 1712–1714 (2001).

Chapter 24
Face Transplantation

Maria Siemionow and Galip Agaoglu

24.1 Introduction

Thousands of patients with severe facial disfigurements due to burns, trauma, and tumor excisions are seeking surgical treatment to reduce their suffering. Unfortunately, the aesthetic outcome of the currently available conventional reconstructive procedures (e.g., skin grafts, flaps) for facial reconstruction is not satisfactory in long-term follow-up. The best result of facial reconstruction was obtained following replantation of total face and scalp avulsion with adequate hair growth on the scalp and normal animation of the facial expression muscles.[1,2]

Advances in composite tissue allograft (CTA) transplantation opened a new era in the reconstructive field. After the first-hand transplant in France in 1998, the success in the field of CTA expands the limits of facial reconstructive procedures beyond the traditional methods.[3] Based on over 7 years experience with clinical CTA transplants the next step for facial reconstruction could be facial transplantation. Similar to clinically applicable CTA transplants, apart from the technical and immunosuppressive issues, face transplantation raises ethical, social, and psychological issues that need to be addressed. Face transplantation should be introduced as a treatment option for patients with severe facial disfigurements whose problem cannot be addressed by autologous tissues. Many studies were performed and published on the technical, immunosuppressive, and ethical issues of face transplantation with both in favor and against this challenging procedure.[4-6] We want to share our studies done on facial transplantation including development of experimental models, dealing with immunosuppressive issues as well as cadaver dissections and IRB proposal.

24.2 Experimental Facial Transplantation

Over the past 15 years, we have used different experimental models of CTA transplants under varying immunosuppressive protocols to induce tolerance for CTAs. For the last 5 years, in preparation for facial allograft transplantation in humans, we have centered our studies on facial skin transplant models to induce tolerance. This included both full face and hemiface transplant models.[7-11]

To confirm the feasibility of the total facial/scalp allograft transplantation, a full facial/scalp transplant model across major histocompatibility barriers was introduced.[7,8] This is the first experimental study to confirm long-term survival of the full-facial allograft transplants in a rodent model. Transplants were performed between semiallogeneic Lewis–Brown Norway (LBN, RT1) and Lewis (LEW, RT1) recipients. The entire facial skin, scalp, and both ears were harvested based on the common carotid arteries and external jugular veins. In the recipient, facial skin, scalp, and external ears were removed. The facial nerve and muscles, the perioral and the periorbital regions were preserved to avoid functional deficits. Bilateral common carotid or external carotid arteries were used to vascularize the entire facial flap. Venous anastomoses were performed to the external jugular and anterior facial veins (Fig. 24.1). The recipient animals were treated with CsA monotherapy in dose of 16 mg/kg/day, which was tapered to 2 mg/kg/day over 4 weeks, and maintained at this level during the follow-up period of over 200 days (Fig. 24.2).

Recently, to improve the survival of facial/scalp allograft recipients, we have introduced a new approach by modifying the arterial anastomoses in the recipients.[9] Single (unilateral) common carotid artery of the recipient was used to vascularize the entire transplanted facial/scalp flap. Different modifications of the arterial anastomoses were performed (Fig. 24.3). With these modifications, postoperative

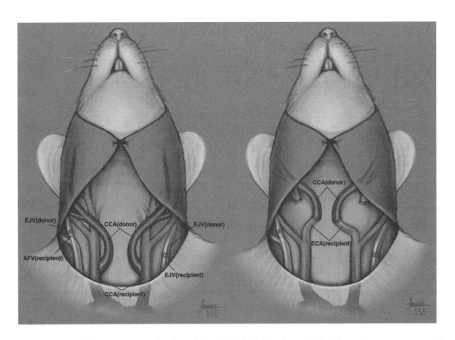

Fig. 24.1 Arterial anastomoses in the original full facial/scalp model. Bilateral common carotid arterial anastomoses in the recipient (*left*). *CCA* common carotid artery, *EJV* external jugular vein, *AFV* anterior facial vein. Bilateral external carotid arterial anastomoses in the recipient (*right*). *CCA* common carotid artery, *ECA* external carotid artery

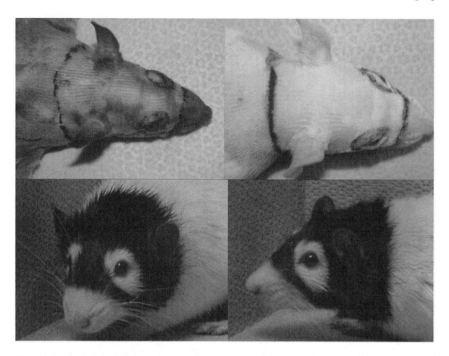

Fig. 24.2 The full-facial allograft transplantation model. Preoperative view of the donor rat with marked facial skin flap (*above left*). Preoperative view of the recipient Lewis rat showing markings of the skin to be excised before the transplant inset (*above right*). Postoperative views of face allograft recipient on low dose of CsA monotherapy at day 200 showing no signs of rejection (*below left and right*)

mortality of the animals was significantly reduced by avoidance of complications associated with bilateral common carotid arterial anastomoses. In this model, facial/scalp allograft transplants were performed between fully allogeneic ACI (RT1[a]) donors and Lewis (RT1) recipient rats. The same CsA immunosuppressive protocol was used as in the previous model and resulted in over 180 days of facial/scalp allograft transplant survival.

To induce operational tolerance across major histocompatibility barrier, we have introduced a less technically challenging hemifacial transplant model.[10,11] Hemifacial allograft transplants were performed between semiallogeneic Lewis–Brown Norway (LBN, RT1) and fully allogeneic ACI (RT1[a]) donor rats and Lewis (RT1) recipients. In this model, hemifacial/scalp flaps including the external ear were harvested based on the common carotid artery and external jugular vein. In the recipient, the anastomoses were performed to the common carotid artery (end to side) and the external jugular vein (end to end). Recipients received CsA monotherapy (16 mg/kg) immunosuppressive protocol which was tapered to 2 mg/kg over 4 weeks and maintained at this dose during the follow-up period. Under this protocol, survival rates of over 400 days in semiallogeneic and 330 days in fully allogeneic transplants were achieved (Fig. 24.4).

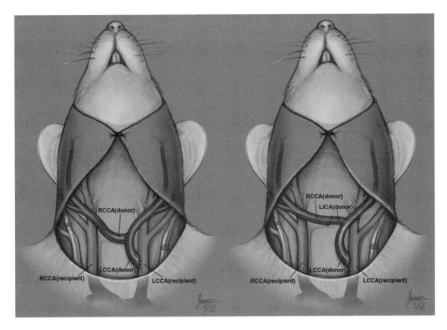

Fig. 24.3 Arterial anastomoses in the modified full facial/scalp model. *Modification 1*. Unilateral arterial anastomoses in the recipient (*left*). *LCCA* left common carotid artery, *RCCA* right common carotid artery. *Modification 2*. Unilateral arterial anastomoses in the recipient (*right*). *LCCA* left common carotid artery, *RCCA* right common carotid artery, *LICA* left internal carotid artery

Our success in both full and hemifacial/scalp transplant models under CsA monotherapy is promising, and taking into consideration the success that has been achieved in the field of CTA transplantation in humans, the next logical step as follow-up of these studies would be development of facial transplantation model in humans.

24.3 Preparation for Human Transplantation

To date, there are only two scalp transplantations described in the literature. The first one was performed between identical twins.[12] The patient had scalp avulsion and was treated initially with skin grafts taken from her identical twin. The twins were HLA identical and had identical blood groups. Two free scalp flaps, based on the superficial temporal vessels, were performed in two separate sessions. Six months after surgery, without any immunosuppressive regimen, the patient presented with adequate hair growth on the transplanted scalp flaps.

The second scalp transplant was recently performed in 72-year-old woman with stage IIIC recurrent cutaneous malignant melanoma on the vertex.[13] Wide excision of the tumor including the scalp, facial/cervical skin, and two ears was performed.

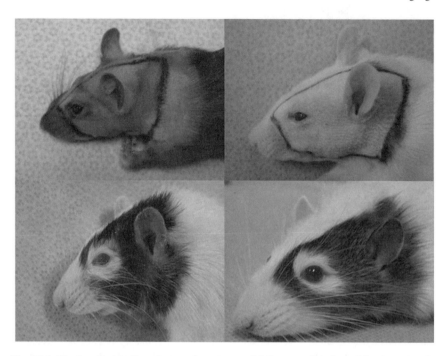

Fig. 24.4 The hemifacial allograft transplantation model. Preoperative view of the donor Lewis–Brown Norway rat showing markings of the facial skin flap (*above left*). Preoperative view of the recipient showing marking of the skin to be excised before inset of the flap (*above right*). Postoperative views of hemifacial allograft recipient at day 400 posttransplant with no signs of rejection on low maintenance dose of CsA monotherapy (*below left and right*)

The defect was reconstructed by CTA, including scalp and both external ears, transplanted from a brain-dead young man. The patient received tacrolimus, mycophenolate mofetil, steroids, and Zenapax as an immunosuppressive protocol. The follow-up of 4 months was presented. This transplant raises many technical, ethical, social, and legal concerns as this elderly cancer patient was not the proper candidate for such extensive treatment requiring lifelong immunosuppression therapy.[14]

For the face transplantation to become a clinical reality, there are many questions which need to be addressed, including technical, immunosuppressive, ethical, psychosocial, and economical issues.

In preparation for facial allograft transplantation in humans, we have performed a series of cadaver dissections.[15,16]

To study the technical feasibility of face transplantation, we have harvested the entire face and scalp including the external ears based on the external carotid arteries and external jugular and facial veins (Fig. 24.5). Methylene blue dye injection revealed integrity of the vascular territories of the harvested facial/scalp flap. We have also measured the total surface area of the harvested facial flaps with and without scalp and the surface areas of the alternative conventional flaps. The mean surface area for total facial/scalp flap with and without scalp was $1,192 \pm 38.2$ and

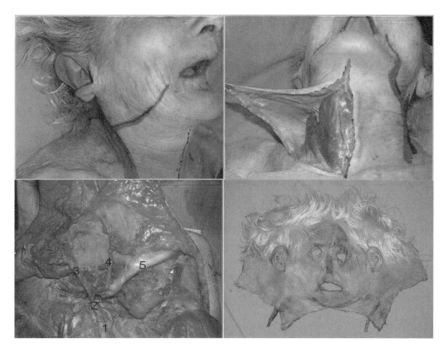

Fig. 24.5 Dissection of the facial/scalp flap from the donor. Following marking of the vascular structure (*above left*) the flap was elevated in subplatysmal plane (*above right*). Elevation of the flap showing arterial network of the flap (*below left*): *1* the common carotid artery, *2* the external carotid artery, *3* the superficial temporal artery, *4* the facial artery, *5* lower border of mandible. The frontal view of the harvested total facial/scalp flap (*below right*)

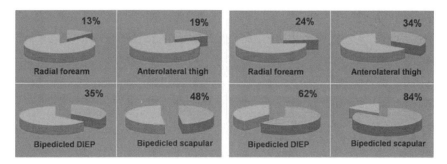

Fig. 24.6 Outline of the percentage of the conventional flaps that covers the surface area of a total facial scalp defect (*left*) and a facial defect without scalp (*right*). *DIEP* deep inferior epigastric perforator

$675\pm22.3\,cm^2$, respectively. It was found that the largest alternative conventional flap (bipedicle scapular–parascapular flap) covered only 50% of the total facial/scalp defect (Fig. 24.6). We concluded that perfect match of facial skin color, texture, and pliability could be achieved only by the tissue of similar characteristics, which can be supplied by facial skin transplantation from the human cadaver donors.[15]

In another cadaver study to simulate clinical circumstances, we have performed mock facial transplantation. Total facial/scalp flaps were harvested from the donor cadavers and transplanted into the recipient cadavers. During flap harvesting from the donor cadavers, we have measured the time of facial/scalp flap harvesting and the length of the vascular pedicles and sensory nerves that were included in the flap. In the recipient cadaver after excision of the facial skin in the form of a monoblock full-thickness skin graft, time of facial flap inset into the recipient was evaluated and the optimal sequences of flap attachment were outlined (Figs. 24.7 and 24.8). We have estimated that the total mean time of facial flap harvest and inset into the recipient cadaver was 5h and 20min, and the best sequences of flap inset and anchoring during this mock facial transplantation are presented in Table 24.1.[16]

Based on these cadaver studies, we have confirmed the technical feasibility of facial skin transplantation and this has further encouraged us to address one of the most debatable issues following face transplantation which is related to "identity transfer." To test this, we have performed a series of cadaver studies to evaluate facial appearance of the recipient cadavers following mock facial transplantation

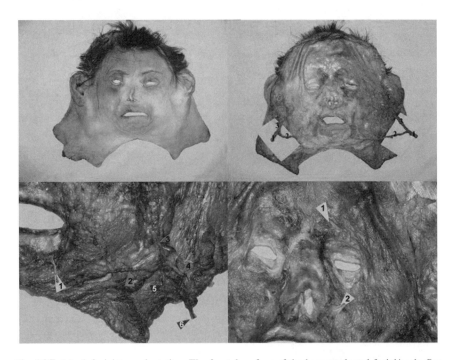

Fig. 24.7 Mock facial transplantation. The frontal surface of the harvested total facial/scalp flap (*above left*). The inverted surface area of the flap (*above right*): *1* the external carotid artery, *2* the facial artery, *3* the superficial temporal artery. The inverted surface of the harvested total facial/scalp flap showing preserved sensory nerves, and arterial and venous pedicles (*below left*): *1* the mental nerve, *2* the facial artery, *3* the superficial temporal artery, *4* the external carotid artery, *5* the facial vein, *6* the external jugular vein. The sensory nerves (*below right*): *1* the supraorbital nerve, *2* the infraorbital nerve

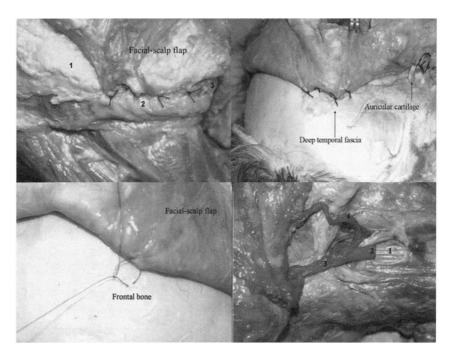

Fig. 24.8 Anchoring of the facial/scalp flap in the recipient cadaver. Fixation to the mandibular ligament region (*above left*): *1* the platysma, *2* the mandibular border, *3* the mentum. Facial flap fixation to the temporalis fascia and suturing of the auricular cartilages of the external ears (*above right*). Flap anchoring to the frontal bone by the suture passing through the tunnel created in the cortical bone (*below left*). The vascular pedicles of the donor facial flap were approximated to their respective vessels in the recipient for future vascular anastomoses (*below right*): *1* the recipient's external carotid artery, *2* the donor's external carotid artery, *3* the donor's superficial temporal artery, *4* the donor's facial artery

Table 24.1 Sequences of mock facial transplantation procedure

1	Transfer of the donor facial flap into the recipient's facial defect
2	Coaptation of the supraorbital, infraorbital, and mental nerves
3	Anchoring of the flap at the region of the mandibular and zygomatic ligaments
4	Anchoring of the flap to the preauricular region, mastoid fascia, and temporal fascia
5	Anchoring of the flap to the frontal bones
6	Closure of the upper and lower gingivobuccal incisions
7	Closure of the upper and lower conjunctival incisions
8	Anastomoses of the external carotid arteries between the donor and recipient
9	Anastomoses of the facial veins between the donor and recipient
10	Coaptation of the great auricular nerves
11	Anastomoses of the external jugular veins between the donor and recipient
12	Closure of the skin incisions

(unpublished data). The appearance of the harvested facial/scalp flaps was also assessed after mounting them on artificial head models made of Glass and Styrofoam. We have found that facial features of the recipient cadavers after facial skin flap transplantation from different donors were a combination of donor and recipient features. In contrast, when the harvested donor flaps were mounted on the artificial head models serving as the recipients, the donor flap took the appearance of the recipient's head model.

Over the past 4 years, there has been a vigorous social, ethical, and psychological debate within the medical community on aspects of face transplantation.[4–6,17] There is, however, an agreement that if this procedure is considered in the future, a team of experts from different specialties should evaluate the potential candidates for the facial transplantation.[18] Since face transplantation would require lifelong immunosuppression, which exposes the recipients to significant life-threatening complications and uncertain benefits, the question was raised if surgeons should proceed.[4]

The French National Ethics Advisory Committee refused an application of plastic surgeons led by Lantieri to perform transplantation of facial subunits, based on inherent risks of the procedure.[19]

Louisville group has outlined the ethical criteria and weighed risk/benefit factors taking into account the physical, aesthetic psychological, and social dimensions of facial disfigurement, reconstruction, and transplantation. They, however, stated that "time has come to move facial transplantation research into the clinical phase."[5] Based on the work of Moore, they emphasized the significance of public discussion as an ethical requirement for any innovative surgery.[5]

Agich and Siemionow,[20] however, stated that none of the work of Moore does clearly argue that open display and public discussion are an ethical requirement for an innovative surgical procedure. They have emphasized that the rights of patients with severe facial deformities to improve their quality of life should be included in any discussion on facial transplantation and the suffering of patients with severe facial disfigurement must be recentered in the public ethical discussions.

The opponents of the transplantation procedure bring an issue of consequences in case of facial flap rejection. They argue that the psychological consequences of graft rejection will be enormous and issues related to facial identity considered an important ethical contraindication.[6,17] It is clear that the psychological consequences of graft rejection would be significant, but to be prepared, in our protocol we have outlined all rescue procedures which will include application of autologous skin grafts to provide face coverage similar or better than the pretransplant condition.[20]

Based on over 15 years of research on the technical and immunological aspects of CTA transplants and the biological evidence that facial transplants work in the experimental setup, we performed a series of cadaver studies presenting feasibility, anatomy, and technical aspects of facial flap harvest. All this data served as the base for an IRB protocol, which was submitted for review and evaluation.

After 10 months of debate on the medical, ethical, and psychological issues related to facial transplantation, The Cleveland Clinic Foundation's Institutional Review Board approved the protocol presented by Dr. Maria Siemionow. This approval permits the Clinic to screen and evaluate patients with severe facial disfigurements, and considers them as potential candidates for facial skin transplantation.[18]

24.4 Future Approaches

At this stage, the appearance of the recipient's face after facial transplantation is difficult to predict. However, computer-based modeling studies suggest that the face would take more of the characteristics of the recipient skeleton than the soft tissues of the donor.[6] Our cadaver studies have shown that it is difficult to asses facial appearance since all the cadavers looked alike as usually have widely open eyes and lack facial expression. The recipient cadaver appearance after mock facial transplantation was neither like the donor nor like the recipient but was a mixture of both. When the harvested flaps were mounted on head models, they looked more like the models (unpublished data). In the future, head models of different size and shape can be used to assess the appearance of facial flaps. In addition computer simulation software can also be used to predict facial appearance after transplantation. The 3D CT scans of different bony skeletons of the faces can be draped with different cadaver facial skin flaps correlation of donor and recipient features can be evaluated.

At this stage, we have substantial anatomical knowledge, microsurgical skills, and immunological expertise to make facial transplantation a clinical reality. However, before we proceed, the risk/benefits of lifelong immunosuppression should be validated, and the ethical and psychological factors should be presented and discussed with potential candidates. The patients with severe facial disfigurements should be informed about all available reconstructive options, including facial allograft transplantation. When the risk and benefits are presented and understood by the psychologically stable candidates, it should be patient's right to choose what is crucial for their life.

References

1. A. Thomas, V. Obed, A. Murarka, et al., Total face and scalp replantation, *Plast Reconstr Surg* **102**, 2085–2087 (1998).
2. B. J. Wilhelmi, R. H. Kang, K. Movassaghi, et al., First successful replantation of face and scalp with single-artery repair: model for face and scalp transplantation, *Ann Plast Surg* **50**, 535–540 (2003).
3. J. M. Dubernard, E. Owen, G. Herzberg, et al., Human hand allograft: report on first 6 months, *Lancet* **353**, 1315–1320 (1999).
4. P. E. M. Butler, A. Clarke, R. E. Aschcroft, Face transplantation: when and for whom? *Am J Bioethics* **4**, 16–17 (2004).
5. O. P. Wiggins, J. H. Barker, S. Martinez, et al., On the ethics of facial transplantation research, *Am J Bioethics* **4**, 1–12 (2004).

6. P. J. Morris, J. A. Bradley, L. Doyal, et al., Facial transplantation: a working party report from the Royal College of Surgeons of England, *Transplantation* **77**, 330–338 (2004).
7. M. Siemionow, B. Gozel-Ulusal, A. Ulusal, et al., Functional tolerance following face transplantation in the rat, *Transplantation* **75**, 1607–1609 (2003).
8. B. G. Ulusal, A. E. Ulusal, S. Ozmen, et al., A new composite facial and scalp transplantation model in rats, *Plast Reconstr Surg* **112**, 1302–1311 (2003).
9. S. Unal, G. Agaoglu, M. Siemionow, New surgical approach in facial transplantation extends survival of allograft recipients, *Ann Plast Surg* **55**(3), 297–303 (2005).
10. Y. Demir, S. Ozmen, A. Klimczak, Tolerance induction in composite facial allograft transplantation in the rat model, *Plast Reconstr Surg* **114**, 1790–1801 (2004).
11. Y. Demir, S. Ozmen, A. Klimczak, et al., Strategies to develop chimerism in vascularized skin allografts across MHC barrier. *Microsurgery* **25**(5), 415–22 (2005).
12. H. J. Buncke, W. Y. Hoffman, B. S. Alpert, et al., Microvascular transplant of two free scalp flaps between identical twins, *Plast Reconstr Surg* **70**, 605–609 (1982).
13. H. Q. Jiang, Y. Wang, X. B. Hu, Y. S. Li, J. S. Li, Composite tissue allograft transplantation of cephalocervical skin flap and two ears, *Plast Reconstr Surg* **115**(3), 31e–35e; discussion 36e–37e (2005).
14. M. Siemionow, G. Agaoglu, Controversies following the report on transplantation of cephalocervical skin flap, *Plast Reconstr Surg* **118**(1), 268–270 (2006).
15. M. Siemionow, S. Unal, G. Agaoglu, et al., A cadaver study in preparation for facial allograft transplantation in humans: Part I. What are alternative sources for total facial defect coverage? *Plast Reconstr Surg* **119**(3), 1114–1115 (2006).
16. M. Siemionow, G. Agaoglu, S. Unal, A cadaver study in preparation for facial allograft transplantation in humans: Part II. Mock facial transplantation, *Plast Reconstr Surg* **117**(3), 876–885 (2006).
17. A. Caplan, Facing ourselves, *Am J Bioethics* **4**, 18–20 (2004).
18. M. Siemionow, G. Agaoglu, Allotransplantation of the face: how close are we? *Clin Plast Surg* **32**, 401–409 (2005).
19. Working Group-Comité Consultatif National d'Ethique (CCNE): Composite Tissue Allotransplantation of the Face (Full or Partial Facial Transplant) (6 February 2004). http://www.ccne_ethique.fr/english/avis/a_082.htm
20. G. J. Agich, M. Siemionow, Facing the ethical questions in facial transplantation, *Am J Bioethics* **4**, 25–27 (2004).

Chapter 25
The Role of Allografts in Lower Extremity Reconstruction

Milton B. Armstrong, Ricardo Jimenez-Lee, and Eddie Manning

25.1 History

Early in the history of lower extremity reconstruction, some basic concepts and principles were defined:

- Incision, drainage, and debridement of dead tissue were advocated by Pierre-Joseph Desault (1744–1795).
- Ollier introduced fracture stabilization with casting.
- Sir Arbuthnot Lane's The Operative Treatment of Fractures was published in 1905.
- Gillies and the concept of plastic surgery were sponsored by Lane in 1915.
- Closed plaster treatment of lower extremity wounds was the standard of car by WWI as described by Orr.
- By 1939, Trueta improved on this by advocating debridement before plaster application with improved results and decreased incidence of osteomyelitis.
- Delayed primary closure was introduced by the end of WWII.
- Presently, the exponential rate of improvements in osseous and soft tissue injury management make the reconstructive approach to the lower extremity a challenging and exciting endeavor.[1–5]

Although the majority of debate over composite tissue allotransplantation (CTA) is centered upon the reconstruction of hands and upper limbs, there is a small but growing body of literature addressing the significance of this modality in correcting lower extremity deformities. One of the first accounts of CTA was depicted by Jacopo da Varagine in AD 1270, in the famous painting of "The Legend of The Black Leg." This illustration was inspired by the replacement of a gangrenous and cancerous leg of a sleeping man with an amputated limb from a recently deceased Ethiopian Moor, conducted by the physician twins Saint Cosmos and Saint Damian in AD 348. More recently and prior to the elucidation of transplant immunology, immunosuppression, or even antibiotics, the first composite knee transplants were performed in humans by Erich Lexer in 1908.[6] Despite the early failure of these grafts, the stage was set for CTA of lower extremity tissues. To this end, the significance of the vascular anatomy of these composite grafts was realized in 1990, when

Chiron et al.,[7] performed the first vascularized allogeneic transplant of a human femoral diaphysis. Unfortunately without immunosuppression these grafts ultimately failed as well. The common cause of failure appeared to be disruption of vascular perfusion, i.e., acute rejection. The advent of immunosuppressive pharmaceuticals allowed amelioration or at least temporization of acute rejection episodes. With these advances we have achieved prolonged viability of vascularized composite tissue allografts of the lower extremity.

25.2 Etiology of Lower Extremity Wounds

Many attempts have been made to define lower extremity injuries to optimize management and outcomes. Multiple prognostic scores are available to the reconstructive surgeon. These should be regarded as tools in the assessment and planning of the approach to each wound, but should not rigidly dictate the final intervention. One might assume that salvage of a limb might not be considered with high trauma scores in any of the scoring systems but this has not been the case. Improvements in tissue engineering have made other tools available to the clinician.

25.3 Management of Lower Extremity Wounds

Management of lower extremity wounds and defects is dependent on etiology.[8] In the case of trauma, the severity and extent of injury translate into a range of management modalities; from closed management of low-energy closed fractures to external fixation of comminuted tibial fractures with free tissue transfer for coverage of a soft tissue defects. Clinical assessment of a wound is the principal determinant of the specific intervention. Other tools are essential in the assessment of these defects, such as the use of angiography in the reconstructive planning of a complex lower extremity fracture with loss of soft tissues where the recipient vessels are in question. Scoring systems are useful in communicating findings and defining strategies when a multidisciplinary team is involved with the patients care. These tools help define the goals and limitations of the operation and rehabilitation improving outcomes.

One of the sequelae of high-energy lower extremity trauma is a chronic infection or osteomyelitis. The zone of injury is very important in the acute setting but takes lesser importance in the face of osteomyelitis, although it should not be totally disregarded. In the inflammatory reaction a chronic infection is easy to underestimate and might prove the undoing of a perfectly planned reconstructive approach. Fibrosis in the surrounding soft tissues is hard to assess preoperatively. Therefore one should backtrack and reassess the cause of the chronic event and plan accordingly.

Color Plates

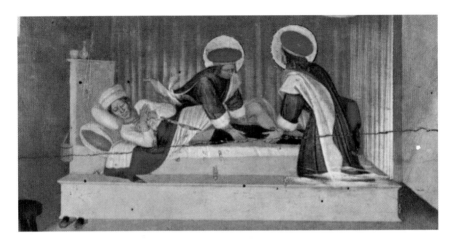

Fig. 2.1 Saints Cosmas and Damian performing a posthumous limb allograft transplant. (With permission from Gordon CR, Nazzal J, Lozano-Calderan SA, et al. "From experimental rat hindlimb to clinical face composite tissue allotransplantation: historical background and current status." Microsurgery 26(8):566–72, 2006.)

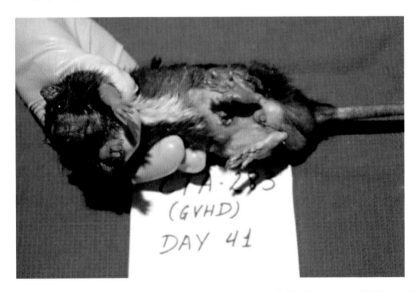

Fig. 19.1 Graft-versus-host-disease in a LEW to LBN CTA/VBMT recipient. LEW to LBN composite tissue allograft/vascularized bone marrow transplant undergoing one-way donor antihost graft-versus-host disease day 41 posttransplant

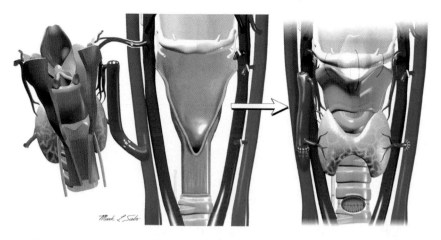

Fig. 23.1 The 1998 surgical technique of laryngeal transplantation. Anastomoses included the donor right internal jugular vein to recipient right facial vein, donor superior thyroid arteries to recipient superior thyroid arteries, and donor left middle thyroid vein to recipient left internal jugular vein. Note that both superior laryngeal nerves were anastomosed, while only the patient's right recurrent laryngeal nerve could be located for anastomosis

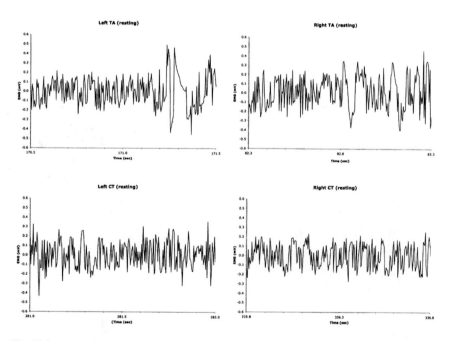

Fig. 23.3 (a) Resting laryngeal EMG tracings of four phonatory muscles 4 years after transplantation. (b) Laryngeal EMG tracings on phonation with "ee" and raising and lowering of pitch (*TA* thryoarytenoid muscle; *CT* cricothyroid muscle)

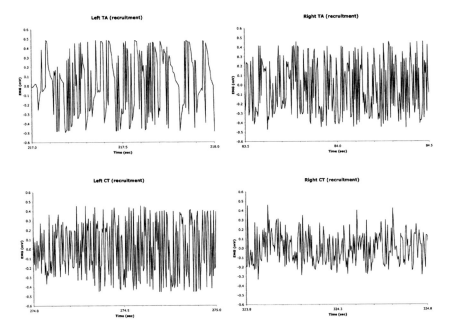

Fig. 23.3 (continued)

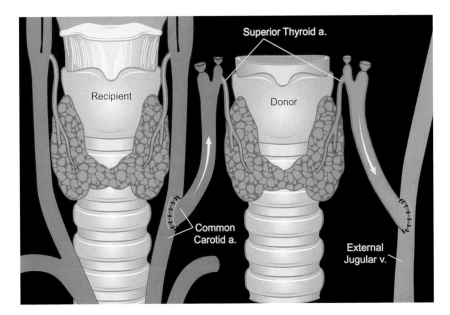

Fig. 23.4 (a) The rat model for laryngeal transplantation. The donor organ is placed in tandem to the recipient's airway and an arteriovenous shunt is used for venous outflow through the left superior thyroid artery.

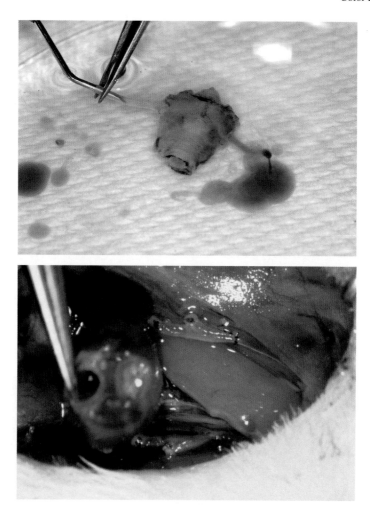

Fig. 23.4 (continued) (**b**) The donor organ being flushed with Wisconsin's solution prior to revascularization (**c**) The donor organ being rotated superiorly in tandem in the left neck of the recipient rat. Arterial and venous anastomoses are shown as blood flow reestablished

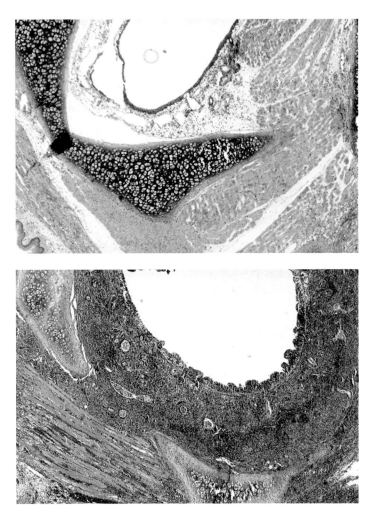

Fig. 23.5 (a) Histologic specimen of rat laryngeal transplant in Lewis to Lewis rat negative control after 15 days following transplantation (×5). Laryngeal architecture including epithelium, minor salivary glands, muscle, and cartilage preserved (b) Histologic specimen of rat laryngeal transplant in LBN-f to Lewis rat after 7 days following transplantation without immunosuppression (×10). Tremendous infiltration of lymphocytes occurs in the subepithelial layer.

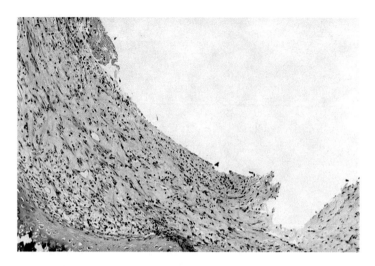

Fig. 23.5 (continued) (**c**) Histologic specimen of rat laryngeal transplant in LBN-f to Lewis rat after 15 days following transplantation without immunosuppression (×10). Laryngeal architecture is lost, with destruction of the epithelium and subepithelial minor salivary glands

Lower extremity defects secondary to oncologic procedures are addressed in an individual basis. These require a close working relationship between the oncologic surgeon and his reconstructive counterpart, yet the guidelines outlined in the scenario of trauma are translatable into the oncologic reconstruction and may provide an empirical basis for surgical planning.

In the face of neoplasms, the defect is dictated by the extent of the oncologic resection but essentially follows the same principles as in the trauma setting. Chronic infection, as in the case of osteomyelitis, follows similar guidelines as trauma except that debridement of affected tissue and the zone of injury may be decreased as compared to the acute setting, yet often require radical resections[9–12] similar to those performed for neoplastic processes. Regardless of the need for soft tissue reconstruction, a stable structural osseous platform and a sensate limb are requirements prior to entertaining a reconstructive endeavor. Loss of neurosensory function in the extremity precludes any intervention given that an insensate limb is of little use to the patient who would be better served by an amputation both from the rehabilitation and socioeconomic standpoint. Most osseous defects are currently addressed by internal or external fixation, depending on the severity of comminution and soft tissue loss. Where indicated vascularized bone flaps, bone grafts, distraction osteogenesis, and/or osseous allografts may be indicated for limb salvage.

25.3.1 Gustilo Classification of Open Fractures of the Tibia[13]

Any eventual reconstruction is dependent on the initial measures taken to address in the defect initially. Debridement and lavage are essential in the initial management of lower extremity traumatic wounds. Bhandari compared high versus low pressure lavage, reporting that high pressure lavage was more effective at an interval of 6 h at mechanically decreasing the bacterial count.

Type	Description
I	Open fracture with a wound <1 cm
II	Open fracture with a wound >1 cm
III	Open fracture with extensive soft tissue damage
IIIA	III with adequate soft tissue coverage
IIIB	III with soft tissue loss with periosteal stripping and exposed bone
IIIC	III with arterial injury requiring repair

Byrd and colleagues[8] have reported decreased complication rate with early or acute (<6 days) treatment of open tibial fractures; with an average complication rate of approximately 18%. After this period complications increased by over a twice that reported on the acute phase (as high as 50%)[9]. Godina's findings advocate that an early intervention with stable soft tissue coverage results in a decreased complication rate. Presently, the standard of care is early debridement of devitalized tissues, osseous stabilization, and soft tissue coverage. Negative pressure dressings, such as the vacuum-assisted closure, may serve as a bridge between debridement and the eventual reconstruction.[11, 12, 13]

25.3.2 Bone Reconstructive Techniques

Bone grafts[14]:

- Defects <3 cm.

Vascularized bone transfers[15–17]:

- Defects >6 cm.
- Common donors:
  - Fibula
  - Iliac crest
  - Scapula

- Prolonged interval between intervention and weight bearing (approx. 2 years). Distraction osteogenesis[18–22]: defects >6 cm.
- After frame placement distraction proceeds at a rate of 1 mm/day until the defect is spanned, this usually takes 1 year.
- This modality has the advantage of an anatomically correct reconstruction; it also advances soft tissue during the process (Cierny).[20]
- Often microvascular tissue transfers are necessary for acute coverage of neurovascular structures and/or bone. Secondary scarring and/or pedicle placement may limit distraction in this setting (Vasconez and Nicholls).[19]
- This procedure is fraught with minor complications such as pintrack infections, joint stiffness, and pain.

25.4 Soft Tissue Reconstruction[10, 23–27]

25.4.1 Local Flaps Versus Microvascular Tissue Transfers

Pedicled local flaps may be inappropriate when treating traumatic lower extremity wounds because of the extent of the zone of injury, in which case microvascular tissue transfer may result in decreased short-term complications. With regard to neoplastic or infectious etiology, zone of injury becomes less of an issue and local tissue flaps become a more viable option.

Thigh[24]:

- Skin grafts on exposed muscle.

- Sartorious with limited inflammatory process or small zone of injury and exposed neurovascular bundle.
- Smaller defects may be covered with gracilis or tensor fascia lata flaps.
- Vertical rectus abdominis myocutaneous or muscle flaps when neurovascular bundle is exposed and there is an extensive zone of injury or severe inflammatory process.

Proximal third or knee[23–27]:

- Defects of 25 cm² in surface.
- Either head gastrocnemius, proximally based Soleus, or bipedicled tibialis anterior.

Middle third[26, 27, 28]:

- Proximally based Soleus
- Either head of gastrocnemius
- Tibialis anterior
- Lower portion of middle third:
  - Flexor digitorum longus
  - Extensor digitorum longus
  - Extensor hallucis longus
  - Flexor hallucis longus

Distal third[27]:

- Microvascular tissue transfer

Foot[28–32]:

- Weight-bearing aspect:
  - Skin grafts if adequate soft tissue
  - Microvascular tissue transfers with skin graft when soft tissue inadequate
  - Toe fillet flaps
  - Local muscle or fasciocutaneous flaps:

    Instep flap
    Lateral plantar flap

- Nonweight-bearing aspect:

Skin grafts

Microvascular muscle transfers are indicated for obliteration of dead space when present and to improve vascularity in the wound. Composite tissue transplantation provides both skeletal and soft tissue support. Serafin and Voci[33] provide an excellent review of composite tissue transplantation. Fasciocutaneous flaps have been reported to be adequate for lower third defects with improved contour reconstruction, yet these flaps fail to fulfill the goal of obliterating dead space. The most commonly used donor muscles are the latissimus, serratus, rectus, and gracilis.

Tissue expansion in the lower extremity is fraught with complications, with infection rates as high as 30%.[34] Tissue expansion may be considered when other options are unavailable.

25.5 Composite Tissue Allotransplantation

Presently there are three published cases of vascularized femoral diaphysis CTA, five total knee joints, and seven nonvascularized peripheral nerve allograft transplants.[35-38] The technical feasibility of vascularized transplantation of lower extremity CTA was well established in animal models over 30 years ago by Reeves.[39] In these studies, total knee joints were transplanted with sufficient vascular pedicles to allow recipient-graft anastamosis and reestablishment of perfusion. Additionally the use of immunosuppressive agents present at that time highlighted the importance of understanding transplant immunology.

The three cases of vascularized transplantation of human femoral diaphysis were published in *Transplantation Proceedings* (1998) by Hofmann et al.[40] from Murnau, Germany. In this study, recipients were matched via blood group compatibilities, vascular anastamosis were performed in an end-to-side manner, osteosyntheses were performed using intramedullary compression nails, and all recipients were treated with immunosuppression therapy. During the induction period (3 days), quadruple therapy was administered. The regimen consisted of Cyclosporine A, Azathioprine, Antithymocyte globulin, and Methyprednisone. At 1-week postoperatively, the immunosuppressive regimen was changed to double therapy with Cyclosporine A and Azathioprine only. All immunosuppressive therapy was eventually withdrawn after 2 years. The grafts remained viable during the study period and full functional status was restored to those individuals.

The first successful vascularized transplantation of a human total knee joint was achieved by the same group. The details of this case were published in *The Archives of Orthooperative Trauma Surgery* (1997).[35] In contrast to the first described human total knee transplant performed by Lexer in 1908, the Hofmann group employed vascular anastamosis, adequate osteosyntheses, and immunosuppression which produced satisfactory results. This group subsequently transplanted two additional total knee CTA, recognizing the same general principles of revascularization, intramedullary fixation, and immunosuppression. Hofmann et al.[35] concluded that preservation of the periosteal vascularity was crucial to the survival of the grafts. To this end intramedullary nailing and fixation are identified as the preferred method of osteosynthesis. Furthermore, the preferred means of establishing recipient-graft vascular continuity were the end-to-side vascular anastamosis.

As noted previously the major obstacle in these cases was overcoming rejection. The subjects in these trials were matched with respect to ABO compatibilities with no regard for HLA mismatch. As a result multiple episodes of acute and chronic rejection were documented. With the use of double therapy immunosuppression (cyclosporine A and azathioprine), these problems were lessened. However, the major detractor of this type of therapy is the necessity for lifelong immunosuppression and the associated adverse effects, i.e., CMV, DVT, recurrent superficial, as well as deep tissue infections.

The complex antigenicity of composite tissue allografts presents a unique challenge to our current understanding of transplant immunology. These grafts are comprised of multiple tissue types, i.e., skin, muscle, tendon, bone, bone marrow, blood vessels, and adipose. It is this broad array of proteins that is believed to make composite tissue allotransplants so much more challenging than orthotopic organ transplantation with regards to immunological tolerance induction. There is published data detailing less complex CTA involving peripheral nerve and vascularized tendon grafts. Mackinnon et al.,[41] from Washington University, published a report in *The Journal of the American Society of Plastic Surgery* (2001), in which they described seven peripheral nerve allografts. The subjects were individuals who sustained injuries that produced nerve gaps greater than that, which could be reconstructed with autografts. They ranged from 72 to 350cm in length. All patients were initially treated with immunosuppression which was subsequently withdrawn after 6 months and once regeneration across the allograft was established. All of the patients regained sensory function but three out of the seven also regained motor function. No neuronal deterioration was noted after discontinuation of the immunosuppression however, one allograft was rejected.

As evidenced by the many successful composite tissue allograft transplantations, the technical challenges associated with these procedures have, for the most part, been overcome. The importance of preservation of the vascular pedicle and restoration of perfusion to these grafts in underscored by the marked increase in the survival as well as function capacity demonstrated in the literature. Currently the major obstacle to the use of CTA remains an adequate alternative means of immunomodulation without chronic immunosuppression.[42] The inherent side effects of current immunosuppressive therapy bolster the argument that these life-enhancing measures may not be appropriate treatment options for those who undergo severely disfiguring or functionally limiting limb alterations. Current dispute seems to favor the use of immunosuppressive therapy only in cases where allografts are used as a life-saving measure. As a result multiple studies are underway to investigate alternative means of immunomodulation to improve tolerance to composite tissue allotransplants.

Elster et al.,[43] at the Naval Medical Research Center in Bethesda, Maryland, are currently investigating a monoclonal antibody directed against CD154. This protein is a costimulatory molecule transiently expressed on T-cells. It is active in the development of an immune response. Once blocked, antigen-specific immune cell downregulation is achieved. The immune system no longer recognizes that specific antigen as foreign. The results appear to be long lasting in both rodent and primate models, with long-term vascularized graft acceptance documented. This therapy though promising is being further evaluated for possible prothrombotic effects. Early clinical trials were suspended after several thromboembolic events were documented in renal transplant patients.

Prabhune et al.,[44] from the University of Louisville, in Louisville, Kentucky, have presented work describing the induction of tolerance via mixed allogeneic chimerism. These genetic mosaics are achieved through total body irradiation and bone marrow transplantation. While this modality has proven to be effective in rodents, large animals, and primates in the induction of donor-specific tolerance, the risks of graft versus host and those associated with massive irradiation and BMT make this an investigative option for now. At least until safer means of myeloablation are developed, it is likely that human trials will not be realized.

One of the most promising investigations in the area of immunomodulation is the induction of donor-specific tolerance through the use of a CD3ɜ immunotoxin and a chemical known as *deoxyspergualin* which eliminates cytokine production by monocytes. Thomas et al.,[45] from the university of Alabama, Birmingham, Alabama, have developed a protocol using these agents together to inactivate both humoral- and cell-mediated immune responses to newly transplanted kidneys and islet cells in the rhesus monkey. They report an 80% long-term survival rate with preservation of immune response to nondonor foreign antigens.

The advent of these investigations promotes a sense of optimism for the future of CTA and its acceptance as a safe and viable modality for the reconstruction of lower extremity defects. To date, we have overcome the mechanical challenges of the surgical technique as well as those associated with maintenance of vascular supply to these grafts. Once the immunomodulation therapies are further refined, CTA is likely to become a common practice in the reconstruction of severe lower extremity defects.

Recently, at the University of Miami/Jackson Memorial Hospital the bilaminate dermal regeneration template known as *Integra* has been used in the management of complex lower extremity wounds in lieu of microvascular tissue transfer. Integra is a tissue allograft composed of silicone sheeting for stability, and a matrix of shark glycosaminoglycan and bovine collagen.[48] This matrix serves as the scaffolding for dermal regeneration. Integra's (ILS) dermal regeneration template is a biosynthetic skin substitute that allows for the early excision and prompt coverage of complex wounds.

Traditionally, Integra (Integra Life Sciences) is used for the treatment of deep partial-thickness and full-thickness skin injuries. The dermal replacement layer is a matrix of bovine tendon collagen and glycosaminoglycan, which serves as a template for the generation of neodermis.[47] The upper layer is a temporary epidermal substitute made of silicone. During neodermis formation, the silicone epidermal layer controls moisture loss from the wound. The silicone epidermal layer is removed once the neodermis has fully developed. A thin epidermal autograft is then applied over the neodermis.

In clinical trials, the Integra (ILS) method has demonstrated excellent take, with satisfactory aesthetics. An early study on artificial dermis by Heimbach confirmed its efficacy for the closure of wounds in burn victims.[46] More recent studies have reported the successful use of Integra (ILS) to aid in the closure of other types of soft tissue wounds, including skin cancer excision sites and degloving injuries.[50,51] In one study, the use of dermal regeneration template to treat degloving injuries appeared to be a viable alternative to full-thickness skin graft and tissue flaps.[48]

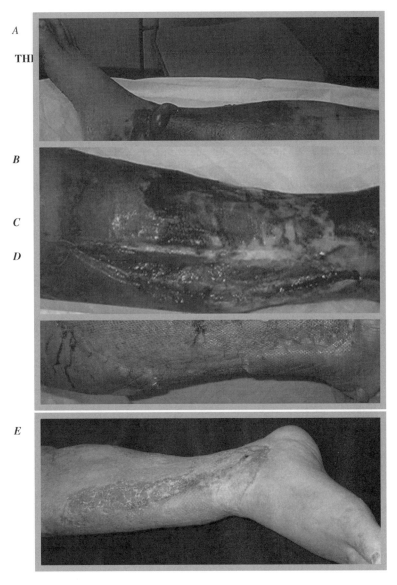

Fig. 25.1 (**a**) wound presentation; (**b**) postoperative after initial debridements; (**c**) Integra placement; (**d**) postoperative day 5, negative pressure dressing removed revealing excellent split thickness skin graft adherence; (**e**) 6-month follow-up

The following case example demonstrates the use of Integra (ILS) in a clinical setting. A sixty-two-year-old diabetic man with a lower extremity wound secondary to necrotizing fasciitis. On initial presentation, the patient displayed signs and symptoms consistent with necrotizing fasciitis of the right lower leg. He required multiple surgical debridements resulting in a complex wound involving soft tissue loss and exposed tibia. The wound required surgical reconstruction and we chose to use Integra[47] (Integra Life Sciences) dermal regeneration template as an aid in the healing and closure of this complex wound. The Integra (ILS) was directly applied onto the bone and the surrounding soft tissue and demonstrated full take. The surgical reconstruction of wounds involving bone can be quite challenging, due to the lack of vascularity in the graft area. Soft tissue transfer often results in a high complication and failure rate. The Integra (ILS) dermal regeneration template was a viable alternative to other grafting techniques to obtain wound closure:

With respect to full-thickness excisions for basal and squamous cell carcinomas, Integra's (ILS) main advantage is immediate closure of large defects over muscle, fascia, and cartilage.[49] Few studies have demonstrated, however, the successful grafting of Integra (ILS) directly onto bone. Engraftment onto bone is more difficult because of the lack of vascularity and risk of infection. Integra (ILS), unlike skin, is acellular and therefore does not require immediate revascularization for successful incorporation into poorly vascularized tissues, such as bone. One study demonstrated the use of Integra (ILS) for radiated scalp wounds. Vascular ingrowth is significantly delayed in irradiated tissues; Integra (ILS) has been successful for the treatment of these types of wounds because of the relatively slow rate vascularization of the dermal template (Fig. 25.1).[50]

References

1. W. E. Burkhalter, Open injuries of the lower extremity, *Surg Clin North Am* **53**, 1439 (1973).
2. P. A. Aldea, W. W. Shaw, The evolution of the surgical management of severe lower extremity trauma, *Clin Plast Surg* **13**(4), 549 (1986).
3. B. French, P. Torneta, III, High energy tibial shaft fractures, *Orthop Clin North Am* **33**, 211 (2002).
4. L. Heller, L. S. Levin, Lower extremity microsurgical reconstruction, *Plast Reconstr Surg* **108**, 1029 (2001).
5. M. M. Tomiamo, Amputation or salvage of type 3b/3c tibial fractures: what the literature says about outcomes, *Am J Orthop* **30**(5), 380 (2001).
6. E. Lexer, Substitution of whole or half-joints from freshly amputated extremities by free plastic operation, *Surg Gynecol Obstet* **6**, 782–809 (1908).
7. P. Chiron, J. A. Colombier, J. Tricoire, et al., A large vascularized allograft of the femoral diaphysis in man, *Int Orthop* **14**, 269–272 (1990).
8. H. S. Byrd, T. E. Spicer, G. Cierny, III, Management of open tibial fractures, *Plast Reconstr Surg* **76**, 719–730 (1985).
9. S. J. Mathes, B. S. Alpert, N. Chang, Use of the muscle flap in chronic osteomyelitis: experimental and clinical correlation, *Plast Reconstr Surg* **69**, 815 (1982).
10. J. P. Anthony, S. J. Mathes, B. S. Alpert, The muscle flap in the chronic lower extremity osteomyelitis: results in patients over 5 years after treatment, *Plast Reconstr Surg* **88**, 311 (1991).
11. J. W. May, Jr., Free latissimus dorsi muscle flap with skin graft for treatment of traumatic chronic bony wounds, *Plast Reconstr Surg* **73**, 641 (1984).
12. J. W. May, Jr., et al., Treatment of chronic traumatic bone wounds. Microvascular free tissue transfer: a 13-yr experience in 96 patients. *Ann Surg* **214**, 241 (1991).

13. R. B. Gustillo, J. T. Anderson, Prevention of infection in the treatment of one thousand and twenty-five open fractures of long bones, *J Bone Joint Surg Am* **58**, 453 (1976).
14. E. P. Christian, M. J. Bosse, G. Robb, Reconstruction of large diaphyseal defects, without free fibular transfer, in Grade IIIB tibial fractures, *J Bone Joint Surg Am* **71**, 994 (1989).
15. G. I. Taylor, The current status of free vascularized bone grafts, *Clin Plast Surg* **10**, 185 (1983).
16. J. Sekiguchi, S. Kobayashi, K. Ohmori, Use of the osteocutaneous free scapular flap on the lower extremities, *Plast Reconstr Surg* **91**, 103 (1993).
17. R. J. Allen, C. L. Dupin, P. A. Dreschnack, et al., The latissimus dorsi/scapular bone flap ("the latissimus/bone flap"), *Plast Reconstr Surg* **94**, 988 (1994).
18. J. E. Alonso, P. Regazzoni, Bridging bone gaps with the Ilizarov technique. Biologic principles, *Clin Plast Surg* **18**(3), 497 (1991).
19. H. C. Vasconez, P. J. Nicholls, Management of extremity injuries with external fixator or Ilizarov devices. Cooperative effort between orthopedic and plastic surgeons, *Clin Plast Surg* **18**(3), 505 (1991).
20. G. Cierny, III, K. E. Zorn, F. Nahai, Bony reconstruction in the lower extremity, *Clin Plast Surg* **19**(4), 905 (1992).
21. G. A. Ilizarov, V. I. Ledyaev, The replacement of long tubular bone defects by lengthening distraction osteotomy of the fragments (1969 classical article), *Clin Orthop Rel Res* **280**, 7 (1992).
22. G. A. Ilizarov, A. A. Devyatov, V. K. Kamerin, Plastic reconstruction of longitudinal bone defects by means of compression and subsequent distraction, *Acta Chir Plast* **22**(1), 32 (1980).
23. R. Ger, Chronic ulceration of the leg, *Surg Annu* **4**, 123 (1972).
24. M. Pers, S. Medgyesi, Pedicle muscle flaps and their applications in the surgery of repair, *Br J Plast Surg* **26**, 313 (1973).
25. J. B. McGraw, Selection of alternative local flaps in the leg and foot, *Clin Plast Surg* **6**, 227 (1979).
26. S. J. Mathes, F. Nahai, *Clinical Applications for Muscle and Musculocutaneous Flaps*. Mosby, St. Louis (1982).
27. J. R. Griffin, J. F. Thornton, Lower extremity reconstruction, Selected Readings in *Plast Surg* **9**(3), 29–31(2003).
28. E. A. Woltering, et al., Split thickness skin grafting of the plantar surface of the foot after wide excision of neoplasm of the skin. *Surg Gynecol Obstet* **149**, 229 (1979).
29. B. C. Sommerland, D. A. McGrouther, Resurfacing of the sole: long term follow-up and comparison of the techniques, *Br J Plast Surg* **31**, 107 (1978).
30. J. W. May, Jr., M. J. Holls, S. Simon, Free microvascular muscle flaps with skin graft reconstruction of extensive defects of the foot: aclinical and gait analysis study, *Plast Reconstr Surg* **75**, 627 (1985).
31. J. W. May, Jr., R. J. Rohrich, Foot reconstruction using free microvascular muscle flaps with skin grafts, *Clin Plast Surg* **13**(4), 681 (1986).
32. T. R. Stevenson, S. J. Mathes, Management of foot injuries with free-muscle flaps, *Plast Reconstr Surg* **78**, 665 (1986).
33. D. Serafin, V. E. Voci, Reconstruction of the lower extremity: microsurgical composite tissue transplantation, *Clin Plast Surg* **10**, 55 (1983).
34. E. K. Manders, et al., Soft-tissue expansion in the lower extremities, *Plast Reconstr Surg* **81**, 208 (1988).
35. G. O. Hofmann, M. H. Kirschner, F. D. Wagner, et al., Allogeneic vascularized grafting of a human knee joint with postoperative immunosuppression, *Arch Orthop Trauma Surg* **116**, 125–128 (1997).
36. M. H. Kirschner, L. Brauns, O. Gonschorek, et al., Vascularized knee joint transplantation in man: the first two years experience, *Eur J Surg* **166**, 320–327 (2000).
37. V. S. Gorantla, C. Maldonado, F. Johannes, J. H. Barker, Composite tissue allotransplantation (CTA): current status and future insights, *Eur J Trauma* **27**, 267–274 (2001).

38. F. Petit, A. B. Minns, J. Dubernard, S. Hettiaratchy, W. A. Lee, Composite tissue allotransplantation and reconstructive surgery: first clinical applications, *Ann Surg* **237**, 19–25 (2003).
39. B. Reeves, Orthotopic transplantation of vascularised whole knee-joints in dogs, *Lancet* **1**, 500–502 (1969).
40. G. O. Hofmann, M. H. Kirschner, F. D. Wagner, et al., Allogeneic vascularized transplantation of human femoral diaphysis and total knee joints – first clinical experiences, *Transplant Proc* **30**, 2754–2761 (1998).
41. S. E. Mackinnon, V. B. Doolbh, C. B. Novak, E. P. Trulock, Clinical outcome following nerve allograft transplantation, *Plast Reconstr Surg* **107**, 1419–1429 (2001).
42. D. W. Mathes, M. A. Randolph, W. A. Lee, Strategies for tolerance induction to composite tissue allografts, *Microsurgery* **20**, 448–452 (2000).
43. E. Elster, J. B. Patrick, A. D. Kirk, Potential of costimulation-based therapies for composite tissue allotransplantation, *Microsurgery* **20**, 430–434 (2000).
44. K. A. Prabhune, V. S. Gorantla, C. Maldonado, et al., Mixed allogeneic chimerism and tolerance to composite tissue allografts, *Microsurgery* **20**, 441–447 (2000).
45. F. Thomas, P. Ray, J. M. Thomas, Immunological tolerance as an adjunct to allogeneic tissue grafting, *Microsurgery* **20**, 435–440 (2000).
46. D. Heimbach, A. Luterman, J. Burke, et al., Artificial dermis for major burns: a multi-center randomized clinical trial, *Ann Surg* **208**, 313–320 (1988).
47. Integra Dermal Regeneration Template – Template Guidelines. Corporate Literature. Ethicon, Inc., New Brunswick, NJ 1–12 (2001).
48. D. Lozano, The use of a dermal regeneration template for the repair of degloving injuries: a case report, *Wounds* **15**(12), 395–398 (2003).
49. J. Prystowsky, D. Siegel, J. Ascherman, Artificial skin closure and healing of wounds created by skin cancer excisions, *Dermatol Surg* **27**(7), 648–655 (2001).
50. D. Gyon, M. Zenn, Simple approach to the radiated scalp wound using INTEGRA skin substitute, *Ann Plast Surg* **50**(3), 315–320 (2003).

Chapter 26
Skin Allografts in Scalp Reconstruction

Peter C. Neligan

Abstract Current techniques for the closure of scalp defects are reviewed. These include allografts, skin grafts, local flaps, regional flaps, and free flaps. Advantages and disadvantages of these procedures are pointed out in the context of the feasibility of allograft reconstruction in the form of composite tissue transplantation.

26.1 Introduction

Reconstruction of large scalp and forehead defects presents a particularly challenging clinical problem. The scalp is a specialized structure consisting of a large hair-bearing surface area with a variable expanse (especially in males) of nonhair-bearing forehead. Integral to the scalp are the frontalis and occipitalis muscles. The former is important as a muscle of facial expression and both work to maintain skin tone in the scalp. It is not unusual to have to reconstruct the scalp…either for purposes of resurfacing, as in elderly patients with squamous cell carcinoma in a milieu of extensive actinic changes, or following trauma. The concept of allograft reconstruction of the scalp is not new. Allografts have been used extensively in the treatment of burn injuries but in this context are utilized as a biologic dressing with the expectation that the graft will reject and be replaced with autologous graft.[1] Similarly allografts have been used in the context of the radiation-compromised wound.[2] Once more, in this situation it has been used as an adjunct in the ultimate healing of the wound. There have also been reports of allogeneic muscle transplantation to reconstruct the scalp. The single report documented transfer of a cadaver rectus abdominis muscle to reconstruct the scalp of a renal transplant patient, already on full immunosuppression who had a large scalp defect secondary to resection of a squamous cell carcinoma.[3] Replantation of the scalp has been reported extensively in the literature.[4] Thomas[5] has reported a case of complete face and scalp replantation. The technical feasibility of scalp and/or face transplantation is not disputed. To date there has been one reported case of transplantation of cephalic and cervical skin along with both ears in a human.[6] As Butler's discussion points out,[6] this case was ill advised as it involved a patient with carcinoma and raises the issue of immunosuppression in a cancer patient. This is very different to the allogeneic muscle transplant cited above since that patient was already on immunosuppression for a renal transplant and the squamous cell carcinoma presumably arose as a consequence of the immunosuppression. Nevertheless, this case report, along with recent reports in the popular press of a partial face transplant in France, draws our attention not only to the issue of soft tissue transplantation, but also to the concept of "spare-part" transplantation. The scalp certainly has features that make it unique enough to be considered a good candidate for allotransplantation.

26.2 Anatomy of the Scalp

The scalp consists of a composite construct of hair-bearing skin under which is a musculoaponeurotic layer consisting of frontalis and occipitalis muscles that are confluent with the galea aponeurotica. Also confluent with the galea is the temporoparietal fascia overlying the parietal region. This area consists of a more complex arrangement of fasciae enveloping the underlying temporalis muscles.[7] The temporalis muscle while being integral to jaw functioning lies under the deep temporal fascia. While loss of the temporalis in isolation has little impact on jaw function, it does have a significant impact on contour. This is evidenced by the temporal hollowing defect evident in situations where the temporalis is removed, or moved elsewhere in the head and neck as a flap.

The forehead is a subsection of the scalp and differs from it in that it is not hair bearing. The frontalis muscle as well as the procerus and corrugator muscles animate the forehead, allowing it to play an important role in communication and facial expression.

26.3 Current Approaches to Scalp Reconstruction

Much of the transplantation debate has revolved around the efficacy of current reconstructive techniques. One of the major criticisms of the recent French partial face transplant has been the fact that none of the standard reconstructive techniques had been attempted on the patient before the transplant. In the current climate, the concern regarding the effects of long-term immunosuppression is not unreasonable. Before contemplating transplantation of the scalp therefore we should first review our current reconstructive techniques. I believe that one of the criteria we should use to determine the advisability of transplantation is to assess the quality and ease of execution of our current techniques. While the simplest and most reliable method of reconstruction should be considered in all cases, there are situations in which the size of the defect, the presence of infection, or previous radiation and surgery may indicate the need for a more radical approach. Scalp and forehead defects may be caused by trauma, burns, benign or malignant tumor resection, osteomyelitis, osteoradionecrosis, or congenital lesions.[8–11] Some of these defects will simply involve skin superficial to the pericranium, while in other defects the entire thickness of the soft tissue of the scalp sometimes even including calvarial bone and dura will be involved.[8,10]

As with all cases, careful evaluation of the patient and potential defect is the first stage in reconstruction. This includes assessment of the location and size of the defect with radiological assessment of the depth as well as evaluation of bony or dural defects.[11] Previous surgery or radiation, or ongoing infection such as osteomyelitis will affect the viability of the skin around the defect. This will reduce the number of options available in terms of using local flaps. The pathology of the presenting lesion is important in planning reconstruction.[8] As already alluded to, the case of posterior scalp transplantation recently reported[6] did not apparently consider that immunosuppression could potentially create additional problems in a patient with a malignant diagnosis.

Current options for scalp reconstruction include direct closure, tissue expansion, skin graft, local flaps, regional flaps, and free flaps. Direct closure is only possible in the smallest defects. Techniques such as galeal scoring can reduce the tension of closure but afford fairly minimal advancement. If the disease process allows the luxury of pre-excisional tissue expansion, one can ensure that there will be adequate scalp to close the defect by pre-expanding adjacent scalp flaps prior to excision of the defect. More commonly we do not have that luxury when we are presented with a traumatic defect or are forced to proceed with excision for a malignant process. In this situation a skin graft can be used as a method of temporary closure. Skin grafting works well in the scalp. And the issue of skin allografts in burn patients has already been discussed. However a skin graft has several disadvantages. These include lack of hair growth and lack of thickness, so that there is usually a visible depression. The use of integra would seem to address this problem as the integra provides a graftable bed that provides elements of an artificial dermis and facilitates a more durable and aesthetically pleasing result. This technique has been used in burn reconstructions,[12] following resection of malignancies[13,14] as well as in radiated scalp wounds.[15] This has also opened up the possibility of microhair grafting. In fact Navsaria et al.[12] have reported microhair grafting in integra without the need of a skin graft. This makes for a very effective reconstruction albeit one that has to be completed in several stages.

Use of a skin graft assumes a vascularized bed so that a skin graft is not always an option in patients in whom the pericranium has been lost, or in patients who have undergone radiation to the scalp. A very useful technique for closing defects that are not amenable to skin grafting is to rotate a local scalp flap into the defect and reconstruct the secondary defect with a skin graft. While this is expedient, it still has the disadvantage of replacing an area of hair-bearing skin with a nonhair-bearing skin graft.

Orticochea[16] reported an ingenious method of closing relatively large scalp defects using three local flaps. There have been several other reports of various local flap combinations used to close scalp defects.[17–19] The advantage is that of replacing like with like and avoiding use of nonhair-bearing tissue. Use of these flaps assumes an otherwise healthy scalp. Previous surgery, previous radiation, or extent of defect may preclude the use of these flaps.

For larger defects, these options are not available and recourse must be made to the use of regional flaps or free flaps. For posterior scalp defects, the Trapezius Myocutaneous flap is a good option[20–22] (Fig. 26.1). Angrigiani[23] has described the dorsal scapular perforator flap as a good option for these defects. It has the advantage of avoiding muscle harvest and therefore minimizing donor morbidity. Both of these flaps have the disadvantage of replacing hair-bearing scalp with nonhair-bearing back skin. However as already described, tissue expansion can subsequently be used to replace the nonhair-bearing skin as shown in Fig. 26.2.

Free flaps are used for larger scalp defects. Usually when a free flap is required for scalp reconstruction, a large surface area is the issue. Several flaps have been used in this situation. Omentum provides a quantity of tissue that can easily cover most scalp defects.[24] However the irregularity of contour is suboptimal in terms of aesthetics. The latissimus dorsi muscle is the largest muscle flap available to us. As

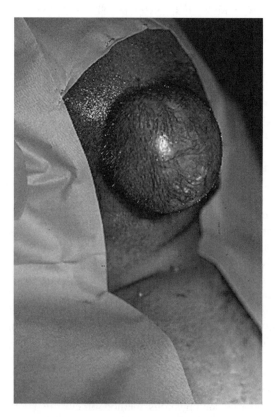

Fig. 26.1 (a) Patient with liposarcoma of posterior scalp and (b) sarcoma resected and defect reconstructed with pedicled trapezius myocutaneous flap

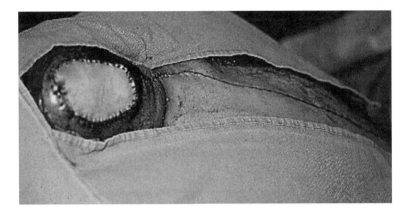

Fig. 26.1 (continued)

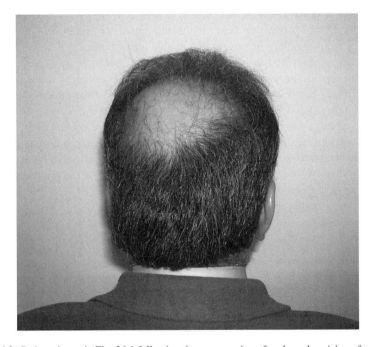

Fig. 26.2 Patient shown in Fig. 26.1 following tissue expansion of scalp and excision of trapezius skin paddle

a myocutaneous flap it is somewhat bulky. As a muscle flap with a nonmeshed skin graft, it provides adequate cover. Furthermore the atrophy of the muscle that ensues following transfer leaves a thin yet durable reconstruction that generally moulds very well to the contour of the cranium. The main disadvantage is the lack of hair as well as the color difference between the grafted muscle and the facial skin.

The circumflex scapular system is another source of tissue for scalp reconstruction. It is particularly suitable for forehead reconstruction where hair growth is not an issue.[25] Color match is usually reasonable though it is variable. However all of these reconstructive techniques fall short of what could be achieved by replacing scalp with scalp. Tissue transplantation could achieve that result.

26.4 Scalp Transplantation

So where does transplantation fit? Certainly we have several options in choosing an appropriate method to reconstruct the scalp. There is obviously no substitute for like tissue.

The technical aspects of scalp transplantation are relatively straightforward. The clear obstacle to universal acceptance of scalp reconstruction is the issue of immunosuppression. This is the debate that is ongoing in terms of "nonlife-saving" transplants. However there are other issues that are less obvious. While we worry about skin color match in reconstructing visible areas, particularly in the head and neck, we have never had to worry about hair color match or hair characteristics. While hair dye is the obvious color solution, it is nevertheless a consideration. Putting a curly patch on someone with straight hair is still probably better than leaving a bald patch. The other issue is that of alopecia. If the whole scalp is being transplanted this is probably less important, but it may be important in the situation where a partial scalp is transplanted. Does male pattern baldness occur in a male scalp transplanted to a female? We do not know the answer to that question but it is one to which we will need an answer. Finally, because of the options currently available to us in terms of scalp reconstruction, I do not think that scalp transplantation will become a reality until such time as it can be achieved with minimal impact on patient health.

References

1. F. Groenevelt, A. J. van Trier, Y. L. Khouw, The use of allografts in the management of exposed calvarial electrical burn wounds of the skull, Ann NY Acad Sci **888**, 109–112 (1999).
2. S. W. Fosko, C. B. Cuono, D. J. Leffell, Allograft skin as an adjunct in the repair of radiation-compromised wound, Arch Dermatol **129**(3), 293–295 (1993).
3. T. R. Jones, P. A. Humphrey, D. C. Brennan, Transplantation of vascularized allogeneic skeletal muscle for scalp reconstruction in a renal transplant patient, Transplantation **65**(12), 1605–1610 (1998).
4. K. Cheng, Microsurgical replantation of the avulsed scalp: report of 20 cases, Plast Reconstr Surg **97**(6), 1099–1106; discussion 1107–1108 (1996).
5. A. Thomas, Total face and scalp replantation, Plast Reconstr Surg **102**(6), 2085–2087 (1998).
6. H. Q. Jiang, et al., Composite tissue allograft transplantation of cephalocervical skin flap and two ears, *Plast Reconstr Surg* **115**(3), 31e–35e; discussion 36e–37e (2005).

7. J. J. Accioli de Vasconcellos, et al., The fascial planes of the temple and face: an en-bloc anatomical study and a plea for consistency, Br J Plast Surg **56**(7), 623–629 (2003).
8. B. S. Lutz, et al., Reconstruction of scalp defects with free flaps in 30 cases, Br J Plast Surg **51**(3), 186–190 (1998).
9. B. Lee, K. Bickel, S. Levin, Microsurgical reconstruction of extensive scalp defects, *J Reconstr Microsurg* **15**(4), 255–262; discussion 263–264 (1999).
10. D. G. Pennington, H. S. Stern, K. K. Lee, Free-flap reconstruction of large defects of the scalp and calvarium, Plast Reconstr Surg **83**(4), 655–661 (1989).
11. R. P. TerKonda, J. M. Sykes, Concepts in scalp and forehead reconstruction, Otolaryngol Clin North Am **30**(4), 519–539 (1997).
12. H. A. Navsaria, et al., Reepithelialization of a full-thickness burn from stem cells of hair follicles micrografted into a tissue-engineered dermal template (Integra), Plast Reconstr Surg **113**(3), 978–981 (2004).
13. E. Komorowska-Timek, et al., Artificial dermis as an alternative for coverage of complex scalp defects following excision of malignant tumors, Plast Reconstr Surg **115**(4), 1010–1017 (2005).
14. J. S. Wilensky, et al., The use of a bovine collagen construct for reconstruction of full-thickness scalp defects in the elderly patient with cutaneous malignancy, Ann Plast Surg **54**(3), 297–301 (2005).
15. D. L. Gonyon, Jr., M. R. Zenn, Simple approach to the radiated scalp wound using INTEGRA skin substitute, Ann Plast Surg **50**(3), 315–320 (2003).
16. M. Orticochea, New three-flap reconstruction technique, Br J Plast Surg **24**(2), 184–188 (1971).
17. J. L. Frodel, Jr., K. Ahlstrom, Reconstruction of complex scalp defects: the "Banana Peel" revisited, Arch Facial Plast Surg **6**(1), 54–60 (2004).
18. L. M. Field, Hairline reconstruction utilizing modified winged V-plastic hair-bearing flaps and focal anastomotic line excisions, Dermatol Surg **22**(11), 937–940 (1996).
19. M. A. Lesavoy, et al., Management of large scalp defects with local pedicle flaps, Plast Reconstr Surg **91**(5), 783–790 (1993).
20. J. R. Lynch, et al., The lower trapezius musculocutaneous flap revisited: versatile coverage for complicated wounds to the posterior cervical and occipital regions based on the deep branch of the transverse cervical artery, Plast Reconstr Surg **109**(2), 444–450 (2002).
21. M. R. Ozbek, N. Kutlu, Vertical trapezius myocutaneous flap for covering wide scalp defects, Handchir Mikrochir Plast Chir **22**(6), 326–329 (1990).
22. M. I. Dinner, B. Guyuron, H. P. Labandter, The lower trapezius myocutaneous flap for head and neck reconstruction, Head Neck Surg **6**(1), 613–617 (1983).
23. C. Angrigiani, et al., The dorsal scapular island flap: an alternative for head, neck, and chest reconstruction, Plast Reconstr Surg **111**(1), 67–78 (2003).
24. A. Losken, et al., Omental free flap reconstruction in complex head and neck deformities, Head Neck **24**(4), 326–331 (2002).
25. P. Neligan, P. Gullane, Head and neck reconstruction. In Perforator Flaps: Anatomy, Technique and Clini*cal Applications*, ed. by Blondeel, P., et al., pp 758–774. Quality Medical Publishing, St. Louis (2006).

Chapter 27
Abdominal Wall Transplantation

David M. Levi and Andreas G. Tzakis

27.1 Introduction

The abdominal wall graft is a composite tissue allograft that has been developed in the context of intestinal transplantation. Some intestinal transplant candidates have severely damaged abdominal walls and/or a loss of domain of the abdominal compartment making closure at the time of transplant extremely difficult. Although a variety of techniques exist to address this problem, some patients are impossible to close. For these patients, the addition of an abdominal wall graft can facilitate closure and restore the integrity of the abdominal compartment.[1]

This chapter focuses on a description of the abdominal wall graft, the indications for its use, technique for procurement, technique and timing of implantation, immunosuppression, graft surveillance and rejection, and some ethical considerations.

Abdominal wall transplants have been performed in a small number of highly selected patients. To date, all abdominal wall graft recipients have been intestinal graft recipients. As clinical results and immunosuppression strategies improve, we may be able to consider transplantation of an abdominal wall as an isolated organ for patients with massive abdominal wall defects. The pool of patients that may need this type of transplant is likely to remain small. However, the lessons learned from this experience are highly relevant to the field of composite tissue transplantation.

27.2 The Abdominal Wall Graft

The abdominal wall graft is a vascularized, denervated, full-thickness portion of the anterior abdominal wall of a cadaveric donor. It is composed of one or both rectus abdominus muscles, their investing fascia, underlying peritoneum, overlying subcutaneous tissue, and skin. The anatomic boundaries of the graft are the costal margin superiorly, the symphysis pubis inferiorly, and the edges of the rectus sheath bilaterally. The size of the graft and consequently the surface area that it can cover vary depending on the size of the donor. The blood supply to the graft is based on

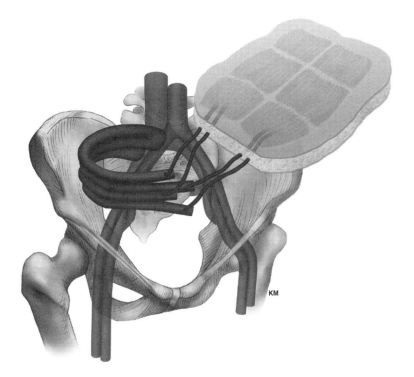

Fig. 27.1 The abdominal wall composite graft

the donor inferior epigastric vessels, left in continuity with the femoral and iliac vessels (Fig. 27.1). This provides a long vascular pedicle, and facilitates implantation and positioning of the graft in the recipient.

27.3 Intestinal Transplantation

To date, all recipients of abdominal wall composite allografts have been patients undergoing intestinal transplantation. Intestinal transplantation emerged has a viable treatment option for selected patients with intestinal failure, the permanent loss of sufficient functional intestinal absorptive surface area to maintain homeostasis. Improvements in perioperative patient management, surgical technique, immunosuppression, and graft surveillance over the past decade have resulted in improvements in graft and patient survival.[2-4]

The composition of the intestinal graft is dictated by the patient's need. The abdominal organs comprising the graft are transplanted in tandem based on the "cluster" principle originated by Thomas Starzl. According to this principle, the abdominal viscera are suspended from a central vascular pedicle or "stem" which includes the celiac axis, superior mesenteric artery, and the corresponding venous drainage; either the portal vein or the suprahepatic vena cava depending on whether the graft includes the liver. Most patients receive an isolated small intestine, a multivisceral graft (en bloc engraftment of the stomach, liver, duodenum, pancreas, and small intestine), or a modified multivisceral graft (stomach, duodenum, pancreas, and small intestine). Each type has its own variations in composition and technique for implantation.

Many patients being considered for intestinal transplantation have severely damaged abdominal walls from prior laparotomies, ostomy construction, traumatic injury, wound infections, enterocutaneous fistulae, and tumor invasion. Additionally, many have previously undergone extensive resections of their native abdominal viscera and as a result have a contracted abdominal compartment. Both of these factors can make closure of the abdomen at the time of intestinal transplantation extremely difficult, if not impossible. Failure to close the abdomen, at the very least, delays the recovery and rehabilitation of the recipient. Moreover, it exposes the patient to potential life-threatening complications including injury to unprotected organs, intraabdominal infection, bleeding, and fistula formation.

Abdominal closure is facilitated by selecting donors that are relatively small, surgically reducing the size of the graft, utilizing synthetic mesh materials, and/or employing plastic surgical techniques to recruit autologous tissue for closure.[5] Using these strategies and techniques, most patients can be closed primarily or several days later. A few remaining patients are impossible to close. For those, the use of an abdominal wall graft transplanted contemporaneously or several days after the intestinal transplant procedure can greatly facilitate coverage of the intestinal graft, restoring the integrity of the abdominal compartment.

27.4 Graft Procurement

The abdominal wall graft is obtained as part of the cadaveric, heart-beating donor, multiorgan procurement procedure.[6] Specific consent is obtained from the donor's family for its procurement and transplantation. The main modification to the procurement procedure involves the mobilization of the graft prior to flushing with cold preservation solution. The procedure begins with a median sternotomy and bisubcostal incisions. Parallel longitudinal incisions are made along the lateral edges of both rectus sheaths from the costal margin to the inguinal ligaments. A transverse suprapubic incision joins the two longitudinal incisions. The femoral vessels are exposed bilaterally (Fig. 27.2).

The other organs to be procured are evaluated and mobilized using standard techniques. The donor is heparinized and the aorta is cannulated. The abdominal wall graft, still attached by its vascular pedicles inferiorly, is wrapped with iced towels and is reflected onto the anterior aspect of the donor's thighs. The other organs are flushed with cold preservation solution and are removed. The aortic cannula is then redirected distally and the previously exposed femoral arteries are clamped. Now the abdominal wall graft is flushed with cold preservation solution. While flushing, the internal iliac arteries can be quickly exposed and clamped thus directing more of the preservation

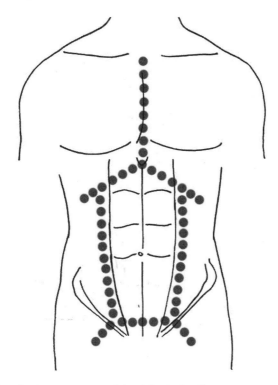

Fig. 27.2 Incisions for the procurement of the abdominal wall

solution into the abdominal wall graft. After flushing, the abdominal wall graft is removed in continuity with the common femoral and iliac vessels attached by a short cuff of distal aorta and inferior vena cava. No attempt is made to skeletonize the major vessels and their numerous branches. Instead the graft vessels are procured with a generous amount of adjoining pelvic soft tissue. The graft is stored and transported in cold preservation solution like any other solid organ to be transplanted.

27.5 Implantation

At the back table, the abdominal wall graft is prepared for implantation. The iliac vessels are cleaned, but the soft tissue around the inferior epigastric vessels is left intact to avoid injury to these small vessels. The open common femoral vessels are ligated as are the fine branches in the soft tissue. If the vascular pedicle is deemed too long and redundant, the external and common iliac vessels can be shortened and reconstructed (Fig. 27.3). Except for the graft vessels, the abdominal wall needs no further preparation.

The abdominal wall graft is implanted as a separate organ after engraftment of the intestinal graft. Not unlike a kidney graft, the abdominal wall can be anastomosed

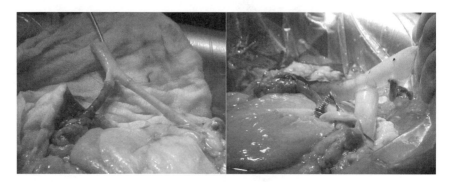

Fig. 27.3 Vascular reconstruction of the iliac arteries (*left*) and veins (*right*) of the abdominal wall graft

to the recipient's common iliac artery and vein. Alternatively, the distal aorta and inferior vena cava can serve as the anastomosis sight. Upon reperfusion, a small amount of bleeding from the skin edge and rectus muscle is a sign of good perfusion. A palpable pulse can be detected in the inferior epigastric arteries.

The abdominal wall graft is incorporated into the recipient's abdominal wall during closure. The graft is mobile and flexible; its position is dictated by the abdominal wall defect of the recipient. The fascial edges of the graft are sewed the fascial edges of the recipient's abdominal wall. Starting inferiorly ensures that the intestine is adequately covered. Care must be taken to avoid kinking or twisting of the graft vessels. Some defects are so large that the abdominal wall graft can be used in conjunction with other techniques to achieve closure.

27.6 Timing

In most cases the abdominal wall graft is procured from the intestinal graft donor and both are implanted contemporaneously. In a few cases, however, the abdominal wall graft was obtained several days later from another donor. This time delay can be clinically advantageous. It may not be certain that the abdominal wall is needed for closure at the time of the transplant. Waiting several days for edema to resolve may permit a delayed primary closure. If an abdominal wall graft is still needed, a larger donor can be sought yielding a larger abdominal wall graft than would have been available from the first donor.

27.7 Immunosuppression/Rejection

All patients that have received an abdominal wall graft are intestinal graft recipients, and thus are subjected to immunosuppressive medications. It is important to note that the regimen for this group is not modified because of the addition of the abdominal wall. Our immunosuppressive regimen for intestinal transplantation has evolved since the program began at the University of Miami in 1994. Historically, the abdominal wall graft has been introduced during the third and most recent era.[4]

The immunosuppressive regimen consists of alemtuzamab (Campath 1-H, Genzyme, Cambridge, MA) for induction, tacrolimus (Prograf, Astellas Pharma US, Deerfield, IL) and no maintenance corticosteroids. The usual dose of Campath (0.3 mg/kg) is administered intravenously on postoperative days 1 and 4. Prograf is usually started in the early postoperative period, depending on renal function, first intravenously then enterally as gastrointestinal function returns with a goal serum trough level of 10 ng/ml. Rejection of the intestinal graft is treated on the basis of the severity of involvement of the terminal ileum. Specific endoscopic features and histologic criteria have been established.[7] The treatment ranges from close surveillance with repeat endoscopy, to corticosteroid bolus and increased baseline immunosuppression, to antibody therapy with OKT-3 (Orthoclone OKT3, Orthobiotech, Bridgewater, NJ) for severe acute cellular rejection.

Abdominal wall graft surveillance is easy because a large surface of the graft is visible that being the skin of the abdominal wall. Rejection of the abdominal wall graft manifests clinically as an erythematous skin rash without native skin involvement. If rejection is suspected based on visual inspection of the graft, a skin punch biopsy can confirm the diagnosis and assist in grading its severity.[8] Histologically, rejection is characterized by perivascular inflammatory cell infiltrates in the superficial dermis. Reactive lymphocytes and red cell extravasation can be observed at higher power (Fig. 27.4). Skin rejection responds well to a brief course of corticosteroids. No abdominal wall graft has been lost to refractory rejection. In the few patients that experienced abdominal wall rejection, rarely the event did correspond temporally with an episode of intestinal rejection. Skin allotransplantation has historically been very difficult both experimentally and clinically due to its immunogenicity. Yet, as part of an abdominal wall allograft, transplanted with an intestinal graft, skin rejection is infrequent and easily managed. The reasons for this paradox are not well understood.

27.8 Ethical Considerations

Composite tissue transplantation, specifically hand and face transplantation, has gained the attention of the general public and the media.[9] The issues raised focus not so much on the science of these procedures but on their ethical and social impact. In other words, the question is not "can" these procedures be performed but "should" they be performed.

Abdominal wall transplantation has not generated the same magnitude of controversy or concern. This may be because of some fundamental differences separating abdominal wall transplantation from hand and face transplantations.

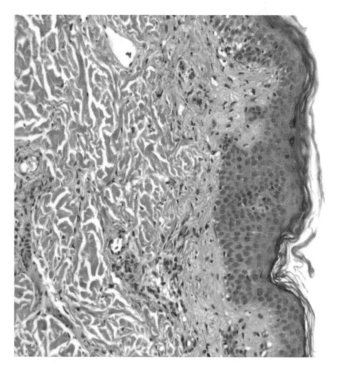

Fig. 27.4 Photomicrograph of a skin biopsy specimen demonstrating acute rejection

Intestinal transplantation is reserved for those patients who would otherwise die as result of their illness. To date, all abdominal wall recipients are intestine or multivisceral graft recipients. The abdominal wall, transplanted in this context, is employed to save the life of the recipient. Hand and face transplantation, no matter how valuable to the recipient, are generally not considered life saving.

Another difference distinguishing abdominal wall transplantation form other types of composite tissue transplants is regarding immunosuppression. The recipient of a hand or face allograft must receive potent immunosuppressive medications and thus is subjected to all the potential toxicity of these agents. Abdominal wall recipients are already subjected to these risks as intestine or multivisceral graft recipients. The immunosuppression regimen is not altered because of the inclusion of the abdominal wall.

Finally, the goals for each type of composite tissue transplant are different, and the goals of abdominal wall transplantation may be more easily achieved. A successful hand transplant must achieve a functional outcome that approximates the sensory and motor capabilities of the normal hand. The functional face allograft must be able to perform the intricate, concerted movements required for normal speech, mastication, and emotional expression. It must also be cosmetically acceptable. The purpose of the abdominal wall graft, while important, is relatively simple. It must remain viable and cover the abdominal viscera.

References

1. D. M. Levi, A. G. Tzakis, T. Kato, et al., Transplantation of the abdominal wall, *Lancet* **361**, 2173–2176 (2003).
2. S. Nishida, D. M. Levi, T. Kato, et al., Ninety-five cases of intestinal transplantation at the University of Miami, *J Gastrointest Surg* **6**, 233–239 (2002).
3. T. Kato, J. J. Gaynor, G. Selvaggi, et al., Intestinal transplantation in children: a summary of clinical outcomes and prognostic factors in 108 patients from a single center, *J Gastrointest Surg* **9**, 75–89 (2005).
4. A. G. Tzakis, T. Kato, D. M. Levi, et al., 100 multivisceral transplants at a single center, *Ann Surg* **242**, 480–493 (2005).
5. I. J. Alexandride, P. Liu, D. M. Marshall, et al., Abdominal wall closure after intestinal transplantation, *Plast Reconstr Surg* **106**, 805–812 (2000).
6. T. E. Starzl, C. Miller, B. Broznick, et al., An improved technique for multiple organ harvesting, *Surg Gynecol Obstet* **165**, 343–348 (1987).
7. P. Ruiz, D. Weppler, S. Nishida, et al., International grading scheme for acute rejection in small bowel transplantation: implementation and experience at the University of Miami, *Transplant Proc* **38**, 1683–1684 (2006).
8. P. A. Bejarano, D. Levi, M. Nassiri, et al., The Pathology of full-thickness cadaver skin transplant for large abdominal defects: a proposed grading system for skin allograft acute rejection, *Am J Surg Pathol* **28**, 670–675 (2004).
9. N. McDowell, Surgeons struggle with ethical nightmare of face transplants, *Nature* **420**, 449 (2002).

Chapter 28
Peripheral Nerve Allotransplantation

Chau Y. Tai and Susan E Mackinnon

28.1 Background and Historical Perspectives

Philipeaux and Vulpian were credited with the first description of peripheral nerve allograft (PNA) in dogs in 1863.[1] While all the allografts failed, their continued work on nerve autografts yielded important observations still true today – they noted that the sensory lingual nerve was able to function as an autograft in the hypoglossal motor nerve, and tested this function using in vivo electrical stimulation.[1] In 1885, Albert reported first two clinical cases of nerve reconstructions, a 3-cm median and 10-cm ulnar nerve gaps, using segments from amputated lower extremities.[2] The follow-up was only 10 days, and Huber subsequently reported graft necrosis of the second case within a week of transplantation.[3] Mayo-Robson reported one early case of successful nerve allograft in 1889 in a 12-year-old girl, who received a 2.5-in. posterial tibial nerve graft from an amputated leg of another patient to the median nerve of her hand.[4] However, subsequent attempts at nerve allotransplantation were met with failures.[5,6]

In contrast to the studies in solid organ and bone marrow (SOT, BMT), using long-term immunosuppression to sustain a nonvital PNA was not heavily pursued. Noting the unique properties in a peripheral nerve – its abilities for manipulation and neuronal regeneration – investigators began researching methods of altering the properties of this allograft to reduce its antigenicity. Attempts at manipulation of nerve allografts to render them more universally usable included radiation, lyophilization, freeze-thaw, and cold storage. However, none of these provided consistent results equivalent to fresh autografts that would permit wide usage.

Further understanding of neuronal regenerative capacities and advances in biomaterials led to the development of multiple conduits to bridge short nerve gaps. Uses of tubulation methods such as vein, artery, silicone, and polyglycolic acid tubes are limited to nerve gaps 1–5 cm.[7] However, large nerve deficits are still without good alternatives when the limited amount of autografts is exhausted.

With better understanding of transplantation immunology and development of better tolerated immunosuppressants, the first clinical case of PNA was performed in 1988 in Toronto, followed by a series of cases reported in the 1990s.[8] These reports solidified the use of PNA as a reconstructive option for large nerve-gap deficits in extremities that would otherwise face the alternative of amputation. Table 28.1 provides a chronological review of clinical nerve allografts reported prior to current immunosuppression.

As its own entity, PNA is a highly viable reconstructive option for selected patients. With the ability for eventual withdrawal of immunosuppression, PNA overcomes the major obstacle that impedes other types of "elective" nonlife-threatening transplantations such as a composite tissue allotransplantation (CTA).

In context of a CTA for an extremity, survival of the nerve allograft component is essential since it is the rate-defining step for return of sensory and motor functions. Fortunately, the nerve appears to be one of the more resilient components, though its importance as the cornerstone for the final success of the composite graft cannot be taken for granted. A transplanted hand without neuronal input is worse than a prosthesis.

28.2 Nerve Regeneration

Injury to a peripheral nerve induces a response that involves the entire cell and its associated glia. After transection, approximately 30% to 60% of the axotomised neurons undergo apoptosis after losing their target-derived neurotrophic support.[9,10] The more proximal the injury, the more marked the central neuronal loss.[11] Surviving neurons undergo compensatory changes and increased gene expression for regrowth[12] while Wallerian degeneration occurs distally. Like most somatic tissues in the body, healing of a severed nerve does result in scar formation that can be detrimental to the final functional result.

28.2.1 Axonal Regeneration

After transection, the severed ends of the axons are sealed by coalescence of endocytosed axolemma in a matter of hours.[13] The injured cell bodies proximally respond by apoptosis or phenotype switching, while the distal portions undergo Wallerian degeneration.[12] Meanwhile, axonoplasmic transport continues at both proximal and distal stumps, and stimulation at the distal stump can still transmit electrical signals for up to 3 days. Evidence exists that another caspase-independent mechanism is responsible for injured axonal degeneration that may be seen in development associated with branch elimination, with implications for treatment of neurodegenerative diseases.[14]

Nerve regeneration begins with axonal sprouting from the sealed proximal stump tips and from the nodes of Ranvier, affected by local presence of laminin and fibronectin.[15] Axonal sprouts are enveloped by regenerating Schwann cells (SCs), and local fibroblasts and perineural cells then ensheath the SC and axonal unit in new-formed minifascicle. Using transgenic mice expressing fluorescent proteins,

Table 28.1 Chronological review of clinical nerve allografts prior to immunosuppression

Authors and year	No.	Treatment	Delay	Graft (cm)	Follow-up	NCS	Motor function	Sensory function	Comment
Albert, 1885	2	None	0	3; 10	10 days; ?				No follow-up; necrotic
Mayo-Robson, 1889, 1917	1	None		3	3 years		Normal by 3 years	Normal in 36h	Success
Burk, 1917	1	None							Rejected
Eden (in Barnes), 1919	1	None		Inlaid	28 days				Rejected
Delagénière, 1924	6	None		>11	>4–5 months		0	0	Rejected
Duel, 1934	6	None (ABO match)		2–4			Excellent	Excellent	Facial nerve
Gosset, 1938	4	Formalin + ETOH		3–5		Twitch			Success (spinal cord grafts)
Seddon, 1944	2; 2	None; Ringer's 14 days		12–19	371–573 days	EMG	0	0	Rejected
Barnes, 1945	8	None	230–526 days	6–25	140–904 days	EMG	0	0	Rejected
Spurling, 1945	8	None	186–456 days	3.2–9	122–265 days	EMG	0	0	Axons regenerated 5–40 mm
Davis, 1950	9	5°C for 0.5–40h		9–15	0.5–16 years	EMG	0	3/9	Failure
Davis, 1950	8	5°C for 0.5–40h		9–15	0.5–16 years	EMG	0	6/9	Central necrosis
Campbell, 1963	24	FRZ + IR + millipore		2.5–13.5	1–2 years		3/24	3/24	14/24 improving, 7/24 failed
Marmor, 1963	2	FRZ + IR		7.5; 13.75	4–5 months		2/2 good	1/2 good	Success
Marmor, 1964	2	FRZ + IR	19; 11 months	7.5; 12.5	6 months; 8 months	EMG	0	2/2	Limited success
Afanassieff, 1967	20	Cialit		2–12	1–5 years		10/20	10/20	
Campbell, 1970	17	FRZ + IR + millipore					10/17	7/17	Poor
Marmor, 1967	18	FRZ + IR	1–84 months	2–9	2–48 months	EMG	2/18	11/18	Unsuccessful
Jacoby, 1970	2	FRZ + IR		2; 3	10–15 months	EMG	2/2	2/2	Lyophilized dura repair

Author, Year	N	Treatment	Storage time	Gap	Follow-up	Method	Result 1	Result 2	Comments
Marmor, 1970	3;25	FRZ + IR ± AZA		8.5–12.5; 7.5–22.5	19–20 months	EMG	0	0; 4/21 good	3/3 failure; 21/24 failure
Gye, 1972	8	Saline (5°C for 2 weeks) + LYO + IR + AZA + PRED		7–23	6–14 months	EMG	0/8	7/8	
Hiles, 1972	2	FRZ + LYO + IR	>6 months	20; 10	2; 2.5 years	EMG	0	2/2	Poor
Jacoby, 1972	57	Chemical + LYO ± IR		4–8			84%		Lyophilized dura repair
Kuhlendahl, 1972	8	LYO + IR			1–15.5 years	EMG	0/85	0/8	Review of Jacoby's patients
Marmor, 1972	4	FRZ + IR + AZA		"large"	2 years		0	0	Unsuccessful
Wilhelm, 1972	17	LYO + IR		3–27	5–12 months	EMG	6/17 good	6/17 S-4	
Morotomi, 1973	2	FRZ + cialit ± IR		4; 9	10; 20 months		Good	Good	
Penzholz, 1973	74	LYO + IR			4 years	EMG	Failure	Failure	Review of German experience
Singh, 1974	13;18	FRZ; LYO + IR		2–9; 4–7	25–33 months; 18–20 months	EMG	7/13 M_{3-5};7/18 M_{3-5}	7/13 good; 5/18 good	
McLeod, 1975	23	Saline (5°C for 2 weeks) + LYO + IR + AZA	2–25 years	10–36	18–36 months	EMG	0 (not expected)	7 good-fair	Success related to degree of proximal disease (leprosy)
Singh, 1975	7	LYO + IR	2–7 months	4–7	18–20 months	EMG	7/7 M_{3-5}	5/7 S1–3	Reasonable
	11		8–46 months	4–7	7–21 months	EMG	3/11 M_{3-5}	3/7 S1–3	Hopeless
Chakĭbrevekovskĭbreve, 1987	12	FRZ							Success but inferior to autograft
Ogleznev, 1990	90	"allostatic"		>4			Improved	Improved	Success

ABO blood group; *AZA* azathioprine; *CsA* cyclosporin A; *EMG* electromyography; *ETOH* ethyl alcohol; *FRZ* freezing; *IR* irradiation; *LYO* lyophilization (freeze drying); *NCS* nerve conduction studies; *PRED* prednisone; *S* short course. Reprinted with permission, modified from Evans et al.[49]

Witzel et al. captured and detailed the paths of regeneration.[16] Sprouting axons travel transversely across a lesion before distal growth, enabling it to select one of many Schwann cell basal lamina (SCBL) tubes available. Thus, even with refined surgical techniques and realignment of fascicular bundles, this pattern of regeneration may intrinsically limit a surgical repair.

The cut distal nerve end exerts trophic effect on the regenerating axon such that growth is directed toward reestablishing continuity with the disrupted end.[17] More specifically, regenerating motor axons preferentially reinnervate distal muscle branches. In a mixed nerve, the multiple axonal sprouts from motor and sensory neurons initially travel down SCBL tubes with equal density. Then, over a long time in terms of months, the "pruning process" occurs and motor innervation that incorrectly contacts a cutaneous target is eliminated.[18] In clinical practice, sensory nerves are often used to bridge a motor nerve defect. Nichols et al. examined the effects of the type of graft, motor, sensory, or mixed, on regeneration of a motor nerve. For approximately equal cross-sectional areas, nerve regeneration in motor grafts was significantly better than seen in sensory grafts.[19] However, there are a limited number of expendable motor nerves in the body for use as autograft, and in large nerve reconstructions the option of allografts is still the most reasonable.

28.2.2 Fate of Schwann Cells

Wallerian degeneration of the distal segment was named in honor of Augustus Waller, who observed the myelin destruction in frogs.[20] After nerve transection and loss of axonal input, SCs in the distal segment continue survival by autocrine signals involving insulin-like growth factor, neurotrophin-3, and platelet-derived growth factor-BB.[21] The SCs proliferate, though the enzymatic digestion and phagocytosis of the myelin sheath are largely the responsibilities of migrant macrophages.[22] After removal of neural constituents, the bands of von Bungner made of viable SCs and basal lamina are ready to accept new axonal input for regeneration.

When axonal regeneration is present, it was thought that SCs within autografts persisted and adopted the function of the missing segment by responding to the axonal signals.[23] Using nerve grafts from same strain, sex-mismatched rats, it was found that the H–Y antigen component in graft SCs was gradually replaced by host, H–Y negative, Schwann cells.[24] Further detailed studies using green fluorescent protein (GFP) transgenic rats then showed that the SC migration is actually bidirectional. Donor SCs migrate along host proximal and distal segments, while host SCs migrate into the donor graft.[25] Kimura's study was done using short graft segments of 8 mm, and tracked changes up to 3 weeks, so the end fate of the allografted SCs is still unclear.

Viable SCs in the distal nerve segment support axonal regeneration through production of trophic factors and are essential in long nerve graft regeneration.[26] Regenerating axons provide the signal to the SCs for myelination. Low expression of neuregulin-1 Type III on the regenerating axon leads to ensheathment by the SC, while high expression leads to myelination.[27] Autologous transplanted SCs injected into conduits can also support axonal regeneration in long grafts that otherwise did not support regrowth.[28] However, long-term maintenance of SCs requires axonal contact, and without it undergo necrosis and replacement by connective tissue over time.[29] Thus, the interplay and communication between SCs and axons are essential in propagation of nerve regeneration, and the exact mechanisms are still under investigation.

28.2.3 Revascularization

The mechanisms of revascularization in a PNA involve neovascularization for large diameter nerves and inosculation for small diameter nerves. Inosculation refers to reperfusion of the existing vasculature within the nerve graft. Best et al. used a 2-cm sciatic nerve graft model in the rat (small caliber nerve graft) and the fluorescent properties of an Evans blue dye injection to study revascularization patterns. They found that epineurial perfusion was consistently reestablished in 48 h, and endoneurial perfusion established by 72 h in an "all-or-none" fashion.[30] Also, the reperfusion patterns were indistinguishable from the contralateral control specimens once established, and the same was found for both autografts and allografts. Meanwhile, capping of the graft ends with Silastic prevented the reperfusion. The authors concluded that inosculation was the primary mechanism for small-caliber nerve revascularization. Studies in the ovine sural nerve correlated with the findings in small-caliber nerve revascularization.[31]

On the contrary, in a larger animal model such as rabbit sciatic nerves, Penkert found revascularization mainly from the surrounding tissues by postoperative day 3. When revascularization was limited to the longitudinal direction, blood flow demonstrated by microangiogram was slower with areas of hypoperfusion especially in the midgraft segments.[32] A more recent study by Prpa et al. controlled graft exposure to the soft-tissue bed in 10-cm canine saphenous nerves (also considered small-caliber) and found no difference in blood flow at 3 days.[33] However, analysis at 7, 14, and 28 days showed better blood flow in nonisolated grafts, with evidence of both lateral and longitudinal revascularization. This study suggests that neovascularization is the primary mechanism for restoration of blood flow in such grafts.

However, in large-caliber autografts such as the ovine peroneal nerve, no patent endoneurial vessels were seen at 7 days.[31] Studies in vascularized nerve grafts models attempt to address the question of revascularization in large-caliber nerves. Settergren and Wood compared blood flow between 10-cm free and vascularized saphenous nerve grafts in dogs and found better flow in the free graft at 4–6 days postoperatively.[34] Analysis of the same model then showed better flow in the vascularized graft at earlier time points (2, 24, and 72 h), especially in the fascicular level.[35] On gross inspection, the vascularized nerve appeared similar to a pristine nerve, while the conventional free graft was discolored and indurated.[35]

In CTA of the hand and forearm where large-caliber nerves are involved, direct revascularization through the nerve's intrinsic and extrinsic vascular tree is probably the primary mechanism. We know from anatomic studies that larger nerves carry a microarterial tree with sufficient flow and perforators to supply the overlying skin.[36,37] The technical aspects of hand CTA leaves the nerves intact with most of its vascular connections except for the proximal end, and specific revascularization of this segment has not been needed.

28.2.4 Long Nerve Regeneration

Current tubulation techniques are limited to short nerve gaps. Biologic conduits such as vein and artery performed poorly when interposed in gaps longer than 3 cm.[38] Nonbioabsorbable silicone tubules have been used though complications such as compression, scar, or tissue reactions have since been reported.[39] Multiple bioabsorbable conduits, poly(L-lactic acid), trimethylenecarbonate-co-epsilon-caprolactone (TMC/CL), alginate/chitosan, are all under investigation.[40–42] Nontubular alginate gel has also been demonstrated to support nerve regeneration for a 5 cm gap in a cat sciatic nerve model.[43]

In general, acellular grafts can only support limited regeneration. Researchers have found that axonal growth stopped after 1–2 cm in a 4-cm freeze-dried nerve grafts in the rat.[44,45] Meanwhile, the addition of SCs to all types of conduits improved nerve regeneration. Successful reinnervation of a 6-cm gap was achieved in rabbit peroneal nerve using a venous conduit filled with SCs.[28] Better nerve regeneration was observed in the synthetic conduits as well.[40,41] However, no one synthetic scaffold has clear advantage to autograft functional results and is limited to small-caliber nerves. Although no "head-to-head" study has been performed between the four commercially available conduits, it is likely that there is a difference between conduits.[46]

The adult human body can provide approximately 120 cm of autograft from expendible sensory branches (30–40 cm from each sural, 20 cm from each medial antebrachial cutaneous nerve, and 5–8 cm from each lateral antebrachial nerve). All of these grafts are of small caliber suited for better revascularization, but require multiple cables to bring meaningful end motor function for large nerve defects. For example, a 30-cm length of sural nerve graft, when divided into four cables to match the caliber of a large upper arm nerve, can only bridge at most a 7-cm gap, assuming no extra length was required to provide a tensionless repair. Thus, PNA remains as an option for nerve reconstructions when autograft capacity is exhausted.

When long nerve autografts or allografts are used, the Tinel sign is followed to the end organ at the expected rate of 1 mm/day. For motor recovery, there is a race in time with the degeneration of motor end plates and the regeneration of the new axon. Thus, whenever possible, local nerve transfers to provide trophic support to the denervated muscle is well justified.[47,48]

28.3 The Nerve Allograft Response

Allograft responses in the peripheral nerve follow principles of transplantation immunology of allorecognition followed by graft rejection. Direct recognition occurs through host T-cell recognition of donor MHC with generation of host lymphocyte migration and activation to the graft (Fig. 28.1).[49]

For several decades, the antigenic components of a PNA were debated. In the 1960s, myelin was thought to be a contributing factor.[50] Later experiments showed equivalent rejection of fresh and predegenerated PNA that was documented to lack myelin.[51] The extracellular matrix was also suspected, but later studies clarified that the acellular SCBLs, with sole composition of extracellular matrix, do not incite a detectable primary immune response.[52-54]

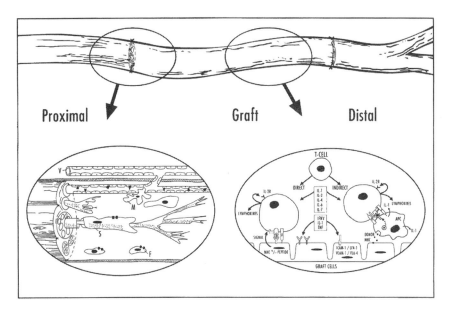

Fig. 28.1 Alloantigen recognition, presentation, and processing in a peripheral nerve allograft. Following nerve grafting, new axon sprouts appear crossing the proximal suture line. Invading host T lymphocytes and monocyte/macrophages encounter graft antigens (black squares and triangles) either directly or indirectly. Graft Schwann (S), fibroblast (F), endothelial or perivascular macrophage (M) cells may provide a source of MHC antigen and/or act as antigen presenting cells (APC). Direct recognition refers to host T-cell recognition of donor MHC (with/without processed peptide in MHC binding site). Indirect recognition refers to host T-cell recognition of donor MHC peptide, processed and presented by host APC (likely a macrophage) in the context of host MHC. Allopeptide recognition requires nonspecific intercellular adhesion molecule pairs (ICAM/LFA, VCAM/VLA, and others) to stabilize MHC binding. T-cell activation may also require auxiliary signals from host or donor APCs. Once activated, T cells, APCs or other nearby cells release cytokines (interleukins (IL), interferon gamma (IFNγ), and tumor necrosis factor (TNF) which can further activate T cells (via IL-2 receptor, IL-2R), upregulate MHC and adhesion molecule expression, and initiate a cascade of infiltration of immunocompetent cells into the graft which can lead to graft destruction. Reprinted with permission from Evans et al.[49]

Since then multiple studies provided evidence that SCs were responsible for eliciting the rejection response. In vitro, SCs presented foreign and exogenous autoantigen to syngeneic T cells.[55] In vivo, simple light microscopy and electron microscopy demonstrated MHC class II expression in PNA undergoing rejection in contrast to autografts undergoing Wallerian degeneration and no MHC class II expression.[56,57] Grafts that have been rendered acellular by lyophilization or freeze-thaw are tolerated without significant in vivo rejection response compared with syngeneic controls using a ^{51}Cr cytotoxicity assay.[58] Meanwhile, fresh or cold preserved allografts with viable SCs all elicit a strong rejection response, with immunogenicity decreasing as the number of SCs decreased with prolonged storage.[54]

Other cells in a PNA are also candidates for serving as the antigen presenting cell (APC). The endothelial and perivascular cells in a PNA have demonstrated increased MHC class II expression at 8–15 days following engraftment.[59] This is consistent with numerous studies in nonnerve grafts demonstrating the graft endothelium involvement in the rejection response. From available evidence, both SCs and endothelium appear to be the mediators of rejection in PNAs.

28.4 Methods of Nerve Allograft Tolerance

To render a PNA immunologically acceptable to the host, multiple techniques were attempted which aimed at reducing the immunogenicity of the graft and/or reducing the host response to the alloantigens.

28.4.1 Decrease Graft Antigenicity

28.4.1.1 Radiation, Lyophilization, and Freezing

Earlier experiments used freezing and radiation to alter the PNA's immunogenic properties.

In the 1960s, Marmor performed experiments in dogs using allografts frozen at −12°F followed by 1.66 Mrad irradiation and subsequent muscle reinnervation was observed. Clinical application followed, and in 1963 and 1964, he reported clinical cases with successful return of sensation in hands using frozen and irradiated homografts for upper extremity nerve defects.[60,61] Unfortunately, these encouraging early results were not obtained in subsequent 21 patients, even with addition of azathioprine.[62] Buch's experiments in guinea pigs and dogs were consistent with these clinical findings. Frozen and radiated grafts examined at 2, 4, and 6.5 weeks showed decrease in inflammatory responses compared with fresh homografts and autografts, but the grafts were ultimately rejected.[63]

After Jacoby's reports of two successful results of disantigenized and disenzymatized grafts from a cadaver, Singh and Lange published their experience with

18 lyophilized nerve grafts in 1975. Results of lyophilization showed good regeneration and functional results for grafts under 4–5 cm and earlier surgery before 6 months postinjury.[64] However, this represented only 32% of this series of patients. Thus, the performance of a lyophilized allograft was not much better than tubulization techniques.

Freezing a PNA renders a graft acellular by killing the SCs (thus removing antigenicity) but preserves the basal lamina architecture to serve as a scaffold for SC repopulation, i.e., SCBL. In rodents, acellular PNA supported reinnervation well across allogeneic and xenogeneic grafts.[65,66] In rabbits, SCBLs allowed regeneration across nerve gaps 3 to 4-cm long. In beagles, regeneration through a 5-cm SCBL was demonstrated, though nerve density was less than that of autograft controls[67]. Similar findings were noted in monkeys, across a 3-cm ulnar nerve graft.[68] In the above studies, the killed SC debris were removed by host macrophages while the basal lamina tubules remained intact, in contrast to fresh allografts where the rejection reaction destroyed both SCs and the basal lamina. On the other hand, Zalewski and Gulati found that freeze-thawed grafts, both isografts and allografts, did not support axonal growth through a 4-cm nerve gap in the rat.[69]

With varied reports of pretreatment methods, different animal models, and different nerve graft lengths, it was difficult to succinctly determine the applicability of PNA pretreatment for clinical practice. Using the ^{51}Cr cytotoxicity assay to provide quantitative data of the degree of reactivity evoked by a specific allograft, Mackinnon et al. compared responses in six groups of pretreatment methods: (1) No pretreatment fresh allografts; (2) 200, 10,000, and 35,000 rad of a single-dose radiation to fresh allografts; (3) predegeneration for 1, 3, 6, or 10 weeks; (4) freezing at −70°C for 2 weeks; (5) lyophilization; and (6) predegeneration, frozen, and irradiated.[58,70] Only the high-dose radiation of 35,000 rad and lyophilization produced inlaid grafts that elicited an index of recognition similar to that of a control fresh isograft. Then, regeneration was assessed through lyophilized and irradiated PNAs and regeneration was simply not comparable to that of fresh isografts.[71]

28.4.1.2 Cold Preservation

Cold preservation has been used for many years for storage of PNA and as a method to decrease its antigenicity. Tarlov and Epstein (1945) found that allografts stored at 5°C for 24–72 h regenerated better than fresh homografts.[72] In a rabbit model, Sanders stored nerves in Ringer's solution at 2°C prior to grafting and found less lymphocytic infiltration and better regeneration versus fresh allografts.[73] This finding was consistent in a sheep model as well and showed time dependence of cold preservation. At 5°C, 6 and 12 h preservations actually enhanced lymphocyte entry into allograft tissue. Longer period of cold preservation of 1 and 3 weeks dramatically reduced lymphocyte migration to levels comparable to that of freeze-thawing pretreatment.[74]

The viability, immunogenicity, and regeneration of PNA are altered by cold preservation. SC viability assessed by DNA synthesis showed marked decrease in nerves stored in University of Wisconsin solution after 1 week, and by 3 weeks dropped to that background level.[54] Intercellular adhesion molecule I (ICAM-1) and MHC class II antigen are molecules known to play an important role in antigen presentation to CD4+ T lymphocytes. Immediate, 2-week, and 7-week analyses using immunostaining showed that class II MHC antigen decreased proportional to storage time, and ICAM I decreased only at 7 weeks of storage.[75] In isografts, axonal regeneration was best in fresh grafts, and increasing storage time led to inferior regeneration secondary to decreasing viable SCs in the graft. On the other hand, for allografts, the longer that grafts were stored, the less rejection was seen. After storage for 7 weeks, regeneration in a 2-cm PNA rat model was comparable to that of isograft.[76] However, the regeneration potential then approaches that of an acellular freeze-thaw PNA as discussed above with limitation in bridging long-nerve gaps. Meanwhile, the SCBL remained intact through freeze-thaw or cold storage preparations.[75]

It is important to note that 7 days of cold preservation at 4–5°C (refrigerator) in University of Wisconsin solution will decrease graft antigenicity but also still have grafts with viable donor SCs necessary for regeneration across long nerve allografts. This 7-day window also allows for careful screening of donor tissue for transmissible agents, preloading of the patient with FK506, and renders the allograft procedure an elective procedure. By contrast with 7 weeks of cold preservation, the allograft is acellular and completely nonantigenic. Such a graft would be an excellent bridge for short ≤3-cm grafts but would require the addition of donor SCs to ensure regeneration across longer grafts.

28.4.1.3 Recellularized Nerve Grafts

From the above findings, it became clear that SCs are desirable in supporting axonal regeneration. More specifically, it is host SCs, or that in autografts, that are useful since allogeneic cells are inevitably rejected. In late 1980s, Gulati showed that cellular nerve grafts can support axonal regeneration beyond that possible by acellular SCBL.[26] Then, by repopulating a 2-cm acellular allogeneic SCBLs with isogeneic SCs, he demonstrated viability of cultured SCs in the SCBL and the ability of the recellularized nerve graft to support axonal regeneration.[77]

Instead of trying to balance donor SC viability while reducing antigenicity and not getting 100% of either goal, researchers can look to acellular SCBLs or other scaffolds as the construct to house autogenous cultured SCs for long-nerve grafts. Strauch et al. previously established a rabbit model using autogenous veins as nerve conduits for nerve regeneration up to 3-cm.[38] With the addition of autologous SCs, excellent regrowth was noted at 6 cm.[28] Similarly, injections of SCs in acellular muscle conduits enabled reinnervation to 5 cm in the rat sciatic nerve.[78] Even for synthetic guides, addition of SCs improved regeneration approaching that of an autograft.[41,79] However, recellularization of acellular grafts still does not meet the gold-standard of fresh autologous grafts histologically and clinically.[80,81] Thus for smaller nerve defects, an autologous source is still preferred.

Revascularization of these tissue-engineered PNAs are critical in supporting SC viability. Fansa et al. compared the revascularization of conduits filled with SCs – control autografts, venous grafts, and acellular muscle grafts.[82] They found that the manipulated grafts had delayed revascularization, but rapid enough that by the day 7 the SCs were nourished by a vascular supply. This was within the window for SC viability as demonstrated by Penkert.[32]

These studies highlighted the conditions of an ideal PNA for optimal nerve regeneration: (1) a basal lamina scaffold; (2) autologous SCs; (3) timely revascularization; and (4) comparable clinical results to fresh autografts. The method of cold-storage is comparatively gentle in tissue handling versus freeze-thaw or lyophilization methods and may offer an advantage in preserving the native vascular tree for revascularization. Reseeding cold-stored (>7 weeks) allografts with autologous cultured SCs has not yet been reported in large animal models, and it would be important to demonstrate the utility of such a graft for possible clinical use.

28.4.2 Decrease Host Immune Response

The other approach to enable PNA acceptance is to manipulate the recipient's immune system via immunosuppression or tolerance induction. However, accepting the risk of immunosuppression for a transplant that is not essential for survival of the patient is still controversial. Fortunately, PNA does not require lifelong immunosuppression since the cellular component is replaced by the host over time, and with usage of safer agents the balance of risk versus benefit can be achieved.

28.4.2.1 Immunosuppression

28.4.2.1.1 CsA

Soon after its discovery in the late 1970s and demonstration of improved efficacy in graft maintenance, cyclosporin A (CsA) rapidly incorporated into multiple transplantation models including nerve allografts.[83,84] Midha et al. used Shiverer mice as donors, whose SCs are deficient in myelin basic protein, and evaluated nerve grafts into normal hosts by immunohistochemistry from week 6 to week 14 under no, temporary, or continuous CsA immunosuppression. It was found that host SCs migrated into the transplanted PNA and eventually replaced the allogeneic SCs in all groups.[85] This observation was confirmed in a longer 3-cm graft in the rat model. Lewis nerves grafted into Buffalo recipients under immunosuppression were then regrafted and accepted by a naïve Buffalo recipient, indicating that the Lewis allograft assumed Buffalo antigenicity under immunosuppression by CsA.[86] Furthermore, withdrawal of CsA was possible after this transition with indefinite survival of the allograft.[86]

CsA still has the disadvantages of systemic immunosuppression including increased infections, solid organ toxicity, and dependence on maintenance of therapeutic levels. If subtherapeutic levels resulted in acute graft rejection episode, CsA is unable to rescue the graft even if therapeutic-levels were resumed.[87] The use of combination therapy to augment efficacy while decreasing side effects of each drug is desirable, and the combination of CsA with anti-ICAM-1 and anti-LFA-1α has been shown to decrease the CsA requirement by sixfold.[88] However, the addition of CsA to costimulatory blockade agents used for tolerance induction abrogated the effects of the latter.[89,90] This is a very important side effect to be aware of as novel agents are tested along with established agents.

28.4.2.1.2 FK506

A more potent calcineurin-inhibitor, tacrolimus (FK506), has been found to have a ten times stronger immunosuppressant effect than CsA.[91] In vitro, FK506 has demonstrated to protect neurons from excitotoxicity and blocked neuronal apoptosis induced by serum deprivation.[92,93] These observations were further elucidated in an acrylamide-induced neuropathy model where administration of FK506 protected axonal loss with markedly increased expression of heat-shock protein 70 that is known to be cellular protective against stress.[94] In studies on pretreatment of donors with FK506, intestinal grafts were found to display lower apoptotic rate and reduced caspase-3 activity, increased heat-shock protein 72 expression, and inhibited NFκB activation.[95] Although the mechanisms have not been fully elucidated, these studies clearly show utility of FK506 in neuroprotection in PNA.

In a sciatic nerve crush injury model, Wang et al. tested FK506 versus CsA (at 10 or 50 mg/kg) and found that both axonal regeneration and functional recovery were improved in the FK506 treated animals in a dose-dependent fashion, with the 5 mg/kg as the optimal dose.[91] Since both drugs share similarity in its immunosuppressant effect by inhibiting calcineurin-mediated activation of IL-2 gene transcription in T cells, the authors hypothesized that FK506 has calcineurin-independent properties that effects nerve regeneration. In a nerve isograft model, Doolabh et al. used FK506 at 1 mg/kg and found functional recovery measured by walking track analysis to be better than controls and CsA (5 mg/kg) groups.[96] At even lower doses of 0.3 and 0.6 mg/kg, administration of FK506 resulted in better regeneration after 6 weeks compared with no-FK506 controls.[97] Furthermore, allografts grafted under FK506 administration also benefited from the neuroregenerative effects. In a cold-preserved PNA, animal studies have demonstrated superior regeneration under FK506 compared with isograft controls without immunosuppression.[98] These studies suggest that FK506 can be used to augment nerve regeneration and improve upon the current benchmark of fresh autologous grafts.

However, in the clinical setting, the mechanism of neurotoxicity associated with FK506 remains unknown. High levels of FK506 has been correlated in some but not all reports of neurotoxicity in transplant patients, but in many cases the side effects improved with reduction or cessation of drug.[99,100] Interestingly, Yamauchi et al. have found that the administration time of FK506, at light phase (8 a.m.) or dark phase (8 p.m.), has an effect on both nephro- and neurotoxicity in the rat, without compromise of the immunosuppressive effects.[101] Since transplant protocols have multiple variables and many of which are difficult to control, it may be some time before clinical and laboratory correlations can be achieved.

Reconstruction of peripheral nerve injuries is often delayed. Therefore, the time sensitivity and the neuroregenerative potential of FK506 was investigated to understand its clinical implications. Sobol et al. found that administration of FK506 0, 3, and 5 days following nerve transection and immediate repair showed enhancement of regeneration at 0 and 3 days but not 5 days compared with untreated controls.[102] Preoperative administration 3 days prior to nerve transection and repair also showed significant enhancement of nerve regeneration,[103] consistent with in vitro findings of Gold and Oltean.[94,95] Thus, in patients with immediate repair of nerve injuries, administration of FK506 within 3 days can enhance regeneration. Alternatively, freshening scarred nerve stumps with a knife produces an acute "new" injury immediately prior to reconstruction. And in planned allograft reconstructions, preloading the patient with FK506 3 days prior to surgery will maximize its neuroprotective effects.

28.4.2.1.3 Costimulatory Blockade

Development of costimulatory blockade for tolerance induction in SOTs opened exciting avenues to explore its use for PNA. In a cardiac transplantation model, using synergy of two costimulatory blockades, anti-CD40L mAb (MR1) and CTLA4-Ig, investigators achieved long-term acceptance of the heart and skin allografts.[89] The use of MR1 alone was sufficient for regeneration of murine PNA, though the effect was a permissive state rather than that of tolerance.[104] This work translated to the nonhuman primate model, but again, donor-specific tolerance was not achieved.[105] Additionally, it was found that application of a skin graft actually abolished the permissive effects of MR1 on PNA regeneration compared with a nerve graft alone.[105] Meanwhile, we know that the quantity of nerve allografts does not change the "antigen load" seen by the recipient.[106] Therefore, properties within the skin graft has clear influence on the nerve graft and is of important consideration in CTAs.

Abrogation of the efficacy of costimulatory blockade for transplant tolerance by CsA is of concern with FK506 as well. In the mouse model where MR1 alone allowed PNA regeneration, addition of CsA at 25 mg/kg/day decreased fiber counts. On the contrary, addition of a low-dose or high-dose FK506 (0.5 or 2 mg/kg/day) did not adversely affect regeneration, and results were comparable to the isograft group.[107] Moffat and Metcalfe also found that tolerance induction by combined CD4/CD8 blockade was not prevented by FK506, while CsA addition to the blockade was toxic to mice.[108]

While CsA abrogated the combined effects of MR1 and CTLA-4Ig in a murine cardiac allograft model, substitution of CsA with rapamycin resulted in permanent engraftment.[109] Meanwhile, rapamycin did not show neuroregenerative effects as demonstrated in FK506.[110] These studies underlined the differences among this class of calcineurin inhibitors, and that effects observed in the older CsA studies cannot be readily translated to FK506 and rapamycin. The positive effect of FK506 on neuroregeneration is desirable in PNA as well as for CTA. Whether it can be used in regimens with combined costimulatory blockade has not been definitively answered.

28.4.2.2 Immune Tolerance

As with other SOTs, achievement of donor-specific immune tolerance for the allograft is the ideal goal to eliminate dependence on immunosuppression for graft survival. Encouraging results of UVB-irradiated donor blood transfusion in prolonging pancreatic islet graft survival led to investigation with intrathymic injections of UVB-irradiated spleen cells (UVB-SC) for tolerance induction.[111,112] Indefinite cardiac allograft survival was achieved, and three of four recipients also accepted second-set transplant of donor pancreatic islet grafts, indicating donor-specific tolerance.[112] This effect was not observed with administration in subcutaneous, intraperitoneal, and intratesticular sites. Portal administration, on the other hand, promoted donor-specific hyporesponsiveness and prolongation of allografts.[113,114]

When applied to PNA, portal-injected UVB-SC also facilitated nerve regeneration when combined with anti-CD4 monoclonal antibody.[115,116] However, the donor-specific "tolerance" achieved by portal injection of UVB-SC is not sustained as the case in intrathymic administration. Pretreated Buffalo rats accepted Lewis PNA with rejection. However, subsequent challenge with a second Lewis PNA resulted in rejection.[117]

Newer costimulatory blockades as discussed earlier are under investigation for tolerance induction. These agents also have side effects, and concerns for increased risk of thromboembolism will likely lead to the "combination therapy" strategy as mentioned. Again, drug–drug interactions must be carefully worked out before clinical application. As of today, tolerance induction to a CTA is still out of reach.

28.5 Clinical Nerve Allotransplantation

The consistent poor outcomes of nerve allografts in the 1940s led to abandonment of clinical use of nerve allograft for many years.[5,6] With the advent of CsA, research in all fields of transplantation made impressive renewals and progresses, including PNA. As detailed earlier, extensive laboratory studies demonstrated the feasibility of long allograft regeneration and the ability to eventually withdraw immunosuppression in PNA. Faced with severe, multiple nerve injuries in the extremities of young patients with years of medical burden ahead of them, Mackinnon explored the use of cadaveric nerve allografts with host immunosuppression for PNA reconstruction beginning in the late 1980s. And in 2001, the long-term outcomes of seven patients who underwent nerve allograft were reported.[118]

This patient series had a mean age of 15 years, with nerve injuries to the upper ($n = 4$) and lower extremities ($n = 3$) that exceeded available autograft reconstruction and had suitable proximal and distal nerve stumps for grafting. After approval through the institutional Human Studies Committee, patients underwent medical screening under the same protocol for solid organ grafts. Smaller caliber long sensory nerve strands were transplanted in multiple cables to allow greater revascularization potential. Mean time of immunosuppression was 18 months. Protective sensation was recovered in six patients, motor recovery achieved in three patients, and subtherapeutic levels of CsA led to one case of rejection.

This series saw the transition from CsA to FK506 use in transplantation, and also noted the improved regenerative capability of neuronal tissues under immunosuppression. An important point to note is to preload the patient with FK506 prior to surgery. Preconditioning by activation of the stress protein response allows cells to subsequently withstand additional metabolic insult from surgical stress.[119] Additionally, rescue of acute rejection has not been successful by simply resuming immunosuppression levels. Therefore, having FK506 on board prior to transplantation prevents the start of the rejection response that is difficult to halt.

Most recently, two young men were recipients of living donor grafts from their mothers and one also from an unrelated patient that serendipitously had unused sural graft segments. These patients were ABO compatible with the recipient. They are currently still under FK506 immunosuppression and final functional outcomes are pending. These historic operation opened exciting possibilities for neural reconstruction. With a time limit of end-target responsiveness to reinnervation, the wait for a compatible cadaveric donor may exceed the window of opportunity for an otherwise reconstructable deficit. The ability to use living donor grafts will help bridge the gap in technology until ready-made long allografts with minimal antigenicity are available for clinical use. Table 28.2 summarizes nerve allograft transplants performed using current immunosuppressants.

These examples clearly demonstrated the feasibility, utility, as well as pitfalls in clinical nerve allotransplantation. The risks versus benefits decisions were carefully considered with the patients and their guardians, as required in any transplantation. Clinical application of PNA is unique in the success to eventually withdraw immunosuppression, a goal still sought after by other SOTs. The following protocol is currently used at Washington University (WU) for clinical PNA.

1. Evaluation by peripheral nerve surgery to determine if the patient is a candidate for reconstruction with nerve allografts or by other methods.
2. If nerve allografts are required, the patient is scheduled with transplant surgery (at WU the lung transplant physician assists with the administration and informed consent regarding immunosuppression)
3. ABO matching is done between donor and recipient. HLA and antibody screening is also performed to see if the recipient is sensitized to donor antigens,

Table 28.2 Nerve allograft patients treated with immunosuppression at Washington University 1992–2006

	Gender/age (years)	Interval between injury and grafting (months)	Injured nerve	Total length of grafts (cm) autograft, allograft	Length of time immunosuppressed (months)
1	M/12	4	Posterior tibial	0, 160	19
2	F/15	8	Median, ulnar	59, 178	12
3	F/3	5	Ulnar, radial	24, 72	18
4	F/22	3	Median, ulnar, radial	44, 226	17
5	M/16	3	Median, ulnar, radial	63, 350	Rejected allografts at 4 months
6	M/24	5	Posterior tibial	28, 112	19
8	M/19[a]	1	Median, ulnar, radial	62, 20	Ongoing
9	M/21[a]	9	Median, ulnar, radial	126, 44	Ongoing

[a]Living-related donor.

especially in cases where the patient has received prior blood transfusions. Since a significant waiting period may be required for a suitable cadaveric donor, living-related donors are used when available and feasible.

4 At harvest, small caliber nerves are selected for transplantation, e.g., sural nerves.
5 Donor nerves are stored in University of Wisconsin solution at 4–5°C with additives as followed: Penicillin G 200 kU/L of UW, regular insulin 40 U/L, and dexamethasone 16 mg/L.
6 The recipient is preloaded with FK506 at least 3 days prior to scheduled surgery, and levels are checked prior to surgery to reach or near therapeutic goal.
7 The same evening after surgery, the patient continues on FK506 and is also started on a purine synthesis antagonist, usually azathioprine. The transplant physician is involved to monitor and titrate immunosuppressions postoperatively to reach therapeutic dosages.
8 We have involved the pain management team to assist with pain control in patients that needed better control. Occasionally, the patient presents to the surgeon already in chronic pain secondary to neuropathy, and the insult of surgery can acutely exacerbate the problem until sensory reeducation occurs.
9 The patient is maintained on two immunosuppressants until good clinical recovery is demonstrated and to allow time for SC replacement by host, usually around 2 years. Steroids were used as the second agent in our early cases, and Imuran is now preferred.
10 Drug levels are routinely monitored, first level checked 5 days after discharge. For patients who live far away, laboratory results drawn near their homes are communicated back to WU Transplant team via facsimile.

28.6 Peripheral Nerve Allotransplantation in CTA

Motor function and sensory restoration in a CTA is dependent on the regeneration and reestablishment of neuronal contacts between the host and the graft. Our understanding of PNA unfortunately cannot be readily extrapolated to the nerve allograft since the distal nerve stump consists of no host signaling mechanisms. In nerve allografts, the donor SCs are eventually replaced by host SCs migrating from both the proximal and distal nerve. In a CTA, however, the distal side is composed entirely of donor (Fig. 28.2). We do not know exactly how the distal regeneration signaling process is affected, or how the host axons and donor motor endplates interact.

There are limited information available thus far from current studies in CTA. In the rat hindlimb CTA model, Maeda et al. showed that quality of nerve regeneration in the allograft CTA were similar to that in isografts using electromyographic, histologic, and morphometric assessments at 8 months.[120] Both groups regenerated similarly but were of decreased quality compared with normal controls. Song et al.

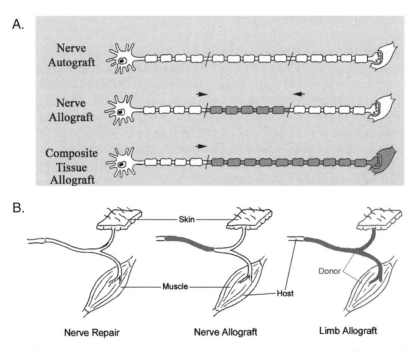

Figure 28.2 Fate of Schwann cells in nerve grafts. (**a**) In autografts, Schwann cells resist without replacement after grafting. In allografts, donor Schwann Cells are replaced from both proximal and distal anastimoses by host SCs. In composite tissue allografts, the fate of the grafted SCs is unknown, or the events that may occur at the motor end plates. (**b**) Interaction of nerve graft with associated tissues. In autogenous nerve repairs, sensory and motor targets are reinnervated. In nerve allografts, the allograft is eventually replaced by host. In composite tissue grafts, the fate of the nerve component is unknown since the target tissues are not of host origin

confirmed these findings at 1-year time point using walking track and electrophysiologic assessments.[121] Using GFP rats, Kimura et al. observed retrograde transmigration of GFP cells at the anastomosed sciatic nerve into host nerve.[25] Detailed descriptions of the nerves were not focused in their hindlimb experiment paper,[122] and it would be very interesting to see the interactions at the motor endplate level from these animals.

In human hand transplants, a number of unexpected observations were seen that are not explained by our current understanding of PNA regeneration. In the first hand-transplant patient, the ulnar and median nerves joined 20 and 21 cm proximal to the wrist crease, respectively. Tinel sign advanced to wrist crease by 100 days, faster than the expected normal regeneration of 1 mm/day.[123] In a 22-year-old man with traumatic circular-saw amputation of his right dominant forearm, functional MRI (fMRI) was used to provide objective clinical recovery of sensory function. This patient showed activation of the somatosensory and motor cortices as early as 10 days postoperatively.[124] Although a purely imaginary effect triggered by mechanical transmission to the upper part of the arm cannot be excluded, the fMRI observations were consistent with the patient's clinical exam. It appears that connections to the somatosensory cortex can be rapidly established prior to known sequence of axonal regeneration.

The relationship of skin rejection in a CTA and its effects on the underlying components has not yet been characterized. At follow-up of 15 months, the first double-hand transplant already experienced two episodes of acute skin rejection requiring increasing steroid doses. From extensive studies in SOTs, acute rejections in the early posttransplant periods are indicators for irreversible chronic rejection in later stages. In PNA studies, the addition of the skin component has been shown to adversely affect a PNA in the primate.[105] We currently do not have the data to know if that applies to CTA as well, and need to proceed cautiously and gather more human as well as large animal long-term data before making CTA a common part of the reconstructive armamentarium.

References

1. E. S. Dellon, A. L. Dellon, The first nerve graft, Vulpian, and the nineteenth century neural regeneration controversy, *J Hand Surg (Am)* **18**, 369 (1993).
2. E. Albert, Einige Operationen an Nerven, *Wien Med Presse* **26**, 1285 (1885).
3. G. C. Huber, A study of the operative treatment for loss of nerve substance in peripheral nerves, *J Morphol* **11**, 629 (1895).
4. A. W. Mayo-Robson, Nerve grafting as a means of restoring function in limbs paralyzed by gunshot or other injuries, *BMJ* **1**, 117 (1917).
5. H. J. Seddon, W. Holmes, The late condition of nerve homografts in man, *Surg Gynecol Obstet* **79**, 342 (1944).
6. R. G. Spurling, W. R. Lyons, B. B. Whitcomb, B. Woodhall, The failure of whole fresh homografts in man, *J Neurosurg* **2**, 79 (1945).
7. S. E. Mackinnon, Surgical management of the peripheral nerve gap, *Clin Plast Surg* **16**, 587 (1989).

8. S. E. Mackinnon, Nerve allotransplantation following sever tibial nerve injury: case report, *J Neurosurg* **84**, 671 (1996).
9. S. Y. Fu, T. Gordon, The cellular and molecular basis of peripheral nerve regeneration, *Mol Neurobiol* **14**, 67 (1997).
10. P. Hu, E. M. McLachlan, Selective reactions of cutaneous and muscle afferent neurons to peripheral nerve transaction in rats, *J Neurosci* **23**, 10559 (2003).
11. J. Ygge, Neuronal loss in lumbar dorsal root ganglia after proximal compared to distal sciatic nerve resection: a quantitative study in the rat, *Exp Brain Res* **478**, 193 (1989).
12. H. S. Xiao, Q. H. Hunag, F. X. Zhang, et al., Identification of gene expression profile of dorsal root ganglion in the rat peripheral axotomy model of neuropathic pain, *Proc Natl Acad Sci U S A* **99**, 8360 (2002).
13. C. S. Eddleman, G. D. Bittner, H. M. Fishman, Barrier permeability at cut axonal ends progressively decreases until an ionic seal is formed, *Biophys J* **79**, 1883 (2000).
14. M. C. Raff, A. V. Whitmore, J. T. Finn, Axonal self-destruction and neurodegeneration, *Science* **296**, 868 (2002).
15. G. Y. Wang, K. Hirai, H. Shimada, S. Taji, S. Z. Zhong, Behavior of axons, Schwann cells and perineurial cells in nerve regeneration within transplanted nerve grafts: effects of anti-laminin and anti-fibronectin antisera, *Exp Brain Res* **583**, 216 (1992).
16. C. Witzel, C. Rohde, T. M. Brushart, Pathway sampling be regenerating peripheral axons, *J Comp Neurol* **485**, 183 (2005).
17. M. J. Politis, K. Ederle, P. S. Spencer, Tropism in nerve regeneration in vivo. Attraction of regenerating axons by diffusible factors derived from cells in distal nerve stumps of transected peripheral nerves, *Exp Brain Res* **253**, 1 (1982).
18. T. M. Brushart, J. Gerber, P. Kessens, Y. G. Chen, R. M. Royall, Contributions of pathway and neuron to preferential motor reinnervation, *J Neurosci* **18**, 8674 (1998).
19. C. M. Nichols, M. J. Brenner, I. K. Fox, et al., Effect of motor versus sensory nerve grafts on peripheral nerve regeneration, *Exp Neurol* **190**, 347–355 (2004).
20. A. Waller, Experiments on the section of the glossopharyngeal and hypoglossal nerves of the frog, and observations on the alterations produced thereby in the structure of their primitive fibers, *Phil Trans R Soc Lond* **140**, 423 (1850).
21. K. R. Jessen, R. Mirsky, Why do Schwann cells survive in the absence of axons? *Ann N Y Acad Sci* **883**, 109 (1999).
22. W. Beuche, R. L. Friede, The role of non-resident cells in Wallerian degeneration, *J Neurocytol* **13**, 767 (1984).
23. A. J. Aguayo, J. Epps, L. Charron, G. M. Bray, Multipotentiality of Schwann cells in cross-anastomosed and grafted myelinated and unmyelinated nerves: quantitative microscopy and radioautography, *Exp Brain Res* **104**, 1 (1976).
24. R. Midha, V. Ramakrishna, C. A. Munro, T. Matsuyama, R. M. Gorczynski, Detection of host and donor cells in sex-mismatched rat nerve allograft using RT-PCR for a Y chromosome (H-Y) marker, *J Peripher Nerv Syst* **5**, 140 (2000).
25. A. Kimura, T. Ajiki, K. Takeuchi, et al., Transmigration of donor cells involved in the sciatic nerve graft, *Transplant Proc* **37**, 205 (2005).
26. A. K. Gulati, Evaluation of acellular and cellular nerve grafts in repair of rat peripheral nerve, *J Neurosurg* **68**, 117 (1988).
27. C. Taveggia, G. Zanazzi, A. Petrylak, et al., Neuregulin-1 Type III determines the ensheathment fate of axons, *Neuron* **47**, 681 (2005).
28. B. Strauch, D. M. Rodriguez, J. Diaz, H. L. Yu, G. Kaplan, D. E. Weinstein, Autologous Schwann cells drive regeneration through a 6-cm autogenous venous nerve conduit, *J Reconstr Microsurg* **17**, 589 (2001).
29. H. J. Weinberg, P. S. Spencer, The fate of Schwann cells isolated from axonal contact, *J Neurocytol* **7**, 555 (1978).
30. T. J. Best, S. E. Mackinnon, R. Midha, D. A. Hunter, P. J. Evans, Revascularization of peripheral nerve autografts and allografts, *Plast Reconstr Surg* **104**, 152 (1999).

31. T. J. Best, S. E. Mackinnon, P. J. Eves, D. Hunter, R. Midha, Peripheral nerve revascularization: histomorphometric study of small-and large caliber grafts, *J Reconstr Microsurg* **15**, 183 (1999).
32. G. Penkert, W. Bini, M. Samii, Revascularization of nerve grafts: an experimental study, *J Reconstr Microsurg* **4**, 319 (1988).
33. B. Prpa, P. M. Huddleston, K. N. An, M. B. Wood, Revascularization of nerve grafts: a qualitative and quantitative study of the soft-tissue bed contributions to blood flow in canine nerve grafts, *J Hand Surg (Am)* **27**, 1041 (2002).
34. C. R. Settergren, M. B. Wood, Comparison of blood flow in free vascularized versus nonvascularized nerve grafts, *J Reconstr Microsurg* **1**, 95 (1984).
35. R. Lind, M. B. Wood, Comparison of the pattern of early revascularization of conventional versus vascularized nerve grafts in the canine, *J Reconstr Microsurg* **2**, 229 (1986).
36. N. Imanishi, H. Nakajima, S. Fukuzumi, S. Aiso, Venous drainage of the distally based lesser saphenous-sural veno-neuroadipofascial pedicled fasciocutaneous flap: a radiographic perfusion study, *Plast Reconstr Surg* **103**, 494 (1999).
37. A. C. Masquelet, M. C. Romana, G. Wolf, Skin island flaps supplied by the vascular axis of the sensitive superficial nerves: anatomic study and clinical experience in the leg, *Plast Reconstr Surg* **89**, 1115 (1992).
38. B. Strauch, M. Ferder, S. Lovelle-Allen, K. Moore, D. J. Kim, J. Llena, Determining the maximal length of a vein conduit used as an interposition graft for nerve regeneration, *J Reconstr Surg* **12**, 521 (1996).
39. M. Merle, A. L. Dellon, J. N. Cambell, P. S. Chang, Complications from silicon-polymer intubulation of nerves, *Microsurgery* **10**, 130 (1989).
40. G. R. Evans, K. Brandt, S. Katz, et al., Bioactive poly(L-lactic acid) conduits seeded with Schwann cells for peripheral nerve regeneration, *Biomaterials* **23**, 841 (2002).
41. N. Sinis, H. Schaller, C. Schulte-Eversum, et al., Nerve regeneration across a 2-cm gap in the rat median nerve using a resorbable nerve conduit filled with Schwann cells, *J Neurosurg* **103**, 1067 (2005).
42. L. A. Pfister, T. Christen, H. P. Merkle, M. Papaloizos, B. Gander B, Novel biodegradable nerve conduits for peripheral nerve regeneration, *Eur Cell Mater* **7**, 16 (2004).
43. T. Hashimoto, Y. Suzuki, K. Suzuki, T. Nakashima, M. Tanihara, C. Ide, Review: peripheral nerve regeneration using non-tubular alginate gel crosslinked with covalent bonds, *J Mater Sci Mater Med* **16**, 503 (2005).
44. J. S. Belkas, S. C. Munro, M. S. Shoichet, R. Midha, Peripheral nerve regeneration through a synthetic hydrogel nerve tube, *Restor Neurol Neurosci* **23**, 19 (2005).
45. S. Y. Fu, T. Gordon, Contributing factors to poor functional recovery after delayed nerve repair: prolonged axotomy, *J Neurosci* **15**, 3876 (1995).
46. S. Y. Fu, T. Gordon, Contributing factors to poor functional recovery after delayed nerve repair: prolonged denervation, *J Neurosci* **15**, 3886 (1995).
47. A. K. Gulati, Evaluation of acellular and cellular nerve grafts in repair of rat peripheral nerve, *J Neurosurg* **68**, 117 (1988).
48. W. Nadim, P. N. Anderson, M. Turmaine, The role of Schwann cells and basal lamina tubes in the regeneration of axons through long lengths of freeze-killed nerve grafts, *Neuropathol Appl Neurobiol* **16**, 411 (1990).
49. P. J. Evans, R. Midha, S. E. Mackinnon, The peripheral nerve allograft: a comprehensive review of regeneration and neuroimmunology, *Prog Neurobiol* **43**, 187 (1994).
50. T. K. Das Gupta, Mechanism of rejection of peripheral nerve allografts, *Surg Gynecol Obstet* **125**, 1058 (1967).
51. J. D. Pollard, J. G. McLeod, Fresh and predegenerate nerve allografts and isografts in Tremble mice, *Muscle Nerve* **4**, 274–281 (1981).
52. A. K. Gulati, G. P. Cole, Nerve graft immunogenecity as a factor determining axonal regeneration in the rat, *J Neurosurg* **72**, 114 (1990).
53. C. Ide, T. Osawa, K. Tohkyama, Nerve regeneration through allogeneic nerve grafts, with special reference to Schwann cell basal lamina, *Prog Neurobiol* **34**, 1 (1990).

54. P. J. Evans, S. E. Mackinnon, A. Levi, et al., Cold preserved nerve allografts: changes in basement membrane, viability, immunogenicity, and regeneration, *Muscle Nerve* **21**, 1507 (1998).
55. H. Wekerle, M. Schwab, C. Linington, R. Meyermann, Antigen presentation in the peripheral nervous system: Schwann cells present endogenous myelin autoantigens to lymphocytes, *Eur J Immunol* **16**, 1551 (1986).
56. F. Lassner, E. Schaller, G. Steinhoff, K. Wonigeit, G. F. Walter, A. Berger, Cellular mechanisms of rejection and regeneration in peripheral nerve allografts, *Transplantation* **48**, 386 (1989).
57. A. D. Ansselin, J. D. Pollard, Immunopathological factors in peripheral nerve allograft rejection: quantification of lymphocyte invasion and major histocompatibility complex expression, *J Neurol Sci* **96**, 75 (1990).
58. S. E. Mackinnon, A. R. Hudson, R. E. Falk, D. Kline, D. Hunter, Peripheral nerve allograft: an immunological assessment of pretreatment methods, *Neurosurgery* **14**, 167 (1984).
59. L. Yu, W. F. Hickey, W. K. Silvers, D. Larossa, A. M. Rostami, Expression of class II antigens on peripheral nerve allografts, *Ann N Y Acad Sci* **540**, 472 (1988).
60. L. Marmor, Regeneration of peripheral nerves defects by irradiated homografts, *Lancet* **1**, 1190 (1963).
61. L. Marmor, The repair of peripheral nerves by irradiated homografts, *Clin Orthop* **34**, 161 (1964).
62. L. Marmor, Nerve grafting in peripheral nerve repair, *Surg Clin North Am* **52**, 1177 (1972).
63. B. L. Buch, Experimental study of radiated vs. fresh nerve homografts, *Plast Reconstr Surg* **45**, 586 (1970).
64. R. Singh, S. A. Lange, Experience with homologous lyophilized nerve grafts in the treatment of peripheral nerve injuries, *Acta Neurochir* **32**, 125–130 (1975).
63. T. Osawa, C. Ide, K. Tohyama,. Nerve regeneration through allogenic nerve grafts in mice, *Arch Histol Jpn* **49**, 69 (1986).
66. T. Osawa, C. Ide, K. Tohyama, Nerve regeneration through cryo-treated xenogeneic nerve grafts, *Arch Histol Jpn* **50**, 193 (1987).
67. C. Ide, K. Tohyama, K. Tajima, et al., Long acellular nerve transplants for allogeneic grafting and the effects of basic fibroblast growth factor on the growth of regenerating axons in dogs: a preliminary report, *Exp Neurol* **154**, 99 (1998).
68. K. Tajima, K. Tohyama, C. Ide, M. Abe, Regeneration through nerve allografts in the cynomolgus monkey (*Macaca fascicularis*), *J Bone Joint Surg (Am)* **73**, 172 (1991).
69. A. A. Zalewski, A. K. Gulati, Evaluation of histocompatibility as a factor in the repair of nerve with a frozen nerve allograft, *J Neurosurg* **56**, 550 (1982).
70. S. Mackinnon, A. Hudson, R. Falk, J. Bilbao, D. Kline, D. Hunter, Nerve allograft response: a quantitative immunological study, *Neurosurgery* **10**, 61 (1982).
71. S. E. Mackinnon, A. R. Hudson, R. E. Falk, D. Kline, D. Hunter, Peripheral nerve allograft: an assessment of regeneration across pretreated nerve allografts, *Neurosurgery* **15**, 690 (1984).
72. I. M. Tarlov, J. A. Epstein, Nerve grafts. The importance of an adequate blood supply, *J Neurosurg* **2**, 49 (1945).
73. F. K. Sanders, J. Z. Young, The degeneration and re-innervation of grafted nerves, *J Anat* **76**, 143 (1942).
74. G. M. Hare, P. J. Evans, S. E. Mackinnon, et al., Effect of cold preservation on lymphocyte migration into peripheral nerve allografts in sheep, *Transplantation* **56**, 154–62 (1993).
75. A. Atchabahian, S. E. Mackinnon, D. A. Hunter, Cold preservation of nerve grafts decreases expression of ICAM-1 and class II MHC antigens, *J Reconstr Microsurg* **15**, 307 (1999).
76. I. K. Fox, A. Jaramillo, D. A. Hunter, S. R. Rickman, T. Mohanankumar, S. E. Mackinnon, Prolonged cold-preservation of nerve allografts, *Muscle Nerve* **31**, 59 (2005).
77. A. K. Gulati, Immunological fate of Schwann cell-populated acellular basal lamina nerve allografts, *Transplantation* **59**, 1618 (1995).
78. G. Keilhoff, F. Pratsch, G. Wolf, H. Fansa, Bridging extra large defects of peripheral nerves: possibilities and limitations of alternative biological grafts from acellular muscle and Schwann cells, *Tissue Eng* **11**, 1004 (2005).

79. F. J. Rodriguez, E. Verdu, D. Ceballos, X. Navarro, Nerve guides seeded with autologous Schwann cells improve nerve regeneration, *Exp Neurol* **161**, 571 (2000).
80. H. Fansa, T. Dodic, G. Wolf, W. Schneider, G. Keilhoff, Tissue engineering of peripheral nerves: epineurial grafts with application of cultured Schwann cells, *Microsurgery* **23**, 72 (2003).
81. H. Fansa, G. Keilhoff, Comparison of different biogenic matrices seeded with cultured Schwann cells for bridging peripheral nerve defects, *Neurol Res* **26**, 167 (2004).
82. H. Fansa, W. Schneider, G. Keilhoff, Revascularization of tissue-engineered nerve grafts and invasion of macrophages, *Tissue Eng* **7**, 519 (2001).
83. A. A. Zalewski, A. K. Gulati, Survival of nerve allografts in sensitized rats treated with cyclosporine A, *J Neurosurg* **60**, 828 (1984).
84. J. R. Bain, S. E. Mackinnon, A. R. Hudson, R. E. Falk, J. A. Falk, D. A. Hunter, The peripheral nerve allograft: a dose-response curve in the rat immunosuppressed with cyclosporine A, *Plast Reconstr Surg* **32**, 447 (1998).
85. R. Midha, S. E. Mackinnon, L. E. Becker, The fate of Schwann cells in peripheral nerve allografts, *J Neuropathol Exp Neurol* **53**, 316 (1994).
86. A. Atchabahian, V. B. Doolabh, S. E. Mackinnon, S. Yu, D. A. Hunter, M. A. Flye, Indefinite survival of peripheral nerve allografts after temporary cyclosporine A immunosuppression, *Restor Neurol Neurosci* **13**, 129 (1998).
87. D. L. Chen, S. E. Mackinnon, J. N. Jensen, D. A. Hunter, A. G. Grand, Failure of cyclosporine A to rescue peripheral nerve allografts in acute rejection, *Ann Plast Surg* **49**, 660 (2002).
88. D. J. Fox, V. Doolabh, S. E. Mackinnon, E. M. Genden, D. A. Hunter, Decreased cyclosporin A requirement with anti-ICAM-1 and anti-LFA-1α in a peripheral nerve allotransplantation model, *Restor Neurol Neurosci* **15**, 319 (1999).
89. C. P. Larsen, E. T. Elwood, D. Z. Alexander, et al., Long-term acceptance of skin and cardiac allografts after blocking CD40 and CD28 pathways, *Nature* **381**, 434 (1996).
90. A. Chandraker, M. E. Russell, T. Glysing-Jensen, T. A. Willet, M. H. Sayegh, T-cell costimulatory blockade in experimental chronic cardiac allograft rejection, *Transplantation* **63**, 1053–1058 (1997).
91. M. S. Wang, M. Zeleney-Pooley, B. G. Gold, Comparative dose-dependent study of FK506 and cyclosporine A on the rate of axonal regeneration in the rat sciatic nerve, *J Pharmacol Exp Ther* **282**, 1084 (1997).
92. T. M. Dawson, J. P. Steiner, V. L. Dawson, J. L. Dinerman, G. R. Uhl, S. H. Snyder, Immunosuppressant FK506 enhances phosphorylation of nitric oxide synthase and protects against glutamate neurotoxicity, *Proc Natl Acad Sci U S A* **90**, 9808 (1993).
93. C. Yardin, F. Terro, M. Lesort, F. Esclaire, J. Hugon, FK506 antagonized apoptosis and c-jun protein expression in neuronal cultures, *Neuroreport* **9**, 2077 (1998).
94. B. Gold, J. Voda, X. Yu, H. Gordon, The immunosuppressant FK506 elicits a neuronal heat shock response and protects against acrylamide neuropathy, *Exp Neurol* **187**, 160 (2004).
95. M. Oltean, R. Olofsson, C. Zhu, S. Mera, K. Blomgren, M. Olausson, FK506 donor pretreatment improves intestinal graft microcirculation and morphology by concurrent inhibition of early NF-κB activation and augmented HSP72 synthesis, *Transplant Proc* **37**, 1931 (2005).
96. V. B. Doolabh, S. E. Mackinnon, FK506 accelerates functional recovery following nerve grafting in a rat model, *Plast Reconstr Surg* **103**, 1928 (1999).
97. H. Fansa, G. Keilhoff, S. Altmann, K. Plogmeier, G. Wolf, W. Schneider, The effect of the immunosuppressant FK506 on peripheral nerve regeneration following nerve grafting, *J Hand Surg (Br)* **24**, 38 (1999).
98. A. G. Grand, T. M. Myckatyn, S. E. Mackinnon, The synergistic effects of cold preservation and FK506 on peripheral nerve allografts. In *Proceedings of the Midwestern Association of Plastics Surgeons*, Chicago, IL, April 7–9, 2000.
99. L. Backman, M. Nicar, M. Levy, et al., FK506 trough levels in whole blood and plasma in liver transplant recipients. Correlation with clinical events and side effects, *Transplantation* **57**, 519 (1994).

100. S. L. Small, M. B. Fukui, G. T. Bramblett, B. H. Eidelman, Immunosuppression-induced leukoencephalopathy from tacrolimus (FK506), *Ann Neurol* **40**, 575 (1996).
101. A. Yamauchi, R. Oishi, Y. Kataoka, Tacrolimus-induced neurotoxicity and nephrotoxicity is ameliorated by administration in the dark phase in rats, *Cell Mol Neurobiol* **24**, 695 (2004).
102. J. B. Sobol, I. J. Lowe, R. K. Yang, S. K. Sen, D. A. Hunter, S. E. Mackinnon, Effects of delaying FK506 administration on neuroregeneration in a rodent model, *J Reconstr Microsurg* **19**, 113 (2003).
103. A. K. Snyder, I. K. Fox, C. M. Nichols, S. R. Rickman, D. A. Hunter, S. E. Mackinnon, Neuroregenerative effects of pre-injury FK-506 administration, *Plast Reconstr Surg*, 118, 360 (2006).
104. M. J. Brenner, T. T. Tung, S. E. Mackinnon, T. M. Myckatyn, D. A. Hunter, T. Mohanakumar, Anti-CD40 ligand monoclonal antibody induces a permissive state, but not tolerance for murine peripheral nerve allografts, *Exp Neurol* **186**, 59 (2004).
105. M. J. Brenner, J. N. Jensen, J. B. Lowe III, et al., Anti-CD40 ligand antibody permits regeneration through peripheral nerve allografts in a nonhuman primate model, *Plast Reconstr Surg* **114**, 1802 (2004).
106. S. K. Sen, J. B. Lowe II, M. J. Brenner, D. A. Hunter, S. E. Mackinnon, Assessment of the immune response to dose of nerve allografts, *Plast Reconstr Surg* **115**, 823 (2005).
107. M. J. Brenner, S. E. Mackinnon, S. R. Rickman, et al., FK506 and anti-CD40 ligand in peripheral nerve allotransplantation, *Restor Neurol Neurosci* **23**, 237 (2005).
108. S. D. Moffat, S. M. Metcalfe, Comparison between tacrolimus and cyclosporine as immunosuppressive agents compatible with tolerance induction by CD4/CD8 blockade, *Transplantation* **69**, 1724 (2000).
109. Y. Li, X. X. Zheng, X. C. Li, M. S. Zand, T. B. Strom, Combined costimulation blockade plus rapamycin but not cyclosporine produces permanent engraftment, *Transplantation* **60**, 1387 (1998).
110. T. M. Myckatyn, R. A. Ellis, A. G. Grand, S. K. Sen, J. B. Lowe III, D. A. Hunter, S. E. Mackinnon, The effects of rapamycin in murine peripheral nerve isografts and allografts, *Plast Reconstr Surg* **109**, 2405 (2002).
111. H. Lau, K. Reemtsma, M. A. Hardy, Pancreatic islet allograft prolongation by donor-specific blood transfusions treated with ultraviolet irradiation, *Science* **221**, 754 (1983).
112. S. F. Oluwole, N. C. Chowdhurg, R. A. Fawwaz, Induction of donor-specific unresponsiveness to rat cardiac allografts by intrathymic injection of UV-B-irradiated donor spleen cells, *Transplantation* **55**, 1389 (1993).
113. S. Yu, Y. Nakafusa, M. W. Flye, Portal vein administration of donor cells promotes peripheral allospecific hyporesponsiveness and graft tolerance, *Surgery* **116**, 229 (1994).
114. T. Kamei, M. P. Callery, M. W. Flye, Pretranspalnt portal venous administration of donor antigen and PV allograft drainage synergistically prolong rat cardiac allograft survival, *Surgery* **108**, 415 (1990).
115. V. B. Doolabh, T. H. Tung, M. W. Flye, S. E. Mackinnon, Effect of nondepleting anti-CD4 monoclonal antibody (Rib 5/2) plus donor antigen pretreatment in peripheral nerve allotransplantation, *Microsurgery* **22**, 329 (2002).
116. E. M. Genden, S. E. Mackinnon, S. Yu, M. W. Flye, Induction of donor-specific tolerance to rat nerve allografts with portal venous donor alloantigen and anti-ICAM-1/LFA-1 monoclonal antibodies, *Surgery* **124**, 448 (1998).
117. T. H. Tung, V. B. Doolabh, S. E. Mackinnon, D. Hunter, M. W. Flye, Immune unresponsiveness by intraportal UV-B-irradiated donor antigen administration requires persistence of donor antigen in a nerve allograft model, *J Reconstr Microsurg* **20**, 43 (2004).
118. S. E. Mackinnon, V. B. Doolabh, C. B. Novak, E. P. Trulock, Clinical outcome following nerve allograft transplantation, *Plast Reconstr Surg* **107**, 1419–1428 (2001).
119. M. Pespeni, M. Hodnett, J. F. Pittet, In vivo stress preconditioning, *Methods* **35**, 158 (2005).
120. N. Maeda, N. Ishiguro, G. Inoue, T. Miura, K. Sugimura, Nerve regeneration in rat composite-tissue allografts, *J Reconstr Microsurg* **7**, 297 (1991).

121. Y. X. Song, K. Muramatsu, Y. Kurokawa, et al., Functional recovery of rat hind-limb allografts, *J Reconstr Microsurg* **21**, 471 (2005).
122. T. Ajiki, M. Takahashi, S. Inoue, et al., Generation of donor hematolymphoid cells after rat-limb composite grafting, *Transplantation* **75**, 631 (2003).
123. E. R. Owen, J. M. Dubernard, M. Lanzetta, H. Kapila, X. Martin, M. Dawahra, N. S. Hakim, Peripheral nerve regeneration in human hand transplantation, *Transplant Proc* **33**, 1720 (2001).
124. C. Neugroschl, V. Denolin, F. Schuind, et al., Functional MRI activation of somatosensory and motor cortices in a hand-grafted patient with early clinical sensorimotor recovery, *Eur Radiol* **15**, 1806 (2005).

Chapter 29
Live-Donor Nerve Transplantation

Scott A. Gruber and Pedro Mancias

29.1 Introduction

We recently reported the first case of live-donor nerve transplantation, performed in November 2000 in an 8-month-old infant with global obstetric brachial plexus palsy (OBPP) and four root avulsion who had undergone prior sural nerve autografting at 3 months.[1] Cross-chest C7 nerve transfer and temporary tacrolimus (TCL)/prednisone immunosuppression were utilized. The purpose of this chapter is twofold. First, we provide the scientific rationale for our decision to develop the research protocol by reviewing the background information available at the time with regard to (1) the current treatment and long-term prognosis for infants with global OBPP; (2) use of the contralateral C7 nerve root as a donor site; (3) prior experimental and clinical experience with peripheral nerve allografting and clinical hand transplantation; and (4) experience with the use of immunosuppressants in pediatric solid-organ transplant recipients as well as in infants and young children receiving these drugs for nontransplant indications. Second, we present the case in detail and discuss the results obtained.

29.2 OBPP

The incidence of OBPP is approximately 1–2 per 1,000 live births in the United States and up to tenfold higher in underdeveloped countries.[2,3] Despite overall improvements in obstetrical care and training, the incidence may be increasing due to increasing newborn birth weight; pressure to decrease the number of C-sections; and increased performance of midwife-assisted and home deliveries. The plexopathy is equally distributed between males and females,[4] and gestational age does not seem to play a role. Vertex presentation accounts for 94–97%; breech presentation 1–2%; and C-section deliveries 1% of the cases.[2] OBPP is most likely the result of direct or indirect compression from delivery instruments or fingers in cases of fetal malposition and cephalopelvic disproportion with subsequent traction/avulsion injury to the nerve roots.[2,5] Upper root palsy (C5 and C6 ± C7 involvement) occurs most frequently; isolated lower root palsy (C8-T1) rarely; and complete (global) lesions (C5-T1) with intermediate frequency.[2,3,6] In one series, however, 51 of 80 patients had global palsy.[2] Ipsilateral clavicular fracture is the most commonly associated injury.[2]

Approximately 80% of patients recover spontaneously within months and with minimal residual dysfunction.[2] Patients without spontaneous recovery, as evidenced by persistent signs of global paralysis (flail arm and Horner's sign) or absence of deltoid and/or biceps contraction, should undergo exploratory surgery by 3 months. The goals of this initial procedure are to (1) anatomically define the extent of injury; (2) resect neuromas; and (3) perform local nerve repair (neurotization) as indicated, either with direct suture or using bilateral nonvascularized sural nerve autografts to bridge the gaps. Autotransplantation of sacrificable peripheral nerves, such as lower extremity sural nerves which are only sensory in function, provides optimal nerve regeneration and has become the gold standard for reconstituting peripheral nerve gaps and deficits in injured limbs. In the patient with brachial plexus injury, priority is given to reconstructing the suprascapular, musculocutaneous, and axillary nerves to achieve stability of the shoulder and elbow function.[2,5]

The nerve graft serves merely as a structural conduit, providing Schwann cells (SCs), endoneurial sheaths, and neurotrophic factors, through which the severed recipient axons regenerate in a proximal to distal direction along the extremity to reach their sensory end organs and target muscles. Sensory receptors are far more resilient and will accept reinnervation after prolonged denervation. In contrast, the total time that the target muscle remains denervated is critical with regard to the functional result achievable following nerve grafting. Generally speaking, best functional results are achieved if the target muscle is reinnervated within 9–12 months from the time of injury. Satisfactory results may still be achieved if the motor endplate is reached in 12–18 months, but if the delay is more than 18 months, the chances for meaningful return of motor function are significantly compromised. Since in the healthy adult, nerves regenerate at a rate of 1 mm/day, the total time interval from injury to reinnervation normally depends on two factors: (1) how soon nerve grafting is accomplished following injury; and (2) the distance across which the recipient axons need to regenerate.

In patients with global OBPP, there is simply not sufficient length of autograft nerve available of suitable quality for achieving wrist and finger function, even if an ipsilateral vascularized ulnar nerve autograft is used. Indeed, with current therapeutic modalities, affected individuals rarely regain useful hand and wrist function, and may be left with socially disabling secondary deformities and hand posturing which produce deleterious medical, psychological, and economic sequelae for the patient and his or her family. Although these deformities can be corrected surgically with aid of tendon transfers, the overall functional gain is never enough to dramatically improve the daily use of the limb.[7] In one series of 20 patients with total OBPP treated with nerve reconstruction, only 20% and 35% regained useful function of the shoulder and elbow, respectively.[8] Of the 17 patients with a totally palsied hand preoperatively, none regained useful movement of the wrist, fingers, or thumbs after primary or secondary surgery. Given these results, the continued search for a new modality of therapy seems justified.

Based on the above, we reasoned that the affected infant's only hope for a complete functional restoration of the upper extremity would be to undergo a second surgical procedure during which nerve allografts, taken from living or deceased donors, are used to traverse the distance between remaining contralateral motor and sensory "donor nerves" and the median, radial, and medial pectoral nerves on the injured side. Examples of suitable "donors" include C7 nerve root (see below), ulnar nerve, thoracodorsal nerve, and medial pectoral nerve on the uninjured side. Ideally, this procedure using transplanted nerve should be performed as soon as possible following the exploration at 3 months to optimize the patient's ultimate chance for achieving the best functional recovery. The fact that

1. Nerve regeneration in the pediatric age group is faster than that in adults
2. The absolute distances which need to be traversed are much less, particularly in the infant
3. The overall "plasticity" of the nervous system in the infant and child is greater than that in adults
4. The immunosuppressive drug TCL, which would be used as the primary agent for preventing rejection of the nerve allograft (see below), is also a nerve growth factor which speeds the rate of nerve recovery and regeneration[9,10]

are all theoretical factors in the patient's favor with regard to achieving an excellent functional result following nerve transplantation for complete OBPP.

29.3 Cross-Chest C7 Nerve Transfer (Adapted from Gruber et al.[1])

Although controversial when first introduced by Gu et al.[11] and Chuang et al.[12] in the early 1990s, multiple investigators demonstrated over the subsequent decade that the contralateral normal isolated C7 root can be safely divided in part or in its entirety and used as a donor nerve for treatment of a posttraumatic complete brachial plexus injury via subcutaneous cross-chest or prespinal transfer.[13–18] In these studies, motor and sensory neurologic deficits of the ipsilateral upper extremity were either never clinically apparent or transient, with complete resolution and/or full functional recovery by 3–6 months, presumably as a result of the presence of considerable crossinnervation with C6 and C8.

29.4 Nerve Transplantation in Animal Models

Many experimental studies have demonstrated regeneration of nerve allografts in rats and mice immunosuppressed with continuous cyclosporin A (CsA) therapy equivalent to that across nerve autografts.[19–22] In the early 1990s, Bain and

Mackinnon demonstrated excellent regeneration and functional reinnervation across short-segment (3-cm) nerve allografts in primates immunosuppressed with CsA, similar to that seen in autograft controls.[23,24] More recently, excellent regeneration through rat nerve allografts has been observed with the immunosuppressant TCL, which not only prevents rejection across a major histocompatibility barrier,[25] but also enhances the rate of nerve regeneration more so than does CsA.[26,27]

A substantial body of experimental evidence supports the concept that immunosuppression is only required on a temporary basis until demonstrable nerve regeneration across the allograft conduit has occurred. Withdrawal of CsA in rat nerve allograft models following reinnervation of end organs results in a modified rejection response, consisting of demyelination and remyelination components accompanied by a transient decrease in function.[28,29] Following initial injury and degeneration, a significant proportion of axons persist and survive in the demyelinated state. Subsequent axonal remyelination and regeneration result in rapid restoration of graft histologic and functional parameters to a level equivalent to that in grafts maintained on continuous immunosuppressive therapy.[28,29] Similar findings have been reported in rat allograft recipients immunosuppressed with TCL.[25]

Consistent with these observations, it has been proposed that the SC, a highly immunogenic component of peripheral nerve, is the main target of the allograft rejection response.[21] Upregulation of major histocompatibility complex (MHC) class II expression on SCs has been demonstrated,[30] along with the ability to act as antigen presenting cells to T lymphocytes.[31] In an adequately immunosuppressed allograft recipient, regenerated host axons become ensheathed by donor SC.[32] Withdrawal of immunosuppression has differential effects on graft constituents, with rejection of donor-derived SCs, survival of demyelinated host axons, and eventual replacement with recipient-derived SCs.[25,33]

Multiple studies in canine, rabbit, and rat nerve transplant models emphasize the importance of genetic relatedness between donor and recipient strains with regard to the incidence, timing, and severity of acute rejection.[34-49] In general, nerves transplanted across minor histocompatibility differences did not reject or rejected late and demonstrated superior regeneration, whereas those transplanted across MHC barriers were acutely rejected and demonstrated no or inferior regeneration. In an outbred rabbit model for example, parent-to-F1 transplants produced the least rejection, followed by same-strain transplants, which, in turn, were superior to grafts between different strains.[49] Moreover, there is experimental data which suggests that the rapidity and severity of the antiallograft rejection response increases as the volume or length of nerve transplanted (i.e., the antigenic load) increases.[50-52] On the basis of this information, clinical transplantation of the relatively short length of nerve allograft that would be required from a related living adult donor, such as a parent, into an infant would provide a one-haplotype matched graft with a theoretically decreased propensity for rejection.

In an attempt to decrease the immunogenicity of nerve allografts, various pretreatment methods, including repeated freeze-thawing, lyophilization, and irradiation, have been investigated, with cold storage emerging as the most successful and clinically relevant.[53–57] In 1993, Mackinnon's laboratory noted that lymphocyte migration into sheep peripheral nerve allografts was reduced down to corresponding autograft levels if the grafts were preserved in University of Wisconsin (UW) solution at 5°C for 7 days prior to implantation.[56] This is the same preservation solution that is used routinely for cold storage of solid-organ transplants. In a follow-up study, Strasberg and Mackinnon demonstrated that cold storage of rat posterior tibial nerve allografts in UW solution for 1 week prior to implantation resulted in better nerve regeneration by all histomorphometric parameters studied when compared with recipients of fresh grafts at the two CsA doses that were studied.[57] Moreover, functional recovery of preserved grafts was equivalent to that of autografts regardless of CsA dose, while functional recovery of fresh grafts was equivalent to that of autografts only in the subgroup receiving high-dose CsA. These data suggest that cold storage pretreatment may decrease immunosuppressive drug requirements while preserving SC viability and maintaining adequate regeneration. Finally, storage of nerves prior to transplantation is clinically feasible; would facilitate elective planning; and would give time for recipient "loading" with immunosuppressive drugs to achieve therapeutic blood levels by the time of the scheduled procedure.

29.5 Peripheral Nerve Allografting: Clinical Experience

Although the first reported account of peripheral nerve allografting appeared in 1885 with sporadic cases documented throughout the twentieth century, the modern era of clinical nerve transplantation began in 1988 when Mackinnon performed the first of two cases utilizing CsA-based immunosuppression. In brief, the two cases are as follows.[58,59]

29.5.1 Case 1

An 8-year-old boy sustaining an extensive left sciatic nerve injury from a motor boat propeller accident received a cadaveric-donor nerve allograft 4 months postinjury (September 1988). The defect was reconstructed using ten nerve allografts, 23 cm in length. Immunosuppression consisted of CsA 100 mg po BID, subsequently adjusted to maintain plasma trough levels 50–60 ng/ml by RIA, and prednisone, 10 mg po qd. The drugs were discontinued 26 months after surgery, when reliable evidence of functional sensibility in the peroneal and posterior tibial nerve distributions was obtained. Independent evaluation of the left foot revealed monofilament pressure thresholds of 5.18 versus 3.84 in the right foot; vibratory thresholds of 1.2–1.8 mm amplitude versus 1.2 mm in the right foot; light touch present with a two-point discrimination of 4 cm; and pinprick sensibility.

29.5.2 Case 2

A 12-year-old boy sustaining a severe posterior tibial nerve injury from a riding lawn-mower accident received a cadaveric-donor nerve allograft 5 months postinjury (September 1993). The defect was reconstructed using eight nerve allografts, 20 cm in length, that were stored in UW solution at 5°C for 1 week prior to implantation. Initial immunosuppression consisted of CsA 150 mg po BID begun 4 days prior to transplantation, with subsequent adjustment to maintain whole-blood trough levels 150–200 ng/ml, and prednisone 10 mg po qd. The CsA dose was decreased to 125 mg po BID at 3 months; 75 mg po BID at 7 months; and discontinued at 17 months posttransplant, 5 months after the Tinel's sign had reached the foot and light touch sensation was present. The prednisone dose was decreased to 7.5 mg po qod at 3 months due to weight gain, and was discontinued at 13 months. Quantitative measurement of return of sensation in the foot, including cutaneous pressure and vibratory thresholds as well as static and moving two-point discrimination revealed that all modalities returned but not equivalent to the uninjured contralateral side. Recovery was qualitatively judged as 7/10 versus 10/10 on the normal side. The patient walked without assistance and was pain-free.

In both cases, the donor and recipient were ABO-blood group compatible; T- and B-cell crossmatches were negative; there was no clinical evidence of acute rejection; there were no significant drug-specific or general systemic side effects from the immunosuppressants except weight gain, which resolved spontaneously; there was no evidence of even transient deterioration of nerve function following withdrawal of immunosuppression; and, perhaps most importantly, there was no motor recovery.

Clearly, if nerve allografting is to restore upper extremity functional deficits in children with OBPP, then motor recovery is essential. From 1993 to 1998, the Washington University group transplanted an additional five patients who sustained traumatic extremity injuries (four upper extremity, one lower extremity) with massive peripheral nerve deficits that could not be reconstructed by conventional means, and ranged from 3 to 26 years of age.[60] In contrast to the previous two cases in which allografts were used exclusively for the reconstruction, allografts were used in combination with autografts in these later cases. Total allograft length varied from 72 cm in a 3-year old to 350 cm for a three-nerve reconstruction in a 16-year old. All allografts were cold-stored in UW solution for 1 week prior to implantation. Initial immunosuppression consisted of CsA (three cases; trough levels 200–300 ng/ml) or TCL (2 cases; trough levels 5–15 ng/ml) in combination with azathioprine (1.0–1.5 mg/kg/d) and prednisone (0.25–0.5 mg/kg/d). Drug doses were tapered and ultimately discontinued when the Tinel's sign had progressed into the distal segment of the reconstructed nerve (12–19 months posttransplant). One graft was lost as a result of failure to timely diagnose and treat acute rejection at a clinic remote from the transplant center when the patient presented with obvious clinical signs in the setting of subtherapeutic immunosuppression. Although one cannot draw any definite conclusions, it is interesting to note that this graft was the one with greatest total length (350 cm). Of the remaining four patients, all have had sensory recovery and three excellent motor recovery (Medical Research Council grade 4/5) with useful function. Again, in contrast to the experimental data, none of the patients showed any evidence of even transient deterioration of nerve function following withdrawal of immunosuppression, and no complications of systemic immunosuppression occurred. When examined in toto, the experience prior to November 2000 indicated that clinical nerve allografting could be safely and successfully accomplished with sensory and motor recovery utilizing a temporary, 1–2-year maintenance immunosuppressive regimen that was comparable to that used for renal transplant recipients without the need for antilymphocyte antibody induction.

29.6   Clinical Hand Transplantation

In September 1998 and January 1999, the first and second successful human hand transplants were performed in Lyon, France and at the Jewish Hospital of Louisville, Kentucky, respectively.[61,62] In both cases, (1) combination TCL, mycophenolate mofetil (MMF), and prednisone maintenance immunosuppression was utilized; (2) the rate of sensory nerve regeneration was faster than that observed in replants, presumably the result of two factors: the controlled nature of the donor procedure and the facilitatory effect of TCL on nerve regeneration; and most importantly, (3) return of intrinsic muscle function within the hand was documented. In the French patient, despite being lost to follow up for 8 months and sustaining a late episode of acute rejection due to noncompliance, activity appeared within the abductor digiti minimi muscle at 12 months; was detected as very weak in the other intrinsic muscles by 16 months; and was present into the first dorsal interosseous muscle by 17 months.[63] In the Louisville patient, there was electromyographic evidence of intrinsic muscle innervation by 1 year, with 3/5 strength thumb adduction at 18 months (Personal communication from Dr. Warren Breidenbach).

29.7   Risks of Immunosuppression

Prior to November 2000, there already was much experience with the use of immunosuppressive agents in the 6-month to 2-year-old age group, not only with solid-organ transplant recipients (kidney, liver, and heart), but also in pediatric patients receiving these drugs for nontransplant indications. For example, low-to-moderate dose CsA had been used in the treatment of steroid-dependent or steroid-resistant nephrotic syndrome for up to 2 years with a low incidence of drug-induced side effects.[64,65] Along these lines, in one study of 28 infant heart transplant patients receiving CsA and azathioprine, both axial and craniofacial growth were not significantly altered when compared with standardized growth and development curves during the time period of evaluation.[66]

The risk of immunosuppressive therapy in our otherwise-healthy infant with OBPP undergoing living-donor nerve allografting using the regimen described in this protocol (next section) could be divided into two categories: (1) drug-specific side effects, and (2) general (systemic) side effects. Some assessment of the magnitude of these risks was made by making comparisons to Mackinnon's series of patients; to the pediatric renal transplant population; and to children with nephrotic syndrome.

The planned total exposure of our patient to prednisone, particularly in the early postoperative period, was an order of magnitude less than that of pediatric renal transplant recipients and several-fold less than that in children who receive steroids for minimal-change nephrotic syndrome (see below). In addition, the intended duration of therapy was at most 18 months, with dose tapering along the way. Moreover, since the incidence of rejection in nerve allograft recipients treated similarly appeared to be low, the likelihood of our patient receiving additional steroid pulse therapy was correspondingly low. Finally, the only steroid-related toxicity reported by Mackinnon's group was weight gain. As a result, although our patient might develop weight gain, fluid retention, and a Cushingoid appearance, the risk for development of other steroid-related complications, particularly growth suppression, osteopenia, and cataract formation, was felt to be miniscule.

In renal allograft recipients, the risk for development of infection (most importantly, CMV) and PTLD is most dependent upon the total burden of immunosuppression to which the patient is exposed.[67] Given the fact that in our nerve transplant patient (1) antilymphocyte antibody would not be used for induction or treatment of rejection; (2) a two-drug, rather than three-drug, maintenance immunosuppressive regimen would be employed with much lower prednisone exposure; (3) the incidence of rejection, the treatment of which would require additional immunosuppressive therapy, was likely to be very low; and (4) immunosuppression would be temporary, the risk for development of a serious opportunistic infection or non-Hodgkins lymphoma was estimated to be much less than that of a renal transplant recipient and altogether very, very low (probably in the range of 1–0.1%, respectively).[68,69] None of Mackinnon's patients developed these complications.

29.8 Case Presentation (Adapted from Gruber et al.[1])

The patient is a Mexican male born to a gravida 1 para 1 mother at 40 weeks gestation in March 2000 with birth weight 3,500 g noted to have a left global OBPP. Surgical exploration at 3 months revealed complete C6-T1 avulsions with a proximal C5 rupture. At this time, the spinal accessory nerve was directly transferred to the suprascapular nerve, and sural nerve autografts were used to bridge gaps from the C4 nerve root to the axillary nerve and from the C5 nerve root to the musculocutaneous nerve (Fig. 29.1).

Live-Donor Nerve Transplantation 415

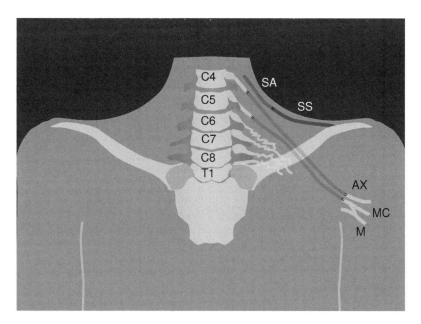

Fig. 29.1 Initial procedure performed at 3 months of age. Surgical exploration revealed complete C6-T1 avulsions with a proximal C5 rupture. The spinal accessory nerve (SA) was directly transferred to the suprascapular nerve (SS), and sural nerve autografts were used to bridge gaps from the C4 nerve root to the axillary nerve (AX) and from the C5 nerve root to the musculocutaneous nerve (MC). The median nerve (M) is shown for reference. Reproduced with permission from Gruber et al.[1]

On presentation to Memorial Hermann Children's Hospital in September 2000, the patient was in the fifth percentile for height and tenth percentile for weight and head circumference, and was developmentally normal. Physical examination of the left upper extremity demonstrated minimal shoulder abduction (MRC 1/5) and elbow flexion (MRC 1/5), with no wrist extension or flexion and no intrinsic hand function. Preoperative EMG testing at 8 months of age revealed absent median, ulnar, and radial sensory responses on the left, with normal responses on the right. The left median and ulnar nerve compound muscle action potentials (CMAPs) showed mildly prolonged distal latencies and severely reduced amplitudes, with normal responses on the right. Needle examination showed 2–4+ fibrillations in the biceps, pronator teres (PT), extensor digitorum communis (EDC), abductor pollicis brevis (APB), and first dorsal interosseous (FDI) muscles. A single motor unit was seen in the FDI and APB muscles, and fast firing motor units of increased amplitude and duration with a moderately reduced interference pattern were noted in the EDC and PT. The biceps had fast firing motor units of normal amplitude and duration with a mildly reduced interference pattern, while the deltoid demonstrated slowed increased insertional activity without fibrillations and a mildly reduced interference pattern with motor units of normal appearance admixed with those displaying polyphasic activity.

A routine preoperative laboratory screen was within normal limits; all serologies were negative; immunizations were up to date; and the patient had no prior blood transfusions. He was felt to be a suitable candidate for living-donor nerve allografting. Approval for the protocol, donor and recipient procedures, as well as the informed consent process, was obtained from The Committee for Protection of Human Subjects of the University of Texas at Houston Health Science Center. A Research Intermediary independent of the transplant team was assigned as an ombudsperson for the patient and his parents involved in the study.

29.8.1 Donor Evaluation and Procedure

The donor was the patient's mother, a 24-year-old Mexican female in excellent health who was ABO-compatible with the recipient. There was no personal or family history of diabetes, or the presence of any disease state which might produce a neuropathy or any kind of metabolic, physiologic, or traumatic injury to the sural nerves to be procured. Physical, neurologic, and complete laboratory examination were within normal limits, with negative serologies. A screening cross match with recipient serum performed prior to initiating donor evaluation, as well as flow cytometry and antihuman globulin final crossmatches performed 2 days prior to the scheduled donor procedure, was negative.

One week prior to the scheduled transplant, the donor underwent a 2-h procedure under general anesthesia on an outpatient, same-day-surgery basis during which open, bilateral sural nerve harvest was performed from the lateral ankle to just above the level of the posterior knee crease. The total nerve length obtained was 80 cm. The nerves were stored at 5°C in University of Wisconsin (UW) organ preservation solution with 100 U/ml penicillin and 100 µg/ml streptomycin added until transplantation. The donor's recovery was uneventful, with transient, mild lower extremity edema. She experienced a limited sensory deficit along the lateral aspect of the foot bilaterally, which did not interfere with ambulation.

29.8.2 Recipient Preparation

TCL 0.1 mg/kg BID as an oral suspension was initiated 1 week prior to transplantation. Twelve-hour whole blood trough levels were obtained on day 4 and day 1 preoperatively to permit dose adjustment as necessary for achieving target trough levels in the 10–15 ng/ml range (IMx Tacrolimus II assay; Abbott Laboratories, Abbott Park, IL) by day 0. Pretransplant immune evaluation revealed the recipient to have 0% panel reactive antibody by both ELISA and flow cytometry (class I and class II) and to be HLA-haploidentical with the donor.

29.8.3 Recipient Procedure

On November 17, 2000, the patient underwent living-related donor nerve transplantation. After complete dissection of the right plexus, electrodiagnostic testing confirmed the traditional overlap patterns of C7 with adjacent roots and identified one of three fascicles of the ulnar nerve that contributed primarily to flexor carpi ulnaris but minimally to function of the ulnar flexor digitorum profundus tendons and intrinsic muscles of the hand. Thus, C7 and the ulnar nerve fascicle were chosen as donor sites. Interfascicular dissection of recipient left median, radial, and ulnar nerves, together with electrodiagnostic testing using bipolar and tripolar electrodes by an experienced neurology team, was performed. In concordance with preoperative EMG studies, one fascicle of the radial nerve and one fascicle of the ulnar nerve that appeared to illicit negligible responses on intraoperative nerve conduction studies were preserved, even though they were felt to represent clinically insignificant axonal continuity. The remaining fascicles of each nerve, as well as the entire median nerve, were chosen for end-to-end reconstruction with donor nerve.

Solumedrol 0.5 mg/kg was given intravenously. The donor nerves were brought on to the operative field, warmed to room temperature, and oriented for a progressive grouping of axonal flow via two subcutaneous tunnels across the chest wall. In the superior tunnel, donor nerve was used to traverse the distance between the anterior component of C7 on the right and median nerve on the left, and between the posterior component of C7 on the right and radial nerve on the left. In the inferior tunnel, donor nerve traversed the distance from the ulnar fascicle on the right to ulnar nerve on the left (Fig. 29.2). All junctions were performed under the microscope without tension using 11–0 nylon suture and sealed with fibrin glue. Sectioning of only 40% of the cross-sectional area of the right C7 nerve root was required.

The patient was then turned to the prone position. Skin incisions above the level of the previous sural nerve harvests were made, and the residual tails of sural nerve identified bilaterally. Six centimeters of the remaining donor nerve graft was joined to the end of each of these tails and directed transversely so as to serve as "marker nerves" for future protocol and as-needed biopsies to rule out acute rejection during the postoperative period. Following the 10-h procedure, the patient was extubated and taken directly from the recovery room to the regular ward.

29.8.4 Postoperative Care and Immunosuppressive Regimen

There were no intraoperative or postoperative surgical complications. The recipient was discharged from the hospital on postoperative day 2, as soon as oral feedings were tolerated. Oral therapy with TCL as a suspension was continued with twice- or thrice-daily dosing as necessary to maintain target trough levels 10–15 ng/ml for

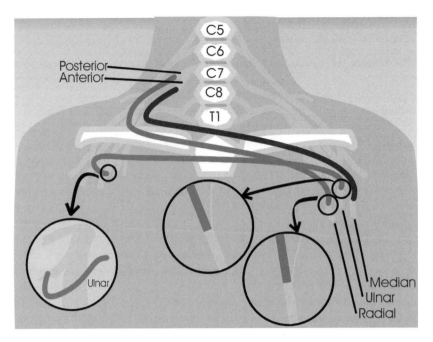

Fig. 29.2 The transplant procedure performed at 8 months of age. Sural nerve allografts were grouped in two subcutaneous tunnels across the chest wall to bridge gaps from the anterior component of C7 on the right to the median nerve on the left; from the posterior component of C7 on the right to the radial nerve on the left; and from one of three fascicles of the ulnar nerve on the right to the ulnar nerve on the left. Reproduced with permission from Gruber et al.[1]

the first 6 months posttransplant; 8–12 ng/ml during months 6–12; and 6–10 ng/ml after 1 year until drug withdrawal. Oral prednisone was initiated at a dose of 0.4 mg/kg/d, with tapering to 0.3 mg/kg/d at 1 week; 0.25 mg/kg/d at 1 month; 0.2 mg/kg/d at 3 months; 0.15 mg/kg/d at 6 months; and 0.1 mg/kg/d at 12 months until drug withdrawal. No antilymphocyte antibody induction therapy nor a third maintenance immunosuppressant was administered. Nystatin and acyclovir were given for 3 months posttransplant, and trimethoprim/sulfamethoxazole was administered until 3 months following drug withdrawal.

Our study protocol called for (1) marker nerve biopsies under general anesthesia at 3 and 6 months or in the presence of clinical signs of rejection, including erythema, induration, swelling, and tenderness along the subcutaneous course of the graft(s); (2) clinical examination and EMG studies at baseline, 3, 6, 9, 12, 18, 24, 36, and 48 months posttransplant to assess functional recovery; and (3) sequential withdrawal of prednisone and then TCL, each over a 6-week period, when electrodiagnostic evidence of nerve regeneration across the grafts occurred, but no later than 2 years posttransplant.

29.9 Results

29.9.1 Graft Rejection and Immunosuppression

Preimplantation biopsies of the donor nerve demonstrated that 1 week of cold storage did not adversely affect its structural integrity, with axon preservation and a normal number and ratio of thick and thin myelinated fibers, a normal ratio of myelinated and unmyelinated fibers, and only mild degenerative alterations of myelin sheaths. The patient had no evidence of acute rejection on clinical examination at any time during his postoperative course. Marker nerve biopsies performed on a protocol basis at 3 and 6 months did not reveal any evidence of acute rejection, inflammation, or fibrosis, with preservation of Schwann cell viability. There were no significant side effects related to TCL or prednisone use. The child exhibited normal growth and development, with weight and height consistently around the 25th percentile. Unfortunately, the patient returned to Mexico at 2 years posttransplant, and was unavailable for further follow-up beyond that time.

29.9.2 Functional Recovery: Sensory Responses

At baseline, the left median and ulnar nerve sensory responses were absent (Fig. 29.3). At 2 years posttransplant, however, sensory responses in the left median, ulnar, and radial nerves did become reliably present. Although the amplitudes of the responses in the left median and radial nerves were only 26% and 17% of their contralateral counterparts, respectively, the left ulnar sensory response was well within the normal range of amplitudes that was recorded for the right ulnar nerve during the study period. Similarly, the distal latencies at 2 years were mildly prolonged in the left median and radial nerves when compared with those on the right side, but were virtually identical in the ulnar nerves bilaterally.

29.9.3 Functional Recovery: Motor Responses

CMAP amplitudes in the left median and ulnar nerves steadily increased from baseline over the 2-year study period, and ultimately reached values that were 55% and 45% of those on the right side, respectively (Fig. 29.4). Distal latencies remained somewhat prolonged on the left when compared with the right side in both nerves throughout the 2-year study period.

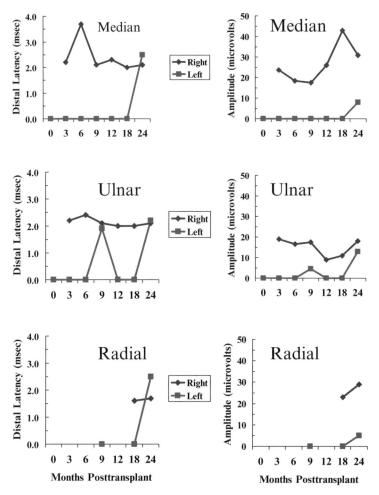

Fig. 29.3 Comparison of sensory responses in the median (*top panels*), ulnar (*middle panels*), and radial (*lower panels*) nerves of the right and left upper extremities at various time points posttransplantation. Studies of the radial nerves were only performed at 9, 18, and 24 months. Reproduced with permission from Gruber et al.[1]

29.9.4 Functional Recovery: Needle Examination

Needle EMG studies of the left upper extremity muscle groups at baseline and throughout the 2-year follow-up period showed persistent active denervation in the form of fibrillations, with distal muscles greater than proximal and a trend toward decreased denervation changes of all muscle groups over time. In the biceps, deltoid, and PT muscles that were the targets of the previously performed autograft procedure, motor unit potentials displayed only mildly reduced interference patterns throughout the study period, with fast firing motor units of essentially normal amplitude and duration. In contrast, motor unit potentials remained

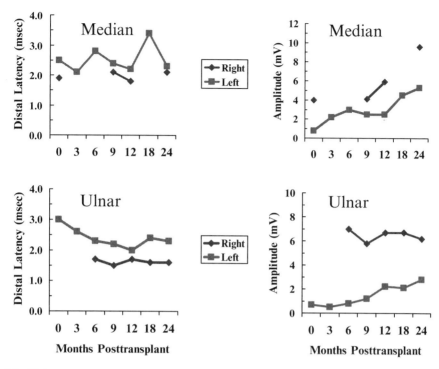

Fig. 29.4 Comparison of motor responses in the median (*upper panels*) and ulnar (*lower panels*) nerves of the right and left upper extremities at various time points posttransplantation. Reproduced with permission from Gruber et al.[1]

moderately to severely reduced in the EDC, APB, and FDI muscles, with fast firing motor units of increased amplitude and duration.

29.9.5 Functional Recovery: Clinical Progress

The patient's motor strength steadily improved in the left upper extremity, primarily in the proximal muscles, but he did demonstrate persistently weak radial nerve-innervated muscles distally. He progressed from very little movement the time of transplantation, to 1–2/5 MRC strength of the biceps at 8 months, and to the point of being able to raise his arm above his head to 120° active range of motion and 4/5 MRC strength in the biceps at 24 months. At this point, he had persistently weak wrist flexion and extension (1/5) and wrist flexion/finger flexion of 4/5. With the use of a wrist dorsal cock-up splint for support, he was able to grasp and release objects with his left hand. Functionally, he could dress himself, including being able to pull his shirt off over his left arm and elbow; feed himself; and grasp objects and release them with his left hand.

29.10 Discussion (Adapted from Gruber et al.[1])

To our knowledge, this is the first reported case of nerve transplantation performed in which the source of the allograft has been a living donor; the recipient has been an infant; the transplant was performed to address multiple nerve root avulsions rather than more distal nerve injury; and the transplant was performed to address a nerve injury acquired at the time of birth rather than a traumatic injury occurring later in life.

During the 2 year follow-up period, we were able to document some return of sensory and motor responses to the left upper extremity on nerve conduction studies which must have derived from the transplant, specifically those observed in the median nerve. However, we did not observe a clinically significant functional improvement in the affected limb which could be definitively attributed to the transplant rather than to the prior autograft procedure. The possible explanation for this may be twofold. First, the transplant procedure may have been performed too late to allow sensory receptors and target motor end plates to be reinnervated within sufficient time to achieve meaningful return of function, despite the shorter absolute distances in the infant, faster baseline rate of nerve regeneration, and the presence of TCL. Perhaps if the transplant had been performed within the month following the initial diagnostic and therapeutic procedure, a better clinical result could have been achieved.[2] Second, 2 years might not be a sufficient follow-up period in which to fully assess the long-term results of nerve allografting for OBPP. Indeed, in the three patients with return of motor function reported by Mackinnon et al.,[60] the only follow-up evaluations reported were at 33, 30, and 41 months, respectively. Along these lines, Birch[70] specifically comments on the slowness of apparent recovery after surgical repair of OBPP, with no evidence of recovery in the hand until 3 years postoperatively. Similarly, Gilbert and colleagues[71,72] have repeatedly emphasized that recovery will last for 3–4 years following surgical intervention in global OBPP cases, and that more than 3 years is required to judge the overall result. Finally, our child's excellent functional recovery from his initial procedure performed at 3 months may well have been accelerated by exposure to TCL beginning 5 months later with the performance of the transplant.

29.11 Conclusion

In summary, the rationale for performing and the 2-year outcome following live-donor nerve allotransplantation for global OBPP with four root avulsion and proximal C5 rupture using cross-chest C7 nerve transfer and temporary TCL/prednisone maintenance immunosuppression are presented herein. Acute rejection was prevented with no observable short-term side effects or infectious complications of the immunosuppressive medications, ipsilateral deficits resulting from the use of the contralateral C7 root as a donor nerve, or untoward effects on growth and development, attesting to the safety of the procedure. Although we did document some return of sensory and motor responses on nerve conduction studies, our failure to observe a clinically significant functional improvement in the affected limb directly attributable to the transplant may have been due to performing the procedure too late and/or inadequate follow-up. We conclude that live-donor nerve transplantation can be performed safely in an infant with OBPP. The results of additional cases performed earlier than in our patient with longer follow-up will need to be evaluated to determine whether the procedure proves to be a viable therapeutic option for treatment of global OBPP with four or five root avulsions.

References

1. S. A. Gruber, P. Mancias, R. D. Swinford, et al., Living-donor nerve transplantation for global obstetric brachial plexus palsy, *J Reconstr Microsurg* **22**, 245–54 (2006).
2. J. K. Terzis, K. C. Papakonstantinou, Management of obstetric brachial plexus palsy, *Hand Clin* **15**, 717–36 (1999).
3. S. M. Shenaq, E. Berzin, R. Lee, et al., Brachial plexus birth injuries and current management, *Clin Plastic Surg* **25**, 527–36 (1998).
4. B. J. Michelow, H. M. Clarke, C. G. Curtis, et al., The natural history of obstetric brachial plexus palsy, *Plast Reconstr Surg* **93**, 675–80 (1994).
5. R. D. Leffert, Brachial plexus. In: Green, D. P., Hotchkiss, R. N., Pederson, W. C. (eds), *Green's Operative Hand Surgery*, fourth edition. Philadelphia: Churchill Livingstone, 1999, pp. 1557–87.
6. J. P. Laurent, R. T. Lee, Birth-related upper brachial plexus injuries in infants: operative and nonoperative approaches, *J Child Neurol* **9**, 111–17 (1994).
7. J. Liu, R. W. H. Pho, A. K. Kour, K. A. Zhang, B. K. C. Ong, Neurologic deficit and recovery in the donor limb following cross-C7 transfer in brachial plexus injury, *J Reconstr Microsurg* **13**, 237 (1997).
8. S. Waikakul, S. Orapin, V. Vanadurongwan, Clinical results of contralateral C7 root neurotization to the median nerve in brachial plexus injuries with total root avulsions, *J Hand Surg* **24B**, 556 (1999).
9. B. G. Gold, T. Storm-Dickerson, D. R. Austin, The immunosuppressant FK506 increases functional recovery and nerve regeneration following peripheral nerve injury, *Restor Neurol Neurosci* **6**, 287–96 (1994).
10. B. G. Gold, K. Katoh, T. Storm-Dickerson, The immunosuppressant FK506 increases the rate of axonal regeneration in rat sciatic nerve, *J Neurosci* **15**, 7509–16 (1995).
11. Y. D. Gu, G. M. Zhang, D. S. Chen, et al., Cervical nerve root transfer from contralateral normal side for treatment of brachial plexus root avulsions, *Chin Med J (Engl)* **104**, 208 (1991).
12. D. C. Chuang, F. C. Wei, M. S. Noordhoff, Cross-chest C7 nerve grafting followed by free muscle transplantations for the treatment of total avulsed brachial plexus injuries: a preliminary report, *Plast Reconstr Surg* **92**, 717 (1993).
13. M. M. Al-Qattan, H. Al-Khawashki, The "beggar's hand and the "unshakable" hand in children with total obstetric brachial plexus palsy, *Plast Reconstr Surg* **109**, 1947 (2002).
14. C. E. Dumont, V. Forin, H. Asfazadourian, C. Romana, Function of the upper limb after surgery for obstetric brachial plexus palsy, *J Bone Joint Surg.* **83B**, 894 (2001).
15. P. Songcharoen, S. Wongtrakul, B. Mahaisavariya, R. J. Spinner, Hemi-contralateral C7 transfer to median nerve in the treatment of root avulsion brachial plexus injury, *J Hand Surg* **26A**, 1058 (2001).

16. Z. Yu, S. Sui, S. Yu, et al., Contralateral normal C7 transfer after upper arm shortening for the treatment of total root avulsion of the brachial plexus: a preliminary report, *Plast Reconstr Surg* **111**, 1465 (2001).
17. C. N. McGuiness, S. P. J. Kay, The prespinal route in contralateral C7 nerve root transfer for brachial plexus avulsion injuries, *J Hand Surg* **27B**, 159 (2002).
18. Y. Gu, J. Xu, L. Chen, Long-term outcome of contralateral C7 transfer: a report of 32 cases, *Chin Med J* **115**, 866 (2002).
19. J. R. Bain, S. E. Mackinnon, A. R. Hudson, et al., The peripheral nerve allograft: a dose-response curve in the rat immunosuppressed with cyclosporin A, *Plast Reconstr Surg* **82**, 447–55 (1988).
20. J. R. Bain, S. E. Mackinnon, A. R. Hudson, et al., The peripheral nerve allograft: an assessment of regeneration across nerve allografts in rats immunosuppressed with cyclosporin A, *Plast Reconstr Surg* **82**, 1052–64 (1988).
21. P. J. Evans, R. Midha, S. E. Mackinnon, The peripheral nerve allograft: a comprehensive review of regeneration and neuroimmunology, *Progr Neurobiol* **43**, 187–233 (1994).
22. J. R. Bain, Peripheral nerve allografting: review of the literature with relevance to composite tissue transplantation, *Transplant Proc* **30**, 2762–67 (1998).
23. J. R. Bain, S. E. Mackinnon, A. R. Hudson, et al., The peripheral nerve allograft in the primate immunosuppressed with cyclosporin A: I. Histologic and electrophysiologic assessment, *Plast Reconstr Surg* **90**, 1036–46 (1992).
24. J. S. Fish, J. R. Bain, N. Mckee, S. E. Mackinnon, The peripheral nerve allograft in the primate immunosuppressed with cyclosporin A: II. Functional evaluation of reinnervated muscle, *Plast Reconstr Surg* **90**, 1047–52 (1992).
25. R. Büttemeyer, U. Rao, N. F. Jones, Peripheral nerve allograft transplantation with FK506: functional, histological, and immunological results before and after discontinuation of immunosuppression, *Ann Plast Surg* **35**, 396–401 (1995).
26. M. S. Wang, M. Zeleny-Pooley, B. G. Gold, Comparative dose-dependence study of FK506 and cyclosporin A on the rate of axonal regeneration in rat sciatic nerve, *J Pharmacol Exp Ther* **282**, 1084–93 (1997).
27. V. B. Doolabh, S. E. Mackinnon, FK506 accelerates functional recovery following nerve grafting in a rat model, *Plast Reconstr Surg* **103**, 1928–36 (1999).
28. R. Midha, S. E. Mackinnon, P. J. Evans, et al., Comparison of regeneration across nerve allografts with temporary or continuous cyclosporin A immunosuppression, *J Neurosurg* **78**, 90–100 (1993).
29. R. Midha P. J. Evans, S. E. Mackinnon, J. A. Wade, Temporary immunosuppression for peripheral nerve allografts, *Transplant Proc* **25**, 532–36 (1993).
30. A. D. Ansselin, J. D. Pollard, Immunopathological factors in peripheral nerve allograft rejection: quantification of lymphocyte invasion and major histocompatibility complex expression, *J Neurol Sci* **96**, 75–88 (1990).
31. H. Wekerle, M. Schwab, C. Linington, R. Meyermann, Antigen presentation in the peripheral nervous system: Schwann cells present endogenous myelin autoantigens to lymphocytes, *Eur J Immunol* **16**, 1551–57 (1986).
32. A. J. Aguayo, G. M. Bray, S. C. Perkins, Axon-Schwann cell relationships in neuropathies of mutant mice, *Ann N Y Acad Sci* **317**, 512–31 (1979).
33. O. Ishida, A. Martin, J. C. Firrell, Origin of Schwann cells in peripheral nerve allografts in the rat after withdrawal of cyclosporine, *J Reconstr Microsurg* **9**, 233–36 (1993).
34. S. E. Mackinnon, A. R. Hudson, R. E. Falk, D. A. Hunter, The nerve allograft response – an experimental model in the rat, *Ann Plast Surg* **14**, 334–39 (1985).
35. A. A. Zalewski, A. K. Gulati, Survival of nerve allografts in sensitized rats treated with cyclosporin A, *J Neurosurg* **60**, 828–34 (1984).
36. A. A. Zalewski, A. K. Gulati, Failure of cyclosporin-A to induce immunological unresponsiveness to nerve allografts, *Exp Neurol* **83**, 659–63 (1984).
37. A. A. Zalewski, W. K. Silvers, A. K. Gulati, Failure of host axons to regenerate through a once successful but later rejected long nerve allograft, *J Comp Neurol* **209**, 347–51 (1982).

38. A. A. Zalewski, A. K. Gulati, Evaluation of histocompatibility as a factor in the repair of nerve with a frozen nerve allograft, *J Neurosurg* **56**, 550–54 (1982).
39. A. A. Zalewski, A. K. Gulati, Survival of nerve and Schwann cells in allografts after cyclosporin A treatment, *Exp Neurol* **70**, 219–25 (1980).
40. A. A. Zalewski, W. K. Silvers, An evaluation of nerve repair with nerve allografts in normal and immunologically tolerant rats, *J Neurosurg* **5**, 557–63 (1980).
41. A. A. Zalewski, W. K. Silvers, The long-term fate of neurons in allografts of ganglia in AG-B-compatible normal and immunologically tolerant rats, *J Neurobiol* **8**, 207–15 (1977).
42. A. A. Zalewski, The effect of allelic dosage on neuronal survival in homografts of ganglia in Ag-B-histoincompatible rats, *Transplantation* **13**, 501–05 (1972).
43. A. A. Zalewski, The effect of Ag-B locus compatibility and incompatibility on neuron survival in transplanted sensory ganglia in rats, *Exp Neurol* **33**, 576–83 (1971).
44. E. Schaller, F. Lassner, M. Becker, G. F. Walter, A. Berger, Regeneration of autologous and allogenic nerve grafts in a rat genetic model: preliminary report, *J Reconstr Microsurg* **7**, 9–12 (1991).
45. R. Singh, The role of histocompatibility matching in the use of preserved nerve allografts, *Clin Neurol Neurosurg* **89**, 129–35 (1987).
46. R. Singh, H. M. Vriesendorp, K. Mechelse, S. Stefanko, Nerve allografts and histocompatibility in dogs, *J Neurosurg* **47**, 737–43 (1977).
47. R. Singh, K. Mechelse, S. Stefanko, Role of tissue typing on preserved nerve allografts in dogs, *J Neurol Neurosurg Psychiatry* **40**, 865–71 (1977).
48. R. Singh, H. M. Vriesendorp, K. Mechelse, S. Stefanko, Cadaver nerve allografts in dogs, *Biomedicine* **35**, 67–70 (1981).
49. Y. Hirasawa, K. Tamai, Y. Katsumi, et al., Experimental study of nerve allografts: especially on the influence of histocompatibility in fresh nerve grafting, *Transplant Proc* **16**, 1694–99 (1984).
50. R. Levinthal, W. J. Brown, R. W. Rand, Fascicular nerve allograft evaluation. Part 2: comparison with whole-nerve allograft by light microscopy, *J Neurosurg* **48**, 428–33 (1978).
51. R. Levinthal, W. J. Brown, R. W. Rand, Fascicular nerve allograft evaluation. Part 1: comparison with autografts by light microscopy, *J Neurosurg* **4**, 423–27 (1978).
52. R. Levinthal, W. J. Brown, R. W. Rand, Preliminary observation on the immunology of nerve allograft rejection, *Surg Gynecol Ob*stet **146**, 57–58 (1978).
53. J. D. Pollard, L. A. Fitzpatrick, A comparison of the effects of irradiation and immunosuppressive agents on regeneration through peripheral nerve allografts: an ultrastructural study, *Acta Neuropathol (Berl)* **23**, 166–80 (1973).
54. S. E. Mackinnon, A. R. Hudson, R. E. Falk, et al., Peripheral nerve allograft: an assessment of regeneration across pretreated nerve allografts, *Neurosurgery* **15**, 690–93 (1984).
55. S. E. Mackinnon, A. R. Hudson, R. E. Falk, et al., Peripheral nerve allograft: an immunological assessment of pretreatment methods, *Neurosurgery* **14**, 167–71 (1984).
56. G. M. Hare, P. J. Evans, S. E. Mackinnon, et al., Effect of cold preservation on lymphocyte migration into peripheral nerve allografts in sheep, *Transplantation* **56**, 154–62 (1993).
57. S. R. Strasberg, M. C. Hertl, S. E. Mackinnon, et al., Peripheral nerve allograft preservation improves regeneration and decreases systemic cyclosporin A requirements, *Exp Neurol* **139**, 306–16 (1996).
58. S. E. Mackinnon, A. R. Hudson, Clinical application of peripheral nerve transplantation, *Plast Reconstr Surg* **90**, 695–99 (1992).
59. S. E. Mackinnon, Nerve allotransplantation following severe tibial nerve injury. Case report, *J Neurosurg* **84**, 671–76 (1996).
60. S. E. Mackinnon, V. B. Doolabh, C. B. Novak, et al., Clinical outcome following nerve allograft transplantation, *Plast Reconstr Surg* **107**, 1419 (2001).
61. J. M. Dubernard, E. Owen, G. Herzberg, et al., Human hand allograft: report on first 6 months, *Lancet* **353**, 1315–20 (1999).
62. J. W. Jones, S. A. Gruber, J. H. Barker, et al., Successful hand transplantation. One-year follow-up, *N Engl J Med* **343**, 468–73 (2000).
63. E. R. Owen, J. M. Dubernard, M. Lanzetta, et al., Peripheral nerve regeneration in human hand transplantation. Abstract presented at the Eighteenth International Congress of the Transplantation Society, August 27–September 1, 2000, Rome, Italy.

64. N. Aksu, M. Turker, H. Erdogan, S. Ozinel, S. Kansoy, Cyclosporin A plus prednisone treatment of steroid-sensitive frequently relapsing nephrotic syndrome in children, *Turk J Pediatr* **41**, 225–30 (1999).
65. K. Kano, K. Kyo, Y. Yamada, et al., Comparison between pre- and posttreatment clinical and renal biopsies in children receiving low dose cyclosporine-A for 2 years for steroid-dependent nephrotic syndrome, *Clin Nephrol* **52**, 19–24 (1999).
66. D. G. Niles, R. D. Rynearson, M. Baum, et al., A study of craniofacial growth in infant heart transplant recipients on CsA, *J Heart Lung Transplant* **19**, 231–39 (2000).
67. S. A. Gruber, A. J. Matas, Etiology and pathogenesis of tumors occurring after organ transplantation, *Transplant Sci* **4**, 87–104 (1994).
68. S. A. Gruber, B. Chavers, K. L. Skjei, et al., De novo cancer after pediatric kidney transplantation, *Transplant Proc* **23**, 1373–74 (1990).
69. S. A. Gruber, K. Gillingham, R. B. Sothern RB, et al., Cancer development in pediatric primary renal allograft recipients, *Transplant Proc* **26**, 3–4 (1994).
70. R. Birch, Invited editorial: obstetric brachial plexus palsy, *J Hand Surg* **27B**, 3 (2002).
71. A. Gilbert, R. Brockman, H. Carlioz, Surgical treatment of brachial plexus birth palsy, *Clin Orthop Relat Res* **264M**, 39 (1991).
72. A. Gilbert, Long-term evaluation of brachial plexus surgery in obstetrical palsy, *Hand Clin* **11**, 583 (1995).

Section VII

Chapter 30
Ethical and Policy Concerns of Hand/Face Transplantation

Rhonda Gay Hartman

30.1 Introduction

Early in the nineteenth century, surgeons in Edinburgh excised a tumor from Robert Penman's lower jaw that had caused severe disfigurement of his face. A remarkable surgical innovation at the time, the patient not only survived but remained in excellent health for many years.[1] Since then, phenomenal strides in composite tissue allograft have revolutionized reconstructive surgery.[2] Success in hand transplantation prepared the way for the first partial face transplant in November 2005.[3] These innovations are intended to optimize quality of life for a small, select group of patients whose "conditions cannot be adequately addressed by conventional reconstructive surgery procedures."[4]

Such surgical achievements are revolutionary, but attendant ethical and policy concerns should be scrutinized as composite tissue allograft progresses. This chapter examines these concerns related to professional responsibility, patients, and donors. While many concerns overlap, distinctions also exist between hand and face transplants because the latter symbolizes identity and image constitutively linked to personhood.[5]

30.2 Innovative Surgery and Professional Responsibility

Composite tissue allograft is a revolutionary advance and therefore experimental. Whether and the extent to which such innovative surgery should be performed are inherent overarching concerns.

30.2.1 Risk-Benefit Assessment

Bound by their Hippocratic Oath, physicians voluntarily act primarily for a patient's benefit. In promoting beneficence (patient's well-being) and minimizing harm (nonmaleficence), physicians owe a fiduciary duty (loyalty) to patients that includes refraining from exploiting the latter's vulnerability for personal or professional gain and avoiding serious risk exposure wherever possible.

Innovative surgeries like hand and face transplants are "nonessential" in that they are life enhancing rather than life saving. While living with a disfigured face or without a hand presents functional and psychosocial difficulties, the condition does not affect general health, unlike a failing heart or liver. In contrast to organ transplant patients, hand and face transplant patients have other viable options including prosthesis and autologous skin graft, respectively.

Risk-replete, nonessential surgeries offer less moral justification for proceeding.[6] Serious risks in the context of both hand and face transplants include toxic side effects resulting from the immunosuppressive drugs that are necessitated following composite tissue allograft. Additionally, the incidence of other adverse effects and long-term outcome are unknown.[7] The justifiability of exposing patients to the risks of elective, life-enhancing surgical procedures when other options exist remains an overriding consideration.[8]

Particularly with regard to face transplant, concerns abound about how to offset and remedy possible tissue rejection or postoperative infection.[9] An early hand transplant failure, for example, was precipitated by the recipient's noncompliance with immunosuppressive drugs because he wanted the transplanted hand to be removed. Removal of infected tissue may not be possible for a face-transplant recipient, who can reject the "new face" at any time[10] and be worse off than having never undergone the transplant. Yet, risk reduction and remedies for tissue rejection could conceivably drive composite tissue allotransplant as a "life-saving" procedure in terms of transforming the direction of patients' physical and mental health that includes an improved self-relationship.[2] Strengthening this are hand-transplant recipients' experiences with immunosuppression that is proving to be comparable to organ transplant patients.[11] Perhaps most poignant is the expression of gratitude from the first partial face-transplant recipient, who touched her tracheotomy tube and whispered "merci."[12]

30.2.2 Developing Standards and Oversight

To sustain continued benefit to patients, physicians must diligently develop standards and proceed under oversight. In contrast to the scientific realm where rigorous testing, refutation, and peer review are staples prior to deeming a hypothesis viable, scientific assessment of surgical innovation preperformance is not a norm within the practice of medicine. As hand and face transplants demonstrate, innovative surgical procedures proceed without rigorous testing and regulatory oversight. A year prior to the first partial face transplant performed in France, the French National Ethics Advisory Committee found that inherent risks of the procedure made it unethical.[13] This prompted criticism of surgeons who seemingly bypassed proven procedures and cut corners to avoid addressing ethical concerns in a rush to be the first to perform these innovations.[14]

Consequently, the "standard" practice emerges later, from informal acceptance by other medical professionals and organizations after the experimental procedure has been performed on patients. For example, published articles reported on the progress of hand transplants along with the lessons learned from the surgeries.[15] This led to the establishment of The International Registry of Hand and Composite Tissue Transplantation, which collects detailed information on every case of hand or composite tissue transplantation, "thereby providing a unique opportunity for participants to keep abreast of the latest developments by sharing their experiences."[11]

Most innovative surgical techniques, including composite tissue allograft, proceed ad hoc, influenced only by the guidelines from national consensus organizations that lack authority to enforce sanctions. In contrast to strict regulation of pharmaceuticals and medical devices as they progress from innovative stages to general use, determinations about whether to progress with innovative surgery rest primarily with doctors without regulatory oversight. In fact, surgeons determine whether it is ethically sound to subject a patient to a procedure with both known and unknown – and in some untried procedures, unknowable – consequences. While patients may be willing to undergo these procedures in the hope of a positive outcome, physicians have responsibilities to ensure safety and not subject patients to medical procedures that endanger them.[16]

Institutional Review Boards (IRBs) frequently provide little patient protection due to inherent conflicts of interests and lack of rigor plaguing IRB review of human subject research. Endemic problems such as overworked boards, lack of expertise, perfunctory inquiry, insufficient surveillance of research protocols, and misrepresentation of adverse events preclude effective IRB review.[17] Complex challenges presented by innovative surgeries undermine the policy of protecting research participants and ensuring informed consent on which IRB regulation is primarily based. Thus, oversight of innovative surgeries should not solely be within purview of institutional oversight.

Collaboration between medicine and society is needed to catalyze support for innovative transplant surgeries as extraordinary procedures for alleviating pain and transforming the lives of a small, select group of persons for whom current reconstructive techniques are ineffective. This joint collaboration should guide the surgical and postsurgical protocols. For example, risk assessment for innovative surgeries such as hand and face transplants implicate not just individual interests but societal judgment about what risk is tolerable and how the risk should be distributed. Oversight of the consent process for innovative surgeries is needed, including calibrating in advance the guidelines and protocols for risk assessment and how it should be communicated to prospective patients.

30.2.3 The Consent Process

Whether a patient has the capacity and capability to make such a medical decision warrants specific inquiry. Disfigured persons are by definition vulnerable, and they are susceptible to influence and increased psychological damage. The consent process implicates this concern of vulnerability, as prospective patients for face transplant are defined by precisely the character trait that renders informed consent inherently suspect. In fact, any concept of informed consent in this context seems counterintuitive; a disfigured patient's euphoric anticipation accompanied by desperation and despair may preclude voluntary, capable decision making. The response of one potential face transplant candidate who, upon simply learning of the mere possibility, resoundingly exclaimed "I want it, I want it!" underscores this concern.[18]

Patient vulnerability can vitiate decisional capability for consenting to any surgical procedure, let alone an experimental one. The very patients for whom composite tissue allograft is advanced experience psychological difficulties borne by their disfigurement; they suffer with conditions that severely impair their overall functioning and quality of life.[19]

Vulnerability stems from a sense of helplessness and disempowerment. The despair and desperation accompanying disfigurement suggest that face transplant patients are susceptible to external influence and exploitability.[20] Yet these concerns may properly be addressed not by means of categorical exclusion from deciding whether to undergo innovative surgery but rather through individual assessment in which physicians expressly weigh these concerns and adjudge degree and type of vulnerability on a case-by-case basis. In that way, the consent process can be tailored to the specific patient.

If, for example, prospective hand or face transplant patients understand the risk of harm and are able to tolerate failure of the surgical procedure, their opportunity to exercise autonomous choice for participating in the surgery could reduce their vulnerability by providing them with an invigorated sense of hope and control.[21] Facially disfigured persons, for example, experience loneliness and isolation more acutely than nondisfigured persons.[22] They also tend to perceive themselves as being on the fringe of humanity, shunned from "human" inclusion.[23] Others' reactions to their disfigurement deepen this perception and sense of exclusion.[24] As one person whose disfigurement resulted from a malignant facial tumor attested, "We don't go out because of the way we look... So disfigured just shut themselves away. They only leave home at night with hoods over their faces. For them, face transplants could mean a chance at a normal life".[25]

The prospect that composite tissue allografts would restore functioning and appearance thereby providing respite from the physical and psychological pain of disfigurement must not be devalued when adjudging whether a patient can capably consent to the surgery. Thus, judgments made about patient vulnerability and any vitiating impact on capable informed consent must be made on individualized bases after careful evaluation about the type and degree of a particular patient's vulnerability.[26]

Composite tissue allotransplant patients should not on the ground of vulnerability per se be begrudged a decision to participate in a risk-inclined procedure that could ultimately temper their physical and psychological pain, as well as benefit others who are similarly afflicted. Cast in this light, values of well-being and autonomy underlying informed medical decision making are not opposed but complementary in this context. Dignity is found in valiance and altruistic spirit, along with meaning derived from being a part of something beyond oneself that cannot be devalued as contributing to personal welfare. Quality of life has been realized by thousands of people today who are beneficiaries of the autonomous judgment of patient pioneers who chose to undergo unrealized risks in transplant surgery.[27]

30.2.4 Patient Selection

As achievements in composite tissue allograft continue, patient selection presents several concerns including resource allocation and human dignity. Hand and face transplants are intended to benefit patients for whom conventional reconstructive surgeries do not provide an adequate remedy. Limited use of face transplant is arguably justified for persons born with facial anomalies or who have been severely traumatized and are featureless, virtually faceless. Such limited use could provide restorative promise and dignity to those suffering with disfigurement without affronting the symbolic value of the face and the shared humanity it represents.[5]

As a repository of physical particulars that comprise personal identity, the human face is the locus of interaction with others and of how others distinguish, recognize, react to, and remember us. Its symbolic value to our common humanity signals a moral significance that exceeds even fingerprint or DNA to individuate us. Broadening the use of face transplant to nonexceptional situations such as for an unsatisfying result from cosmetic surgery affronts human dignity. Misuse of facial transplant would denigrate the sanctity of personhood found in the donative tissue.[5]

Due to the absence of regulatory oversight, surgeons exercise broad discretion in selecting among patients for receiving a transplanted hand or facial tissue. Any expansion of patients beyond those currently designated for these procedures implicates concerns relevant to allocation of scarce resources. Emerging anecdotal evidence suggests that public support of composite tissue allograft does not coincide with donative inclination,[28] thereby raising the justifiability of eliminating patients from allotransplant consideration by differentiating conditions which results from vanity choices rather than from trauma or disease, akin to the influence of alcoholism on liver transplant candidate selection.[29]

Medical determinants alone are not sufficient for selecting patients to receive face transplants. What degree of "disfigurement" justifies the surgery? While a universal concept of disfigurement exists, degrees of disfigurement are nonetheless influenced by systematic and subjective elements.[30] More precise standards must be adopted for narrowing discretion in making this determination.

Another central determinant must be the psychological state of the prospective patient. This is so, because the ability to cope with stressors of intensive postsurgical care indicates transplant success and survival. These stressors are intensified with composite tissue allograft that not only will necessitate ongoing compliance with complex immunosuppressive regimens but also adjustment and acclimation to transplanted tissue that has unique visual significance. Integration of another's tissue into one's self-image, especially for face-transplant recipients, may also be difficult. Added pressures of media scrutiny and public curiosity compound these difficulties during recovery.[31]

Ethically responsible development of surgical guidelines and oversight must consider the distinct concerns related to both the composite tissue allograft recipients and the donors. Concerns presented by composite tissue allograft move beyond professional responsibility to psychological implications and policy considerations for the transplant recipients as well as for the tissue donors.

30.3 Recipient-Related Concerns

Composite tissue allograft patients face substantial risks. In addition to tissue mutations, significant risks of infection and rejection require vigilant postsurgical compliance with immunosuppressive drug regimens that may contribute to diabetes and malignancy among other problems. Although immunosuppression following hand transplantation is less of a concern than originally anticipated, possibility for noncompliance exists nevertheless.[15]

The effect and extent of, as well as remedy for, facial tissue rejection remain unknown. Facial allotransplanation is unique. A hand-allotransplant recipient is able to endure a second transplant or a prosthetic replacement. Furthermore, a larger supply of donor hands than facial tissue is likely given the nature of harvest and meanings ascribed to the donative tissues. Whether a second face transplant is possible and whether the patient would be worse off than having never undergone the allotransplant command exploration.

In addition to the physical risks are the inestimable psychological implications. Surgeons maintain that a face-transplant recipient would neither look like one's former self nor the donor; rather, a transplant recipient would adopt altogether a new facial identity.[9] A face-transplant recipient could be shocked by a drastic result but this unfamiliar facial identity is not necessarily deleterious to someone who has undergone the horror of disfiguration. In the realm of human repertoire, nonfacially disfigured persons willingly undergo risky "extreme makeover" surgical procedures to reinvent themselves and reshape self-outlook.[32] For someone with a disfigured or featureless face, any hope for regaining "normalcy" is immeasurable. The sense of isolation experienced by disfigured persons and an opportunity to regain normal appearance should not be underestimated. The initial appreciative response from the first partial face-transplant recipient captures this sense of inestimable emotional respite and renewed hope.[12]

Compounding other psychological implications could be the recipient's perception of a stranger's engrafted presence, making the recipient feel uncomfortable or even violated. As research suggests, if organ-transplant recipients perceive that their personality or attitudes have changed because they have received in their body an organ from another person,[33] even greater adjustment difficulty may result when the transplanted tissue is visual. This could complicate emotional acclimation postsurgery (and compliance with antirejection drugs), as well as interpersonal relationship with others who provide sustained psychological support for the patient, pre- and post-transplant.

30.4 Donor-Related Concerns

Procuring tissue from a deceased donor presents numerous concerns. These include dignified treatment of the deceased, donative decision making, and the psychological impact on persons related to the donor due to the visual, intimate aspect of the donor tissue.

30.4.1 Dignified Treatment of the Deceased

When asked about harvesting tissue from deceased donors, a prospective face-transplant recipient replied, "they wouldn't lose anything."[18] Or would they? What may be lost is the survival of the donor's personal identity and image, distinguishing facial tissue from other donor tissue.[5] Anecdotal evidence highlights loss or transfer of identity as the major concern among prospective donors.[28]

How we know and conceptualize a person is connected to his or her face, and removal of the deceased's facial tissue symbolically strips away that identity. The identity attached to a person survives postmortem, both legally and in the memory of others. Psychological impact on survivors is not discounted in society and law, evidenced by common law and statutory provisions that afford legal recourse for acts committed against a deceased that outrage sensibilities, consecrate image, or are otherwise averse to the surviving dignity interests of the deceased.[34]

Social norms assign dignitary interests to the deceased that transfer to the living and give expression to humanity. This abiding sense of dignity for the deceased expressed through social norms that shape law and law's reciprocal impact further segues into treatment of human remains. Laws that regulate exhuming a buried body and restrain personal choice for disposition of the body illustrate this.[35] Conscriptions of personal choice are grounded in societal views and values about treatment of the deceased that preserve sanctity of human existence that a deceased body represents.

From criminal sanctions for corpse abuse to grave robbing that inspire revulsion toward using human remains in ways that diminish the life once embodied,[36] an underlying fundamental value suggests that respect and dignity afforded the dead transfer to the living. Demonstration of dignity and respect both underlies and influences intuitive judgments about treatment of the deceased (and, by extension, ourselves). Thus, in striking contrast to organ harvest, careful attention is warranted regarding the process for harvesting hand and face tissues along with a concern for mutilation of a corpse.

30.4.2 Donor's Family and Loved Ones

Physicians must consider the impact of donation on family members and loved ones and approach discussions about donation with sensibilities to the survivors. At a time of profound personal loss, psychological impact on survivors may be acute in ways not necessarily found with solid organ donation given the nature and meaning of the donative tissue. Although the human hand has individuated, identifiable fingerprints, donation of facial tissue may have greater impact on the survivors. The donor's constitutive sense of identity and connection found in the human face would be lost metaphysically through harvest of the tissue and may impair loved ones' ability to grieve.

The surviving image of the decedent in the minds of others should not be undervalued. The face is arguably central to that image and the affection inspired by it for survivors, which reasonably provides a source of strength and support particularly at a difficult time. Survivors may identify themselves through the recipient in ways that connect intimately with memory of the deceased. To the extent that connectedness with the deceased is linked to a comfort found in genetic similarity, resemblance seen in the donative tissue may deepen that sense of loss in quite a personal way.[5]

Knowing the decedent's tissue has been retrieved for use by another may cause a survivor to detach emotionally from the deceased, impacting psychological and emotional ability to engage in the bereavement process. The memory of the deceased and related feelings could plausibly be marred with resentment that the person permitted procurement of such an intimate part of self, including strong religious reasons important to the survivor that could disgrace that person in the mind of the survivor and degrade the memory that impacts the survivor throughout life. These reasons suggest that the legal model used for solid organ donation is not necessarily transferable to visual, identifiable donative tissue for hand and face transplants.

In the absence of any premortem expression of intent from the donor, family may be ill at ease with any donative request for the deceased's facial tissue; thus, attempts to increase tissue supply in the absence of any clear expression of intent by the donor through request to family would likely be counterproductive. Unlike organs, the human face is vested with identity of the deceased and such request at the emotional time of death could inspire resentment, even repulsion. Survivors' perception of pressure to authorize donation of this nature and a sense of repugnancy inspired by such a request could galvanize sentiment against donation generally, including organ donation.

Thus, greater uneasiness would seem to inhere when considering whether to have facial tissue or hands, rather than a solid organ, removed upon death. Fears of mutilation or dismemberment are not insubstantial barriers to family resistance of procurement of any part of the deceased and constitute the most difficult barrier to overcome in donation discussions.[37]

30.4.3 Donor Intent and Incentive

The British Association of Plastic Surgeons has reminded surgeons to consider the donative nature of the tissue used in hand and face transplants.[38] Under principle provisions of the Uniform Anatomical Gift Act, persons have the right to designate prior to death whether their bodies or organs are to be given for transplant.[39] Personal wishes are paramount; in the absence of any express wishes by the decedent, however, the next of kin may decide.

Some anecdotal evidence suggests that public view in favor of hand and face transplants is not altogether indicative of desire to donate tissue needed for transplant.[28] While some similarity may be found to cadaveric organ donation in that public sentiment favoring organ transplant is accompanied by a lack of donative expression, the personal fulfillment derived from donation in the context of organ transplant may prove inapposite to nonessential transplant surgeries. Unlike organ transplantation where persons die awaiting selection for an available donor organ, that same withering-on-the-vine awaiting donor tissue is not present in the context of hand and face transplants. However, if composite tissue allografts prove to be optimal as a surgical technique that restores physicality to patients and transforms their lives then altruistic donations may increase.[2]

Despite public sentiment favoring organ transplant and policy encouraging altruism that underlies legal proscription of cadaveric organ markets, the lack of salvageable organs is the leading cause of death in transplant surgery.[40] The National Organ Transplantation Act prohibits commercial markets in transplantable organs with criminal sanction.[41] Premised on a policy of altruistic intent, federal funding for nonprofit regional organ procurement organizations and a transplant network are provided by NOTA.[41] Underlying these laws is the notion that donations of the body should constitute a gift, rather than a good, and derive from altruistic desire to give of oneself for the welfare of another.[42]

In the absence of a clear application of NOTA to composite tissue allografts, hands and faces could well command a market price due to their value to recipients.[43] Should composite tissue allotransplant surpass current reconstructive methods, ensuring a supply commensurate with need could plausibly give rise to tissue markets.[44] While the unsavory notion of markets in visual, identifiable tissue such as the face or hand seems antithetical to moral and ethical sensibilities, it is not unimaginable that success in composite tissue allograft could result in tissue markets,[45] whereby tissue of a certain color or texture, or from an attractive source, could be lucrative. Yet, viability of a market in human tissue for allotransplant does not compel the conclusion that such tissue should constitute a marketable commodity.

On closer examination, any commercial value attached to tissue used for allotransplant may be equally or more disturbing than for organ transplant. Differentiating tissue in terms of individual perception of appeal versus function debases both the donation and the restorative promise that transcend any quantifiable commercial value. Should composite tissue allograft prove superior to other reconstructive techniques for the hand and face, ensuring a suitable means to increase supply may be difficult due in part to meaning attached to the donative tissue that dissuades even altruistic intention, coupled with a personal sense of losing a critical part of one's identity at death. Thus, arguments against any market in tissue for allotransplant may be powerful due to the profound aspect of humankind the donative tissue represents.

Aside potential marketability, attempts to increase supply could also be made by presuming consent to procurement of hands or facial tissue at death in the absence of express objection by the donor. Such presumptive consent, however, both places a burden on a person affirmatively to opt out and requires persons to acquire information about that particular tissue donation during life. While presumptive consent would likely increase tissue supply due in large part to persons not knowing enough – or anything – about it for informed choice whether to opt out, it would ignore wishes of the deceased and the family. As a method for increasing cadaveric organ supply, presumed consent has not been embraced because absence of donor intention is not necessarily predictive of a person's wishes and deprives a person the virtue of autonomous choice and generosity.[46]

While these reasons resonate in the context of facial transplant, additional reasons such as affronting personal identity bound up in the human face that in all probability was not contemplated by the deceased strongly argue against presumed consent for harvesting facial tissue. It cannot be assumed that the decedent even contemplated donation of something as personal as facial tissue to justify a stance that the decedent's silence on the subject should constitute acquiescence to donation. There is also the sense that harvesting something so intimately connected with self as a person's face without express consent demeans dignity for the whole of humanity. These reasons distinguish facial tissue apart from gametes or cadaveric organ contexts – in which presumed consent has also not attracted support.[47] Giving facial tissue upon death entails losing an intimate part of one's self, rather than giving it for creating or sustaining life.

Indeed, if donating facial tissue upon death represents something intimately bound up with one's unique persona, requiring express donative consent ensures that the donor considered the personal meaning in such a donation. This is underscored by preference afforded autonomous wishes in other areas, such as end of life care and disposition of one's remains.[48] The importance attached to expressed wishes segues into acceptable means for a person's informed decision making about donating their tissue at death and adequate evidence of that intent.

As with cadaveric organ donation, education and appeals to altruism could increase supply. There could also be private and public establishment of procurement organizations and networks designed to discuss hand and facial tissue procurement with families. However, it is questionable whether, in the absence of a donor's express consent, any person – however closely connected – should be permitted to authorize a tissue donation when the donor's wishes are not known. In other words, in the absence of the donor's express consent, the presumption not to harvest hands or facial tissue should prevail to safeguard surviving interests of the deceased.[5]

The premise that express consent is preferable especially when donation involves that part of the human body central to individual identity and vital to shared humanity strengthens why the donor's express consent should be required prior to harvesting facial tissue rather than permitting consent from family. Requiring personal authorization rather than presumed acquiescence or consent by a surrogate furthers societal respect for individuality bound up in visual, intimate tissue and dignity for the whole of humanity.

The importance attached to a donor's express wishes strongly suggests that clear and convincing expression of the decedent's donative wishes should be required. Advance directives, as expressions of intent, are analogous. Some laws require clear and convincing proof of autonomous wishes for refusing life-prolonging care, rejecting a standard of preponderance of the evidence as insufficient and unreliable for ascertaining individual intent about integrity of the body.[49]

The donor's express consent prior to death should be required for harvesting facial tissue and hands. The existing model of consent used in the context of solid organ harvesting affording family members an ability to consent in the absence of any indication from the deceased seems inappropriate and inapposite. Particularly, the intimate nature of facial tissue – and personage it represents – distinguishes it from transplantable organs and thus implies that only a donor's clear, premortem expression of intent should suffice. Because the nature of donation is intimately bound up with one's persona and powerfully symbolic of self-giving, donation of facial tissue – and to some extent donation of hands as visual, identifiable tissue – should result solely from personal meaning found in this gift of the body.

30.5 Conclusion

Composite tissue allograft signals an extraordinary era in reconstructive surgery. How it proceeds and is used deserves discerning, deliberative inquiry. This inquiry calls for finely-grained scrutiny of the ethical and policy concerns. Risk allocation, the decision-making process, and oversight of surgical innovation are chief among these concerns. As discussed in this chapter, ethical and policy concerns related to the recipient include physical risks and psychological effects. Donor-related concerns involve premortem intent and the tissue procurement process, along with impact on the decedent's survivors.

Professional responsibility is central to these concerns. Consistent with their commitment to the Hippocratic Oath, surgeons must maximize benefits and minimize harm to patients. Responsible practice is also critical for shaping the public's perceptions about the ways in which reconstructive surgical resources should be used and for sustaining the public's trust in surgeons and the public's desire for new advances without the necessity of undue constraints. To the extent that advancement in composite tissue allograft necessitates donor tissue that is visual and identifiable, constituents of individual identity and image are implicated, particularly in facial tissue donation. Thus, collaboration between society and medicine that involves informed, incisive inquiry about the ethical and policy concerns raised by composite tissue allograft is crucial for catalyzing progress.[50]

References

1. M. H. Kaufman, M. T. Royds, The Penman Case: A Re-evaluation, *Journal of the Royal College of Surgeons of Edinburgh* 45 (1), 51–55 (2000).
2. S. Hettiaratchy, M. A. Randolph, F. Petit, W. P. A. Lee, P. E. M. Butler, Composite Tissue Allotransplantation – A New Era in Plastic Surgery? *The British Association of Plastic Surgeons* 57, 381–391 (2004).
3. L. K. Altman, French, in First, Use a Transplant to Repair a Face, New York Times, December 1, 2005.
4. F. Petit, A. Paraskevas, A. B. Minns, W. P. A. Lee, L. A. Lantieri, Face Transplantation: Where Do We Stand? *Plastic & Reconstructive Surgery* 113 (5), 1429–1433 (2004).
5. R. G. Hartman, Face Value: Challenges of Transplant Technology, *American Journal of Law & Medicine* 31 (1), 7–46 (2005).
6. P. A. Clark, Face Transplantion: Part II-An Ethical Perspective, *Medical Science Monitor* 11 (2), RA41–RA47 (2005).
7. S. Baumeister, C. Kleist, B. Dohler, B. Bickert, G. Germann, G. Opelz, Risks of Allogeneic Hand Transplantation, *Microsurgery* 24 (2), 98–103 (2004).
8. J. Martin, Hand Transplantation: A Future Clinical Option, *Acta Orthopaedica* 76 (1), 14–27 (2005).
9. P. J. Morris, J. A. Bradley, L. Doyal, M. Earley, P. Hagan, M. Milling, N. Rumsey, Facial Transplantation: A Working Party Report From the Royal College of Surgeons of England, *Transplantation* 77 (3), 330–338 (2004).
10. L. K. Altman, A Pioneering Transplant, And Now an Ethical Storm, New York Times, December 6, 2005.
11. M. Lanzetta, P. Petruzzo, R. Margreiter, J. M. Dubernard, F. Schuind, W. Breidenbach, S. Lucchina, S. Schneeberger, C. van Holder, D. Granger, G. Pei, J. Zhao, X. Zhang, The International Registry on Hand and Composite Tissue Transplantation, Transplantation 79 (9), 1210–1214 (May 15, 2005); X. F. Aheng, G. X. Pei, Y. R. Qui, L. J. Zhu, L. Q. Gu, Serial Monitoring of Immunological Parameters Following Human Hand Transplant, Clinical Transplantation, 18(2), 119–123 (2004).
12. Associated Press, Woman Says 'Merci' After Face Transplant, New York Times, December 2, 2005.
13. X. Bosch, Surgeon Denied Ethics Approval for Face Transplantation, *The Lancet* 363, 871 (2004).
14. C. S. Smith, As a Face Transplant Heals, Flurries of Questions Arise, New York Times, December 14, 2005; L. K. Altman, A Pioneering Transplant, And Now an Ethical Storm, New York Times, December 6, 2005; E. Check, Surgeons Seek Go-Ahead to Perform First Face Transplant, *Nature* 431, 389 (September 2004).
15. M. Lanzetta, P. Petruzzo, G. Vitale, S. Lucchina, E. R. Owen, J. M. Dubernard, N. Hakim, H. Kapila, Human Hand Transplantation: What Have We Learned?, *Transplantation Proceedings* 36, 664–668 (2004).
16. F. Petit, A. Parcskevas, L. Lantieri, A Surgeon's Perspective on the Ethics of Face Transplantation, *American Journal of Bioethics* 4 (3), 14–16 (2004).

17. A. M. Capron, Ethical and Human-Rights: Issues in Research on Mental Disorders that May Affect Decision-Making Capacity, *New England Journal of Medicine* 340 (18), 1430–1434 (1999).
18. D. Jones, Soon I May Have My Life Back, Daily Mail (London), June 27, 2004 (Interview with Jacqui Saburido).
19. I. Fukunish, Relationship of Cosmetic Disfigurement to the Severity of Posttraumatic Stress Disorder in Burn Injury or Digital Amputation, *Psychotherapy and Psychosomatics* 68 (2), 82–86 (1999).
20. C. Levine, R. R. Faden, C. Grady, D. Hammerschmidt, and L. Eckenwiler, The Limitations of 'Vulnerability' as a Protection for Human Research Participants, *American Journal of Bioethics* 4 (3), 44–49 (2004).
21. L. K. Altman, Patient Opted for Transplant as Method to Mend Face, New York Times, December 2, 2005.
22. M. T. Miliora, Facial Disfigurement: A Self-Psychological Perspective on the 'Hide-and-Seek' Fantasy of an Avoidant Personality, *Bulletin of the Menniger Clinic* 62 (3), 378–394 (1998).
23. F. Coull, Personal Story Offers Insight into Living with Facial Disfigurement, *Journal of Wound Care* 12 (7), 254–258 (2003).
24. R. Newell, I. Marks, Phobic Nature of Social Difficulty in Facially Disfigured People, *British Journal of Psychiatry* 176, 177–181 (2000).
25. P. Gorner, Surgery's Next Step: Face Transplants, Chicago Tribune, June 12, 2005 (Interview with Christine Piff).
26. N. S. Jecker, Protecting the Vulnerable, *American Journal of Bioethics* 4 (3), 60–62 (2004).
27. C. Barnard, C. B. Pepper, One Life (Macmillan 1969).
28. C. Siebert, Making Faces, New York Times, March 9, 2003.
29. A. H. Moss, M. Siegler, Should Alcoholics Compete Equally for Liver Transplantation, *Journal of the American Medical Association* 265 (10), 1295–1298 (1991).
30. C. B. Terwee, F. W. Dekker, G. J. Bonsel, S. H. Heisterkamp, M. F. Prummel, L. Baldeschi, W. M. Wiersinga, Facial Disfigurement: Is It in the Eye of the Beholder? A Study in Patients with Graves' Ophthalmopathy, *Clinical Endocrinology* 58 (2), 192–198 (2003).
31. C. S. Smith, As a Face Transplant Heals, Flurries of Questions Arise, New York Times, December 14, 2005; E. H. Morreim, About Face: Downplaying the Role of the Press in Facial Transplantation Research, *American Journal of Bioethics* 4 (3) 27–29 (2004).
32. R. La Ferla, N. Singer, The Face of the Future, New York Times, December 15, 2005.
33. M. A. Sanner, Transplant Recipients' Conceptions of Three Key Phenomena in Transplantation: the Organ Donation, the Organ Donor, and the Organ Transplant, *Clinical Transplantation* 17, 391–400 (2003).
34. E.g., In re Tri-State Crematory Litigation, 215 F.R.D. 660 (N. D. Ga. 2003); Christensen v. Superior Court, 820 P.2d 181 (Cal. 1991); Colorado Revised Statutes Section 18-13-101 (2003); Pennsylvania Statutes Annotated title 18, Section 5510 (West 2004).
35. E.g., In re Moyer's Estate, 577 P.2d 108 (Utah 1978); Ohio Revised Code Annotated Section 517.23 (West 2004); New York Public Health Law Section 4200 (McKinney 2004).
36. E.g., Indiana Code Annotated Section 35–45–11–1 (Michie 2004); New Hampshire Revised Statutes Annotated Section 644:7 (1996); Oregon Revised Statutes Section 166.087 (2004); Tennessee Code Annotated Section 39–17–312 (2003).
37. M. Verble, J. Worth, Fears and Concerns Expressed by Families in the Donation Discussion, *Progress in Transplantation* 10 (1), 48–55 (2000).
38. S. P. Kay, Editorial, Give and Take, *The British Association of Plastic Surgeons* 57, 379 (2004).
39. Uniform Anatomical Gift Act, 8A U.L.A. 19 (1993) (amended 1987).
40. United Network for Organ Sharing, Waiting List Deaths and Death Rates, at http://www.unos.org/SharedContentDocuments/Waiting_list_deaths_and_rates.pdf; R. A. Epstein, Organ Transplant: Is Relying on Altruism Costing Lives? American Enterprise (November–December 1993).
41. National Organ Transplantation Act, 42 U.S.C. Sections 273–274 (1994).

42. E. D. Pellegrino, Life or Death: The Issue of Payment in Cadaveric Organ Donation, *Journal of the American Medical Association* 265 (10), 1302–1306 (1991).
43. H. Hansmann, The Economics and Ethics of Markets for Human Organs, *Journal of Health Politics, Policy & Law* 14 (1), 57–85 (1989).
44. J. D. Mahoney, The Market for Human Tissue, *Virginia Law Review* 86 (2), 163–223 (2000).
45. M. Sandel, What Money Can't Buy: The Moral Limits of Markets, in 21 The Tanner Lectures on Human Values 89 (G. B. Peterson ed., 2000).
46. P. Ramsey, The Patient as Person: Explorations in Medical Ethics (Yale University Press, 2nd ed. 2002).
47. E.g., Virginia Code Annotated Section 54.1-2986(B) (2004).
48. E.g., California Health & Safety Code Section 7100.1(a)(1) (West 2004); Minnesota Statutes Section 149A.80 (2003).
49. E.g., Cruzan v. Harmon, 760 S.W.2d 408 (Mo. 1988), aff'd sub nom, Cruzan v. Director, Mo. Dep't of Health, 497 U.S. 261 (1990).
50. R. G. Hartman, The Face of Dignity: Principled Oversight of Biomedical Innovation, *Santa Clara Law Review* 47 (1), 55–91 (2007).

Chapter 31
Ethical Debate on Human Face Transplantation

François Petit

In 1998, the first clinical cases of hand and composite tissue allotransplantation (CTA) opened a new era in the practice of reconstructive surgery. Some had suggested that face (allo)transplantation could be the next step to benefit patients whose conditions cannot be addressed by conventional techniques of reconstructive surgery using autologous tissues. The first human face transplantation has finally been performed on November 2005, and the results seems extremely encouraging.

The author intended to review the current status of science and ethics regarding human face transplantation. The main issues fall into three categories: (1) the surgical challenge of the procedure, specifically regarding vascular viability and functional recovery of the graft; (2) the risks of side effects from lifelong immunosuppression necessary to prevent graft rejection; and (3) the ethical debate and the consequences of the procedure on the population. Although face transplantation might one day be performed "routinely" and extend the boundaries of reconstructive surgery, there are still many obstacles that need to be overcome first.

31.1 Introduction

The world's first human hand allograft performed in Lyon, France in September 1998 launched the practice of composite tissue allotransplantation (CTA) for reconstructive surgery.[1] To date, more than 20 patients have received hand transplants including bilateral hand allografts, or other anatomic parts such as larynx and knee joints.[2,3] Early results of these first clinical cases demonstrated partial functional recovery while the immunosuppressive treatment could prevent graft rejection with no major complications. Although these operations will need to be evaluated in the long term, as time and experience evolve, it becomes clearer that CTA extends the boundaries of reconstructive surgery to patients with tissue defects that cannot be adequately reconstructed with autologous tissues. Some suggested that face transplantation could be the next step.

In the aftermath of the first hand transplant performed in the USA in January 1999, J. Barker, a member of the transplant team, predicted that "the first face transplant will probably be done within a year." More recently, P. Butler, from London, opened the debate on human face transplantation and, at the November 2002 meeting of the British Association of Plastic Surgeons, announced that his team was working on and "will be able to do this within the next six to nine months." The first human face transplant was actually performed in Amiens, France on November 27, 2005, by a team led by Professors J. M. Dubernard and B. Devauchelle.

In this updated chapter with the more recent news (see also our previous publications),[4,5] we seek to review the current status of science regarding the prospect of face transplantation, and to detail the reasons why and how the first human face transplantation has been performed.

31.2 Surgical Challenge

Hand transplantation was an immunological but not a surgical challenge, since surgeons have mastered microsurgery and refined the technique of limb replantation through experience for nearly 40 years. Facial transplantation paints a rather different picture. The vascular anatomy of the face is well known but its surgical application to the harvesting of a free facial flap remains uncertain; this situation is never encountered in clinical practice. Only two cases of total face (i.e., facial skin with scalp) replantation have been reported for traumatic defects.[6,7] The main concerns are vascular reliability of the facial "flap," donor–host tissue discrepancy, and nerve regeneration across the transplanted face. The first step of the transplantation procedure is the harvesting of the facial flap from a brain-dead donor, and the critical step of the harvesting is the dissection of the vessels. Vascularization of the entire facial flap would rely on the terminal branches of the external carotid artery, superficial temporal artery, and internal maxillar artery, for the upper third and the deep structures of the face, and on the facial artery for the central and lower part of the face. The ophthalmic artery, a collateral branch of the internal carotid artery, contributes to the vascularization of the periorbital area. Venous drainage of the face relies on the external, the internal, and the anterior jugular vein, which drain, respectively, the superficial temporal, the facial, and the inferior labial and chin vein. Thus, the transplantation of the whole face would involve all of these vascular systems which should be dissected proximal enough to insure vascularization of the entire facial flap and to enable anastomosis to the recipient's counterparts. Any compromise of vascularity could lead to large necrosis of the transplanted face. Such risk may be decreased by transplanting only part of the face, for example, the central part that is being perfused by the facial vessels only. Central facial tissue defects are sometimes observed after suicide attempts with guns. The defect commonly involves the nose, the superior maxilla, the lips, the mandible, and the chin. Its coverage usually requires the free transfer of autologous tissues such as fibular and forearm flaps. Despite many revision procedures for shaping the flap, the functional and aesthetical results of the reconstruction usually remain poor.

For such major and complex tissue defects, allotransplantation offers a unique and preeminent advantage by restoring "like with like."

A successful face transplantation would also depend on the ability for the recipient to look normal, i.e., to display a face that moves and looks as the recipient. Motion of the transplanted face will depend on the healing of the muscular sutures and on nerve regeneration along the facial nerve across the graft. We learned from hand and peripheral nerve allograft recipients that nerve regeneration across the graft is potentially faster than the known rate of 1 mm/day.[8,9] This observation was attributed to the favorable effect of tacrolimus (FK506) on axonal regeneration, as previously observed in animals and humans.[10,11] We must point out that successful nerve regeneration does not necessarily imply an effective muscular mobility. Hand transplant recipients could regain early muscular activity in the graft because muscles were not transplanted nor deinnervated, but only reattached from the recipient's proximal forearm to the donor's distal tendons within the graft. Functional activity of the intrinsic muscles took much longer to recover. Muscles within the transplanted face would regain motion through the facial nerve. If the facial nerve is being dissected proximally (close to its emergence from the stylomastoid foramen) to include all branches, regeneration will take a very long time and will unlikely enable muscular activity within the graft. It is more suitable to include only branches of the facial nerve into the flap and to move the anastomosis level more distally, thereby shortening the regeneration time. Functional recovery of the graft and anesthetic appearance of the recipient surely are the key determinates for a successful face transplant. An unfavorable anesthetic result could be due to unanesthetic scars, malposition of the graft, or any donor–recipient mismatching: dimensions, skin (color, shininess, thickness, hair, pilosity, etc.), facial skeleton, etc. Cosmetic requirements must be added to immunological hurdles and thus makes any search for a donor even more challenging in the context of organ and tissue donor shortage.

The 38-year-old woman who received the world's first face transplant had been waiting only a few months. She had been bitten by her dog near Amiens, France in May 2005. All the soft tissues of the nose, both lips and the chin have been taken away during the bite. They were not in a replantable condition. The wound was covered with dressings to delay the retraction of the tissues. The patient could hardly eat and talk for a few months. During that time, Prof. B. Devauchelle, head of the department of maxillo-facial surgery in Amiens, contacted Prof. J.M. Dubernard in Lyon to build a joined team to assess the possibility of performing a face transplant to benefit this woman. The agreement from the health administrations were obtained within months. The details of the procedure were defined regarding its surgical aspects and immunosuppressive protocols. The patient was registered into the waiting list for a compatible donor. A compatible donor was detected in Lille in November 2005. The first human face transplant was performed on November 27, 2005.

We consider face transplantation a true surgical challenge because of technical obstacles and uncertainty over the functional and anesthetic results. The risks of technical failure inherent to any procedure performed for the first time had to be carefully weighed. Little data existed in experimental research at this point. To our knowledge, no research protocols on face transplantation had been published or were under evaluation.

31.3 Immunosuppression and Rejection

Just a few years ago, the concept of face or any other CTA would have sounded like an illusion. Back in the early times of transplantation, immunosuppressive treatments were few and deleterious and could hardly overcome the immunological rejection of any transplanted tissue or organ. The introduction of cyclosporine in the early 1980s was a major breakthrough, which was later followed by new immunosuppressive agents such as tacrolimus, monoclonal antibodies, mycophenolate mofetil, and rapamycin. In organ transplantation, current immunosuppressive protocols using these agents now lead to more than 90% graft survival after 1 year, with few side effects for the recipient.[12]

In contrast to solid organ allografts, composite tissue allografts such as the face may include diverse tissues (skin, muscle, tendons, nerves, bone, vessels) that express various levels of antigenicity and contain some immunocompetent tissues (bone marrow, lymph nodes) that may alter the immune response.[13,14] Due to its highest antigenicity within all the tissues, skin has long been regarded as a major obstacle to CTA.[15] Immunosuppression protocols were either too toxic or inefficient to transplant composite tissue allografts including a skin component in humans.[16–18] A few clinical cases of CTA not including skin were performed in the 1990s: digital flexion system,[19] peripheral nerves,[9] femoral diaphyses and knee joints,[20] and larynx.[21] The French hand transplant team started with a single-hand transplant, with the concern that the immunosuppression regimen would not be able to counteract the skin antigenic load carried by a double-hand allograft. Early results of these operations proved that current immunosuppressive agents are able to prevent acute rejection and to maintain the survival of different "components" of CTA, including skin. However, there has not been sufficient time to determine the effects of any chronic rejection of hand allografts.

On the basis of the experience from previous CTA procedures, the immunosuppressive regimen for the first face transplantation started by an induction treatment with tacrolimus, mycophenolate mofetil, and prednisone for the first 15 days. Antithymocyte globulins were also added in the perioperative period. This regimen was followed by a maintenance combination therapy of tacrolimus (adjusted to blood concentration of 5–10 ng/ml), mycophenolate mofetil (75–30,00 mg/day), and prednisone (10–25 mg/day). Tacrolimus is a modern variant of cyclosporine that inhibits calcineurin. It also has a neuroregenerative effect that makes it particularly useful in nerve transplants.[10,11] Its main side effects are nephrotoxicity and hyperglycemia. Steroids bring about antiedematous and anti-inflammatory effects on tissue healing that make them also useful in the initial phase of CTA. To prevent their side effects, the dosage of steroids should be tapered if possible. Mycophenolate mofetil, a modern variant of azathioprin, is an antimitotic agent that interrupts lymphocyte cell division. Its main side effects are hematological and digestive toxicities.

Long-term graft survival depends upon adequate and indefinite immunosuppression. Thus, the postoperative follow-up of the recipient must insure that the immunosuppressive treatment is not over- or underdosed. Compliance of the patient with his/her treatment must be assessed with blood concentrations and should be repeated at each visit. Signs of rejection should be investigated, especially in the first 6 months postoperatively. On the recent face transplant, the earliest signs of rejection were visible on the skin surface of the graft as erythema, rash, and pinpoint swelling. Skin biopsies were performed to confirm the diagnosis of rejection. With an increase in systemic immunosuppression, the rejection could quickly be reversed.

Long-term side effects of the immunosuppressants fall into three categories: opportunistic infections (cutaneous, fungal, and tinea infections, and CMV and herpes virus recurrences), metabolic disorders (diabetes, Cushing's syndrome), and malignancies (basal cell and squamous cell carcinomas and Epstein–Barr virus B cell lymphoproliferative disorders). These side effects are a major limiting factor in tissue allotransplantation for correcting physical or functional disabilities. They have led many surgeons to oppose using CTA to "only" improve the recipient's quality of life. Also, current immunosuppressive treatments do not prevent the long-term functional deterioration of some organ allografts, a process called "chronic rejection."[22] It is still too early to know if composite tissue allografts will be subjected to this phenomenon, but this is a serious threat for the long-term functional recovery of these allografts.

Successful development of strategies reducing the risks associated with immunosuppression is critical for composite tissue and face transplantation. Various approaches in research are currently being evaluated[23]: (1) Specific tolerance induction in the recipient by reprogramming its immune system; (2) Genetic matching of the donor and the recipient; and (3) Development of new drugs and new immunosuppressive protocols. While progress in these approaches would benefit tissue and organ transplants, CTA entails additional constraints due to its composition of many highly antigenic tissues, the difficult selection of the grafts, and the need for minimizing the associated morbidity. Although these new approaches hold great promises, the widening of CTA awaits further progress in the field.

While a kidney or a hand transplantation is a reversible procedure by nephrectomy or amputation, in case the treatment has to be stopped, face transplantation is not. A failure or a complication either from the surgery or from the medications could generate disastrous consequences for the patient. He/she would be converted from a stable, nonevolving situation of physical and functional disability with psychological repercussions, to an unstable extensive wound with possible serious physical and psychological consequences. Thus, while the success of the procedure is imperative, it is not assured; and this should have been at the core of the ethical debate which followed the first face transplant, rather than arguing about the inevitable mediatization of the procedure.

31.4 Ethical Debate

Years after its "announcement," the prospect of face transplantation was still stirring up an inflamed debate in the medical community. While a few transplant and plastic surgeons opened the discussion on the surgical and immunological aspects of this procedure,[4,24] its ethical aspects have mostly been retained by professional "ethicists" whose positions have been released through governmental ethical agency's formal statements (the Royal College of Surgeons in UK, and the Comité Consultatif National d'Ethique in France).[25] The *American Journal of Bioethics* published an interesting contribution on the ethics of face transplantation,[26] followed by open peer commentaries.[5] We added a few comments and focus on the aspects we consider still remain the most relevant at this time. We had no doubts that human face transplantation would one day be performed. We still did not know when, where, for, and by whom, but these were irrelevant details. The main issue was not even success or failure of the procedure, but rather the ethical conditions surrounding it. An ethical face transplantation that would eventually lead to failure will be remembered as an honorable attempt (as were all the other first organ transplantations). An unethical face transplantation that would eventually lead to a technical success will be looked at as a "trick" made by mercenaries of science. Two months postoperatively (on February 6, 2006), the patient gave a press conference, to get a break from the journalists chasing her. Whoever could see the patient has been astonished by the quality of the aesthetic result. The graft looks as if it had always been hers. The scars were merely visible. Regarding the functional aspects, although the lips still lack some mobility, the patient could sustain a long speech with no help. These results appeared extremely encouraging.

At this point, for doctors, the rationale of the ethical debate falls into different questions: the scientific interest and challenge carried out by the procedure (Have we led modern science far enough to perform it now?); the expected benefit for the patient (Could this procedure improve an individual's life?); and the repercussions on people's consideration for this kind of medicine (Is the procedure going to affect people's opinion of doctors in general, and the practice of transplantation in particular?). In answering these questions, little help should be expected from the media. The prospect of face transplantation has been initially turned into sensationalism by mass media. Photos of potential candidates for a face transplantation have been posted in magazines and on the Internet, their mutilated faces being reinforced by their dreary story revealed with tearful details. This kind of "scientific reality-show" with exhibition of patients diminishes the potential values of these procedures. Face transplantation should be considered as a medical solution to provide relief to suffering for a few number of patients. This suffering comprises physical distortions and functional disabilities that lead to social exclusion and psychological repercussions. From our point of view, three ethical aspects should mostly been taken in account:

31.4.1 On the Recipient

One should be aware that, while the rationale for such procedure is quality of life, it would also threaten the recipient's life. However, plastic surgeons know that, in some rare cases, the health conditions of the patient are so miserable that he/she would accept a potentially shorter life if his/her quality of life could improve. This debate is not specific to disfigurement. Regarding hand transplantation, the French ethic committee has admitted that amputation of both hands could justify a double-hand transplantation. In such rare cases, the handicap is so important that the potential benefits of transplantation outweigh the risks from the procedure and from lifelong treatments. Once again, we strongly believe that plastic surgeons are the right people to assess the risks and benefits of a face transplantation, not only because they have the best knowledge of the technical aspects of the procedure, but also because they deal everyday with patients' distress related to physical and aesthetic disabilities. They should not give up this great responsibility to "ethicists" who lack this clinical experience.

31.4.2 On the Donor

In most societies, whatever the culture and the religion, great respect is due to the dead body to accomplish the rituals for the gateway to "life after death." In the aftermath of the death of the loved ones, rituals should be respected to help get over the mourning. One can imagine how difficult it could be for relatives to proceed to the rituals and deal with a picture of a disintegrated body in mind. Thus, the issue related to the donor also lies into an imperative duty: restoration of the donor body's integrity. When we started considering face transplantation as a potential solution and then announced our plans to the French Transplant Agency (Etablissement Français des Greffes), one of the prerequisite they raised was restoration of the donor's face. We are still looking for a fully satisfactory solution.

31.4.3 On the Population

The prospect of a face transplantation brings up the Frankenstein's myth. Careful approach should be made not to frighten or repulse the population. The mass media take great responsibility by systematically turning this topic into sensational news; face transplantation is NOT a weapon of mass distraction… Over the recent years, transplant teams observed a decline of organ donation and now have to deal with a shortage of organs. If the population's response to face transplantation (especially if seen as "unethical") was the worsening of organ shortage, it would have a terrible impact on the practice of transplantation, one of the greatest achievements of modern medicine. As for any other medical procedure, face transplantation needs to be performed with adherence to strict medical and ethical guidelines: professional competency, clear therapeutic objective, and informed consent of the patient. We must be well prepared and a great amount of tact is needed to face the questions and doubts that already rose among potential donor's families and the population.

It is now the moral responsibility of each and every doctor involved in teams preparing for more face transplants to question his/her own soul and conscience and answer a strong "YES" to the following questions before attempting the procedure: Is face transplantation the most appropriate solution for my patient ? Is my patient's relief my only motivation for practicing this procedure? Would I recommend it if it was for a lovedone?

31.5 Conclusion

Face transplantation has now been performed. It should be pursued as a potential solution for a small and selected group of patients with conditions that cannot be adequately addressed by conventional reconstructive surgery procedures. The current concern lies in the scientific context surrounding the project. More experimental studies and discussion should be held among the plastic surgery community. Any attempt to proceed with face transplantation without adequate scientific foundation would place in jeopardy the progress that has been made in reconstructive surgery.

References

1. J. M. Dubernard, E. Owen, G. Herzberg, et al., Human hand allograft: report on first 6 months, Lancet 353, 1315–20 (1999).
2. J. M. Dubernard, E. R. Owen, M. Lanzetta, N. Hakim, What is happening with hand transplants, Lancet 357, 1711–2 (2001).
3. F. Petit, A. B. Minns, J. M. Dubernard, et al., Composite tissue allotransplantation and reconstructive surgery: first clinical applications, Ann Surg 237, 19–25 (2003).
4. F. Petit, A. Paraskevas, A. B. Minns, et al., Face transplantation: where do we stand? Plast Reconstr Surg 113, 1429–33 (2004).
5. F. Petit, A. Paraskevas, L. A. Lantieri, A surgeons' perspective on the ethics of face transplantation, AJOB 4, 14–6 (2004).
6. A. Thomas, V. Obed, A. Murarka, G. Malhotra, Total face and scalp replantation, Plast Reconstr Surg 102, 2085–7 (1998).
7. B. J. Wilhelmi, R. H. Kang, K. Movassaghi, et al., First successful replantation of face and scalp with single-artery repair: model for face and scalp transplantation, Ann Plast Surg 50, 535–40 (2003).
8. E. R. Owen, J. M. Dubernard, M. Lanzetta, et al., Peripheral nerve regeneration in human hand transplantation, *Transplant Proc* **33**, 1720–1 (2001).
9. S. E. Mackinnon, V. B. Doolabh, C. B. Novak, E. P. Trulock, Clinical outcome following nerve allograft transplantation. *Plast Reconstr Surg* **107**, 1419–29 (2001).

10. H. Fansa, G. Keilhoff, S. Altmann, et al., The effect of the immunosuppressant FK 506 on peripheral nerve regeneration following nerve grafting, J Hand Surg [Br] 24, 38–42 (1999).
11. V. B. Doolabh, S. E. Mackinnon, FK506 accelerates functional recovery following nerve grafting in a rat model, Plast Reconstr Surg 103, 1928–36 (1999).
12. N. R. Parrott, Immunosuppression: "What's new?" In J. L. R. Forsythe (Ed.), Transplantation Surgery, London: Harcourt Publishers; 2001, pp. 101–32.
13. W. P. Lee, M. J. Yaremchuk, Y. C. Pan, et al., Relative antigenicity of components of a vascularized limb allograft, Plast Reconstr Surg 87, 401–11 (1991).
14. W. P. Lee, P. E. Butler, M. A. Randolph, M. J. Yaremchuk, Donor modification leads to prolonged survival of limb allografts, Plast Reconstr Surg 108, 1235–41 (2001).
15. D. Steinmuller, The enigma of skin allograft rejection. Transplant Rev 12, 42–57 (1998).
16. J. N. Jensen, S. E. Mackinnon, Composite tissue allotransplantation: a comprehensive review of the literature – part 1, J Reconstr Microsurg 16, 57–68 (2000).
17. J. N. Jensen, S. E. Mackinnon, Composite tissue allotransplantation: a comprehensive review of the literature – Part II, J Reconstr Microsurg 16, 141–57 (2000).
18. J. M. Jensen, S. E. Mackinnon, Composite tissue allotransplantation: a comprehensive review of the literature – part III, J Reconstr Microsurg 16, 235–51 (2000).
19. J. C. Guimberteau, J. Baudet, B. Panconi, et al., Human allotransplant of a digital flexion system vascularized on the ulnar pedicle: a preliminary report and 1-year follow-up of two cases, Plast Reconstr Surg 89, 1135–47 (1992).
20. G. O. Hofmann, M. H. Kirschner, Clinical experience in allogeneic vascularized bone and joint allografting, Microsurgery 20, 375–83 (2000).
21. M. Strome, J. Stein, R. Esclamado, et al., Laryngeal transplantation and 40-month follow-up, N Engl J Med 344, 1676–9 (2001).
22. J. S. McGrath, K. M. Rigg, Chronic rejection. In J. L. R. Forsythe (Ed.), Transplantation Surgery, London: Harcourt Publishers; 2001, pp. 283–320.
23. F. Petit, A. B. Minns, S. P. Hettiaratchy, D. W. Mathes, et al., New trends and future direction of research in composite tissue allotransplantation, J Am Soc Surg Hand 3, 170–4 (2003).
24. P. J. Morris, J. A. Bradley, L. Doyal, et al., Facial transplantation: a working party report from the Royal College of Surgeons of England, Transplantation 77, 330–8 (2004).
25. http://www.ccne-ethique.fr.
26. O. Wiggins, J. Barker, M. Cunningham, et al., On the ethics of facial transplant research, AJOB 4, 1–12 (2004).

Chapter 32
Psychosocial Issues in Composite Tissue Allotransplantation

Barckley Storey, Allen Furr, Joseph C. Banis, Michael Cunningham,
Dalibor Vasilic, Osborne Wiggins, Serge Martinez, Christopher C. Reynolds,
Rachael R. Ashcraft, and John H. Barker

32.1 Introduction

On December 23, 1954, a team of doctors in Boston led by Dr. Joseph Murray, a plastic surgeon, transplanted a kidney into a dying, 23-year-old man in the first successful long-term transplant of a human organ. At the time, some hailed this revolutionary medical advancement as "a miracle of medicine" while others accused Dr. Murray and his team of "playing God," saying the surgery should not have been done.[1] Ethical debates have accompanied medical advancements throughout history and this is particularly true for transplantation medicine. In the 50 years that have passed since that first successful kidney transplant, organ transplantation has improved extensively and saved the lives of more than 400,000 people in the United States alone. Murray's work is celebrated today as one of the greatest advancements in modern medicine.

The recent introduction of composite tissue allotransplantation (CTA), particularly in the form of hand and face transplantation, has both rekindled many of the same debates that have long accompanied transplantation and ignited new controversies, many of which are psychosocial in nature. Of primary interest in recent studies is the well-known risk versus benefit debate, which has accompanied transplantation medicine from its outset that centers on the question of the risks posed by the lifelong immunosuppression required to prevent rejection vis-à-vis the benefit of receiving a new organ. Indeed, our research has shown high levels of risk acceptance for certain CTA procedures, and we contend that this willingness to accept risk is due to the psychosocial dynamics involved in hand amputation and facial disfigurement. The purpose of this chapter, therefore, is to explore the psychosocial dynamics of CTA giving special attention to face transplant.

C. W. Hewitt et al. (eds.), *Transplantation of Composite Tissue Allografts.*
© Springer 2008

32.2 CTA and Risk Acceptance

CTA is currently being investigated as a reconstructive modality in several clinical situations including the repair of large tissue defects involving amputated extremities and disfigurement of the head and neck region. Beginning in the late 1990s when teams in Europe and the USA started planning the first human hand transplants, a heated debate has ensued as to whether the benefits of these nonlife-saving procedures justified the risks posed by the immunosuppressant drugs required to prevent graft rejection. At the center of these discussions have been issues like posttransplant quality of life and life expectancy as well as patient preference and risk acceptance for these procedures. The fundamental argument has centered on the ideological differences between the risks individuals are willing to accept to receive a "life-saving" morbidity-reducing treatment (heart and liver transplant) versus a "nonlife-saving" quality-of-life-enhancing treatment (kidney transplant and CTA procedures, such as hand transplant).

In an attempt to address this question, we developed the Louisville instrument for transplantation (LIFT), a questionnaire-based instrument designed to assess two forms of risk, the primary risk of reduced longevity due to the toxicity of immunosuppressant drugs and the risk of transplant rejection, on six transplant procedures (face, hand, double hand, hemiface, larynx, and foot transplantation).[2] Our primary interest in the LIFT studies was to compare the perception of risk among individuals who have already received a donated organ (kidney) and live with the day-to-day realities of immunosuppression risk to individuals who may be appropriate candidates for CTA surgery. Research groups included 150 healthy volunteers, 42 renal transplant patients, 21 arm/hand amputees, and 14 foot/leg amputees. (Data on a fifth group, individuals with facial disfigurement, a sixth group, patients who have had their larynx removed, a seventh group, physicians who treat patients on immunosuppressive medications and an eighth group, plastic surgeons who treat facially disfigured patients are currently being analyzed and prepared for publication as well.)

Remarkably, all groups ranked the transplant procedures in the same order of acceptance, hence the same order of risk-versus-benefit. Individual would accept the greatest amount of risk for transplantation of the face, followed by hemiface, then significantly lower for two hands and kidney, followed by larynx, then significantly lower for single hand, and finally, significantly less for the foot.[3,4]

These findings indicate that real-life exposure to immunosuppression does not reduce risk acceptance for CTA. Of note here is the fact that kidney transplantation, a nonlife-saving procedure, is considered standard treatment in contemporary medicine and the associated risks are universally accepted as justifying the benefits of this treatment. Furthermore, these findings suggest that candidates for CTA not only understand and accept the risks of immunosuppression to which they would be exposed, but also perceive the potential benefits of these CTA procedures, including the face, which at this time remains as yet unrealized. We have concluded from these researches that certain CTA procedures, particularly double hand and face transplantation, convey benefits to a recipient that are perceived to be worth the risks of immunosuppression.

32.3 The Face in Social Interaction and the Psychosocial

32.3.1 Consequences of Disfigurement

Of all physical handicaps, perhaps none is more socially devastating than facial disfigurement. Rather than the sympathy or pity typically evoked by an amputated limb, a crutch, or a wheelchair, facial disfigurement elicits anxiety, fear, and a wish to remove it from one's sight.[5,6] In the words of a patient suffering with facial disfigurement: "I've spent fifteen years being treated for nothing other than looking different from everyone else. It was the pain from that, from feeling ugly, which I'd always viewed as the great tragedy in my life. The fact that I had cancer seemed minor in comparison."[7]

The face is a complicated and highly subjective part of the human body that serves as a main point of interface between internal biopsychological motivational states and social sentiments in relationships with others. While the face is obviously central to individual identification and sexual attraction, it also bears clues to our gender, ethnic, and age identities, as well as other markers of social status. Furthermore, the face symbolically communicates emotions such as fear and anger, shame and embarrassment, and happiness and joy. While we use our faces to send symbolic messages, we also interpret these expressions in others and use the interpretations to assess a person's internal state, motivation, and so forth. "Reading" facial expressions provides critical information for understanding a social situation and impugning individual characteristics such as honesty, competence, or fear. In short, much of human interaction is communicated through and given meaning by facial expression and appearance.

As the locus of human symbolic communication, especially in interpersonal relationships, interpretations of facial (and all other) communication are interpreted following certain social rules. Essentially we are describing a symbolic feedback model in which a person has an idea or emotion, encodes it into words or gestures, which in turn are then decoded by the message recipient into meaning. Social rules greatly influence this process. The meaning of eye contact, for example, varies culturally and situationally. Whereas in some social settings, direct eye contact means engagement and caring attention, under other conditions eye contact implies provocation and challenge. We translate what we see in the faces of others and assign a symbolic concept to give meaning to the expression.

Disfigurement of the face interrupts both signaling and receiving symbolic exchanges between people. When the face is judged to be abnormal in appearance, the norms governing the social and psychological interpretations of facial communication may become ambiguous or perhaps even frightening at some level of consciousness. Therefore disfigurement enters into interpersonal social exchanges and forces people to negotiate new rules of social engagement.

Disfigurement interferes with aspects of facial appearance and functionality used to send symbolic messages, thereby leaving facial cues ambiguous. Because social conventions do not provide rules for interpreting a disfigured face, making sense of disfigured facial communication is likely influenced by stereotypes, categorical information that compensates for the lack of genuine interpretive information. The startle responses of others who encounter disfigured people may be due to the rarity of seeing disfigured faces and not knowing how to act[8] and trying to avoid embarrassment.[9]

Consequently it is not surprising that research shows that the most common problems experienced by people with visible facial differences are rooted in social interactions with others. Robinson's (1997) review of research on disfigured people indicates that difficulty in meeting new people, making new friends and relationships, and dealing with stares, hurtful comments, and intrusive questions are common, everyday experiences.[10] As a result, disfigured people commonly respond to the social environment with a fear-avoidance style: social interactions are threatening and therefore should be avoided.

According to symbolic interaction theory in sociology, we take cues about ourselves from how others react to us. We interpret how others act toward us and use that information to form self-esteem and identity. If these interpretations are sufficiently reinforced, we internalize, or incorporate into our sense of self, the messages we receive from others and interpret in our own idiosyncratic way within the context of particular sociocultural norms and values.

One commonly reported problem of facial disfigurement is stigmatization.[11,12] Stigmatization is a social dynamic in which a person is labeled deviant by virtue of some socially agreed-upon characteristic or "mark" that essentially defines the person in social interaction. Once a stigmata is successfully attached, a person experiences prejudice and discrimination, stereotyping, and, frequently, isolation.

Because of the import of the face in human social exchanges, disfigurement of almost any type typically leads to stigmatizing. Consequent to being the target of stigmatization, individuals with facial disfigurement are often treated with less social respect and are powerless when compared to individuals without the perceived abnormality.[13]

This theoretical orientation places into perspective the clinical and survey research that consistently has reported an association between that perceived facial deformity and psychological stress and a less than acceptable quality of life.[13,14] Facially deformed individuals are frequently shut-ins, hiding from social relationships taken for granted by others, and confront a number of psychological problems such as social anxiety, lowered self-confidence and esteem, negative self-image, depression, and even suicidal ideations.[10–12,14] These conditions often become mutually reinforcing and lead an individual into further isolation and anxiety in relating to other people. The more that disfigured people confront startled responses, avoiding glances, and other off-putting messages in the social world, the more likely they are to avoid social interactions altogether and develop a sense of self that reflects this social rejection.

Although studies of the psychosocial impact of facial disfigurement paint a picture of despair and hopelessness, not all people whose cancer, trauma, or congenital state has rendered their faces noticeably different from standards of normality experience such outcomes. Literature reviews conducted by Moss[15] and Robinson[10] indicate not everyone who is disfigured fails to cope and lead isolated lives.

It is at this juncture that one of the theoretical conflicts of face transplantation plays out. One perspective against performing face transplants rests on the notion of civil rights and acceptance of those who differ from standard cultural and social norms and values. In sociology, minority group status is defined as a group whose primary and defining characteristic (e.g., race or sexual orientation) distinguishes it from a group that does not have the characteristic and is more powerful. This distinguishing "mark" is stereotyped and identifies an individual as a member of a group whose "place" in society is subordinate to others and whose social entitlements are restricted. We usually think first of racial and ethnic groups as minorities, but sociologists also include other disenfranchised groups such as the physically disabled as a minority.

At the core of the expansion of civil rights has been the willingness of the more dominant group to accept the defining characteristic of the minority. As in the case of race and ethnicity, greater social acceptance of disability has led society to take collective action to protect the civil rights of the physically different. These actions have brought about improvement in access to public places and opportunities for the disabled. From this history comes the argument that face transplantation is no more appropriate than changing the color of one's skin; it is society's responsibility to accept disfigurement, not the disfigured people's to try to appear "normal."

Although the Louisville team accepts this perspective as an ideal for which society should strive, the team's work is grounded in a second theoretical stance. Unlike race, which is an inherent and immutable characteristic assigned social meaning, disfigurement is a function of trauma or disease that has social meanings. As argued earlier, when people react negatively or in a startled way to a person whose face is perceived as disfigured, the disfigurement is interfering with usual social symbolic communication and identity, which, by definition, is attaching some sort of negative social meaning to the face. These conflicts influence not only interpersonal relationships, say in mate selection for example, but also in participation in the economy. Discrimination in labor markets, housing, and education are everyday realities for many disfigured people.

We contend that acceptance of disfigurement will be slow in coming because of the centrality of the face in basic human emotion, expression, and identity. Therefore it is our position that face transplantation will serve as a tool to remedy a medical condition that has highly undesirable social and psychological sequelae for most who experience it. For these people, waiting for society to accept differences in facial appearance is too protracted to be of benefit.

32.4 Discussion

The human face and facial transplantation have long captured the interest and imagination of scientists, the media, and the lay public. This is not surprising since our faces are unique parts of our anatomy that we associate with special qualities that make us uniquely human. Our face is much more than the anatomical location where our olfactory, auditory, and visual organs are situated. We use facial expressions to communicate with the world around us, and our face is the window through which others see and come to know us. We communicate these feelings in our spoken language with terms like "let's face it," "face to face," "maintain face," and "face value." It is this great importance we attach to our face that makes facial disfigurement such a devastating condition.

As the introduction of solid organ transplantation provided an effective treatment for end stage organ failure and in doing so revolutionized the field of transplant immunology, facial transplantation could revolutionize the field of reconstructive surgery for severe facial disfigurement. Face transplantation provides an excellent alternative to current treatments for the thousands of individuals suffering facial disfigurement caused by burns, trauma, cancer extirpation, or congenital birth defects. That risk acceptance is very high for face transplantation among people already taking immunosuppression to prevent kidney rejection and those who are candidates for CTA suggests that the social and psychological consequences of disfigurement are of such severity that the risk is worthwhile.

Face transplantation is not without critics who assert that such procedures should not be performed until advances in transplant immunology make it possible to reduce or eliminate the risks. The critics thus view facial transplantation as subjecting patients to high risks that are unnecessary in view of the availability of established reconstructive procedures. The critics understand that an improvement in the disfigured person's quality of life can probably be gained from a successful face transplant. Nevertheless, they do not view this benefit as justifying the risks of the immunosuppressive therapy.

Disfigured persons, however, may view the prospect of a face transplant differently. They may perceive the choice of not having the transplant as equivalent to their willing acceptance of a terrible loss, namely, the loss of a normal facial appearance and of the quality of life that such a normal appearance afforded. Such voluntary acceptance of the loss proves immensely difficult because they know first hand the misery involved in their present disfigurement. They perceive the face transplant, on the other hand, as an opportunity – even with its admitted risks – of returning to a normal appearance that they previously enjoyed. Given this choice, patients find it extremely difficult to voluntarily acquiesce in the lifelong loss. They are thus willing to run the serious risks to have the chance to return to their earlier status quo, namely, a normal facial appearance and the quality of life that it offers.

32.5 Conclusion

As the world awaits the outcomes of the first face transplants, we are witnessing how advances in surgical techniques and immunosuppressant drugs have turned what was once a subject for Hollywood scripts into medical and, perhaps equally importantly, social reality. With the technical aspects of the procedure developed and tested over time, the last hurdles to widespread use of this new treatment are primarily social and psychological in character.

As one of several teams exploring the possibilities of performing face transplantation, we contend that the psychosocial and ethical factors are as important as the surgical and immunological questions.[16,17] As part of the research protocol for performing this new reconstructive treatment, we have promoted an academic and public dialogue on the social and psychological implications of face transplantation surgery, and encourage continued discussion on this important subject.

Acknowledgments The authors acknowledge Ramsey Majzoub, MD, Pascal Brouha, MD, Federico Grossi, MD, Claudio Maldonado, PhD, Marieke Vossen, MD, Gustavo Perez-Abadia, MD, Johannes M. Frank, MD, PhD, and Moshe Kon, MD, PhD for their contributions to the research described in this chapter. The authors would like to thank Drs. Peter Krause and Fredrick Bentley for their assistance in recruiting subjects for the studies described here. Finally the work described here was funded in part by grants from Dr. Joseph C. Banis and the Jewish Hospital Foundation in Louisville, Kentucky.

References

1. J. E. Murray, *Surgery of the Soul: Reflections on a Curious Career*. Portland OR: Watson Publishing International, Book News. Inc., 2004.
2. M. Cunningham, R. Majzoub, P. C. R. Brouha, L. A. Laurentin-Perez, D. K. Naidu, C. Maldonado, J. C. Banis, F. Grossi, J. M. Frank, J. H. Barker, Risk acceptance in composite tissue allotransplantation reconstructive procedures: Instrument design and validation, *Eur J Trauma* **30**, 12–16 (2004).
3. P. Brouha, D. Naidu, M. Cunningham, A. Furr, R. Majzoub, F. V. Grossi, C. G. Francois, C. Maldonado, J. C. Banis, S. Martinez, G. Perez-Abadia, O. Wiggins, M. Kon, J. H. Barker, Risk acceptance in composite tissue allotransplantation reconstructive procedures. *Microsurgery* (In Press) (2005).
4. R. K. Majzoub, M. Cunningham, F. Grossi, C. Maldonado, J. C. Banis, J. H. Barker, Investigation of risk acceptance in hand transplantation, *J Hand Surgery* (In Press) (2005).
5. A. Lefebvre, S. Barclay, Psychosocial impact of craniofacial deformities before and after reconstructive surgery, *Can J Psychiatry* **27**, 579–583 (1992).
6. F. C. McGregor, Facial disfigurement: Problems and management of social interaction and implications for mental health, *Aesth Plast Surg* **14**, 249–257 (1990).
7. L. Grealy, *Autobiography of a Face*. New York: Harper Collins Publishers, 1995.
8. E. Langer, S. Fiske, S. Taylor, B. Chanowitz, Stigma, staring and discomfort: A novel-stimulus hyptotheses, *J Exp Soc Psychol*, **12**, 451–463 (1976).
9. N. Rumsey, R. Bull, The effects of facial disfigurement on social interaction, *Hum Learn*, **5**, 203–208 (1986).
10. E. Robinson, Psychological research on visible differences in adults. In Lansdown, R., Rumsey, N., Bradbury, E., Carr, A., and Partridge, J. (eds.), *Visibly Different: Copying with Disfigurement*, pp.104–111. Boston: Butterworth-Heinemann, 1997.
11. E. Robinson, N. Rumsey, J. Partridge, An evaluation of the impact of social interaction skills training for facially disfigured people, *Br J Plast Surg* **49**, 281–289 (1996).
12. E. M. Ye, Psychological morbidity in patients with facial and neck burns, *Burns* **24**, 646–648 (1998).
13. T. Pruzinsky, Social and psychological effects of major craniofacial deformity, *Cleft Palate Craniofac J* **29**(6), 578–584; discussion 570 (1992).
14. N. Rumsey, A. Clarke, P. White, M. Wyn-Williams, W. Garlick, Altered body image: appearance-related concerns of people with visible disfigurement, *J Adv Nurs* **48**(5), 443–453 (2004).

15. T. Moss, Individual variation in adjusting to visible differences. In Lansdown, R., Rumsey, N., Bradbury, E., Carr, A., and Partridge, J. (eds.), *Visibly Different: Copying with Disfigurement*, pp.121–130. Boston: Butterworth-Heinemann.
16. J. H. Barker, M. Vossen, J. C. Banis, The technical, immunological and ethical feasibility of face transplantation, Editorial, *Int J Surg* **2**, 8–12. 2004.
17. O. P. Wiggins, J. H. Barker, S. Martinez, M. Vossen, C. Maldonado, F. Grossi, C. G. Francois, M. Cunningham, G. Perez-Abadia, M. Kon, J. C. Banis, On the ethics of facial transplantation research, *Am J Bioeth* **4**(3), 1–12 (2004).

Chapter 33
Composite Tissue Transplantation in the Twenty-First Century

Kirby S. Black and Charles W. Hewitt

33.1 Introduction

There are many ways you could have reached this last chapter on composite tissue transplantation. Perhaps you have read the book from cover to cover and you're now anticipating the exciting climax. Or you might have picked it up at the latest scientific meeting and turned here to see what wild predictions would be made. Maybe you are studying the subject and wondering what the next exciting research project will be.

In this chapter, we hope to convey both the excitement of composite tissue transplantation's future and the realities of this exciting field's directions. To do so requires a grasp of history. Because the field of composite tissue transplantation broadly encompasses various disciplines of surgery, several areas of medicine, and a broad array of pharmacology and immunology, a detailed history of all these would not fit into this entire volume. Instead, we will attempt to lay out a brief summary of the history that has led us here in an attempt to see where that history points us. As historians are fond of saying, we want to learn from the past. We want to find out what has been successful, what hasn't worked, and gain some hints as where to focus our efforts. But let us start with a flight of fantasy, looking to the future as it might one day look back on us.

33.2 In the Future

33.2.1 April 15, 2045; Orange County Regional Composite Tissue Transplant Center

Grand rounds seminar series; Limb and face transplants; review of the center's first 1,500 transplants; Robert Harrison MD, Center Director

This presentation will review the outcomes of the first 1,500 face and limb transplants in the Orange County regional composite tissue transplant center, beginning in 2039. As has been well reviewed in previous literature, the advent of immunologic tolerance discovered in 2012 has opened immense opportunities in reconstructive surgery. Combining a level 1 trauma center with a composite tissue transplant center has provided the capability for lifesaving and life-restoring services. The center is proud to be a leader in this new field of immediate reconstruction. We have focused on the optimum outcomes as well as the fastest recovery times.

With the recent focus on cost containment, we have demonstrated a 10% decrease in hospital stay every year since our inception. Currently, an above the knee or above the elbow CTA is reconstructed and discharged after an average of 6 days. Our rehabilitation program includes the most up-to-date nerve and muscle growth stimulation equipment. We are also proud of our restoration to normal life duties time which averages 47 days. Our close connection with the regional tissue procurement groups has allowed us to utilize the latest in tissue preservation technologies, thereby giving us the greatest opportunity for the physical matching of tissue to the recipient.

Because many facial injuries also have ocular damage, we're proud to be adding an ocular transplant program starting next year. We feel this will bring the same rapid restoration of sight after facial transplantation as we have seen in our limb transplant program. We also continue to be excited about our elective surgery programs, focusing on existing limb and facial trauma reconstruction. Although restoring function in a CTA performed on an already healed amputation or facial reconstruction takes an average of an additional week, we still see the same excellent outcomes with restoration of full function. Last week we were honored to have Mr. Sam Goodall as our guest. Many of us know Sam as the recipient of the first facial transplant in 2014, when he was only 15 years old.

With all these accomplishments, we still look forward to the time when the new technologies investigating self-regeneration will come to fruition. The stem cell programs started early in this century have had enormous payoffs, and we look forward to tissue regeneration in the next 5–10 years.

33.3 A Short Course of History

"HISTORY repeats itself. Historians repeat each other." Philip Guedalla, 1889–1944, (British writer).

This above fictional account may seem far-fetched until we stop and review the significant advances in the field of transplantation in the last century. The intent of this chapter is to help the reader understand not only where we have come from, but also where we are headed to. The possibility of bringing this type of restoration to a patient who has lost a hand or leg, or suffered facial disfigurement, is the core of composite tissue transplantation.

It is always amazing to consider how often history seems to repeat itself. There have been a number of excellent review articles that analyze the history of plastic and reconstructive surgery. There have even been excellent reviews of the mythology of ancient cultures regarding composite tissue transplantation. One thing many historians agree on is that the attempt to reconstruct individuals with extensive facial and extremity wounds has been driven in a large part by problems associated with war. Several ancient papyruses from Egypt teach reconstructive procedures for those injured in battle. These procedures were adopted first by the Greeks and later by the Romans. Independently, the Chinese and Hindus also investigated methods of reconstruction.

There are also accounts of more significant transplants with mythologies like the reconstruction of Osiris, the transplantation of a leg by Cosmos and Damien, and of course, literature's famous Frankenstein creation. Mankind has long dreamed of being able to do reconstruction on a grand scale, but only now is that possibility becoming a reality.

As we approach modern times, some major milestones have been better understandings of the disease processes that lead to tissue loss, and newly developed surgical techniques and instrumentation. The most important achievement was a greater understanding of the immune system, which gave hope for controlling the inevitable rejection response against transplanted tissue. There has been a better understanding of the underlying pathophysiology of the healing process as well: neurological, vascular, musculoskeletal, and cutaneous systems.

The advent of new immunosuppressive drugs ushered in this whole new realm of possibilities, beginning with the discovery of azathioprine and prednisone in the 1960s. There followed a brief experimenting with anti-T-cell antibodies, but the real breakthrough came with Jean Borel's discovery of cyclosporine, which helped to rewrite our understanding of the immune system. This included T-cell-mediated responses, B-cell-mediated responses, and macrophage responses. Cyclosporine ushered in the New World of drugs that would bring ever more specific agents for control of the immune response.

It would be exciting to say there have been great advances in postoperative patient care, but even surgeons in ancient Egypt understood the importance of controlling infection and keeping the tissues closely approximated to allow the body to proceed with its normal healing process. These medical practitioners had even developed ointments with rudimentary antibiotic properties.

This leaves us with the question: What are the next steps as we go forward in this saga? This is not about surgical advances or improvements in postoperative care, rather, it is about the continued understanding and discovery of ways to specifically control the rejection response, and eventually learning how to induce lifelong tolerance to the new transplant.

Xenotransplantation continues to be a possibility for the world of organ transplantation, but it appears to be of limited value in the discussion of composite tissue transplantation, for it would be unthinkable to reconstruct a patient's missing hand or facial defect with anything other than human tissue. In addition, there is rarely a shortage of human tissues that can be made available for reconstruction.

However, the future is made up of small steps, some so minute as to be almost imperceptible. And there is no telling what branch of science will lead to the big steps. Attempts to help World War II pilots with facial burns led to Medawar's discovery of neonatal tolerance; the search for a new antifungal drug led Jean Borel to the discovery of a new class of immunosuppressant, beginning with cyclosporine. Vigilance is the key to these new discoveries: a constant attentiveness to new ideas from fresh sources.

33.4 Looking Forward

"For my part, I consider that it will be found much better by all parties to leave the past to history, especially as I propose to write that history myself."
   Winston Churchill, 1874–1965; British Statesman, Prime Minister
   So, in looking into the future, it seems clear to this writer that the major near term events necessary to continue to push forward the field of composite tissue transplantation will involve new pharmacologies and procedures that would induce a state of acceptance of the transplanted tissue for the remainder of the patient's life.
   Several areas under investigation show much promise. This book deals specifically with the current state of affairs with hemopoeitic chimerism and the induction of tolerance through the use of vascularized bone marrow transplants. This was proposed some time ago by the authors of this text, and it is surprising how little progress has been made in this area in the last 15 years. Certainly, there is the threat that this hemopoeitic chimera could take a wrong turn and create a state of life-threatening graft versus host disease. However, the possibility of such disease already exists with current bone marrow transplants.
   It is exciting to see the progress that has been made in musculoskeletal transplants. The work by the authors in this text book point out that it is possible to have successful results despite great challenges.
   Possibilities for reconstruction in the future take us into exciting and almost fictional-sounding scenarios. Consider the individual with nonlife-threatening but severely disfiguring facial burns. With older technologies, this patient would be subjected to many surgeries for reconstruction of the important functional components of the face, such as eyelids and nasal passages, but without much hope of restoring normal facial appearance. This can have a devastating and lifelong impact on the patient's social acceptance and ability to reintegrate into society.
   The possibility of facial transplants also was explored some time ago by these authors. The surgical techniques necessary for this type of procedure have existed for some time now, as the creation of a free flap [whole face] has been in existence since the late 1960s. With the advent of cyclosporine, the possibility of providing longer-term survival has been in existence since the late 1970s. So why has no one considered attempting one of these reconstructions?
   The answer lies in each surgeon's estimation of risk benefit. With facial disfigurement or even the loss of limbs, the patient is not in a life-threatening situation. With today's technology and pharmacology there is certainly not a 100% guarantee that the transplant would not be rejected, that the drugs may not have

significant side effects, and lastly, that if the tissue were to reject, it might have a life-threatening effect on the patient.

Risk benefit is something that has plagued physicians since the time of Galen in ancient Greece, and even earlier. In ancient Mesopotamia, laws carved in a black obelisk at the center of town stated that a physician was ultimately responsible for the outcome of his patient. If the patient died due to a physician's treatment, that physician was to be put to death as well.

In addition to risk benefit, we also need to consider the definition of reconstructive surgery. For the most part, reconstructions are performed as quality-of-life, not lifesaving, procedures. This puts a whole new spin on the potential for transplantation. It has been argued in the past that organ transplantation is lifesaving and therefore warrants putting the patient's life at risk with procedures and new drugs. However, with the development of kidney dialysis, it could be argued that kidney transplantation is a quality-of-life, not a life-sparing, matter.

This article will not resolve that dilemma, which has been part of medicine ever since recorded history. What we can do is point out the possibilities of composite tissue transplantation, given the advent of new pharmacologies and immunologic manipulations. What do we have to look forward to in the twenty-first century? The hope is that our understanding of the immune system in the specifics of tissue rejection will become so complete that we can effectively manipulate the patient's immune system to accept new tissue and still have a normal immune response against all other pathogens. With immune response under control, the possibilities now exist for the reconstruction of massive tissue defects, including whole limbs and facial reconstruction, and even things as mundane but life-impacting as baldness. The immediate future is exciting, and the future lies with our understanding of the immune system.

Soon there will be programs with fellowships in composite tissue transplantation. In these fellowships, surgeons will extend their knowledge not only of surgical procedures but also of manipulations of the immune response such that they can be caregivers in this exciting New World of composite tissue transplantation.

33.5 What About Regeneration?

Newts do it. And frogs, when they are young, do it. Most other vertebrate species don't.

Limb regeneration is a fascinating subject. The poor newt has been subjected to many an amputation so that the wonder of limb regeneration can be studied. Theories abound as to how the newt manages the regeneration of an entire limb.

Obviously humans do not regenerate limbs, or there would be no need for this text book. However, we can regenerate other complex structures like skin, bone, liver, and the hemopoeitic system (blood). In fact, many of the components that make up a limb – muscle, nerve, skin, and bone – can replicate the cellular structure, but not the complex shape and function of the entire limb.

There is hope that the study of stem cells will shed new light on this amazing area. Some developmental biologists believe that the immune system is involved in either helping or hindering limb regeneration. Studies on this topic have contradicted each other. The thought is that the highly specific defense mechanism of the mammalian immune system stresses wound closure instead of regeneration. Although an interesting line of thought, naturally occurring or disease-related defects in the immune system and wound healing have not brought about any reports of spontaneous limb regeneration in any mammals.

However, humans do not lack the ability to regenerate. Orthopedic surgeons depend on bone remodeling every time they use a bone graft or substitute. By placing the bone in the appropriate locations the osteoblasts move in and reform the area to the bony shape necessary for the function. The liver also regenerates, and is what allows living related liver transplants; in that the liver of the donor will regenerate to its original size.

So what is next with regeneration? Clearly there are control mechanisms that construct our limbs appropriately in the womb. These mechanisms can sometimes malfunction and produce polydactyl and multiple limbs. The goal would be to replicate the limb development process in postfetal individuals. A recent report indicates that mice with some immune deficiency enjoy a modest amount of regeneration (holes punched in ears and amputated toes) and that the ability to regenerate can be imparted to another individual through fetal liver cell transfer.

It is a small beginning, but a beginning nonetheless.

33.6 Back to the Future

In conclusion, let us take a leap forward to the end of the present century and speculate as to what will be discovered.

33.6.1 *August 15, 2100; Keynote Address to the Society of Interplanetary Surgeons*

As president of the Earth-based delegation to the 60th annual meeting of the society of interplanetary surgeons, I welcome the Mars-, moon- and space-based delegations as well. We are especially thankful to the Mars-based group for making the 2-day trip to join us.

I have been asked to review the progress made over the past hundred years in the area of reconstruction and restoration of musculoskeletal function after traumatic injury.

Several of us in the audience today were in our medical school training at the turn of the last century, and can remember the crude methodologies that were available at that time. The goal in those days was to establish protocols for the transplantation of tissues. I know that for many of you these words seem archaic, but in simpler terms this meant using tissues from a cadaver to restore limited function after injury.

One of the big obstacles at the time was overcoming the immune response directed against these tissues. Another huge challenge was surgically reconnecting the neuromuscular components to provide even a modicum of function. This area of surgery progressed very slowly until the advent of Protocol 43 in 2012, which established a consistent and safe form of immunological tolerance.

It was during the early part of this last century that interest swelled in the study of stem cells. Again, although the early studies were crude, they led to a better understanding of how to control cellular differentiation and regeneration of major structures such as the hand or leg. The groundbreaking work in 2039 led to the first in situ regeneration studies in man. The cellular microenvironment modification protocols continued to advance the regenerative powers of local tissues. It was in 2056 that Professor Ramses discovered the genetic recombination protocol that moved us into the phase of massive tissue regeneration. We weathered a serious setback in the decade of 2060–2070, after the Ionian Institute incident which involved 30 grotesque mutations during the regeneration process. Dr. Hilber's work in 2069 finally overcame the obstacles to massive tissue regeneration.

As you all know, our current results of tissue regeneration after massive trauma are excellent, and this technology has been made a part of every medical unit in the interplanetary healthcare system.

More recent research has focused on enhancing healing potential for all humans while still in the womb. Dr. Poole's techniques, currently in trials, show that children have an 80% faster healing rate as well as some small inherent regenerative powers. Dr. Poole will be speaking on this at tomorrow's session, and he has indicated to me that he will also speak on how this technique is expected to extend our lifespan by another 70 years through the efficient healing and repair expected in the organ systems.

One note of caution: there have been rumors that some of these technologies have been used to create extra limbs on certain individuals to enhance their productivity. The Society and the interplanetary governments have strict rules regarding such misuse of technology. Another caution is the repeated changing of a person's facial appearance to meet new fashion trends. There have been several small studies done to demonstrate the safety of the regenerative protocols if used less than ten times. However, some illegal clinics have been changing facial appearances as often as one per week for years on end. A word to the wise: I've seen several of these patients firsthand, and they have all the appearances of a cellular-based leprosy with tissue slough and loss.

However, if these technologies are used in the prescribed fashion, they are extremely safe and effective. I can attest to this since the loss of my arm during the civil war of 2082, several years ago. As you can see, not only is my arm functional but I was back in my practice after only 3 weeks of regeneration and rehabilitation.

If our predecessors at the turn of the last century had seen where the technology would lead, they would truly be amazed. Thank you very much.

Index

A

Abdominal wall
  allotransplantation, 20, 21
  composite graft, 377
  graft, 376
Abductor pollicis brevis (APB), 417
Acquired immunological tolerance, 107
Activation induced cell death (AICD), 74
Adeno-associated viruses (AAVs)
  nonpathogenic human parvoviruses, 99
  viral vectors, 98
Adenoviruses, double-stranded DNA genomes, 98
Adnexal structures, 45, 46
Alemtuzumab (CAMPATH-1H), humanized antibody, 182
Alloantibodies and hyper acute rejection, 57
Alloantigen, 391, 392
Allogeneic donor cells, pretransplantation infusion of, 96
Allogeneic recipients
  BMC distribution in, 286, 287
  BMC phenotypes in, 287, 288
Allogenic antigens, 58
Allograft, 72–75, 77, 79
  blood transfusion, 96
  cardiac, 101
  components, relative antigenicity of, 55
  immunogenic organ, 90
  limb replantation, 262
  liver, 101
  rejection, 57
  survival optimization, immunosuppressive agents, 152
Allotransplantation, cadaveric vascularized digital flexor tendon unit, 155
Almost tolerance, 108

Amputation level, 220–222. *See also* Prospective hand recipient and donor criteria
AMR. *See* Antibody-mediated rejection
Antibodies
  anti-CD20, 183
  anti-CD25, 181
  anti-CD52, 182
  biologicals, 176
  clinical use of, 177–179
  muromonab-CD3, 177
  used in clinical transplantation, 176
Antibody-based immunosuppressive agents, 179–186
Antibody-mediated rejection therapies, 178, 179
Anti-CD3 antibody (Muromonab-CD3), 180, 181
Anti-CD52-specific monoclonal antibody, 111
Antigen-presenting cells (APC), 58, 76, 78–80, 109, 392
  B7-2 expressed on, 95
  DCs as, 80
  donor-derived, 92
Antilymphocyte serum (ALS), 80, 81, 136
Antirejection agents (antibodies), 178
Antithymocyte globulin (ATG), 156, 157, 177, 179, 201
APC-borne MHC-peptide complexes, 111
APCs. *See* Antigen-presenting cells
Apoptosis, 112, 113, 385
Azathioprine, immunosuppression, 156

B

Basiliximab, chimeric antibody, 181
Bilaminate dermal regeneration template, 364
Bilateral hand transplantation, 211–213. *See also* Hand transplantation

Bilateral lung transplantation, 18
Biologic conduits, nerve regeneration, 390
BM lymphocytes, responsiveness in il-BMTx recipients, 284
Bone allografts
   antigenicity of, 63, 64
   cellular and humoral response to, 63
   rejection of, 63
Bone–artery–few veins–tendon–nerve–remaining veins (BAVTNV), 224
Bone marrow
   cells, 280
      labeling for BMC distribution studies, 281, 282
      released from il-BMTx in allogeneic recipient, 286, 287
      responsiveness to phytohemagglutinin (PHA), 284
      secretion in limb transplant, 280
   chimerism in, 260
   immunomodulatory role for, 256
   serum liver enzyme test, 276
   stromal cells, 261
      chimerism of, 262
   transplantation, 72, 74, 79–81, 92, 255
Bone marrow cells (BMC), 280
Bone reconstructive techniques, 360

C

Cadaveric vascularized laryngeal allograft, transplantation, 156
Calcineurin inhibitors
   immunosuppression with, 124–135
   molecular action, 123, 124
   short-term immunosuppression, 135–146
Campath-1H, antibody, 111
Cartilage in CTA
   MHC antigens, distribution and antigenicity, 62
   rejection, 63
CD28-B7 costimulation, blocking, 112
CD154–CD40 costimulatory pathway, blocking, 112
CD4 cells, 75, 80
Cellular microchimerism, 280
Chemokine antagonists, 99, 100
Chimeric animals
   immunosuppression, 257
   peripheral and flow cytometry, 259
Chimeric models, of transplantation tolerance, 110
Chimerism and skin allograft tolerance, 257

Chimerism (genetics)
   bone marrow, 259
   donor-specific tolerance, 258
   macrochimerism
      flow cytometry, 255
   microchimerism
      polymerase chain reaction (PCR), 255
   PCR-flow assay, 258
Chronic rejection, 159–161
   cumulative inflammation and scarring, 159
   evaluation methods, 160
   high graft survival rate, 160
   loss of allograft, face transplantation, 161
   manifestations, 159
   patient age and donor source, 160
Clinical hand transplantation, 415
Clinical nerve allotransplantation, 398–400. *See also* Peripheral nerve allograft (PNA)
   protocol used, 399, 400
Combination drug therapy, 152. *See also* Calcineurin inhibitors
   and graft survival, 154, 155
Combination with cyclosporin A (CSA), 168–171
Composite tissue allografts (CTA), 166. *See also* Calcineurin inhibitors
   alemtuzumab (CAMPATH-1H), 182
   AMR in, 179
   antibody therapies in, 174, 176–179
   antigenicity of, 363
   with bone marrow, 81
   chimerism and tolerance in, 258
   clinical efficacy, 90
   component tissues rejection in, 264
   face transplantation
      ethical debate, 449
      facial flap harvesting of, 446
      true surgical challenge, 447
   hand transplantation, 211
      immunological challenge, 445
   hindlimb, GVHD develop in, 276
   human face transplantation
      ethical debate, 445, 446
   immune reaction, 73
   immunogenicity of, 80
   LEW to LBN, 275
   limb transplantation, 262
   locoregional immunosuppression, 166
   long-term immunosuppression, 256
   Muromonab-CD3 as treatment option in, 181

Index

psychosocial issues in, 454
  risk acceptance, 455
  social interaction and psychosocial face, 456–458
rat hindlimb, 274
rat model for, 263
rejection, 113, 114
risk acceptance
  immunosuppressant drugs, 455
social interaction and psychosocial face
  disfigurement consequences of, 456–458
source of antigen, 72
stromal cell, 262
survival, in animals, 124–134
survival, in large animals
tissue transplantation, 274
tolerance induction in, 135–146
transplantation, 82, 255
vascularized bone marrow transplant, 256
Composite tissue allotransplantation, 3
  antigenic strengths of components of, 66
  blood vessels, 65, 66
  cartilage in, 62
  chronic immunosuppression effects, 56
  clinical trials, 13–17
  germ layers and immunosuppressive regimen, 56
  hand transplantation, 17
  historical background, 13–17
  human skin rejection in, 44
    classification system, 45, 46
    graft loss and adnexa, 45
  and immunomodulation investigations, 364
  Langerhans cells, activation and migration, 60
  muscle tissue, 61
  NHP model, 46, 47
  pharmalogical research, 15
  reperfusion injury and endothelial trauma, 44
  technical challenges associated with, 363
  tendons in rejection of, 62
  tissue component of, 66
  total knee joints, 362
Composite tissue allotransplantation (CTA), 107, 113, 114, 125, 385
Composite tissue transplantation
  limb and facial trauma reconstruction, 463
  orange county regional composite tissue transplant center
    face and limb transplants, 462, 463
    surgery, 462
  in twenty-first century

interplanetary surgeons society, 467, 468
orange county regional composite tissue transplant center, 462, 463
regeneration, 466, 467
short courses, 463–465
Compound muscle action potentials (CMAPs), 417
Corticosteroids, 381
Cortisone and azathioprine, 27, 28
Costimulation and T cells activation, 58
Costimulation blockade, 77–79, 82
  CD28, 95
  CD40-CD154, 184
  with immunosuppressive drugs, 78
  pairing of, 96
Costimulatory molecule
  CD154 (CD40L), upregulation of, 78, 79
  CD28 receptor, 95
  role of, 95
Costimulatory signals, blockage of, 99, 101
Cross-chest C7 nerve transfer, 411
Cryopreserved human tracheal homograft, 325, 326
CsA. See Cyclosporine
CsA-based immunosuppression, 413. See also Peripheral nerve allograft (PNA)
  in treatment of nephrotic syndrome, 415
CsA–CyP complexes, 30
CTA. See Composite tissue allotransplantation
CTA See Composite tissue allografts
C6-T1 avulsions with C5 rupture, left global OBPP, 416, 417
  donor evaluation and procedure, 418
  functional recovery
    and clinical progress, 423
    and motor responses, 421, 422
    and needle examination, 422, 423
    and sensory responses, 421
  graft rejection and immunosuppression, 421
  postoperative care and immunosuppressive regimen, 419, 420
  recipient preparation and procedure, 418, 419
CTLA4Ig in costimulatory blockade, 112
Cyclophilin (CyP), 30, 123
Cyclosporine
  calcineurin action inhibition, 30
  composite allograft using, 30, 31
  immunosuppressive effects, 28
  for limb allografts, 30, 32, 38, 39
  mechanism of action of, 30, 31

Cyclosporine (cont.)
  selective action of, 29
  structure of, 28, 29
  tracheal transplantation, 315, 316
Cyclosporine A (CsA), 114, 123, 153, 263, 411
  immunosuppressive effects, 28
Cyclosporine immunosuppression, 155, 156
Cylindrocarpon lucidum, 28
Cytokines, 110, 111
Cytotoxic lymphocyte antigen-4 (CTLA-4), 185, 186
Cytotoxic T lymphocytes (CTL), 80

D

Daclizumab, humanized antibody, 181
Dendritic cells (DCs), 76, 77, 80–82
  allogeneic, 94
15-deoxyspergualin (DSG) therapy, tolerance, 111
Dermal dendritic cells (DDCs), 60
Dermal lymphocytic infiltrate, hand transplant recipients, 50
Desensitization agents (antibodies), 178
Desensitization treatments, immunoglobulin (IVIg), 178
Disability of Arm, Shoulder and Hand (DASH), 244
Distal interphalangeal (DIP) joint motion, 199, 201, 203, 205, 206
DNA transfer
  nonviral methods of, 98, 99
  viral methods of, 98
Donor bone marrow cells (DBMC), microchimerism, 82
Donor-specific tolerance, 91, 97, 100, 102, 185
Donor-specific transfusions (DST), 79, 96, 97
  chimerism, 274
  graft survival, 96, 97
  immune suppression, 97

E

Embryonic pre-albumin 1 (Epa-1), 59
Endothelial cells (ECs)
  and allograft rejection, 65
  irradiation doses and graft survival, 314
Epithelial repair, 313
Erythematous rash, 45
Everolimus, immunosuppressant, 343
Extensor digitorum communis (EDC), 417

F

Face transplantation, 346
  donor-related concerns, 437
    deceased, dignified treatment of, 437, 438
    donor intent and incentive, 439–441
    donor's family and loved ones, 438, 439
  ethical debate, 449
    donor issue, 451
    recipient's life, 451
  facial/scalp allograft
    arterial anastomoses in, 347
    operational tolerance induction, 348
  flap shaping, 446, 447
  hemifacial allograft transplants
    common carotid artery and external jugular vein, 348
    CsA monotherapy, 349
  innovative surgery and professional responsibility, 431, 432
    consent process, 433–435
    developing standards and oversight, 432, 433
    patient selection, 435, 436
    risk-benefit assessment, 431, 432
  population's response, 451
  preparation for human
    cadaver study, 350, 351
    donor and recipient cadavers, 352
    mock facial transplantation, 352–354
  true surgical challenge, 447
First dorsal interosseous (FDI), 417
FK506 binding proteins (FKBP), 123–125, 146, 157, 158, 396, 397
Flexor tendon allotransplantation, 19
Fluocinolone acetonide (FA), 169
Forkhead/winged helix transcription factor, Foxp3, 75–77, 81
Free tracheal autograft transplantation, 326. *See also* Tracheal allograft transplantation
French National Ethics Advisory Committee, 354
Full facial transplantation, 21, 22

G

Gene therapy
  chronic rejection, 97
  vectors, 98, 99
Glucocorticoid, in immunosuppression, 169

Index

Graft
  costimulatory molecule, 78
  drugs, 73
  and host, immune balance, 257
  lymphoid organs, 80
  rejection or acceptance of, 80
  transient chimera, 74
Graft harvest procedure, 267, 268
Graft immunogenicity, and reducing
    technique. *See also* Nerve allograft
  cold preservation, 393, 394
  radiation, lyophilization, and freezing, 392, 393
  recellularized nerve grafts, 394, 395
Graft-*versus*-host disease (GVHD), 14, 82, 110, 125, 145, 212, 230, 255, 257
  acute and chronic, 276
  chimerism, 274
  gastro-intestinal, 277
  lichenoid inflammation, characterization, 276
  severity of, 260
  viral hepatitis, 277
  without immunosuppression, 269
Graft-*versus*-host reaction, 280
Green fluorescent protein (GFP), 388, 402
GVHD. *See* Graft-*versus*-host disease

H

Hand transplantation, 17, 157, 158, 431, 437, 438
  acute rejection, 198
  allograft dysfunction, 157
  analysis of hand allograft function, 158
  Bunnell, Sterling, contributions, 195
  Carroll test score, 158
  case studies in
    Austria, 200, 203
    Belgium, 200
    China, 203–206
    France, 206–208
    Italy, 208
    USA, 198–200
  chimerism, 256
  donor-related concerns, 437
    deceased, dignified treatment of, 437, 438
    donor intent and incentive, 439–441
    donor's family and loved ones, 438, 439
  immunosuppressive complications, 157
  induction therapy, 211

  for induction therapy, 157
  innovative surgery and professional
      responsibility, 431, 432
    consent process, 433–435
    developing standards and oversight, 432, 433
    patient selection, 435, 436
    risk-benefit assessment, 431, 432
  in Innsbruck
    chimerism, 243, 244
    criteria for patient selection, 237
    disseminated erythema and papulous lesions, 241, 242
    donors and surgery, 238, 239
    grading for skin rejection, 242, 243
    imagery analysis, 246
    immunosuppressive protocols and prophylaxis, 240
    inclusion/exclusion criteria, 236, 237
    papilloma virus-associated skin lesions, 241, 242
    patient, selected to hand/forearm transplantation, 238
    pretransplant evaluations, 237, 238
    principal goals to satisfactory outcome, 247–250
    rehabilitation, postoperative, 239, 240
    scoring systems, for function, 244, 245
    uniform hair regrowth, 244
  Lyon (France) case study of, 211–213
  patient selection for, 196
  recipient-related concerns, 436, 437
  recipients, 196–198
  systemic immunosuppression and side effects, 197, 198
  transplantation *vs.* replantation, 158
  wrist, fingers, and thumb, mobility of, 208, 209
Hand-transplant donors and recipients, selection, 220–222
Hemifacial allograft transplants
  common carotid artery and external jugular vein, 348
  CsA monotherapy, 349
Hemilaryngeal transplantation, 342
Hemopoietic cells, in bone graft, 280
Heterotopic tracheal allograft transplantation, 18
Heterotopic tracheal transplant models, 313
Hindlimb transplantation model
  allotransplantation of, 262, 263
  chimeric rats, 258
  grafts, 256
  in mouse, 264

HLA antibodies, 238
HLA matching. *See* Human leukocyte antigen matching
Homeostasis, 377
Horner's sign, global paralysis, 410
Host immune response, reducing technique, 395. *See also* Nerve allograft
  immune tolerance, 398
  immunosuppression, 395–398
    costimulatory blockade, 397, 398
    cyclosporin A (CsA), 395, 396
    FK506, 396, 397
Host-specific tolerance, mechanisms, 274
Human femoral diaphysis, vascularized transplantation of, 362
Human hand transplant tissue biopsies, blood vessels antigenicity, 65
Humanized antibody
  aclizumab, 181
  alemtuzumab (CAMPATH-1H), 182
Human leukocyte antigen matching, 197, 362
Human marrow stromal cells, allogeneic peripheral blood proliferative response, 261
Human skin rejection in CTA
  adnexal structures, 45, 46
  characterization of, 45
  classification scheme for, 44, 46
Human trachea
  cervical part, 311, 312
  fibro-muscular membrane and cartilaginous rings, 311
  histology of, 312
  thoracic part, 312

I

IA immunosuppressive drug delivery, 170
il-BMTx. *See* in limb-bone marrow transplantation
IL-15 cytokine, T-cell apoptosis inhibition, 113
IL-2 receptor
  α chain of, 93
  directed antibodies, 181
  T-cell expansion, 95
  Treg cells, 94
Immune system homeostasis, 112
Immune tolerance, 108
  immune mechanisms implicated in central tolerance, 109, 110
  peripheral tolerance, 110–113
Immune tolerance induction, 107

Immunodominant donor MHC, injection of, 81
Immunogenic tissue and rejection response, 44
Immunomodulation, investigations in, 364
Immunophilins, 30
Immunosuppressant drugs, toxicity of, 455
Immunosuppression
  agents, 73
  cytokines, 100, 101
  drugs, 90
  immune tolerance, 175
  metabolic disorders, 449
  protocol, 211, 213, 448
  removal of, 97
  risks, 415, 416
  T cells, 94
  treatment, 211, 212, 448
Immunosuppressive agents, 15
  cell division, blockade of, 26
  6-mercaptopurine, 27
Immunosuppressive therapy, 201
  and graft rejection, 16
  risk, 416
  side effects of, 363
  tracheal transplantation, 315, 316
Indirect tracheal graft revascularization techniques, 324. *See also* Tracheal graft revascularization techniques
  omentum wrapping, 321, 322
  vascular carrier, 322, 323
Induction agents (antibodies), 177
Induction therapy, 156
  alemtuzumab (CAMPATH-1H), 182
  immune responses, 91
  immunosuppression, 90
  physiologic mechanisms of T-cells, 91, 92
in limb-bone marrow transplantation
  allogeneic elimination effect, 286
  BMC distribution, in allogeneic recipient, 286, 287
  BMC, released from, 281, 282
  BM lymphocytes, responsiveness of, 284
  donor DNA distribution, 289
  donor immune cells in recipient lymphoid tissues, 289
  effect on syngeneic irradiated/ nonirradiated recipient BMC and LO cellularity, 282–284
  hemopoietic cytokines and graft BMC, 283
  microchimerism in immunosuppressed recipient, 288, 289

Index 473

MLN lymphocytes, in vitro responsiveness of, 284
peripheral blood cell subsets, analysis of, 285, 286
recipient lymphoid organs (LO), histological evaluation of
BM lymphocyte, 285
T cells and B-cell, repopulation of, 284
recipient tibia cell yield, 283
Integra (ILS) method
for basal and squamous cell carcinomas, 366
skin injuries, treatment of, 364
Integumentary musculoskeletal transplants, 37
Intercellular adhesion molecule I (ICAM-1), 394
Interferon γ, 124
Interleukin-2 (IL-2), 123, 124
Intestinal graft donor, 380
Intestinal transplantation, 377
abdominal wall graft
immunosuppressive regimen, 380, 381
implantation, 379, 380
surveillance, 381
time delay for, 380
closure of abdomen, 378
ethical and social impact, 381, 382
graft procurement, 378, 379
incisions for, 379
vascular reconstruction
of iliac arteries and veins, 380
Intra-arterial (IA), 167
Ipsilateral clavicular fracture, 410
Ischemia-reperfusion model, 36

J
Joints motions, wrists, 312

K
Kendall coefficient of concordance, 45

L
Langerhans cells (LCs), 60
Laryngeal allograft transplantion
animal models of, 334, 341
case study, 332, 334
and immunosuppressive therapy, 20
and laryngectomy, 341, 342
reinnervation of, 341
surgical technique of, 333

LEA29Y in costimulatory blockade, 112
Lewis-Brown Norway donors and Lewis recipients, 144, 145. *See also* Composite tissue allografts (CTA)
Limb allotransplantation, 13, 14
bone marrow cells, 280
to immunosuppressed recipient, 288, 289
in rat, 263
in syngeneic irradiated/nonirradiated recipient, 281–283
tissues in, 264
Liposarcoma, 372
Locoregional immunosuppression, CTA, 166
IA infusion, 170, 171
local immunosuppression, 167, 168
topical therapy, 168–170
Long-term prevention of rejection, 152
Louisville hand transplant program, 217
American patients, outcomes in
acute rejection and immunomonitoring, 230, 231
allograft survival, 228
function, 229
psychosocial status and complications, 231, 232
assessment and clinical diagnosis, 228
Carroll and Semmes Weinstein monofilament testing, 227
donor procurement, 224
immunosuppressive regimen, 225, 226
International Registry Score (IRS), 228
Moore's criteria, ethical guidelines, 219, 220
patient profiles, 218
postoperative management, 226
crane extension outrigger splint, 226, 227
psychosocial evaluation, 228
recipient and donor selection, 220, 221
insurance and/or financial security, 223
medical screening, 222
psychiatric consultation and informed consent, 223
thematic apperception tests, 223
recruitment of recipient, 222
scientific rationale for, 218, 219
technical aspects of hand transplantation, 224, 225
Louisville instrument for transplantation (LIFT), 455
Lower extremity limb transplantation, 20
basic concepts and principles, 357

Lower extremity wounds
  bone reconstructive techniques, 360
  debridement and lavage, 359
  etiology of, 358
  Integra (ILS) method for management of, 364, 365
  management of
    defects, 359
    open tibial fractures, gustilo classification of, 359, 360
    reconstructive planning and scoring systems, 358

M
Macrochimerism, 144
Maintenance therapy, as immune suppression, 91
Major histocompatibility complex (MHC) and molecules, 73, 107, 135, 136
  antigenes, 97
  class I and class II expression, 169
  donor-derived, 92
  gene transfer, 100
  MHC class II expression, PNA, 392
  MHC genes, 113
  mismatch, 92
  peptide bound, 94
  role in antigen presentation to CD4+ T lymphocytes, 394
Major histocompatibility (MHC) antigens and allorecognition, 57, 58
  expression in human endothelial cells (ECs), 65
Medawarian principle, 175
Metacarpalphalangeal (MP) joint motion, 199, 201, 203, 205, 206
Methylprednisolone, 156
Mixed chimerism, 82
MLN lymphocytes, in vitro responsiveness in il-BMTx recipients, 284
Mock facial transplantation procedure, 352–354
Monoclonal antibodies (mAb)
  alemtuzumab (CAMPATH-1H), 182
  anti-CD20, 183
  hybridoma clones, 180
  react against a single elldefined epitope, 177
Motor function and range of motion (ROM), 199
Motor recovery, muscle function, 213
Mouse model, in transplantation research
  advantages of, 264
  tolerance, 265

Muromonab-CD3
  blocks mitogenic, 180
  induction agent, 177, 178
  toxicity, 180
Muscle tissue
  allotransplantation, 61
  rejection pattern of, 62
Mycophenolate mofetil (MMF), 15, 16, 123, 132, 153, 415
  and CsA for composite tissue allotransplants, 32
Mycophenolic acid (MPA), 153

N
Nerve allograft. *See also* Peripheral nerve allograft (PNA)
  alloantigen in PNA, 391
  methods of tolerance, 392–398
  response in peripheral nerve, 391, 392
Nerves, antigenic status of, 64
Nerve transplantation, in animal models, 411–413
Neuregulin-1 Type III, axon, 389
NF-kB signal pathways, 109
NHPs. *See* Nonhuman primates
Noncellular microchimerism, 289
Nonhuman primate models
  CTA rejection studies, 48
  dermal lymphocytic infiltrate, 50, 51
  human-specific immunosuppressants, testing of, 48
  sensate osteomyocutaneous forearm flap allografting, 48, 49
Nonhuman primates, 46, 108, 114
Nonspecific immunosuppression, adverse sequelae, 153
Nonviral methods, gene therapy, 98

O
Obstetric brachial plexus palsy (OBPP), 409–411, 416
Omentum wrapping. *See also* Tracheal graft revascularization techniques
  heterotopic 2-stage procedure, 322
  orthotopic 1-stage procedure, 321, 322
Open tibial fractures, gustilo classification of, 359
Organ procurement organization (OPO), 224
Orthotopic tracheal transplant model, 313

Index

Osteochondral allografts, immune responses against, 63
Osteomyelitis, 358

P

Partial face allografts, 21
Peripheral nerve allograft (PNA), 413–415
  nerve regeneration, 385
    axonal regeneration, 385, 388
    clinical nerve allografts, 386, 387
    long nerve regeneration, 390
    mechanisms of revascularization, 389, 390
    in motor grafts, 388
    Schwann cells, fate of, 388, 389
    transplants and immunosuppressive agents, 18, 19
Peripheral nerve allotransplantation, 384
  in CTA, 401, 402
Peripheral nerves, antigenicity of, 65
Peripheral tolerance, 110. *See also* Immune tolerance
  costimulatory blockade, 111, 112
  cytokines modulation, 113
  regulatory T cells, 112
  T-cell depletion, 110, 111
Perivascular inflammatory cell infiltrates, 381
Plastic surgeon(s), 6
Pneumocystis carinii, 125
Pneumocystis carinii pneumonia, 156
Polyclonal antibodies
  CMV infection rates, 180
  derived from, 177
Polymerase chain reaction (PCR), 255
Polypeptides, biologicals, 176
Posttransplantation, 211, 212, 214
Prednisolone, intra-arterial (IA) infusion, 167
Prednisone, for immunosuppression, 413–416, 420, 421
Prodrug, 30
Programmed cell death 1 (PD-1), 95
Pronator teres (PT), 417
Prope tolerance, 108
Prospective hand recipient and donor criteria, 220
Proximal interphalangeal (PIP) joint motion, 199, 201, 203, 205, 206

Q

Questionnaire-based instrument, risk assess, 455

R

Range of motion (ROM), 225
Rapamycin
  FK506 and, 398
  T cells regulation, 112
  wit calcineurin inhibitors, 126
Rat laryngeal transplant model, 337
  donor organ and in vitro irradiation, 338
  everolimus (immunosuppressive agent), 343
  survivability and graft evaluability, 335
Rat limb allografts, 14
Recipient lymphoid organs (LO), histological evaluation of
  BM lymphocyte, 285
  T cells and B-cell, repopulation of, 284
Renal allograft recipients, risk for development infection, 416
Reperfusion injury and endothelial trauma, 44
Rescue therapy, rejection episode, 91
Rituximab, chimeric murine, 183

S

Saints Cosmas and Damian, 13, 14, 38, 39. *See also* Limb allotransplantation
Scalp anatomy, 370
Scalp reconstruction, 369
  circumflex scapular system, 374
  current options for, 371
  dorsal scapular perforator flap, 372
  free flaps, 372
  galeal scoring, 371
  largest muscle flap, 372
  long-term immunosuppression, effects of, 370
  microhair grafting, 371
  osteomyelitis, 371
  posterior scalp transplantation, 371
  scalp and forehead defects, 371
  trapezius myocutaneous flap, 372
Scalp transplantation, issue of alopecia and skin color match, 374
Schwann cell basal lamina (SCBL), 388, 391, 394
Schwann cells (SCs), 385
  class II expression on, 412
  fate in nerve grafts, 401
  immune response activation, 65
Sensate osteomyocutaneous forearm flap
  disection and perfusion of, 48
  rejection signs in graft of, 50
Sensory evoked potentials (SEPs), 126
Sentinel skin graft, 302, 305, 306

Sirolimus (rapamycin) drug, 123
Skin
　allotransplantation, 381
　antigenicity of, 59
　dendritic cells (DCs), 59
　　migratory property, 60
　rejection
　　pathology of, 60, 61
Soft tissue reconstruction
　local flaps *vs.* microvascular tissue transfers
　　foot and skin grafts, 361
　　thigh, 360
Solid organ transplantation (SOTs), 113
　acute rejection in, 180
　AMR in, 178
　chimerism in, 260, 261
　with donor allogeneic BMT, 259
　malignancies, 91
　tolerance of, 259, 260, 261
Split tracheal transplantation, 322. *See also* Omentum wrapping
Sterling Bunnell Traveling Fellowship, 195
Sternum transplant model, 265–267
　donor operation of, 265
　left and right artery to sternum, 267
　left and right superior vena cava (SVC), 266
Streptomyces tsukubaensis, 123
Stromal cell, plasticity of, 261, 262
Suppressor T cells, 112
Synergism, 170
Systemic immunosuppression
　in hand transplantation, 197
　side effects, 198

T

Tacrolimus (TCL). *See* FK506 binding proteins (FKBP)
T cell/APC interactions, 111
T-cell receptor (TCR), 111
　complex activation of, 58
T cells (Tregs)
　activation, 77–80, 92, 95, 180
　antibodies, 75
　antigen-specific activity, 76, 77, 95
　central tolerance, 256
　costimulatory blockade, 94–96
　depletion, 74
　growth factor receptor pathways, 92
　host-specific tolerance, 274
　immunologic tolerance, 255, 256
　mediated responses, 464
　prevention of, 77
　proliferation of, 76
　receptor (TCR/CD3), 94
　regulatory activity, 75, 83
　　generation of, 92–94
　　induction of, 94
　tolerance, 74, 75, 76, 92, 93
TCL/clobetasol, in hand transplant, 170
TCL, immunosuppression, 411, 412, 414, 415, 418, 419, 421, 424
Tendons, antigenicity of, 62
Thoracic duct lymphocytes (TDL), migration of, 281
Th1/Th2, allograft tolerance, 113
Tissue allograft, 364
Tissue transplantation, 370, 374
TKA. *See* Total knee arthroplasty
Tolerance induction
　in CTA, strategies for, 114–116
　gene therapy for, 97
　strategies for, 77
Tolypocladium inflatum, 28, 123
Total knee arthroplasty, 301
Trachea. *See* Human trachea
Tracheal allograft transplantation
　cadaveric human homograft
　　cryopreserved, 325, 326
　　fresh, 323, 324
　clinical trials, 18
　cryopreserved, 315
　desquamation methods, 314
　detergents, use of, 314, 315
　endothelium-dependent vasodilatatory responses, 314
　free, 326, 327
　immunosuppressive therapy, 315, 316
　reepithelialization, 313, 314
　T-cell tolerance, 316
　tracheal cartilage and ciliated mucosa, 312, 313
　tracheal reconstruction and replacement techniques, 309, 310
　tracheal resection limits, 310
　using Co γ irradiation, 314
Tracheal graft revascularization techniques
　direct, 317
　　composite tyro-tracheal allograft, 318
　　orthotopic tyro-tracheal allograft, 319, 320
　　tyro-tracheal allotransplantation with venous drainage, 318, 319

indirect
    omentum wrapping, 321, 322
    sternohyoid muscle wrapping, 323
Tracheal mucosa, 312
Transforming growth factor-β(TGF–β), 124
Transplantation tolerance
    alloantigens, 97
    central and peripheral, 92
    peripheral Tregs, 93
    response, 92
    T-cell, 73, 91
    Tregs in, 76
Transplanted limb, as BMC source, 280
Transplant immunology
    antigens, 74, 79
    immuno suppression, 72
    T-cell activation, 77
    tissue, 73
    tolerance, 72, 73, 91
Trimethylenecarbonate-co-epsiloncaprolacton (TMC/CL), 390. *See also* Biologic conduits, nerve regeneration
T suppressor cells, 76, 77
Tubulation techniques, 390. *See also* Peripheral nerve allograft (PNA)
Tumor necrosis factor receptor (TNFR), 184
Tyro-tracheal allotransplantation with venous drainage, 318, 319. *See also* Tracheal graft revascularization techniques

U
UVB-irradiated spleen cells (UVB-SC), 398

V
Vascularized bone marrow transplant (VBMT), 255, 256
    bone marrow chimerism in, 262
    femoral artery and vein anastomosed, 267
    femoral isolated
        graft harvest procedure for, 267, 268
    graft-*versus*-host-disease in, 275
    gross clinical aspects of, 275, 276
    hindlimb
        GVHD develop in, 276
        immunologic effect of, 264
    in limb transplant, 263
    nutrient vessels
        isolation of, 269
    sternum transplant, 265–267
Vascularized knee transplantation, 19
    back-table allograft preparation, 298
    bone allograft procurent, 296, 298
    case studies, 300–303
    follow-up (transplanted patients), 299, 300
    histocompatibility and immunosuppression, 299
    history of, 295
    indication for, 295
    recurrence of infection, 304
    rejection and ischemic necrosis, 304, 305
    transplantation procedure, 298, 299
Vascularized limb allograft, 56
    host immune system activation
        cellular response, 57, 58
        humoral response, 57
    reject components of, 58, 59
Vascularized skin, 44
Vascular rejection, 305

W
Wistar Furth (WF), 145